MW01027725

The Canon of Medicine

(*al-Qānūn fī'l-ṭibb*)

Avicenna
(Abū ᶜAlī al-Ḥusayn ibn ᶜAbd Allāh ibn Sīnā)

Adapted by
Laleh Bakhtiar

from
Translations of Volume I by
O. Cameron Gruner and Mazar H. Shah
Correlated with the Arabic by Jay R. Crook
with Notes by O. Cameron Gruner

Series Editor
Seyyed Hossein Nasr

GREAT BOOKS OF THE ISLAMIC WORLD, INC

Printed in the United States of America.

Library of Congress Cataloging-in-Publication Data

Ibn Sina, Abu Ali al-Husayn ibn Abd Allah
The Canon of Medicine (*al-Qanun fi'l tibb*)
1. Islam. 2. Medicine. I. Title.

ISBN: 1-871031-67-2

Cover design: Liaquat Ali
Cornerstones are Allah and Muhammad connected by *Bismillāh al-Raḥmān al-Raḥīm* (In the Name of God, the Merciful, the Compassionate).

Logo design by Mani Ardalan Farhadi
The cypress tree bending with the wind, the source for the paisley design, is a symbol of the perfect Muslim, who, as the tree, bends with the wind of God's Will.

Published by
Great Books of the Islamic World, Inc.

Distributed by
KAZI Publications, Inc.
3023 W. Belmont Avenue
Chicago IL 60618
Tel: 312-267-7001; FAX: 312-267-7002
email: kazibooks@kazi.org

CONTENTS

Dedicated to my parents

Abol Ghassem Bakhtiar, M.D.
and
Helen Jeffreys Bakhtiar, R.N.

Foreword

God's last plenar revelation to present humanity came in the form of a book, al-Qur'an, which for Muslims is also *the* book and is in fact known also as *Umm al-kitāb* or Mother of All Books. While the peerless majesty of the revelation reduced the first generation of Muslims to silence, the echo of the Noble Book and its encouragement of acquiring knowledge could not but result in a culture which cherished books and honored scholars. This unmistakable emphasis of the Noble Quran on knowledge, combined with the synthetic power of Islam to absorb the learning of older civilizations to the extent that they conformed to the doctrine of unity (*al-tawḥīd*), gave rise to a vast and diversified intellectual life which for the past thirteen centuries has produced millions of works dealing with nearly every field of knowledge from the religious sciences, theology and philosophy to the natural sciences, from law to music, and from poetry to politics.

Islamic civilization was a lake into which flowed streams from many civilizations: Greek, Roman, Egyptian, Mesopo- tamian, Byzantine, Persian, Indian and even Chinese. In this lake the various elements became synthesized into a new body of water which itself became the source for numerous tributaries that have watered the various lands of *Dār al-islām*. Furthermore, Islamic civilization created works which had profound influence upon at least three major civilizations outside of the Islamic world: the Far Eastern, the Indian and the Western besides creating numerous masterly works whose influence has remained confined within the Islamic world. Such works in both categories contain a precious message for humanity as a whole and need to be made known by the world at large today.

Most treatises in Islamic civilization were written in the language of the Quranic revelation, Arabic, followed by the only other universal language of Islamic civilization, Persian. But important works have also been written in Turkish, Urdu, Bengali, Malay, Swahili, Berber, and numerous other languages including Chinese and, during this century, even English and French. Nor have all the works in Arabic been written by Arabs nor all the works in Persian by Persians. Numerous treatises in Arabic were written by Persians and later Turks, Indians, Berbers and Black Africans while many books in the Persian language were composed by Indians, Turks and Central Asians. The body of works written within the confines of Islamic civilization belongs to the whole of that civilization and in classical times, in fact, important books became known rapidly from Morocco to India and later Southeast Asia.

The Great Books of the Islamic World series seeks to make some of the most important works produced in Islamic civilization, primarily in Arabic and Persian, available in English so that these treasures of Islamic thought can be appreciated by those who do not possess the facility to benefit from them in the original languages. The audience to which the series addresses itself is predominantly the Western English reading public, but the series is also meant for Muslims themselves who have facility with the English language and also for non-Muslim and non-Westerners who are now becoming ever more knowledgeable in English and who might wish to gain deeper knowledge of the Islamic intellectual universe.

We hope that with the help of God, Exalted is His Majesty, this series will be successfully completed and that by providing a clear and readable translation of some of the great masterpieces of Islamic thought in English, this series will be able to create better understanding of Islam in the world at large and make accessible some of the treasures of traditional thought which, although Islamic in genesis, belong to all human beings who are interested in true knowledge in whatever form it appears. *wa mā tawfīqunā illā biʾLlāh*

Seyyed Hossein Nasr
Washington DC, June, 1997

PREFACE

Praise belongs to God that we have been given permission to publish this great work of Avicenna—written almost 1000 years ago—in a textbook format, as Avicenna had intended, without the incumberance of notes in the middle of the translation. However, the notes of O. Cameron Gruner, invaluable in themselves in that they show the connection to scholastic philosophy and the works of St. Thomas Aquinas, appear in the endnotes.

Parts of the English text which is before you had been prepared by O. Cameron Gruner, M.D. and Mazhar Shah, M.D. O. Cameron Gruner, M.D. had closely followed the Latin translation while Mazar Shah, M.D. had followed the Urdu translation. Both were compared by Jay R. Crook with the critical edition of *al-Qanun fi'l-tibb* published by the Institute of the History of Medicine and Medical Resarch in association with VIKAS Publishing House, Pvt., Ltd., 1982, and appropriate changes were made where the English text strayed from the meaning of the Arabic text.

Esmail Koushanpour, Ph.D. and Jenny Koushanpour provided invaluable medical and technical help with the translation. The spelling of medical terminology, which differed in the two translations, was checked with *Stedman's Medical Dictionary*, 22nd edition, illustrated and published by the Williams & Wilkins, Co. Baltimore, 1972. This dictionary has been completely revised in the 22nd edition by a staff of thirty-three editors covering forty-four specialities and sub-specialities.

Laleh Bakhtiar, Ph.D.

INTRODUCTION

BY LALEH BAKHTIAR

In the Name of God, the Merciful, the Compassionate

I. BIOGRAPHICAL SKETCH

The "Prince of Physicians," Abū ʿAlī Sīnā (Avicenna) (b. 370/980) was born in Bukhara. By the age of ten he had learned the entire Quran as well as grammar and then began the study of logic and mathematics. Once these subjects were mastered, he studied physics, metaphysics and medicine. By the age of sixteen he had mastered all of the sciences of his day except metaphysics. While he had read Aristotle's *Metaphysics* over and over again and had even memorized it, he could not understand it until he read al-Fārābī's commentary on it. Avicenna was then eighteen years old.

He was favored by the ruler of Bukhara because of his mastery of medicine, but when he was thirty-two, he was forced to migrate because of the political situation in his home town area. He migrated to Jurjan on the southeast coast of the Caspian Sea in an attempt to join the court of the well-known Qabus ibn Wushmgir. This never materialized as the ruler had died in 1013 during Avicenna's travels to Jurjan. Avicenna then retired to a village near Jurjan where he was to meet his disciple-to-be, al-Juzjani.

Al-Juzjani was devoted to Avicenna and was to write commentaries upon his works as well as to preserve copies of all of the master's writings. It was in Jurjan in 1012 that Avicenna wrote the beginning of his great medical text, *The Canon (al-*

Qanun) on medicine. Avicenna remained in Jurjan for two or three years before moving to Rey in 405/1014 or 406/1015, a city near present day Tehran and from there to Hamadan in the northwest Iran. He became a minister in the Buyuid Court of Shams al-Dawlah as well as the court physician. Once again Avicenna was obliged to migrate because of the unstable political conditions in Hamadan so he moved to Isfahan where he enjoyed a fifteen year period of peace, writing many of his major works at that time.

Eventually, however, he was forced to migrate once again and moved back to Hamadan where he died in 428/1037.

II. Avicennian Corpus

One of the leading scholars on Avicenna and the editor of this series, Seyyed Hossein Nasr, has written the following:

> The writings of Avicenna, of which nearly 250 have survived, if we take all his short treatises and letters into account, range over nearly every subject known to the medieval world. These works are mostly in Arabic, but occasionally in Persian, as for example, the *Dānish namāh-i ᶜalāī* (*The Book of Science Dedicated to Ala al-Dawlah*), which is the first philosophic work in modern Persian. Avicenna's Arabic style in his earlier works is rather difficult and uneven; and it was only during his long sojourn in Isfahan-when under the criticism of certain literary experts, he began to study Arabic literature intensely-that his style became polished and perfected. The works written later in life, especially the *Ishārāt wa 'l-tanbīhāt*, testify to this change.
>
> Aviennna's philosophical works include his Peripatetic masterpiece *al-Shifāᵓ* (*The Book of the Remedy*), the Latin *Sufficientia*, which is the longest encyclopedia of knowledge ever written by one man, his *Najat* (*The Book of Deliverance*), which is a summary of the *Shifāᵓ*, *ᶜUyūn al-ḥikmah* (*Fountains of Wisdom*), and his last and perhaps greatest masterpiece *Ishārāt wa 'l-tanbīhāt* (*The Book of Directives*

and Remarks). In addition he wrote a large number of treatises on logic, psychology, cosmology, and metaphysics. There are also the "esoteric" works pertaining to his "Oriental Philosophy" of which the *Risalāh fi'l-ᶜishq* (*Treatise on Love*), the Trilogy *Ḥayy ibn Yaqẓān* (*The Living Son of the Awake*), *Risālat al-ṭair* (*Treatise of the Bird*) and *Salāmān wa Absāl*, the last three chapters of the *Ishārāt*, and *Manṭīq al-mashriqīyīn* (*The Logic of the Orientals*), which is a part of a larger work now lost, are the most important.

In the sciences, also, Avicenna composed many small treatises dealing with particular problems in physics, meteorology, and so on, as well as sections contained in the larger compendia, especially the *Shifāᵓ*, in which is found the most complete exposition of his views on zoology, botany, and geology, as well as psychology, which in Peripatetic philosophy—and contrary to the view of the later schools like the Ishrāqīs-is considered as a branch of physics or natural philosophy. As for medicine, Avicenna composed the famous *Qanun*, or *Canon*, which is perhaps the most influential single work in the history of medicine and is still taught in the East today, the *Urjūzah fi'l-ṭibb* (*Poem on Medicine*), containing the principles of Islamic medicine in rhyming verses easy to memorize, and a large number of treatises in both Arabic and Persian on various diseases and drugs.

In addition to his philosophical and scientific works, Avicenna wrote several poems in Arabic and Persian of which *al-Qaṣīdat al-ᶜainiyah* (*Ode on the Soul*) is deservedly the most famous. Moreover, he wrote several religious works which include not only treatises on particular religious subjects, such as the meaning of fate and free will, but also commentaries upon several chapters of the Quran. This latter category is particularly important because it was primarily in these commentaries that Avicenna sought to harmonize reason and revelation along lines already begun by al-Kindī, al-Fārābī, and the Ikhwān al-Ṣafāᵓ, continued after him by Suhrawardī, and finally

> brought to its fruition by Mīr Dāmād and Mullā Ṣadrā. These writings add an important dimension to the already multidimensional corpus of Avicenna's literary output and emphasize the richness of a collection of writings which range from observational and even experimental science to ontology, from mathematics to gnosis and metaphysics, and from logic to commentaries upon the Sacred Book.[1]

III. The Theory and Practice of Islamic Medicine

The traditional concept of medicine[2] differs profoundly from the view held in the modern world because in the traditional view, the spaces—meridians, channels—within the body and what flows through them are of more significance in causing illness than the shapes or organs, members themselves. That is, the emphasis is on that which flows through the channels as the "place" of the soul.

A clear parallel can be seen in traditional Islamic architecture where space is considered to be one of the most direct symbols of Being and it is primordial, all-pervading and, in Islamic cosmology, the locus of the Universal Soul. Space is also structured. Whether one is referring to the macrocosm or the microcosm, they each contain three divisions: body, soul and spirit.

> Traditional man tends towards a mode of comprehension which provides a metaphysical interpretation of life, an interpretation that precedes and goes beyond all external perception. This mode of comprehension, or initial interpretation, affects all of man's perceptions because it begins by situating him in the universe. Initially this interpretation determines his awareness of cosmic space as an externalization of the macrocosmic creation which is analogous to his own microcosmic self. This traditional Hermetic concept forms part of the world view incorporated into the Islamic perspective, a view in which the universe is composed of a macrocosm and microcosm, each con-

> taining three great divisions: the body (*jism*), the soul (*nafs*) and the spirit (*ruh*).[3]

Depending on one's perspective, one is either drawn from the body through the soul to the Divine Spirit in the external world or from the body inward through the soul to the Hidden Treasure or Divine Spirit within.

> Two interpretations of this concept arise which, although apparently different, are essentially the same. In the first, God as Manifest (*al-Zahir*), is the reality of universal externalization. From within the concentric circles of the macrocosm, there is an outward movement from the earth as corporeal manifestation through an all-pervading soul to the enveloping heavens, viewed as the seat of the Divine Spirit. In the second, complementary view of God as Hidden (*al-Batin*), there is an inward movement within the microcosm of man, beginning with his physical presence and moving towards his spiritual center, the Hidden Treasure. The two schemes correspond to each other, at the same time that one is the reverse of the other.[4]

In this structured space, the human being knows where he or she is. Direction is meaningful.

> It is only with reference to the heavens that the apparent indefiniteness of space can be given direction. In this way space acquires a qualitative aspect. The order of the spheres and the movements through the six directions of north, south, east, west, up and down constitute the primary coordinate system within which all creation is situated. All traditional sciences share this common frame of reference.[5]

The concept of place (*makan*) follows a meaningful direction or orientation. A sense of place consists of both a container (*jism*, body) and the contained (soul, spirit, breath).

> [The concept of place] does not have a tangible existence, but exists in the consciousness of the beholder who visually perceives physical boundaries while his intellect perceives [the soul] and spirit as 'contained,' defined within the boundaries.[6]

Within this structured, oriented concept of space as the place of the soul, all of creation contains both active and passive possibilities. The idea of time in motion arises from the active aspect of space while seen in its passive aspect, it is manifested in matter or form which is directly a product of this movement. This concept—that the soul (space) and not the body (shape) should lead in the healing art—is central to an understanding of traditional medicine.

> The esoteric theory of causation describes this motion as the movement of the soul towards the Divine Spirit through space. Thus the locus of time and form is space, which simultaneously manifests its active and passive aspects through motion.[7]

This perspective is the basis for traditional medicine which looks for the simultaneous movement systems which create a continuous flow based on number—three main faculties, three major organs, three souls, four elements, four humors, nine temperaments, and which interact in space, the place of the soul, with the organs, tissues, membranes, etc.

Finally, we come to the concept of rhythm in time which is best described in terms of traditional music based upon the poem with which Jalal al-Din Rum begins his masterful *Mathnawi*.

Hearken to this Reed forlorn,
Breathing, even since twas torn
From its rushy bed, a strain
Of impassioned love and pain.

The Secret of my song, though near,

None can see and none can hear.
Oh, for a freind to know the sign
And mingle all his soul with mine!
'Tis the flame of Love that fired me.
'Tis the wine of Love inspired me.
Wouldst thou learn how lovers bleed.
Hearken, hearken to the Reed![8]

The continuity and harmony of music is well appreciated and may serve to elucidate another aspect of the spiritual meaning of time-form continuity. The reed, in Jalal al-Din Rumi's poem, contains the bifold characteristics of place. Physically, the reed exhibits a *zahir* or external form which is passive to its hollow interior or *batin*, wherein lies the active spirit of the instrument. The music of the reed is symbolically seen as the externalization of an interior movement, just as musical tones work through wind instruments from the inside out. He who hears the music is aware of the inner space and the harmonious encounter of its motion with its outer shell. This interaction, in the traditional view, represents a spiritual synthesis which regards the reed's *zahir* as the body and its *batin* as the spirit, which, through the music of the soul, yearns to return to the reed bed from whence it was plucked, must as man yearns to return to the One from whom he was issued.[9]

The concept of motion associated with the creation of time and space is explored also by Ibn Arabi in his discourses on initial creation and the subsequent manifestations, viewed as the 'Breath of the Compassionate.' Here 'the universe is annihilated at every moment and re-created at the next without there being a temporal separation between the two phases. It returns back to the Divine Essence at every moment while in the phase of contraction and is re-manifested and externalized in that of expansion. . . Creation is renewed at every instant and its apparent 'horizontal' continuity is pierced by the 'Vertical Cause' which integrates every moment of existence into its transcendent Origin.'[10]

Because of the concentration of traditional Islamic medicine on what flows through the inner spaces, it becomes a dynamic system. That is, the whole is present and operative in each individual locus in which each individual locus knows, so to speak, its position in the whole, its relation to center. The dynamic qualities of the elements can be understood as manifestations of an orderly action of faculties (drives, energies, powers) within a given system. The elemental qualities of our body's system are part of a dynamic field and each elemental quality, as it presents itself, gives expression to the exact constellation of faculty that is present at the point at which the element is situated, a dynamic quality that permits the elemental qualities to become the conveyors of meaning; that makes temperaments out of the succession of elements.

Thus, we have introduced the traditional concepts of the soul and its place in space with the traditional components of space: structured (body, soul, spirit), oriented (six directions), sense of place (container/contained), positive space continuity (what flows through space creates shapes), time-form simultaneity (active as motion, passive as form), and rhythm in time (breath, pulse). Now let us turn to Avicenna. He begins *The Canon* with a definition of the science of medicine:

> §**7** Medicine (*tibb*) is the science by which we learn the various states of the human body in health and when not in health, and the means by which health is likely to be lost and, when lost, is likely to be restored back to health. In other words, it is the art whereby health is conserved and the art whereby it is restored after being lost.

Avicenna insists that the human body cannot be restored to health unless the causes of both health and disease are determined. In catagorizing the causes, he uses Aristotle's system:

> §**12** Medicine deals with the states of health and disease in the human body. It is a truism of philosophy that a complete knowledge of a thing can only be

obtained by elucidating its causes and antecedents, provided, of course, such causes exist. In medicine it is, therefore, necessary that causes of both health and disease should be determined.

§**13** Sometimes these causes are obvious to the senses but at other times they may defy direct observation. In such circumstances, causes and antecedents have to be carefully inferred from the signs and symptoms of the disease. Hence, a description of the signs and symptoms of disease is also necessary for our purpose. It is a dictum of the exact sciences that knowledge of a thing is attained only through a knowledge of the causes and origins of the causes—assuming there to be causes and origins. Consequently our knowledge cannot be complete without an understanding both of symptoms and of the principles of being.

§**14** There are four causes—material, efficient, formal, and final. On the subject of health and disease, we have the following:

The Material Causes

§**15** The material (*maddi*) cause is the physical body which is the subject of health and disease. This may be immediate as the organs of body together with their vital energies and remote as the humors and remoter than these, the elements which are the basis both for structure and change (or dynamicity). Things which thus provide a basis (for health and disease) get so thoroughly altered and integrated that from an initial diversity there emerges a holistic unity with a specific structure (or the quantitative pattern of organization) and a specific type of temperament (the qualitative pattern).

The material cause, then is the physical body, as viewed from the traditional perspective. It consists of the organs, the breath, the humors and the elements. We begin with the elements as Avicenna does.

The Elements

The primary constituents of the human body in traditional medicine are called "the elements." They are the basic building blocks for the science of medicine.

The four elements—earth, air, fire, and water—are the simplest particles of all that is material. They are the simplest particles of our bodies. To each of them are joined two qualities. Earth is dry and cold; water, cold and moist; air, hot and moist; and fire is hot and dry. Earth is contrary to air and water to fire. Union is possible because water serves as a means between earth and air and air as a means between water and fire. The elements, like musical tones, possess an inclination not only to ascend and descend, but also to move in a circular direction. Each element is joined by one of its qualities to that which is below and by the other to that which is above it. Water to earth beneath by coldness and to air above by moisture; air to water beneath by moisture and to fire above by heat; fire to air beneath by heat and to earth toward which it declines by dryness; earth to water above by coldness and to fire which declines toward it by dryness. Two of the elemental qualities are active and two passive. Active are hot and cold. Passive are dry and wet. The resulting qualities, the ideal combination, is an equitable one.

Quality results from the opposing qualities of the elements, a mixture of hot, cold, wet and dry. Balance comes when the strength of primary qualities are equal to these qualities—an average of these qualities. In medicine, it does not depend upon exactly equal but "equitable," meaning that the quality and quantity of the elements are distributed in such a manner that the resulting pattern or equilibrium of the body as a whole or if its parts is the one most appropriate for that person.

When one quality predominates over the other, the body is not well suited to the needs of the soul. The proportion in which the elements are united with the body has an influence upon action. Slow and heavy moving signifies a predominance of cold and dryness (earth); fearfulness and sluggishness, of cold and wetness (water); cheerfulness, of heat and wetness (air); and sharp, angry violence, of heat and dryness (fire).

All physical forms consist of elemental qualities prefigured in the physical process. If something changes in the element, something must have changed in the physical process. The two stand to each other in the strict relationship of cause and effect.

As phenomena of the external world and, in traditional medicine, the inner world, consist of the elements and their qualities, as well. Different elemental qualities are always based on the different properties of the elements (higher, lower, lighter, heavier, colder, hotter, etc.). The distinguishing characteristic of the elements is that they differ like two colors, red and green, and like two shades of a single color, light and dark blue or like shapes rough and square. The property is a characteristic of such a nature that it both distinguishes different elements from one another and at the same time orders them in definite ways.

The dynamic quality of the elements is that they have direction. The elements point one to another—attract and are attracted—and are therefore directional forces. Elemental motion has its origin not in differences of properties but in differences of dynamic quality as conveyors of motion.

The Humors

The humors are the primary fluids of the body which move through inner space. These humors affect the function of the body and are themselves influenced by the states of motion and rest of the human being.

Food and drink are transformed into innate heat through the digestive process. The humors arise in the second stage of digestion in the liver. This process produces four humors which sustain and nourish the body and move through the channels or meridians: sanguineous (blood), serous (phlegm), bilious (choler, yellow bile) and atrabilious (melancholy, black bile) corresponding to air (hot and wet), water (cold and wet), fire (hot and dry) and earth (cold and dry). These are subject to variation in quantity and in degree of purity.

Illness results from either a quantitative or qualitative change of humor. In a "normal" state, the humors are assimilated by the organs and completely integrated into the tissues. In an "abnormal" state, due to improper digestion, the material is unsuitable for assimilation and therefore eliminated by the body. Surpluses may be eliminated by exercise, bathing, coition, purges and laxatives.

The sanguineous humor (blood), which is an equal temper, exceeds the others in proportion to quantity, is hot and moist, sweet and red. It imparts strength and color to the body and serves for the engendering of the drives. Located in the heart, it relates to Leo, Aries and Sagittarius in the Zodical constellations.

The serous humor or phlegm, next to blood in quantity, is watery, cold, moist and white. It moderates the strength, heat, and thickness of blood, nourishes the brain, and moistens and nourishes such part of the body as are concerned in motion. If blood fails, heat dissolves the serous humor into blood. Cancer, Pisces and Scorpio, as Zodiacal signs, relate to serous humor.

The bilious humor, least in quantity, is hot and dry, yellow or red and bitter. A part of it passes from the liver to the gall-bladder and a part, flowing thence with other humors, moderates moisture and makes the blood subtle so that it may pass easily through straight ways. The bilious humor prevents the body from becoming heavy, sleepy and dull. It penetrates and opens passages and feeds members of the body in which the fiery element predominates. Zodiacal signs are Gemeni, Aquarius, and Libra.

The atrabilious humor is earthy and gross, thick, black and sour. A part of it passes to the spleen and a part remains with the blood. This humor feeds the bones, the spleen and other parts of the body which are gross or "melancholy" in nature. It tempers the two hot humors (sanguineous and bilious) and serves to stay and retain the floating spirits that arise from blood. The atrabilious humor thickens the blood and thus prevents it from flowing too freely through the veins and arteries. Within the Zodaic this humor is related to the three signs Tarus, Virgo, and Capricorn.

From the natural predominance of a humor in the human

being spring definite characteristics of physique and conduct. Those dominated by the sanguinious humor are cheerful, courageous, kind and ingenious. Their blood, if subtle, makes the wit keen. As fatness increases, blood diminishes. The serous humor dominating is visible in people who are easily provoked, given to treachery and vehement in action; fierce in assailing but inconstant in sustaining the assault; inclined to envy, pride, prodigality and wrath. If the serous humor is corrupt, they are subject to evil passions and dreadful nightmares. Those with a predominance of bilious humor are generally slothful, given to bodily pleasures, sleepy, idle, dull of wit, heavy and slow. They love delicate food and drink. Those dominated by the atrabilious humor are hard to please, obstinate, suspicious, sorrowful and given to fearful thoughts.

The humors are exceedingly variable in quantity and quality. The sanguineous reigns from 3 am to 9 am; bilious from 9 am to 3 pm; serous from 3 pm to 9 pm and atrabilious from 9 pm to 3 am. The sanguineous humor increases in the spring. The heat of summer dissolves superfluities, wastes the humors and opens the pores. The breath escapes from the body with exhalations, moisture and vapors. The bilious humor is in ascendancy. Autumn breeds the serous humor. Winter thickens the humors, constrains the sinews and sends natural heat inward. The atrabilious humor increases and makes people sluggish.

The active elemental qualities—cold and heat—form the humors. When heat is equable, the sanguineous humor forms; when heat is in excess, bilious humor forms; when in great excess so that oxidation occurs, atrabilious humor forms. When the cold is equable, serous humor forms; when cold is in excess so that congelation becomes dominant, atrabilious humor forms.

In addition to this, there are three souls within the human form:

> . . . namely, the vegetable, animal and rational, all of which descend from the world above and each of which possesses its own faculties. The more refined the mix-

> ture of the humors the greater the perfection and the more complete and perfect the possibility of receiving the soul. Moreover, in each man, health means the harmony of the humors and illness the disruption of the balance of the constitution. Of course the harmony is never perfect in any person, but relative to his own constitution, health means the re-establishment of the balance of the humors. Diagnosis for such disorders as fever are, in fact, based on searching for the way in which the balance of the humors has been upset. But for diseases which show overt signs, the most notable sign or signs are made use of it for disgnostic purposes and often the disease receives the name of the leading sign connected with it.[11]

Flowing in the space intermediate between the physical body and the force of life, is a placeless space, a space that, as a whole, has a direction and must have a center, the position toward which it is directed. Health or lack of it is is out from this center.

The Breath

The breath acts as the link between the body, soul and spirit. It is the breath which makes the perfect equilibrium of the elements possible.

> **§486** God created the left side of the heart and made it hollow in order that it should serve both as a storehouse of the breath and as the seat of manufacture of the breath. He also created the breath to enable the drives of the "soul' to be conveyed into the corresponding members. In the first place the breath was to be the rallying-point for the faculties of the soul and in the second place it was to be an emanation into the various members and tissues of the body (whereby these could manifest the functions of those drives).
>
> **§487** Now He produced the breath out of the finer particles of the humors and out of igneity and at the same time produced the tissues themselves (the visible body) out of the coarser and earthy particles of these humors. In other words, the breath is related to

the attenuated particles as the body is related to the coarser particles of the same humors. Just as the humors are intermingled to produce a temperamental "form," whereby the members of the body are enabled to receive a physical appearance, impossible were they separate, so the attenuated portions of the humors, being intermingled into a temperamental form, enable the breath to receive the powers of the soul—impossible were the humors separate.

§**488** The beginning of the breath is as a divine emanation from potentiality to actuality proceeding without intermission or stint until the form (preparation, state) is completed and perfected. Each member, though derived from the self-same substance of the humors, nevertheless has its own particular temperament—for the proportional qualities of the (denser portions of the) humors and the form of their commixture are peculiar to each member. Similarly, although derived from the same attenuated portions of the humors, nevertheless each of the three breaths (natural, animal and vital) has its own particular temperament, because the proportional quantities of the more attenuated portions of the humors and the manner of their commixture are peculiar to each breath.

§**489** Although the body consists of several organs, there is one from which they all originally arose. As to what this organ actually was, there are various opinions. The fact remains that one organ necessarily came to light before other organs could arise out of it. Exactly the same is true in the case of the breaths. There is one single breath which accounts for the origin of the others. This breath, according to the most important philosophers, arises in the heart, passes thence into the principal centers of the body, lingering in them long enough to enable them to impart to it their respective temperamental properties. Lingering in the cerebrum it receives a temperament whereby it is capable of receiving the drives of sensation and movement; in the liver, it receives the drive of nutrition and growth (vegetative drives); in the generative glands it acquires a temperament which prepares it for receiving the drive of generation (reproduction).

The breath is similar to the spirit and is of three kinds:

(1) The vital spirit, hot and dry, has its center in the left ventricle of the heart, preserves life, causes the body to grow, move and reproduce, and travels through the arteries. (2) The psychic spirit, cold and wet, has its center in the brain, causes sensation and movement and moves through the nerves and is the source of movement and reason. (3) The natural spirit, hot and wet, has its center in the liver, is concerned with the reception of food, growth and reproduction and travels through the veins.[12]

Traditional medicine is first concerned with the rhythmic continuity of the breath itself and then the synthesis of breath as "time in motion" or "active space" and organs or members as "passive possibilities of space" of matter and form. Harmonic order brings together those two concepts of breath and organs which appear to be opposite but which inwardly contain one another and are therefore complements. The synthesis is achieved because the breath occupies a continuous space defined by passageways, meridians, channels which move through the shapes of organs, bones, muscles. Movement coalesces breath and organs into a unity.

The Organs

The humors in turn act as the constituent elements for the members or organs of the body which "are derived primarily from the commingling of the humors, just as the humors are derived primarily from the commingling of the aliments and the aliments are primarily composed of commingled elements. The organs are divided into simple ones having homogeneous parts such as flesh, bones, and nerves, and compound organs such as the hands and face. The organs are the instruments by which the passions and actions of the mind are achieved and act as its servants.

The primary elemental quality of an organ is based on its nutrient while its secondary quality is determined by what it excretes.

Hot organs consist of the vital force and heart, blood, liver, flesh, muscle, spleen, kidneys, breasts, testicles, muscular coats of arteries, veins, skin of palm (which is evenly balanced).

Cold organs consist of phlegm, hair, bones, cartilage, ligaments, serous membranes, nerves, spinal cord, brain, solid and liquid fats and skin.

Moist organs consist of phlegm, blood, sold and liquid fats, brain, spinal cord, breast, testicles, lungs, liver, spleen, kidneys, muscles, and skin.

Dry organs consist of hair, bones, cartilage, ligaments, tendons, membranes, arteries, veins, motor nerves, heart, sensory nerves, skin.

The Efficient Causes

> §**16** The efficient (*failiya*) causes are capable of either preventing or inducing change in the human body. They may be external to the person or internal. External causes are: age, sex, occupation, residence, and climate and other agents which effect the human body by contact whether contrary to nature or not. Internal causes are sleep and wakefulness, evacuation of secretions and excretions, the changes at different periods of life in occupation, habits and customs, ethnic group and nationality.

The efficient causes are clear and vary with each individual. Whereas the elements, humors, breath and organs as the material cause are all from nature, the efficient causes develop out of the nurturing process.

The Formal Causes

> §**17** The formal (*suriyah*) causes are three: temperaments (*mizajat*) (or the pattern of constitution as a whole) and the faculties or drives (*qawa*) which emerge from it and the structure (the quantitative patterns).

Temperament

Temperament arises from the elements and humors and it determines the way in which the soul functions. Each animal and each organ of the body has a temperament of its own.

> **§51** The Almighty Creator has bestowed upon every animal and every one of its organs the most appropriate and the best adapted temperament for its various functions and passive states.
>
> **§52** Since the verification of this truth is a matter for philosophers and not physicians, we may accept that the human being has been bestowed a most befitting temperament and most appropriate faculty or drives for the various active and passive states in the body. Similarly, every organ and member is endowed with the proper temperament appropriate to its own functional requirement. Some He has made more hot, others more cold, others more dry and others more moist.

The temperament is "equable" when the contrary qualities are in perfect equilibrium, and out of harmony or "inequable" when the temperament tends toward a particular quality. Therapeutics, then, are based on the allopathic principle of contraries. That is, "cold" diseases can be cured by "hot" remedies and vice versa.

Avicenna then explains this method further:

> **§43** It is worth remembering that when a medicine is referred to as being evenly balanced, it does not mean that its temperament is the same as of a human being, or that it is even similar to it, for it would then be like a human being. It merely means that such a medicine, after being acted upon by the innate heat [metabolized] fails to produce any material change in the normal state of the body, and that its pharmacological actions remain within the limits of normal human temperament. In other words, when this medicine is given to a normal person, it does not

> produce any appreciable change or imbalance in the body. When it is said that a drug is hot or cold, it does not mean that the physical quality of the drug is particularly hot or cold or that it is colder or hotter than the human body. If this were so there would follow the unwarranted inference mentioned above that an evenly constituted medicine is the one which has exactly the same temperament as the human body. It means just that such a medicine produces a greater amount of heat or cold than what was originally present in the body. A drug which, for example, is cold for the human being may be hot for the scorpion, or the medicine which is hot for the human being may be cold for the serpent. In fact it may also mean that the same medicine may be less hot for one person than for another. This is the reason why physicians are advised to change their medicine when it fails to produce the desired result.

The growth and decay of the human body is dependent upon the human temperament. Growth depends upon the heat contained in the sperm which is gradually used up. Meanwhile, the moisture lessens in quantity and quality, thus preserving the innate heat at a constant level up to the old age. Ultimately, however, the moisture of the body comes to an end, and the innate heat ie extinguished, thus causing the death to which everyone is destined and which depends upon the original temperament of the human body.

The correspondences between the various orders of reality and the temperament have been summed up in the following:

> The uniqueness of the temperament of each individual indicates that each microcosm is a world of its own, not identical with any other microcosm. Yet, the repetition of the same basic humors in each constitution bears out the fact that each microcosm presents a morphological resemblance to other microcosms. Moreover, there is an analogy between the human body and the cosmic order, as shown by the correspondence between the humors and elements.

> There is in the Hermetico-alchemical natural philosophy, which was always closely tied to medicine in Islam, a basic doctrine of the correspondence between all the various orders of reality: the intelligible hierarchy, the heavenly bodies, the order of numbers, the parts of the body, the letters of the alphabet which are the "elements" of the Sacred Book, etc. The seven cervical and the twelve dorsal vertebrae correspond to the seven planets and the twelve signs of the Zodiac, as well as to the days of the week and the months of the year; and the total number of discs of the vertebrae, which they consider to be twenty-eight, to the letters of the Arabic alphabet and the stations of the moon. There is, therefore, both numerical and astrological symbolism connected with medicine, although the closeness of the relation has not been the same during all periods of Islamic history, nor among all the medical authorities. But the correspondence and "sympathy" (in the original sense of the word "*sympathia*") between various orders of cosmic reality form the philosophical background of Islamic medicine.[13]

The Faculties or Drives

The body also possesses faculties which originate the functions of various organs. The major faculties are (1) the vital (*hayawaniyah*), responsible for preserving the integraity of the breath, sensation, and movement of the heart; (2) the natural (*tabiiyah*) governing the nutritive powers of the liver and the reproductive powers of the generating organs; and (3) the animal (*nafsaniyah*) controlling the brain and the rational faculty.

The powers of the various members are due to the vital faculty[14] which provides the body with its inner force. The vital faculty is that which appears in the breath at the very moment at which the breath develops out of the rarefied particles of the humors.

Between the human body as a whole and the individual points as its parts there is a relationship—the whole being given with and active in the part and the part being aware that it is part and directly announcing its relation to the whole.

Whenever we encounter a phenomenon showing this relationship between whole and parts we may assume, that a force, an ordered action of forces, is the basis. This is the role of the faculties which we can only know through their effects. They work through the physical body without ever touching it.

The Final Causes

§18 The final (*tamamia*) causes are the actions or functions. They can be understood only from a knowledge of both the faculties or drives (*qawa*) and the vital energies (breaths, *arwah*) that are ultimately responsible for them. These will be described presently.

Conclusion

The power of traditional Islamic medicine is in realizing that space leads and forms shapes; shapes then interact with space and space with the breath/inner light with which every human being has been endowed. What he or she does with that determines the extent of their completion and perfection.

O. Cameron Gruner's Preface to the First Edition

Preface to the First Edition, 1930

The Purpose of the present treatise is two-fold:

(1) To furnish a translation of the First Book of *The Canon of Medicine* of Avicenna. The section on Anatomy has been omitted in favor of the first half of the *De viribus cordis*.* This assists in the second object of the treatise. (2) To present a study of the mystical philosophy (*tasawwuf*) especially showing where this and modern biological knowledge are reciprocally illuminative.

The words of the late Professor E. G. Browne may be quoted here, "Even if we rate the originality of [Islamic] medicine at the lowest, I venture to think that it will deserve more careful and systematic study." Furthermore, the Thomistic philosophy of human nature is especially discussed and its applicability to the medicine of the future is definitely enunciated.

A grateful acknowledgement is made to the School of Oriental Studies, London Institution (University of London) for signal help in the acquisition of the Arabic, Persian, and Chinese essential to the purpose of the treatise.

* Note: In order to present a more complete translation here, we have included the complete section on anatomy omitted by Gruner, using the Shah translation of *The Canon* (see §125-446).

O. Cameron Gruner's Remarks

Introduction

During the past fifty years,[1] the popular imagination has been stirred by a succession of important discoveries in the domain of medicine and surgery. The triumphs of the latter field have been spectacular to a degree. Those of medicine have been much less conspicuous, chiefly because the mind must inquire into them before it can properly appreciate them. How much does not humanity owe to the steadily continued researches in bacteriology, and the painstaking observations which have revealed the life-cycles of many of the parasites to which tropical and other diseases are due and to the whole procedure of immuno-therapy, the just pride of scientific as distinct from clinical medicine, and the outcome of all these researches?

As compared with all this, the speculative subtleties of former times appear both futile and unworthy of resuscitation. But the ancient system was not as valueless as is so generally supposed. Taking as an adequate criterion the first book of *The Canon of Medicine* of Avicenna, which is here presented [almost in its entirety], and is fairly representative of the whole work, we find in its pages references to many departments of human knowledge—(though it might be objected that all these departments of knowledge are now separate sciences, each requiring its own professorial staff, its own literature, and journals and that they are not mentioned under the special names with which we are familiar, their existence in those days cannot be denied) cosmology, anatomy, physiology, and psychology; the: various branches of clinical medicine-etiology, semiology, diagnosis, and prognosis; the departments of therapeutics-hygiene, dietetics, balneology, and climatology, in addition to materia medica, pharmacology, and pharmacy. Moreover, the reader is presumed to be conversant with logic, criteriology, and metaphysics.

The presence of obvious literal errors in the work must not lead us to commit the more serious mistake of overlooking the fact that it is entirely built up upon a sound philosophy of human nature, which is as vitally important today, though largely ignored in former times. The traditional medicine was concerned essentially with the given patient now before us; whereas now it is simply essentially with the given patient now before us; whereas now it is simply the science of diseases which it is our duty to diagnose accurately, prevent if possible, and treat on lines capable of wholesale application. To Avicenna, the determination of the constitution of the patient was of the very first importance, because on it depended the character, course, and duration of his illness, and upon that again depended the choice of remedies.

After all, from the patient's point of view, the real object of consulting a medical man is to be restored to a state of well-being. It is little comfort to be virtually told that 85-90 percent of cases of his complaint are cured by the treatment adopted in his case, only to find that he proves to be one of the remaining 10-15 percent for whom there is little or nothing to be done. True, his sighs are drowned in the shouts of the fortunate, and fail to reach the clinical laboratory, surgical wards, consulting room or research councils.

If, in the interests of these few, chance leads us to the pages of this traditional work, it would seem that suggestions occur in it which enable us to understand their plight, and thereby help them to understand it also. Even if the enemy is not put out of action, his enmity is less evident when he is understood.

It has been the aim of this treatise to elaborate Avicenna's central theme by references to the various philosophies extant in his time—Sufi, Vedantic, Buddhist, Chinese; to Persian writings subsequent to his time (Rumi, Sadi, Shabistari, etc.); and to views presented by various modern philosophies, including western theosophy.

But these various directions of thoughts are not drawn upon in order to elaborate a composite system after the fashion of theosophical eclecticism. On the contrary, readers accustomed to various modes of thought are invited across a bridge leading from their various starting-points, across the chasm of modernism, until they reach the concise teaching of Thomistic philosophy, wherein all other aspects of the one truth receive their proportionate places. The inclusion of ideas from writers whose ideas appear to be altogether of the by-ways may torment a few, but may also help a few to see the: greater thing, and thereafter be content to stay upon the broad highway to which the several paths have converged.

Science has been removed from its usual role of master, and has been pressed into service, and that service is to illuminate the subject of human nature. To quote a recent paper,[2] "Under the great swelling flood that represents the growing complexity of modern medicine, let us not allow ourselves hold fast to that great life-saving conception of the essential unity of the human body. Let us oppose fearlessly those currents of medical thought that tend to isolate—arbitrarily and to the detriment of true knowledge—the various segments of this one great subject. Let us welcome all methods, all discoveries, that help the one man in charge of the one patient to broaden the base of his attack, to widen the sweep of his beneficent vision." These words were possibly expressed with a different object, but apply well to the theme of this treatise.

The old teaching about "constitution" should undergo a mutual inter-growth with the knowledge of modern science, pervaded throughout with the fundamental teaching of Thomistic philosophy, when there would emerge the beginnings of a possible system of modern scholastic medicine—thoroughly logical, plain, free of mystery, free of materialism, but not ignoring the so-called "occult" and metaphysical; with the knowledge of the nature of the constitution of the individual patient as its central and dominant theme. Were the whole medical training along such lines, the student would be able to approach his clinical instruction thoroughly aware that the individuality of the patient comes first, and that the ailment from which he suffers is but part and parcel of one single story, and not merely an accidental superposition. But the student would constantly need guidance to ensure his over-riding the disregard or ignorance, if not actual rejection, of scholastic principles which characterizes the concrete modern teaching of pathology in its various departments.

The following brief survey of the most important teachings of *The Canon* reinterprets them under three headings: (1) the general notion of the nature of the human being; (2) the notion of the constitution of any individual when in health; (3) the notion of the nature of the state of disease. These together provide that clear mental idea of "the patient before me" which is essential before I can effectively treat him.

TEACHINGS OF *THE CANON*

THE GENERAL NOTION OF THE NATURE OF A HUMAN BEING

The following three propositions belong to it: (1) the human being (*MF*)[3] is composed of matter and a principle of life, the two together making him "he" or "she," he or she is "a single substance endowed with a natural tendency to realize and maintain the conditions of its organization." (2) This principle of life comprises three main groups of potential and actual activities—the vegetative, the sensitive and the rational. This multi-potentiality of the principle of life is represented in the expression "bundle of life." (3) The organs of the body are the material manifestations (the actualities) of the several potentialities The vegetative organs belong to the "vegetative soul," the sense-organs and appurtenances belong to the "sensitive soul." The intelligence and will belong to the "rational soul," which has not literal organs but acts through the instrumentation of the organs of the vegetative and sensitive systems. All these components belong intimately together apart from macroscopic or microscopic boundaries it.

These propositions are further defined by the following negative statements: (1) the human being is not a collection of molecules and forces; he manifests chemical, electric, and other phenomena, which are not causes, but effects. (2) The organs are not distinct from the powers they exhibit. (3) The brain is not the producer of thought.

The remarkable action which the human being achieves by his complicated mechanical contrivances are distinct from himself, whereas in the human being the mechanism and the manipulator are the self same. Even when there is as grave mechanical interference with organs as occurs in hemiplegia, or in the cortical lesions of insanity, the rational soul remains untouched, though no longer able to communicate its activities to the outer world. To quote from St. Thomas, "The intellect, being a power that does not make use of a corporeal organ, would in no way be hindered in its act through the lesion of a corporeal organ, if for its act there were not required the act of some power that does make used of a corporeal organ."[4]

Thought is produced by the activity of the rational souls; the changes in the brain—whether chemical, cytological, or otherwise—are not causes, but the visible effects of the activity. (4) There is no bridge over the gulf between rational life and thevegetative sensitive life; the distinctions are radical. (5) The life-principle is not subject to the laws of inheritance, those which govern matter; it is not divisible into organs, or parts, or elements. As soon as it ceases to operate, it is left behind the material body, which though apparently the same is actually quite different from the animate person recently before me.

The Notion of the Constitution of Any Given Individual When in Health

This notion should be made as tangible as possible.[5] The constitution may be expressed in terms of a number of formula to be taken together—a series of "notes," some of which are constants, and others variables. In this formula, the qualities are represented by the initials of their corresponding names; the quantities are represented by index numbers from 1 to 5, to stand for slight, moderate, normal, marked, and very marked, and very marked respectively.

The Constants

I. The body: (1) general physique [good, poor, robust, spare, strong, delicate]; (2) dominant "element" [example: $E^2W^2F^5A^3$] for earth, water, fire and air; (3) dominant "humor," shown in the humoral formula [example: $S^3L^1B^5A^8$] for sanguineous, serous (lymphatic), bilious, and atrabilious]. This formula is really descriptive of the "temperament," but the latter word bears a different meaning in modern popular usage. (4) The absolute or relative strength or weakness (functional capacity) of the several organs; hypo, hyper-function. [example: $V^4T^4M^20^3N^11G^3$, for vegetative (i.e. alimentary), thoracic (i.e. respiratory and circulatory), muscular (including skeletal), osseous (including genito-urinary), nervous (including sympathetic system) and glandular (including haemopoietic, endocrine, and hepatic) types. (5) The emotional make-up, or formula [example: $G^3L^2T^1I^5$ (*gaudium, laetitia, timor, ira*),[6] from which the dominant passion and its modifiers are noted. The modern use of the word "temperament" belongs here.

The difference in capacity is partly explained by considering the time-factor,[7] and partly as a fundamental difference.[8] All the material brought to an organ, whether nutritive, or excretory, is not at once taken up in its entirety; only a certain proportion is removed and the remainder passes on, so that the blood has its composition at a certain level. The modern threshold values recognize this fact. The time-factor is of very great importance.

II. The mind: here comes the description of the disposition, the type of mind, or mental make-up.[9] Mental capacity may be expressed in terms of the relative or absolute strength or weakness of the various faculties, enumerated under "talents" (which are simply developments of particular faculties above the average).[10] "The better the disposition of a body, the better the soul allotted to it which clearly appears in things of different species: and the reason thereof is that act and form are received into matter according to matter's capacity thus because some men have bodies of better disposition, their souls have a greater power of understanding . . . . This occurs in regard to the lower powers of which the intellect has need in its operation, because those in whom the imaginative, cogitative and memorative powers are of better disposition, are better disposed to understand."[11]

The mental attitude towards things, which emerges from the character, is also to be noted, for sometimes this may explain the cause of the illness (i.e., wanton exposure to infections in spite of warnings), and will show whether the patient is suppressing relevant facts, will respond to treatment, or is secretly concerned with some fear or doubt which is the real object of his visit to the doctor. Moreover, knowledge of this aspect of character will safeguard the physician himself, either by making him aware of the patient's possible cynical opinion about a profession he is unfortunately obliged to deal with, or, more important, by enabling him to avoid offering advice which is palpably foolish to an intelligent patient.

The Variables

The degree of vitality: this is also spoken of as the strength of innate heat in the text;[12] (2) deviations from the functional capacities normal to the individual; (3) the nature or degree of "resistance." In terms of *The Canon*, this would be expressed in the "humoral formula," and in terms of "obstructions" of various kinds. These account for the "soil" which renders declared disease: (a) possible; or (b) amenable to alteration by artificial means.[13]

Foreign though such data are to modern clinical work, they are often actually employed in ordinary conversation, as when one describes a person as sanguine, or bilious, or phlegmatic, or as of saturnine temperament. Some adjective descriptive of the emotional make-up is not infrequent in case reports degrees of vitality are spoken of seriously by the laity, diplomatically by the practitioner.

In so far as they provide a simple means of codifying tentative knowledge upon complex and elusive individual characteristics which it is our duty to notice, the data are all worth consideration.

The Notion of the Nature of the State of Disease

The vegetative processes associated with digestion and absorption of food may be first briefly referred to. The picture of the whole nutritive cycle is comprehended in the idea of the "liver."[14] We trace the food constituents through the columnar cells of the intestinal mucosa, across the areolar tissue into the vascular roots of the portal and lacteal system; then into the liver unit itself (comprising phagocytic secretary cells, fundal cells, cubical excretory cells, and the hepatic arterioles and lymphatic clefts related to the sinusoids); then into the general blood-stream, and finally out of the body through various organs, including the goblet cells of the intestinal mucosa, the bile-ducts, the pancreas, etc. The extra-hepatic portion of the cycle is nearly co-terminous with the rest of the body.

To complete this picture we first remember the relation between the quality of food and the quality of chyme; then we consider how the ultimate components of the food travel (N-compounds, glucose, fat, phosphorus, sulphur, iron, and the like)—during rest, exercise, sleep, etc. and according to the character of the diet as a whole, the fluids taken, and the state of the bowels, etc. We may realize that they are manifested in the blood in the form of alkaline tide, viscosity, fibrin-content, and the various morphological changes revealed by blood-examination. We picture also the innumerable chemical interchanges and physical transformations in various parts of the cycle; the formation of waste-substances, and the factors on which the whole of the processes depend.[15] In brief, then our picture of the body is that of a complex of tubes and channels —potential as well as actual—which vary in size from the obvious alimentary-canal, air-passages, and great blood vessels, down to the finest ramifications of the latter, the cavernous tissues—both macroscopic and microscopic—the serous cavities, and the intracellular channels. All these form one continuous labyrinthine system, through which we may trace the ingested food materials, the metabolic, secretory and excretory products. As long as these channels are patent throughout, and As long as these various subs stances (including the "breath of life") can flow freely through them, and the vital energy has a free play outward, so long is the body in a state of health.

But as soon as there is a continued interference with the freedom of movement, even though it be merely an ebb and flow that is affected, in any part of the canalicular system, then a state of disease arises, culminating in histological anatomical changes. Hence, when we observe a case of illness, we may be sure there is some "obstruction" in some channels in some part of the body—not necessarily in that where the symptoms occur (i.e., the nasal discharge of "cold in the head," the bronchial expectoration in bronchitis, the serous effusion into the pleura, the respiratory phenomena in an attack of asthma, are manifestations in the respiratory system of obstructions elsewhere).

The next addition to the picture of the sick person's state is furnished by the causes of the obstruction. Avicenna considered these under two groups, the '"material" (i.e. those in which "matter" is concerned) or "humoral diseases" and the non-material. To the latter group would belong cases of gross obstruction, such as by compression from without, or such as by obstruction with calculi and those in which there is a functional disorder—hypo-function, hyper-function, dysfunction. For instance, in renal disease, the loss of functional capacity may render the-normal ebb and flow of substances disorderly.[16]

The group of humoral diseases is predominant in Avicenna's pathology, and if we bear in mind what the "humors" really are, this position becomes quite reasonable. Perverted metabolism is associated with changes of physical state in the fluids of the body. Limpid fluids may become viscid, viscous substances may become mobile or "tenuous." In the ancient work, these chemical changes were thought of, not in "equations," but under interchanges between the imponderable elements, as being subject to the laws of *uruj, nasul, jalal, jamal, qada, qadr*,[17] the rhythm, phases and rate of movement of the "breath" and the fluctuations of degrees of innate heat. Concrete examples are such as: precipitation of urates in tissues, altered reaction of tissue juices in rheumatoid arthritis, cardio-renal disease, tuberculosis; variations of content of Ca, Na, Mg, etc., in the tissue-water, so that the flow from tissue to blood and vice versa is impeded.[18]

The Canon often insists on the presence of "superfluities" as a cause of "obstructions" of the canalicular system not only in the tangible four humors, but also in regard to the "breath."[19] In the latter case, the substance of the breath (i.e. water-vapor) ceases to be "bright," and "clear," and its odor becomes offensive, and its freedom of flow is impaired .

Finally, adding from modern knowledge, there are the changes in the fluids of the body produced by bacterial or putrefactive breakdown—whether this begins in intestinal stasis or arises in the course of specific bacterial infections. There are then obstructions not only in the old sense, but in the form of the successive histological lesions consequent—vascular, nutritional, and inflammatory. Materials are deposited more or less permanently (irreversible reactions), as i.e., solid odema, collagenous tissue, scar formation, fibrosis, and hyalo-fibrosis, adipose tissue, hyperplastic formations. Loss of anatomical patency is super added to loss of functional perviousness.

Clearly, whereas we give first place to the bacterial invasion, Avicenna gave it to the habits of life. He was deeply impressed by the obvious fact that the quality of food determines the kind of chyme, and that the kind of chyme determines the quality of the freedom of flow through the diffuse canalicular system of the body. As they accumulate in the stagnating tissue-juices they come to exercise a noxious action; they come to be beyond the capacity of the third and fourth digestions (tissue-digestion), and with their stagnation, the ever-circulating bacteria (taken up with the food) also settle and multiply and wandering-cell infiltrations gather together. The beginnings of disease are laid down. The functional disturbance has been succeeded by anatomical lesions.[20]

Finally, Avicenna enlarges his view of humoral disease by noting the influence of many extracorporeal factors[21] as well as the period of life, not to mention "the decree of God."[22] Thus, one and the same kind of food taken at the "warm" period of life in the "warm" season may contribute more to the formation of a given humor than at another.

If we knew the patient's formula, and how the climactic and other conditions are likely to affect it, and whether they are compatible or not with susceptibility to the agents at work, our composite picture of the patient's state would be of great value, and illnesses often inexplicable would lose their mystery. How much more efficient might not the treatment be, if the remedial measures in contemplation were selected to harmonize with them?

No doubt only a fanatic would note the barometer, thermometer, humidity, hours of sunshine, wind-direction and velocity, the character of previous seasons, the clues afforded by then migration so insects, rodents, and birds, the presence or prevalence of certain parasites in a district, and the many other points noted in Part Three[23] before prescribing the regimen for the patient. But it would seem that some Eastern physicians of bygone times conscientiously strove to learn from such factors.

The Guides to the Diagnosis of the State of the Patient

The patient before us is as a manuscript written in some highly complex language which it is our business to decipher. The alphabet is furnished by the several colors, the simple observations of size, shape, consistency, contour, texture, and the like. The vocabulary consists of the external features both in repose and animation, and of the physical signs as taught today. The grammar lies in the "general guides" (sphygmology, urinoscopy, examination of feces and blood). The language is to be translated into: states of natural (vegetative), sensitive, and emotional instinctive drives, functional capacities, plethora, obstructions, solutions of continuity, etc. that is, the state of the whole composite, in all aspects. This task can only be accomplished imperfectly at the best, even by the most skilled and most learned. Our silent teachers, or guides, the "indications" always enable us to ascertain something, and we must perforce be content with that on the present occasion and be determined to use this experience as the guide to better success on the next.

One of the guides suggested in *The Canon* lies in one's own state of health. Properly to interpret what we observe, we must ourselves have no disharmony of functions arising from errors of diet, no deposit in the urine, no weight in the bowels, no obstructions in our own brain, no mental fatigue, no emotional pre-occupation, no rigid notions regarding etiology or prognosis; there must be clear channels for the breath, and the breath must be under the control of the will. It must be kept pure by recollection, by devotion, and observance of prayer. The reason for this is that under such conditions, long persevered, we are enabled to receive an "impression" from the patient. We become aware of his atmosphere, aura, or personality in the form of an idea of his degree and kind of vitality. But unless this impression is registered rapidly, namely at the first approach of the patient, it will be confused and illegible by reason of the mutual inter-impression of one's own vitality with his. In another idiom, we observe "with the eye of a Taoist." In our own idiom, we make use of sound reasoning power, common sense, and a certain kind of "intuition," or "clinical sense."

The guides furnished by general observation of the patient are, in brief: (1) external features in repose: (a) colors of face, hair, skin, eye (sclerae, iris); (b) odors and savors; (c) form of the body: (i) as a whole; (ii) in detail. The features, the hands, the limbs; the relative proportions (length, breadth, and thickness) of nose, cheeks, upper lip, lower lip, chin, mouth, ears, orbit, eyebrows, forehead, etc.; the character of the neck, shoulders, etc. (2) Features when animated: (a) expression, gaze, look, facial gestures (vivacity, sleepiness, languidness); (b) deportment or attitude,[24] gestures, carriage, specific acts or mannerisms, definitely morbid movements or defective movements. (c) voice: tone of voice, manner of speech (clear, loud, or the opposite); clues to the physical and mental type, and the degree of energy and vitality.

Space does not allow of any attempt to furnish precise details of the external signs of functional capacity of internal organs. The principle is exemplified thus: the lower part of the nose is part of the respiratory system, and shares in the degree of development of the whole system; therefore wide nostrils with well-formed aloe go with good development of the whole respiratory function, whereas narrow delicate nostrils and small alae refer the observer to some other system as well-developed. Large mouth, thick lips, large masseters, and generally well-developed lower part of the face go with good development of the digestive tract throughout. Moreover, development or capacity above the average in one system denotes relative weakness and functional deficiency in another system. The subject is extensive.[25]

Our general guides differs noticeably, from that revealed in *The Canon*. To follow Avicenna, (1) when one places the hand on the pulse, one absorbs oneself in it, without the distraction of a watch, until one has found out how it runs minute after minute. Even if it misses, without an intermission of the heart, because the patient gives a twitch of the finger or begins to talk, one learns even from that. The study of the circulation is more than the study of the heart's action. (2) When one examines the urine, even with all the apparatus of modern chemistry, we must remember that it is first and foremost the guide to the state of digestion—especially its "second stage" (that in the liver) as well as in the "third" stage (that in the small vessels). We are misled by the search for albuminuria and glycosuria, for many would make these abnormalities into diseases. Thus, the number of persons in whom albuminuria is not evidence of renal disease far outnumber those in which it is; the presence of such a substance in the urine should lead to the questions: is some substance not being dealt with? If so, why? Can only the kidney handle it? To follow a useful rule, the real trouble is remote. It may lie in the brain, in the emotional state (cf. Graves' disease, i.e., pentosuria, cystinuria, alkaptonuria also break the current ideas about urinalysis.[26] (3) As regards the guide furnished by the feces matter, again, our knowledge is much greater than was Avicenna's and we do not apply it in his terms. We are apt to lose ourselves in fat analyses, nitrogen estimations, occult blood tests, B. coli classifications. Negative results in each case are taken to mean nothing of note, regardless of the continual secretory and excretory changes proceeding in the intestinal mucosa, and the vitality of nerve-ganglia, etc. Essential and definite derangements may occur without conspicuous deviations from the restricted standards usually laid down.

The guide furnished by an examination of the brood may be spoken of as the most notable modern addition to Avicenna's three general guides. The data obtained from it—physical, physicochemical, cytological, serological—are very numerous, but are lost more often than not by restriction to the diagnosis of the various "blood-diseases." When properly applied, all the data obtained from the blood inform us of the functional state of all the organs and of the existence of the main groups of pathological state.[27]

TREATMENT

"The healing art, as it is described in books, is far inferior to the practical experience of a skilful and thoughtful physician." (Rhazes).

"Many are healed by the action of nature without the art of medicine."[28] "Man teaches by outward ministration, but God by inward operation: even so the physician is said to minister, to nature when he heals."[29]

Application of the principles of *The Canon* to modern practice would seem superfluous. The common ailments, especially those of minor surgery, are nowadays treated in stereotyped fashion, which appears to be beyond improvement. It is not with such cases that reference to *The Canon* is suggested. It is the general principle which may be reviewed in the mind, and lines of treatment such as were once in vogue may be quite usefully applicable in a few cases which do not well respond to modern methods. Moreover, the conscience of even the most careful may not be altogether clear in regard to the immemorial rule: " *tutto, cito, et jucunde*."

The subject may be briefly considered under two headings: plan of treatment; methods of treatment.

The Plan of Treatment

The choice of a plan of treatment depends on the view which is taken as to the cause of the illness. It is no new or modern thing to say "treat the cause." The distinction between new and old is in regard to the idea of the nature of the cause. In these days nearly every illness is ultimately due to an infection or intoxication, and the aim of treatment is to destroy the one and render the other innocuous. To Avicenna, illness was primarily an abnormal state of condition, to which many factors contributed. The scheme of treatment must, therefore, envisage them all. To facilitate this, the practitioner of those days would advisedly mentally review the whole of the second part.[30]

Indeed, if we scrutinize the subject more closely, it will appear that Avicenna's plan is after all very proper. For, even if we could attack the microbic cause specifically, there would still remain the lesions which it has produced, and the lowering of the vitality (=interferences with the flow of vital currents, in Paracelsus' idiom)[31] A condition remains to be combated; the condition is uppermost as far as the patient is concerned. Even in those relatively few cases in which the disease is bound up-with a particular organ, so that the name of the disease is according (i.e., gastric ulcer, cerebral hemorrhage), it is the condition we have to face. The cause, even when known, has done its work, and gone.

It is true that many other interpretations of disease and corresponding plans of treatment are put forward in various quarters from time to time, especially by the intellectually anarchistic. This occurrence is partly the outcome of the arbitrary attitudes towards patient and friends sometimes exhibited by some of the representatives of academic medicine and would be best met by frank and courteous enquiry into lay opinions. Not everyone subscribes to the restrictions of medical ethics, and the patient is too often treated as if illness *ipso facto* at once deprives him of ordinary intelligence. After all, he seeks medical help for a distinct object, and remuneration for the services is presumed, so that he is entitled to go elsewhere, at his own choice, if unfortunately in his particular case the plan and method of treatment proves unsuccessful. But this view is not subscribed to by those who assume that the whole of the knowledge needed for every case is comprehended within the orthodox teaching of the day, and that every individual possesses.

The Methods of Treatment

Even the methods of treatment set forth in *The Canon* are still resorted to at times. No doubt, we would do well to follow them more frequently. Thus, systematic purgation is often called for, but not carried out as radically as of old. Cupping is still of value for such conditions as lumbar myositis, acute hemorrhagic nephritis, and those diseases amenable to autohaemolysins. Venesection is sometimes effectively applied for cases of high blood-pressure, threatened apoplexy; it is incidentally used in the course of obtaining blood-tests.

Drug Treatment

The steady decline of drug treatment in modern medical practice is evidenced in several directions: (1) the steady removal, in successive editions of the British Pharmacopceia of herbal remedies which are supposed to have no action because laboratory animals appear to be unaffected by them; (2) the infrequency with which medicines are ordered for hospital patients; (3) the penalization of panel practitioners for "over-prescribing"; (4) the desire on the part of many lay persons to banish "drugs" as being "unnatural."

Inconsistencies are frequent. There is the strange perversity which (through legislation) denies facilities for the use of the few drugs whose potency is quite unquestionable. There is the subterfuge of resorting to placebos (which often cost no more than the bottle containing them). Those among the lay who decry drugs are pleased to employ herbal remedies. Where there is a popular demand for the latest remedies, this is met by a never-ending stream of new synthetic and other preparations, and costly manufactured products, which also the medical world submits to. Truly the mind ever seeks in the relatively inaccessible, and the expensive, that which lies all the time, and without price, at our feet. It describes as progress that which better knowledge would render superfluous.

The truth is that we know far too little about the herbal remedies of *The Canon*. To begin with we forget that they cannot be efficient without careful attention to the conditions of their cultivation (soil, climate, season, etc.), the times proper for their collections, the details of their preservations and the laws governing the formation and circulation of the active principles during the life-cycles of the various plants. We do not individually know how to identify adulterations, whether accidental or deliberate. We leave to wholesale manufacture that which was once properly undertaken individually since personal artistic skill may be the real condition for pharmacological efficiency. We adopt the short cut of standardization of drugs as the remedy for the loss of potency inevitable after neglect of such various factors. But even if the purity and potency of remedies be granted, by recourse to the best sources they must be employed with deliberate care.

As Avicenna shows in the second book of *The Canon*, there must be a knowledge of the constitution or individuality of the plants which yield the drug; harmony with the constitution of the patient must be aimed at. Out of a number of drugs of like action, some will accord better with one person as constitution than with another's. One remedy may soothe and ease without its specific action being at all diminished whereas another performs its work harshly and unpleasantly; another may be overpowered by the personal factor. The scope of the subject is great and its study with intent to serious practical application, should not require an apologia.

Such considerations as these open the door of romance. The discovery that all nature is a living whole, always at work, earnestly, steadily, continuously developing an fidea, would arouse a new and intensely absorbing interest—that of watching the unseen worker, though His hands are not to be discerned, that which He does is ever proceeding before us as a continual motion-picture, and we may become aware not only of the merely superficial fact of the movements, but also of the purpose unfolding.

Watching the medicinal trees and shrubs and herbs in this way, and seeing their properties by their forms, and colors and odors, and their changes in character with the changes of the seasons, and alternations of drought and plenty (variations of rate of growth, of activity of flowering and fruiting), how great is the wonder of the work of nature! We note how substances are being elaborated into plants which we, wanting their help, know how to take at the crucial moment—now we must draw the resin; now we must take these flowering tops, and so on. But we are not the only watchers. The bees have been waiting, the birds, the slugs, the ants, the herbivora all these and many others wait to draw from such supplies that which is applicable to their several requirements. Nature itself also waits for all these things to be collected from its treasury. Everything has been worked out; the interactions are arranged for they all belong to the purpose of the Designer; and He Himself is waiting for that over which He incessantly broods, with entire and complete intention. He too waits to draw out of Creation that which was His object in making it.

No doubt it is true that few of the ancient physicians entered fully into this inner life of the world of which they formed a part. Few even of those who learned *The Canon* by heart may have applied it effectively at all times and on all occasions; few may have meditated sufficiently to consider the soul-life of the patient they were called upon to help. But the life was there then, as it is here now. It could be read then, as it should be now. The entry to the infinite treasure-house of nature was not locked then, and it is not locked now. Indeed, the entry was not merely through one door, there was a portal of entry on every side. Doors so large as to be discernible from afar; doors so small that few could find them; but even through the smallest there was the same ability to enter the treasure-hall. Travelers in those days might fear imagined ogres, jinn, and terrifying guardians to counter talismans; but the keys of safety were everywhere in hand, for all these beings were amenable to caresses the caresses of a heart which approached them with reverence and affection, asking questions but never injuring; always treating everything within the treasury (for it is living) as gently as one should approach to watch a sleeping babe.

It is for us ourselves not to pass these things by. If we did nothing more than study the *materia medica* of those days to see what products were available, we should have ample material for thought, and become cognizant of the links between that age and this. The drugs are still cultivated, and still used in the East in the manner of the past, and the history of their names adds to our understanding of their uses. While it is true we can supply our needs through an order to the apothecary based on information imparted to us through various intermediaries, we may some day find that in doing so we have omitted to look inside the treasure-house. To go back to the old paths, watching nature and studying the uses of the living plants, is not to lose the definite therapeutic effects we seek. Far from it; and there is the added insight into that universal life which needs transference from the inexhaustible abundance of nature at large into the thirsting lack of the patient in particular. It would then be not simply as a "relaxation" from the exacting labors of the city that one would go abroad into the country-side. It would be for the purpose of retiring to watch, and meditate upon the manifestations of the quiet persistent surging life of creatures below the level of man, thereby to learn something of the secret through which the equilibrium of health is to be restored to the needy and also oneself—to receive from the fountains of life.

Dietetic Treatment

In these days, this form of treatment is increasingly to the fore. But whereas modern thought is in terms of food-values and the like, *The Canon* insists (and rightly) on the necessity for studying physiological and psychological incompatibilities in regard to each component of the diet, and for selecting the various articles of food according to their constitution, so that they shall be in harmony with the constitution of the patient.

Regiminal Treatment

The term "regimen" has a wide range. This has already been sufficiently indicated at the end of Part Three.[32] The consideration of the specific constitution of the patient, of his present state, and of the conditions which are likely to arise during the various successive phases of his illness, must pervade every detail of the prescription of the regimen, to ensure that the correspondences between the state and the various measures adopted shall throughout be as harmonious as possible.

In this way, the great importance of individual artistry in treatment is constantly insisted on, by contrast with the prevalent stereotyping of therapeutic methods, whether in regard to state regulated practice in its various branches, or in the provision of medical relief on a wholesale scale, or in the efforts to subject as much as possible to the output of team-work. The atmosphere thus created helps the student to realize that the last word has not been said when the clinician's discourse over the hospital bed is ended, and the protocols, and therapeutic orders have been set upon the bed sheet.

The following may be quoted here, from Bauer:[33] "It is true, there is a difference between the pure medical science and the art of its practical application at the patient's bedside. This art is somewhat more, indeed, than this application; it requires more than a complete knowledge of all scientific details; it is and will be always an art which never will be transformed into an exact science, as the complete understanding of one person's psychophysical machinery never will permit us to understand a second man's personality just as well by a pure analogy, because of the practically infinite variability of the individual constitution. The individual analysis must start always anew, and what science of the human constitution may help, is only to establish certain groups of more or less pronounced common characteristics . . . it will never replace entirely the doctor's art to . . . take the individual particularities of his patient into consideration . . . in constructing his diagnosis and in applying the fitted treatment."

The clinical handling of a case is guided from time to time by the experience which has been concentrated into aphorisms. Like many; ancient medical works, *The Canon* abounds in these also, and some of them will not doubt be found among the modern collections of aphorisms which are available. In this way, too, it may be true to say that the conduct of a modern case sometimes receives the personal guidance of the wisdom of the past.

PROGRESS

Progress[34] is a relative term. The common error is to assume that it is an end in itself. Things which can be described as "up to date," or cast aside as "out of date," do not belong to the real basis of human life. The idea of progress is associated with the introduction of mechanical improvements of all kinds; with mass production of manufactured articles; with the standardization of existence. In the domain of medicine, it is more particularly associated with an increasing knowledge of concrete facts, with specific discoveries in etiology and treatment; and with a new nomenclature.

To illustrate the relative character of "progress" one may call to mind that many discoveries and inventions are simply actualizations of ideas previously current among thinkers, but perhaps not noticed at the time, or even repudiated or attacked as heretical. Further, as to the changes in nomenclature which occur as time goes on: because our language and idiom is different, many are apt to think the old statements were necessarily incorrect. In medieval books dealing with *materia medica*, they said for instance: "dissolved in vinegar, the action is so-and-so," whereas we say simply: acetum, action and uses: . . . In chemistry, they might say "fire produces *YZ*," whereas we says "on heating *Z*, the result is *Y* and *X*." In medical text-books there are innumerable diseases which are not mentioned in old works; and some diseases of the old books do not appear in modern ones. This is partly explained by the undoubted fact that we have diseases which once did not exist, whereas other conditions, very common in those days, certainly never occur now. The methods of teaching are different. In these days we convey information much more quickly and readily by diagrams, charts, tables, styles of print, not to mention experiments,.and moving-pictures. This fact does not prove that the learning of those days, acquired so laboriously, was faulty.

That which is called "progress" is also sometimes merely "fashion." The search for an elixir of life, for instance, has not ceased in the least. The gland therapy for restoring youth is perhaps the most conspicuous of modern variants of ancient research. Cupping and venesection were habitually used solely with the idea of "keeping fit" they have given place to the vogue of athletics and sport. New treatments for various conditions are introduced from time to time, and seem to be great advances because they are often conspicuously successful at first. How often do they not give place to still newer methods, and perhaps finally pass into entire oblivion? The fashion changes, and the old, is supplanted.

It will be suggested that knowledge is not simply "acquaintance with an assemblage of facts" and that facts in the aggregate do not suffice to constitute "truth."[35] There is a tendency to extol the acquisition of facts, as "adding to the sum of knowledge," and as being evidence of "progress." There are different forms of knowledge: human, angelic, divine. The perfection of knowledge is wisdom. There are different forms of truth: scientific, logical, moral, ontological, philosophical, theological, etc. But as to "Ultimate Truth," this is humanly unattainable, as may be illustrated by the accompanying diagram.

The observer and the thing observed are shown in plan, as being separated by a straight semi-transparent screen. The letters *A* to *I* represent the position of as many observers. For the purpose of illustration these are supposed to be of different nationalities and not necessarily acquainted with one another's language; they also belong to different periods of life (childhood, youth, etc.). The observer at A may be supposed only to be able to see the part of the object marked *A*; the observer at *B*. similarly, may only be able to see the part marked *B*. and so on. But even if any of the observers could see several parts, evidently there still remain some areas which are out of the range of vision of all persons, as marked *K. L, M*. No one can comprehend the whole, under the restrictions given.[36]

This conception may be applied to the interpretation of terms applied even to familiar objects. In studying *The Canon*, for instance, it is not enough to know the dictionary equivalent of an Arabic or Latin word, for the full meaning is not always adequately conveyed thereby. The word "*akhlat*" may be taken as an example. It is rendered humor, humour, body-fluid, juice. The impression conveyed by each equivalent varies according to ideas commonly associated with the word and the circumstances under which we first heard it. The conception of the word humor was necessarily different in the mind of the ancient Greek physician, of the Hindu sage. of the erudite Chinese, of the alchemist of the Middle Ages, of the characters in Shakespeare, of the modern laity, of the student of esotericism, and of the modern bio-chemist.

It has been said that we shall reach Truth by whatever road we take. But this is not so. There is really only one path which will take us there direct. All the others are devious and arduous, and in t he end only bring us to the confines of Truth. We may trace out every separate road as outlined for us by as many separate thinkers of the past or present; we may pursue the highway which modern science has opened out; we may decide also to study the tracks with which we are furnished by nature itself. But even after all these have been slowly and laboriously surveyed by spiritual insight, the best we can attain is but the fringe of Reality.

*****

The following list gives those of the Simples discussed in the Second Book of *The Canon* which are still in use. Those marked with an asterisk are pharmacopeial; many of the others are found in the Catalogue of Messrs. Heath and Heather, Ltd., St. Albans.

A. Acacia gummi,* aconiti radix,* acorn, adeps,* agrimony, amygdala,* aloe,* alumen* (native), (ambergris), ammoniacum,* amylum* (from rice), anethi fructus et oleum,* anisi fructus et oleum,* antimonium,* anthemidis flores et oleum,* Armenian bole, asafetida,* ash-tree, asphalt.

B. Barberry bark, banana, barley, bay-tree and berries, beech-tree (bark), beeswax (cera*), betony, bile (fel bovinum*), bistort (black hellebore), bone-marrow, borax* (impure), bran, brown sugar, brooklime, white bryony root, black bryony root, bugloss, buttermilk.

C. Calamint, calamus, calx,* calcii hydras,* chamomile, camphor,* canesugar, cannabis indica,* cantharides,* capsici fructus,* carui fructus et oleum,* cardamomi semina,* carrot, cascara, cassiae fructus,* castor oil,* catechu,* cayenne pepper, chirata,*, chicory, cinchonae rubrae cortex,* cinnamoni cortex et oleum,* cloves and oil,* cochlearia armoracia, cocoanut, colchici cormus et seminal colocynthidis pulpa,* colophonium (" resina,"*), conii folia, convolvulus turpethum,* copper and copper sulphate (impure), coral, coriandri fructus et oleum,* cotton (gossypium,* and gossypii radicis cortex*), couch-grass-(kiticum), creasotum,* proton oil,* cubebae fructus et oleum,* cucurbita semina praep* (cyperus rotundus, cypress-turpentine tree fruit).

D. Dates, dried and fresh; dragon's blood.

E. Egg-plant, elecampane, elaterium, embelia.*

F. Foeniculi fructus; ferrum*; filix mash fuller's earth.

G. Galls, garlic, gelatinum,* gentianae radix,* germander ginger,* glycyrrhizae radix,* gold, grapes (unripe), green vitriol, groundpine, gum tragacanth.

H. Hartstongue fern, hellebore, hemlock,* hyoscyami folia,* honey, humulus lupulus flowers,* horehound, hydrargyrum.*

I. Iron-rust, isinglass, ivy.

J. Jalapa,* alapae resina,* juniper berries, and oil.*

K. Kaolin.*

L. Lard (=adeps*), lavender, lead carbonate and oxide, lemon, lime ("calx") linseed and oil (long pepper, lote tree, lupin).

M. Mace, maidenhair, marsh mallow, mandrake root, manna, marjoram, meadow sweet, mercury (=hydrargyrum*), mistletoe, gmouse-ear, mugwort, myrobalanum,* myrrh.*

N. Naphtha, nigella, nine, nutmeg,* nux vomica* (or, wintercherry ?).

O. Oakbark, olive oil,* opium,* orange-peel,* orangeflower water,* orpiment, oxymel*; many essential oils.

P. Parsley, pearl barley, pearlashes, pellitory root, pennyroyal, pepper (confectio piperis*), pepper-mint oil,* pepsin (tripe), pine resin ("retina,"*), pix liquida,* polygonum root, pomegranate bark, poppy (white), black poplar bark, red poppy petals (rhoeados petala*), pterocarpi lignum,* pyrethri radix.

Q. Quicklime (= calx), quillaiae cortex.*

R. Rapeseed, rhubarb rhizome,* rice, rosemary, rue.

S. Saffron flowers, sage, sal ammoniac (crude), santoninum,* scammony root and gum,* sealingwax, seaweed, sennae folia et fructus,* sesame oil,* sevum praeparatum,* silver, soapwort, sodium chloride,* sorrel, southernwood, spearxrıin t (ol. menth, virid.*), sponge, stavesacre seeds,* styrax praeparatus,* stramonii folia,* sulphur,* fsunbul.

T. Talc, tamarindus,* taraxaci radix,* thyme, tin, tragacanth,* truffle, tumeric, turpethum.*

V, Valerianae. rhizoma,* verbascum, verdigris (copper acetate), vervain, viola odorifera.

W. Walnut, water-cress, white water-lily root, wax, whey, white lead, willow bark, wormwood (= absinthe).

Z. Zinci oxidum* (but impure); zingiber.*

The Relation Between *The Canon* and Modern Thought

Considerations[37] are not wanting which entitle *The Canon of Medicine* of Avicenna to an esteemed position in modern thought. In the first place, there is the outstanding intellectual culture of the [Islamic] Empire—during the period of history to which Avicenna belongs. Secondly, in the case of much of his teaching, it may be said that the difference from ours is largely only that his speech is alien and is apt to be misunderstood. In these days, the great complexity of the language with which we express our scientific thought corresponds with the intricacy of the instruments wherewith facts are elicited. Thirdly, many of the advances of modern times offer the solutions to the very theorems and propositions of former times. Finally, ideas are to be found in his work which provide suggestions for useful research in the future.

The importance of idea over material achievement is not to be forgotten. The achievements of any age are subject to decay with the lapse of centuries but the ideas which gave rise to them remain living through all cycles. Therefore to propose a real place for Avicenna in modern thought is not to propose a return as it were to old architecture, or the costumes of long ago. It is rather to render accessible today the picture which he painted and so enable it to renew its still vital message. It is to play over again the music which he expressed and enable perhaps one or two to rejoice in it. And this without obscuring the issue by discussing nationality or schools of thought or evolution of ideas or technical methods.

If it appear to some a fault that the master appears to have used passages from other works and this without full acknowledgment, it should be remembered that after all a painter may use pigments which someone else has manufactured and is allowed even to employ other persons (usually pupils) to execute certain portions of his picture. Indeed, even after his decease, it is not improper that some may have been entrusted with the delicate task of touching up faded portions of the canvas which he bequeathed.

The place for Avicenna in modern thought is gained when it is agreed that he shall be viewed as one who entered this world entrusted with a mission independently to express for that age, by means of those various tools which he then found in it, the wisdom which is unchanging and impersonal. So also there is the need today that this same wisdom should be re-expressed for this age by means of the new data which lie to our hands.

The Intellectual Culture Contemporary with Avicenna

Carra de Vaux, in his monograph *Avicenna*[38] furnishes particularly striking comments, as follows:

"The more we investigate the enormous literary output of the [Islamic] empire and come into intimate appreciation of the master minds of the middle epoch and of antiquity, the more we become aware of their sincerity.

"We should, we think, offer our salutations to these great personalities of that day whose works and lives were equally encyclopedic.

"Our own times do not show more worthy figures; we complacently assume that there are no more worthy than ourselves because science, so greatly developed today, cannot be held all within one single head. That may be. But it is only right to admit that science has less unity and harmony today than formerly it had; that it is less pure than it was under the grand peripatetic discipline. Our attitude towards that is neither humble nor sincere.

"In these days we are concerned too much to have our name blazoned forth than to grasp a great extent of science. We are more anxious to uphold the profession than to have a passion for study; we seek titles and reputation rather than real knowledge; and in order to appear more specialized than our ancestors wet expose ourselves to the judgment of posterity as having smaller minds and fettered souls."

As to the state of civilization in the western Saracen empire we have the very illuminating description of Ameer Ali,[39] "The Muslims covered the countries where they settled with networks of canals. To Spain they gave the system of irrigation by flood-gates, wheels and pumps. Whole tracts of land which now lie waste and barren were covered with olive groves, and the environs of Seville alone, under Muslim rule, contained several thousand oil factories. They introduced the staple products, rice, sugar, cotton, and nearly all the fine garden and orchard fruits, together with many less important plants, like ginger, saffron, myrrh, etc. They opened up the mines of copper, sulphur, mercury, and iron. They established the culture of silk, the manufacture of paper and other textile fabrics; of porcelain, earthenware, iron, steel, leather. The tapestries of Cordova, the woolen stuffs of Myrcia, the silks of Granada, Almeria, and Seville, the steal and gold work of Toledo, the paper of Salibah, were sought all over the world. The ports of Malaga, Carthage, Barcelona and Cadiz were vast commercial emporia for export and import. In the days of their prosperity, the Spanish Muslims maintained a merchant navy of more than a thousand ships. They had factories and representatives on the Danube. With Constantinople they maintained a great trade which ramified from the Black Sea, and the eastern shores of the Mediterranean into the interior of Asia, and reached the ports of India and China, and extended along the African coast as far as Madagascar.

"In the midst of the tenth century, when Europe was about in the same condition that Caffraria is now, enlightened Moors, like Abul Cassem were writing treatises on the principles of trade and commerce. In order to supply an incentive to commercial enterprise, and to further the impulse to travel, geographical registers, gazetteers, and itineraries were published under the authority of the government, containing minute descriptions of the places to which they related, with particulars of the routes and other necessary matters. Travelers like Ibn Battuta visited foreign lands in quest of information, and wrote voluminous works on the people of those countries, on their fauna and flora, their mineral products, their climate and physical features, with astonishing perspicacity and keenness of observation.

"The love of learning and arts was by no means confined to one sex. The culture and education of the women proceeded on parallel lines with that of the men and women were as keen in the pursuit of literature and as devoted to science as men. They had their own colleges;[40] they studied medicine and jurisprudence, lectured on rhetoric, ethics, and belles-lettres and participated with the stronger sex in the glories of a splendid civilization. The wives and daughters of magnates and sovereigns spent their substance in founding colleges and endowing universities, in establishing hospitals for the sick, refuges for the homeless, the orphan and the widow."

Cordova was the most celebrated western university of the Empire at the time of Avicenna. This is well known as an instance of the high degree of culture of the day. Ameer Ali speaks of "that wonderful kingdom of Cordova, which was the marvel of the Middle Ages, and which when all Europe was plunged in barbaric ignorance and strife alone held the torch of learning and civilization bright and shining before the western world."[41] The greatness of the city is indicated by its population which is given by Haeser[42] as 300,000, and by Campbell[43] as one million; and by the library of "about 200,000" volumes.

To see the city today, traversed as it can be from wall to wall, within half an hour on foot, and to read of an extent of "twenty-four miles one way and six in the other"[44] shows that the word "kingdom" conveys a truer idea of its greatness. To read of "innumerable libraries, 3,800 mosques, 60,000 palaces and mansions, 200,000 houses inhabited by the common people, 3700 baths, 80,000 shops, besides hostels and caravanserais" is to wonder how so much can have come to be now represented by so little ("every dwelling-place, even if it has been blessed ever so long, will one day become a prey."[45] Nevertheless, the "grand mosque" alone, which is still at any rate externally intact (and interiorly is still surely one of the wonders of the world despite its mutilation) stands sponsor for the rest; and no doubt many of the existing imposing buildings—now devoted to very different uses—stand for the palaces and mansions. As to the literary treasures, these have been traced at least in part from Spain to Fez, as shown by Horne,[46] with the Roud El Qartas as his authority; and he then points to years of pilfering from the library of the great mosque of El Karouiyan at Fez, as having scattered these works forever.

A study of the street names, and even the place names and current dialect in "Moorish Spain" today also confirms the story of past greatness. But the mystical knowledge displayed in the dispositions of the decorative designs and their poetic inscriptions on the walls of the Alhambra halls, state-rooms, and private apartments can leave no doubt of unsurpassed artistic power where every sense impression was deliberately drawn on. Lights and shadows and colors changing with the-hours of the day; musical effects of simultaneous diversity of disposition of flowing water; perfumes; courting of the prevailing breezes; interior architectural form; and furnishings, animate and manufactured—all these were combined for the achievement of a perfect representation of (divine, over and above human) beauty.

Among the Chinese? The bearing of Chinese philosophical thought on the subject of Avicenna lies in the fact that we here meet with a notable example of intimacy of relation between world conception and medicine. The writings which are so carefully studied today by so many sinologists were extant at the time of Avicenna, and are still held in the highest esteem by Chinese thinkers. The modern Chinese philosopher is supposed to say to the westerner, "What is the reason for which you deem yourselves our betters? Have you excelled us in arts or letters? Have our thinkers been less profound than yours? Has our civilization been less elaborate, less complicated, less refined than yours? Why, when you lived in caves and clothed yourselves with skins, we were a cultured people . . . ."[47]

The attitude towards western learning so displayed may be blamed by many, but is certainly praised by those who have studied the philosophy most deeply. As long ago as 1876 we read conclusive evidence.[48] If some students discuss their philosophy with a certain cynicism,[49] others[50] see into the justice of their conceptions. As Caruso remarks: "We need not be blind to the many errors and absurdities of the ancient occultism to understand and grant the truth that underlies its system."[51] These words are exactly applicable to *The Canon of Medicine* of Avicenna.

It should be added that errors and absurdities are apt to be ascribed to ancient authors which really arose from misunderstandings and ignorance on the part even of contemporary pupils. The subsequent generations perpetuated the errors, and even in these days the attempt to represent the real meaning of ancient texts by translations exposes one to unexpected extraordinary pitfalls. Our idiom is so diverse from the technical Chinese.

THE NATURE OF THE KNOWLEDGE PRESENTED BY *THE CANON*

The Canon is a precis and not a sum-total of Avicenna's knowledge. Numerous passages occur in *The Canon* which show that this is the case, that it is a series of notes or skeleton outlines of thought not too lengthy to be memorized by his students[52] much as they would memorize the Quran. Thus, "to the full extent necessary, and yet with apt brevity,"[53] "do not place in medicine what does not belong to it,"[54] "having discussed the equable temperaments sufficiently,"[55] "I purposely omit reference to certain other problems relative to the fluids of the body just as much as is necessary to enable you to practice medicine intelligently."[56] Many passages also refer to others of his own works for further details, to avoid confusing the purely medical issue of *The Canon*. These philosophical works are gradually becoming more widely known.

"Generally speaking, the saying of the saints and sages are terse, presenting only the germs of truth; these are developed by later teachers and then expanded and added to. We must see to it, however, that we get at the original meaning of the saints and sages."[57]

"Books are only words and the valuable part of words is the thought therein contained. That thought has a certain bias, which cannot be conveyed in words, yet the world values words as being the; essence of books. But though the world values them, they are not of value; as that sense in which the world values them is not the sense in which they are valuable."[58]

To say that a work is the product of the age in which an author lives is certainly often an error, for it is to confuse the person's insight with the tools (the language at his command) available to express himself with. Similarly to work out the relation between a literary work and the religious belief of the author, as for instance to show the relation between Islamic science and the Quran carries the same fallacy with it. The Prophet said, "Every soul when born is a faithful follower; it is afterwards that he becomes unfaithful"—which is to say that the form of religious belief is a secondary implantation, whereas the spirit of a sincere life can be traced to the original being.

Avicenna's medicine, like Indian medicine, has been traced to the Greek system. But it has been proved that the great works of Charaka and Susruta were available in Arabic, under the title of *Kitab shawshura al-Hindi*, from the 7th century.[59] Similarly, the view that the Chinese borrowed their philosophy of the five elements from the Turks has been sufficiently disposed of by Forke.[60] It is beside the purpose of this treatise to take up such questions.

The common notion that progress or stagnation in secular knowledge has a causal relationship with a certain religion is typically voiced in his address on "Medicine and the Church" by Sir Farquhar Buzzard.[61] The comment to make is: "*post hoc sed non propter hoc*." The advances in the science of medicine, as in all other sciences, are surely a part of the divine plan for mankind whereas the collateral abandonment of religious fundamentals remains a human responsibility.

The word "canon" (*qanun*): equivalent words: code of laws; series of principles; tao.[62] Principle is defined as "something antecedent, which exercises a real positive influence upon the consequent" = causes (four kinds, Avicenna) = reasons.

In view of this it is clear that *The Canon* is not properly to be regarded as an "encyclopedia" of the knowledge of the time, or to be contrasted, for instance, with the now classical "Osler."

The word "knowledge": knowledge is not simply an assemblage of "facts" nor is it to be made synonymous with "truth"—certainly not Absolute Truth, of which all human knowledge falls short although one single word is capable of containing or implying all knowledge, as in mathematics a single term may be equated with an infinite number of terms summed together. But even the mathematical sciences can only afford approximate truth.[63] We may recall the words, "If he attain to all knowledge, he is far off still."[64]

Facts, as St. Thomas[65] explains, are what our intellect regards as external objects—and as we judge of them only in terms of our sense organs—these objects may be different. God knows them as they are. Our intellect depends on our imagination and that depends on our senses. Our senses only convey discrete fragments which we gather into one continuous impression regardless of intervening points." We live as it were in a network only the nodes of which are evident to the senses.

Mystical Insight

There is a distinction between knowledge gained in the ordinary manner and that gained by "mystical insight" (*kashf*). The writer of *Gulshan-i-raz*'s[66] advises his readers to follow this, saying:

> Straightway lift yourself above time and space,
> Quit the world and be yourself a world for yourself.
> And

> The moment we are enlightened within

> We go beyond the voidness of a world confronting us.
> —Seng-ts'an, quoted by Susuki.[67]

As this "opens up all of a sudden a world hitherto undreamed of, it is an abrupt and discrete leaping from one plane of thought to another."[68]

> Real science is seeing the fire directly,
> Not mere talk, inferring the fire from the smoke.
> Your scientific proofs are more offensive to the wise
> Than the urine and breath whence a physician infers.[69]

"Man looks at the surface of the ocean. Yet he is so small that he cannot even be compared to one of its drops, limited as he is in intellect and in his knowledge. It is only to those who, having just touched creation, bow to God, forgetting their limited self, that God has remained. These through whom God has spoken are the only beings who have been able to give any truth to the world."[70]

"The mind is not like a horizontal door which haste be made larger by force. You must clear away the obstructions arising from creaturely desire and then it will be pure and clear with no limit to its knowledge. Heng Ch'u said, 'When the mind is enlarged it can enter into everything throughout the universe.' He who praises God knows about Him."[71]

This attitude towards nature is to be claimed for Avicenna on the plain evidence of his other writings including the *al-Najat* which appropriately appears in the Arabic version of *The Canon* printed at Rome in 1593 and of the *Libellus* on the powers of the hearts and is included in the Latin edition of *The Canon*, 1595.[72]

The acquisition of knowledge by this process demands nothing more than a keen observation of the life around us and was as much within his reach as ours. Such knowledge is not too restricted to one period of history, one language, or to one or two universities. And if it should seem that because our civilization is so different his opportunities were much less, we may pause to reflect that the difference between our age and his is chiefly one of mechanical appurtenances and phraseology; and that even to this day we need not travel far (i.e., the old streets of Cordova and Granada or more definitely, to northern Africa) to see much the same sort of scenery as he was accustomed to, much the same sort of life as is drawn in the 1001 Nights. In any case, what is human life, at bottom, but a matter of buying and selling, receiving and giving, seizing and relinquishing, constructing and demolishing, acquiring learning and losing it, seeking power and breaking it, bidding and forbidding, giving in marriage and seeking to obtain in marriage, birth and death.

The significant phrase "seeing into one's own nature,"[73] in which most admirable work occur many passages by way of explanation) gives a graphic description of that which gives Avicenna his superiority. *The Canon* is simply the medical garb in which the one Truth is expounded. It is for us also to perceive it in whatever idiom it might be described—western, eastern, Islamic, Confucian or Buddhist, for example.

It would then seem as if the mind were now able to float as it were round all the concepts the human being has ever given to the world, or round all the most familiar events of one's daily life, and perceive clearly that which can never be set forth in words. We should then also quote the words."[74] I perceive of it that it is something, but what it is I cannot perceive. Only it seems if I could conceive it, I should comprehend all truths.

Further than this, to find that some of the statements in *The Canon* are certainly erroneous and that modern investigations have placed us at an infinitely greater advantage, does not invalidate the work as a whole. Its possibilities for suggesting thoughts of real value today are more realized the more one reads between the lines, and the present treatise does not claim to exhaust them.

"Let not the authority of the writer offend thee, whether he be of title or great learning, but let the love or pure truth entice thee to read."[75]

Insight into eternal truths. A person may: (1) glimpse them; (2) understand them moderately; (3) understand them fairly thoroughly. But in describing them to another, he may explain them: (i) imperfectly (no one can explain them properly!); (ii) inadequately or incompletely; (iii) wrongly because of: (a) imperfect education; (b) educational bias; (c) religious or anti-religious bias; (d) inherently erroneous methods of thought; (e) restriction to logic. Such truths, again, may be denied by persons being told of them, for because in their turn they misunderstand, or understand only in part, either through careless attention, and (a) to (e).

Insight Versus Intuitional Knowledge

A note should here be made that the term "insight" as used here bears a rather different meaning to that pertaining to the term "intuitive knowledge," which St. Thomas[76] ascribes solely to the angelic mind, and defines as "the attainment of the truth of a thing at a single glance without the aid of reasoning."[77] On the other hand this mode of perceiving truths need not be disallowed a rudimentary commencement among the powers of the human soul, just as the "brute" mind must be allowed to contain rudiments of those high mental capacities which characterize the human being. Throughout all orders of creation, the lower are endowed with the scaffolding for the manifestation of successively more exalted capacities of the higher.

The Basic Difference between The Canon and Modern Medicine

The Canon treats of:

I. Speculative Medicine

Certain fundamental principles (cosmology, psychology, metaphysics)

II. Practical Medicine

A. Application of Speculative Medicine to the study of (i) health; (ii) disease (tendency, predisposition, threshold stage, declared disease; (iii) cessation of life.

B. Actual treatment of "disease" by: (i) regimen, (ii) drugs, (iii) operative interference.

Modern Medicine consists of:

A. Principles of Medicine: The application of the facts of

chemistry, physics, anatomy, biology to the systematic description of innumerable "diseases" classified as far as possible on the basis of the microbic theory; symptomatology; etiology; diagnosis.
B. Practice of Medicine
(a) Laboratory work.
(b) Therapeutics, Pharmacology and Dietetics.
(c) Surgery.
(d) Gynecology and Obstetrics.
(e) States of Medicine: Hygiene in all its branches.
(f) Psychological Medicine: Treatment of insanity.
(g) Legal medicine, etc.

Modern medicine is based on the conception of the universe as a conglomeration of dead matter out of which, by some unexplainable process, life may become evolved in forms. To Avicenna the whole of the universe is the manifestation of a universal principle of life, acting through the instrumentality of forms. Or, again, in modern medicine, the forms are the source of life; to Avicenna they are the product of life. Space itself is an aspect of the one life.[78]

In this way the difference between Avicenna's conception of "principles," and that of modern medicine is easily shown. To the school boy "science" would consist of (a) bookwork and (b) laboratory work which his teachers would insist is the basis of (a). Similarly, the medical curriculum begins with lectures, although these are more and more inclined to become laboratory demonstrations; and goes on to laboratory and hospital work.

In short, Avicenna's medicine, and all ancient and traditional medicine, is intimately bound up with philosophy, to wit, that of human nature—a philosophy which proves to be virtually identical with "modern scholastic philosophy," no doubt partly because the Quranic account of the origin of the human being tallies with the Christian.

Modern medicine, on the other hand, assuming the title and rank of a positive science, emphatically discards and excludes it. Hence we read: "the physiologist" (said Burdon Sanderson) "can pursue philosophy if he has a turn for it, but must understand that the moment he enters the field of philosophy he leaves his tools behind him." For "it is unfortunate that the limitations of scientific thought were often ignored by men of science in their writings . . . the result diverts those who know, but befogs the unsuspicious reader who will probably put the blame on his intelligence."[79]

"According to positivism, science cannot be as Aristotle conceived it, the knowledge of things through their ultimate causes, since material and formal causes are unknowable, final causes are illusions, and efficient causes are simply invariable antecedents, while metaphysics under any form is illegitimate."[80] Or, expressed more boldly, "philosophy" is considered to be the exact antithesis of the truth which modern medicine gives us, and is therefore inherently inadmissible to medicine.

The ignorance which accounts for this attitude is only met by insisting on proper definitions of terms. The following apply here:

Philosophy is "the science which is concerned with first causes and principles; it is the profound knowledge of the universal order, and the duties which that order imposes on the human being.[81]

Again, philosophy is the true perception and understanding of cause and effect. Metaphysics is "that portion of philosophy which treats of the most general and fundamental principles underlying all reality and all knowledge."[82] Psychology is "the science which treats of the soul and its operations" and, therefore, clearly, must be the real foundation of medicine.

It is in modern scholastic philosophy that the student finds ample exposure of the fallacy in positivism and its cognates, enabling him to detect the difference between false and true, expressed with enough force of logic to satisfy the most meticulous. This queen of all the sciences amply proves positivist science (including medicine) to be incomplete knowledge when taken alone. The knowledge of movement or change must be supplemented by mathematical and metaphysical viewpoints.[83] Such men as Albertus Magnus and Roger Bacon were convinced of the necessity of linking the sciences with philosophy.[84]

When medicine has in this way become ennobled it reaches

its highest degree of perfection, in that it penetrates to the very depths of reality,[85] admitting this knowledge to need, even then, a further complement to make it complete-namely, knowledge in relation to God ("Christian wisdom").

"Sapientia est scientia qua considerat causas primas et universales causas. Sapientia causas primas omnium causarum considerat."[86] *"Ille qui cognoscit causam altissimam simpliciter, qua est Deus dicitur sapiens simpliciter, in quantum per regulas divinas omnia potest judicare et ordinare."*[87] *"Non acquiritur studio humano, sed est deursum scendens."*[88] *"Cum homo per res creatas Deum cognoscit, magis videtur hoc perti nere ad scientiam, ad quam perti net formaliter, qu am ad sapientiam ad qu am pertinet materialiter: et e converso cum secundum res divinas judicamus de rebus creatis, magis hoc ad sapientiam quam ad scientiam pertinet."*[89]

As St. Thomas said in his day, "they think that nothing exists besides visible creatures." [N.B.:"Creatures" are (a) animate; and (b) inanimate]. "They think that things proceed not by the divine will but by natural necessity."[90] So even in those days time and fortune were expended on researches which sound philosophy would have shown to be inherently futile.

We may reflect for instance on the reiterated search for a location of the soul, which the pioneer anatomists prosecuted, and also on the commonly repeated announcement to successive students of anatomy that the pineal gland is now no longer regarded as the site of the soul. There is the sub-conscious suggestion to the student that scientific research has effectively disposed of the medieval belief in the soul, whereas history only proves that the revolt against the precise teachings of the Council of Trent necessarily came to naught.[91] The very definition of "soul" which this council laid down makes a search for its location ludicrous.

Special Differences Between The Canon and Modern Medicine

Conceptions Known to Avicenna

NOT NOW RECOGNIZED

There are four main conceptions belonging to *The Canon*, but not recognized by modern medicine. To use St. Thomas' words, they can be shown to be "not impossible";[92] that is, the discoveries of modern science do not abrogate them.

These conceptions are relative to: (1) the nature of the human being as a whole; (2) the constitution; (3) the "breath"; (4) the "elements." Each of these is dealt with in some detail under the corresponding sections of *The Canon*, but some of the salient points are suitably referred to at this stage.

The varieties of views on conception of the nature of the human being as a whole, which people in every country and race exhibit both in conversation and in literature, numerous though they are, are capable of classification under one of three headings: (1) The Platonic view—regards the human being as "soul within a body," while admitting "soul" to be indefinable, and beyond the power of location. This view, widely supposed to be "Christian," is well known as "pagan" to students of folklore. (2) The scientific or rationalistic and modern view—takes the physical body as the fundamental, seeing in it the outcome of known or at least knowable forces. The facts of anatomy, physiology, etc., convey their own inevitable conclusions. This view makes its immediate appeal. From the first lesson the pupil is able to feel a grasp of some tangible knowledge, whereas the alternative third view entails a long study before the intricacies of abstract philosophy can be mastered. The difference between experience and "poring over books" is only too obvious. The possibility of interweaving the two methods is not on the horizon.

In its answer to "religion," this scientific view has no objection to raise to its votaries retaining a private belief in the Platonic view, if their temperament demands it. But this "pious belief" must not be allowed to vitiate procedure when scientific research is undertaken.

This modern conception regards the body as an aggregate of "spare parts" which are "assembled" well, or ill; can be repaired, or remedied. According as the assembling is good or bad, and, according to the "fuel," so is there health, or susceptibility to infection by organisms. The kind of assembling is a matter partly heredity and partly of environment.

The following remarks in a review on a recent article in *Science*.[93] They present the idea in technical language:

"Physiology finds the organism to be a nexus of physicochemical determination; differing only from non-living systems in its complexity. . . . Speaking of freewill, one argument against indeterminism is that the energy balance sheet of a man shows us there is no creation of energy within the body. To assume will-power we conflict with Newton's first law. . . . The ultra microscope alone suggests indeterminism, and even this may be only because we do not know enough about Brownian movement, etc. Protoplasm is a heterogeneous system. In heredity sub-microscopical units determine the details of inheritance—but an event originating in an ultra-microscopic particle can spread to the whole cell or organism. On this view, a human action appearing entirely spontaneous and voluntary to the actor and spectator would exhibit itself as a succession of mechanically determined events capable of study and prediction in all its microscopic details. But traced inward it would ultimately resolve itself into certain ultramicroscopic events in the interior of the nerve-cell." But "even the freedom of the ultra-microscopic particle may be no more than a subtler kind of determinism beyond the reach of present analysis."[94]

It may be noted, in passing, that the doctrine of vitalism is really only another form of rationalism, as will appear when the scholastic doctrine is duly investigated.

The third view—scholastic, Thomistic-presented by modern scholastic philosophy has the Aristotelian basis. Its soundness is best appreciated by careful study prolonged until the prevalent inadequate and illogical conceptions of the universe are clearly exposed. Briefly, the view is expressed in the words: "the human being is a material body vivified by a life-principle, the two together constituting the rational human soul." As St. Thomas says, "It is not my soul that thinks, or my body that eats, but 'I' that do both."[95] In other words, again: The body and "soul" form one complete whole—one "single being."[96]

It is this view which underlies the whole *Canon*, and is expounded in connection with the corresponding parts of the text. It is this view that makes the ancient work fall in line with the most "modern." Its consequences are far-reaching. The external configuration of the body, including the physiognomy, is a reflection of the functional capacity of the internal organs and general make-up of the individual. The character, talents, physical form, shape of individual features, general development, and indeed every detail of the physique, length of limbs, of fingers, cutaneous markings, contour of the eyes and ears, etc., ark all part and parcel with the functional conformations of the viscera, and the mental characters; a study of the visible will inform of the nature of the internal conformation.[97]

The idea that from a study of external features and general habit one should deduce conclusions as to functional capacities[98] is generally opposed by academic medicine; as is voiced by F. Muller when he says, "We must steadfastly avoid drawing any far-reaching conclusions about the functional behavior of the organism from a study of the external characters of the body."[99]

While it may be urged that the external features are usually misread, it may also be admitted that even the customary "physical examination" of a patient does not yield uniform results when practiced, as it necessarily is, by persons of varying talent. Surely, the remedy is to exert greater care. We may, for instance, observe how a skilled weaver will detect the site of a flaw in the "set-up" of a loom by a mere glance, whereas a novice discovers it only after laborious search.

On the other hand, the biochemical tests for functional capacity of organs—so much the vogue and so much exploited, and so duly impressive on patients and their friends—are clearly inadequate in the light of the scholastic doctrine. It is true that the attempt to force the intangible to yield to mathematical formula rules and weights and measures (as, for instance, in blood-cholesterol analysis is sincere enough, to judge by the time, energy and money expended so freely).

But what is to be the verdict once it is realized that the

anatomical organs are not functionally discrete or amenable to distinctive "specific" tests? A just appreciation of the intimacy of relation inherent in the conception of the human being insisted on here suffices to show the futility of those labors and studies whether made upon man or upon the various orders of animals taken instead.

More than this, there is the conception that the internal organs belong to one another beyond the anatomical limits. The heart, to anatomy, is a circumscribed organ; to Avicenna it is part of a force occupying the whole body. "The human heart is both corporeal and incorporeal."[100] So, again, the liver is simply a visible portion of a "liver" whose operation pervades the whole body.[101] Or to combine modern with ancient knowledge, the physical heart, the arterial vessels, and the sympathetic nervous system, including the connections between this and the sensorium and that which corresponds to the "sensitive soul" in its emotional aspect, for instance—all this is one great composite; and its state is also reflected in many subtle indications which offer themselves to the keen observer of the patient.

The modern research on diseases of the brain and insanity is based on the assumption that the material brain is the source of all nervous activities, which are correlated with definite biochemical, physicochemical and even structural changes in brain substance. Mental disease is the outcome of similar changes The Platonists would consider mental disease as apart from the "soul." The Thomistic view leads to much more subtle conclusions, capable of lasting influence.

The Doctrine of "The Constitution"

The term "constitution" conveys different ideas to different minds. The laity regard the term as synonymous with "temperament" or "make-up," at least in part, and consider a description of a patient as haying a nervous temperament, a delicate constitution, etc., quite adequate. With this goes the conviction among the lay that the medical curriculum leaves the graduate fully able to " understand his constitution" whereas in actual fact the subject is never discussed. The study of physique is quite superficial and is admittedly made solely to establish a diagnosis of specific "diseases." Hence the term, in conversation, is actually nothing more than platitudes.

To modern medicine, regarding the body as corporeal, constitution is a matter of physique, resistance to disease, mode of reaction to various stimuli (including psychic stimuli). Classifications of varieties of constitution on this basis are afforded by various writers in all countries—i.e., a classification into athletic, leptosomic and dysplastic; into arthritic, endocrine, lymphatic, asthenic, infantilistic, chlorotic, etc. (current medical journals).

In *The Canon*, Avicenna establishes "constitution" in terms of humors, temperaments (hot, cold, dry, moist) and "elements" (whose proportions are set. for every individual). If we go further, and apply to this term the method which Rumi,[102] the great Persian sage demanded of students of the Quran, we shall not regard a patient's constitution as understood until we have studied the matter much more intimately.

Know the words of the Quran are simple,
But within the outward sense is an inner secret one.
Beneath that secret meaning is a third,
Whereat the highest wit is dumbfounded.
The fourth meaning has been seen by none
Save God, the Incomparable and All-sufficient.
Thus they go on, even to seven meanings, one by one,
According to the saying of the Prophet, without doubt.

"I know," said Tawaddud, the lady most learned, "the sublime Quran by heart and have read it according to the seven, the ten, and the fourteen modes."[103]

Therefore, to draw a lesson for our study out of these indications, we shall see that the aim in view is to formulate a person's constitution out of a number of components, none of which must be omitted from the series. To express the whole picture many modern aspects must be studied—histological, biochemical, psychological, without neglecting factors (metaphysical, etc.) accepted by the ancients but almost forgotten today. For instance, the past events in the ancestral history of the patient must be included and all the factors coming into play even from the time of quickening may not be overlooked.

The insight afforded by the true conception of the nature of the human being in this way leads us on to an understanding of individual constitutions which should be amply satisfactory.

The Doctrine of "The Breath"

This subject is discussed in the course of the text.[104] The term "breath" found in Eastern writings is taken as the exact equivalent of Avicenna's conception, and is understood properly only when the "elements" are understood.[105]

Equivalent terms: life-principle; *hayat*; the breath of life; *virtus vitalis*; *spiritus*; vitality; *Hu* (in Persian mysticism; *Hu* in Chinese is not the exact equivalent although being used more for the act of expiration unless there is a mystical sense attached to the term); *Ch'i*; *nafas* (also used for "soul," "individuality").

It may be conceded that many of these words are used synonymously with much confusion in consequence. Thus the old doctrine of vitalism—supported by vitalists—is not the antithesis of, but strictly speaking, another form of rationalism. In Paracelsus we read "the first matter of the elements is nothing else than life. The soul of the elements is the life of all created things. . . . There is again a difference between the soul and the life. Fire if it lives, burns. But if it be in its soul, that is; in its element, it lacks all power of burning."[106] Errors of this kind are avoided by a careful study of the scholastic philosophy.

The Doctrine of "The Elements"

This is fully entered into at the end of the corresponding chapter in the translation.[107] The conception of the universe in terms of four, or five, elements has been found among all peoples. To argue in favor of the doctrine almost compels an attempt at harmonization of its different forms (Aristotelian, Indian, Persian, Chinese, for instance). Suppose a number of people each set out to paint one certain landscape; that each is of different nationality; that each is restricted to a certain limited number of pigments; that each is a true artist. The final picture presented by each will be striking and inspiring. But it would be out of place to begin and compare stick with stick and stone with stone. If we understand, we shall learn from each, The modern futurist may excite ridicule in lets attempts to depict a landscape in terms of psychic forces, which he claims to discern, but to the mind of a student his work would have a different effect. These varying forms of one conception are amenable to intelligent understanding.[108]

Carus writes, "An explanation of the universe which derives all distinctions between things, conditions, relations, etc., from differences of mixture must have appeared very plausible to the ancient sages . . . even today Western scientists of reputation attempt to explain the universe as a congeries of force-centers, acting either by attraction or repulsion in analogy to positive and negative electricity. On the ground of this fact the educated Chinese insist with more than a mere semblance of truth that the underlying idea of the Chinese world conception is fully borne out and justified by the results of Western science."[109] Elsewhere the intimacy, in fact unity, between this philosophy and everyday life is referred to as the justification for so often quoting Chinese thought in expounding Avicenna.[110]

Conceptions Known to Modern Medicine; but Not to Avicenna

Among the most important of these are: (1) the anatomy of the circulation of the blood. (2) the rate of that circulation. (3) The details found in *The Canon*'s anatomy; the microscopic anatomy; such complexities as form the theme of Bayliss' *Physiology*. These details might be expressed as those of "the mechanics of the body." (4) Interactions in the tissues: chemical and cellular metabolism. (5) In pathology: the microbic theory; the endless and always increasing number of "diseases"; the laboratory diagnosis of dysfunction of organs; (albuminuria was, of course, unknown); symptoms as evidences of disordered reflexes. (6) In treatment: the use of antisera and specific antisubstances of organisms; hypodermic medication; complex drug treatment has passed out of vogue; surgery.

Considerations which suggest that these instances of ignorance are not as grave as is supposed, and do not invalidate the standing of ancient medicine in regard to actual practice.

Circulation of a kind was propounded in the case of the "breath," the elements, and the body-fluids, though not along anatomical channels. The Chinese recognized a process of "revolution," a succession of cyclical changes an ebb and flow. Indeed, it is suggested in Duhalde[111] that the Chinese knew of the circulation of the blood itself some hundred years BC.

Wieger,[112] discussing whether the Chinese knew of the circulation of the blood twenty centuries before Harvey or not, decides truly that "their knowledge of the circulation of the blood in the human microcosm was intuitive, not experimental, conjectured in imitation of the circulation of the vital principle in the universal microcosm, in which they believed. They guessed the fact, and they never verified it. . . . During more than twenty centuries, the how of the guessed circulation never worried their mind. The yin-yang circulates in a ring, the five agents do the same, the blood the same. That is all . . ." But if a doctrine which is common to Taoism and esotericism [that of microcosm and macrocosm] is allowed to be valid, the words "intuitive knowledge" cannot be made synonymous with "conjecture," "guess."

The rapidity of the changes was certainly not realized. The Chinese apparently believed that the circulation was completed only fifty times in one day. There is however room for fallacious. Lest there should be over-satisfaction with ourselves, it may be suggested that the rapidity of the movement of the lymph was not realized before about 1908, and is perhaps not fully realized by many practitioners today; the rapidity of passage of food-materials down the small intestine was not known until the advent of the "bismuth" meal. The circulation of nerve-impulses is not yet admitted.

The capillaries of the liver are referred to[113] in the body in general.[114] True, what Avicenna calls capillaries are larger than those we see with the microscope. But he knew that the blood passes from large trunks into the liver, traverses "capillaries" in the liver, and re-emerges by large trunks.

Interactions in the tissues were conceived of as taking place with an ebb and a flow (which is correct); lymph exudes into the tissue-spaces. Interactions take a considerable time (true). Digestion goes on within the blood-vessels in various parts of the body.

Fermentation was the counterpart of bacterial growth as we know it. The term is used sufficiently specifically in the text.[115] Diseases were regarded chiefly as parts of a process; and there were but few processes (which is quite true: nine processes).[116] Urinalysis was carried out in order to assess the functional state of the liver.[117]

Modern medicine claims its title to superiority by its successes, and judges the medicine of the past by its failures. But what would the judgment be if this method were reversed? Suppose we accepted the verdict of those among the laity (who are not so few) who are dissatisfied with their experiences of orthodox medicine and have turned to the "unqualified" of one kind or another, or those of other countries who prefer their native doctors still, or even those Europeans who have experienced triumphant success from native doctors, aver modern methods had failed? After all the ancient medicine is still practiced from Cairo to Calcutta, and a medicine not very different holds sway through the Far East. The late Sir Charles Pardy Lukis[118] is quoted as saying "Many of the empirical methods of treatment adopted by hakims are of the greatest value, and there is no doubt whatever that their ancestors, ages ago, knew many things which are nowadays being brought forward as new discoveries.[119]

DRUG-TREATMENT

The complexity of prescriptions of former times has given place to simple and short ones, and the tendency is to discard them altogether. But the reasons for the ancient method are given in the Canon, and Avicenna's choice of remedies depended on a careful consideration of the constitution of the remedies, as well as of the patient and his idiosyncrasies. Thus, certain ingredients would be allowed or disallowed in a given standard confection according to the nature of the particular patient. " The presence or absence, and the amount, of nardus, ginger, fennel-seed, anise, piper, cyperus rotundus, must be according to the season, and the age of the patient.[120]

F. Hartmann[121] describes the accuracy of native diagnosis[122] as "disconcerting," and describes certain forms of treatment (auto-chemotherapy, Bier treatment) as being practiced in a manner only different in outward appearance from the technique which we pride ourselves as being absolutely the "latest." "No wonder," he says, "that the Chinese are proud of their art, considering how long they have known that which we have only recently discovered." (These words can be fully endorsed, if only from a study of the Chinese classic on the pulse, Wan K'an t'ang, 80 volumes, discussed under the heading "The Pulse" in the present treatise.[123] Among other ancient Chinese medical works-first seen by the present writer in the very extensive collection in the Library of McGill University-reference may be made to the astonishing accuracy of representations of medicinal and other plants, and the almost dramatic representations of various diseases states in the *I tsung chin ch'un* by Hung Chou, extant in Avicenna's time. This work was reprinted between 1904 and 1924 and an older edition is in the Library of the School of Oriental Studies).

The cynical mind cannot be upheld which passes off the reputed successes during the Middle Ages as coincidences, and overlooks the modern crowded out-patient departments as evidences of the limitations of our current therapy and theory; nor can the skeptic be much noticed who denies miraculous cures rather than admit scientific theories to be in any sense inadequate.

Nevertheless, it is obvious that the principles of *The Canon* could not be taught over a hospital bed or in the out-patient department. It is true that they cannot cater for the wholesale requirements of the hospital or clinic. It should be clear to the candid that our modern technique does not avail for 100 per cent of cases; for those who do not benefit at least an experiment with other systems of treatment should not be denied. If the fault is laid at the feet of over-strenuous routine work, the more leisured may yet find an advantage in a system which puts the details of a person's constitution in all its aspects into the forefront, where there is no question of teaching it either to classes or even to possibly indifferent individuals. The words of Paracelsus may be recalled, where he says: a the doctor who loves his art does not undertake twenty cases but five, knowing that no one person can conscientiously treat more than a certain number. No one person could ever make the whole world sound."

Knowledge Common to Avicenna and Modern Medicine

A perusal of the text of *The Canon* will show many passages which apply quite well, without explanation, in these days. Thus, the following may be specified: the close relation between emotions and physiological states (shown to be even closer than modern research has realized); the classification of people into sanguine, phlegmatic, bilious, saturnine, frigid, "hot"; the physiology of sleep; and how posture may remedy insomnia.

Choice of Location for Dwellings

Health resorts. Climactic influences on health and illness-Plethoric maladies. Dietetics. Hydrotherapy. Regiminal treatment. The uses of counter-irritation. Bier treatment. The introduction of remedies into the urethra. The use of vaginal tampons. The use of anesthetics by the mouth (medicated wines: scopolamine). Testing the strength of a drug by animal experiment (Vol. 5) The treatment of insanity by malaria.[124]

No doubt the great difference between the ancient and modern is one of outlook, which accounts for the difference of topic. That which appeared interesting and even important in those days is passed over by modern physiology and pathology. Each century has its own interests. The mistake made is to suppose that the older interests were "wrong," "incorrect," "useless"; and to label them as "out of date." True, fashions of all kinds come to be out of date, but the epithets "right," "wrong" do not apply.

The more carefully we observe modern science the more evident does it become that just its terminology and subject of conversation is different Things are seen from new angles, and things only surmised at then are amenable to tangible description now. In fact, there occur moments, even at this day, when suggestive thoughts might be drawn from *The Canon*, to help in studying the individual, tedious, or baffling case, especially where the practice is far distant from the laboratories and appliances of modern medicine.

Of Interest to the Scholar

The present translation is based on the Latin versions published at Venice in 1608 and 1595, supported by a study of the Arabic edition printed at Rome in 1593 and the Bulaq edition. It is true that as E. G. Browne pointed out, " The Latin *Qanun* swarms with barbarous words which are not merely transcriptions, but in many cases almost unrecognizable mistranscriptions of Arabic originals,"[125] and that Hirschberg and Lippert[126] regard the Latin as almost unintelligible, though they admit the "slavish adherence" of the Latin to the Arabic. Campbell[127] states that there was a "society of translators" at Toledo, about 1130 A.D., "whose method of translating from Arabic to Latin was to put the Latin equivalent over the Arabic words, disregarding the sense of the original." It is true that in many passages the obscurity is similar to the effect which would result if one were at this day to render idiomatic French word for word into English.

It is important to point out that the Latin of Volume I is very different from that of Vols. III-V; so different that the translation must have been the work of different persons. While the criticisms are justified with regard to these three volumes, they do not apply to the first, whose Latin is very close to the Arabic, and hardly to be improved. The difficulty really is that the Arabic itself is so condensed that the meaning can only be clearly represented in English by the use of many more words, whether to help out the meaning itself, or to make a presentable reading.

It may well be said, as did E. G. Browne, "He who judges Arabian Medicine only by the Latin translation will inevitably undervalue it and do it a great injustice. Indeed it is difficult to resist the conclusion that many passages in the Latin version of the Qanun of Avicenna were misunderstood or not understood at all by the translator, and consequently can never have conveyed a clear idea to the reader."[128]

The following aids to clearness have been utilized: (1) the study of Avicenna's other works, and of contemporary philosophical writings, in the existing translations. (b) The study of various Latin terms as understood by modern scholastic philosophy in its exposition of the medieval nomenclature. (c) The use of modern terms when there is no reasonable doubt of their referring to the same idea, though the literal term in the Latin is obsolete. The careful study of the original Arabic has here been of special importance, for words in the Latin version, which are evidently technical there, become merely colloquial when translated into English, whereas in the Arabic version, such words at once take on their proper character in the Arabic-English and Persian-English dictionaries (d) The use of tabulation of the matter. There are instances where this proves possible without omitting even a single Arabic word. (e) The use of paraphrase for certain passages. These are marked (p). A certain freedom of rendering has been inevitable in view of the importance of bringing the meaning of the text to the reader's notice without subjecting him to the need of reflecting deeply on passage after passage-as is requisite with the original Arabic (to have dealt with the work from the point of literature would have entailed giving the preference to safeguarding against likely criticisms at the hands of pure scholarship).

The main purpose of this treatise will now be seen to center in the idea that in the ancient philosophy there is material capable of useful application to-day. The selection of the work of Avicenna is not intended to provide an apologium for that one author, but is specially appropriate for these reasons: (i) his acknowledged excellence; (ii) his greater accessibility among medieval medical writings; (iii) a certain indefinable charm of expression peculiar to himself; but above all, (iv) the fact that his central theme is a conception of the nature of the human being really identical with that of Thomistic philosophy, and in these days specially stressed and developed by "modern scholastic philosophy." As these are related, so might Avicenna be related to a modern scholastic medicine, which would aim at reasons for health and ill health far deeper than those given by the microbic and cognate theories.

With Mercier,[129] "We do not regard the Thomistic philosophy . . . as a boundary which sets limits to personal activity of thought . . . but make use of his" (in this case, Avicenna's) "teaching as a starting-point from which we may go further afield."

With Maher,[130] we ". . . resuscitate and" (apply to medicine) ". . . a psychology that has already survived four and twenty centuries, and has had more influence on human thought and human language than all other psychologies together. My desire, however, has been not merely to expound, but to expand this old system . . . to make clear to the student of modern thought that this ancient and traditional psychology (and medicine) is not so absurd, nor these old thinkers as foolish, as current caricatures of their teaching would lead one to imagine. . . . To trespass (on the soul) . . . . is assumed by (many writers) to be the gravest of professional delinquencies."

Therefore Avicenna is allowed once more to present his theme. To the questions we are constrained to ask of him, we find our answers: (1) in his other writings; (2) in contemporary literature; (3) in the writings of modern Eastern thinkers; (4) in the works of St. Thomas; (5) in modern scholastic philosophy. If some truths are crudely expressed or perhaps faultily explained, it is our privilege to re-express and re-explain with those aids.

Those who may have failed to identify one single Truth under different garbs are not obliged to accord these garbs an unfriendly reception upon the stage of our modern world. To recall a favorite Indian metaphor, the danseuse has so robed herself, and displays such diversities of art that under the ever-changing colored beams of light it is difficult to believe there can be only one and the same artiste before us. Should it prove impossible to verify this, at least the very exhibition of the art should serve so to refresh that we can resume our work and ambitions with an added zest now confident that the future realization of our desires is not so intangible as at first appeared.

I deemed life was tranquillity and rest,
I find it but a never-ending quest;
And I, who sat in quietude and peace,
Toil on a journey that shall never cease
(Shamshad)
Why should the Cosmos turn its wheel of worlds
If not to search for Thee eternally?
Why should the tireless Sun arise each morn
If not to look for Thee?
(Zauq)

How can I win that Hidden One
Who sits within the secret place,
For even in my very dreams
She wears the veil upon Her face.
(Jurat)

For long, throughout the world, I sought for Thee,
Through weary years and ages of unrest—
At last I found Thee hidden in my arms
Within my breasts.
(Zauq)

That which is spread before us, beneath the unceasing surge and change of the crowded life of the thoroughfares of great cities, as well as beneath the panorama of nature herself, was surely understood by those who insisted " there is no second Cause," and by Chu Hsi in saying "the innumerable laws (of nature) all proceed from one source."[131] In this the thought is not pietistically of a Creator, but of a living Reality met (passively or receptively) or encountered (actively or contestingly) by us all at all times. That Reality must be understood before we handle the problem of our patient with real efficacy.

In the intention of this work, then, there comes into consideration that greater art of medicine—not an ethical Hippocratic ideal, but something of the divine—an art as real to Avicenna, philosopher, poet, musician, the worker among the great and the small, aware of the dramatic in life, as it should be to us. So we step out of the world of the modern critic, the scholar, and the medical historian, indeed of modern medicine itself, into one in which we stand, as it were, hand in hand, with the great Master of the East—almost with his very eyes gazing upon and scrutinizing this ever open book of life of ours—divested of the false notions of "progress" and "time." His language is thus no longer alien—and, incidentally, he lives again!

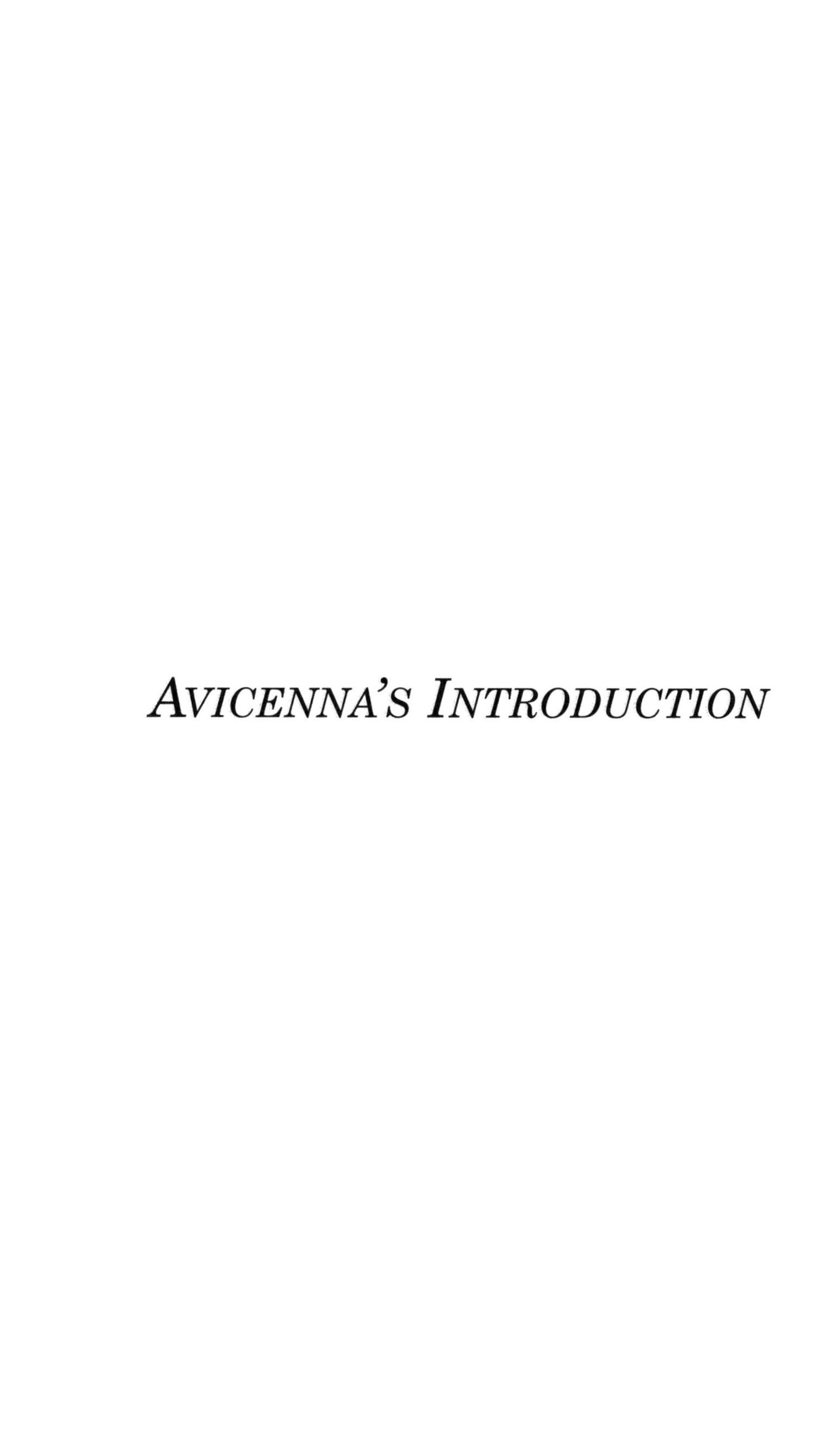

AVICENNA'S INTRODUCTION

Avicenna's Introductory Words

§1 In the first place we render thanks to God, for the very excellence of the order of His creation, and the abundance of His benefits. His mercies are upon all the prophets. Secondly, is at the request of one of my special friends [was it al-Juzjani?], one whom I feel most bound to consider, that I prepare this book on medicine, setting forth its general and particular laws to the full extent necessary, and yet with apt brevity.

§2 My plan is to deal with the general aspects of each of the two divisions of medicine—the speculative and the practical. Then I shall treat of the general principles applicable to the diagnosis of the properties of the simples, following this with a detailed account of them. I shall, then, take up the disorders which befall each individual member, beginning with an account of its anatomy, and that of its auxiliary. The anatomy of the several members and their auxiliaries is dealt with in the first book. Having completed the account of the anatomy, I shall show how the health of the member is to be maintained.

§3 This subject being completed, I proceed to a general discourse about general diseases: their causes, the signs by which they are recognized, and the modes of treatment. After this, I pass on to the special diseases and will point out in as many cases as possible: (1) the general diagnosis of their characters, causes and signs; (2) the special diagnostic features; (3) the general rules of treatment; (4) the special methods of treatment by (a) simples; and (b) compounded medicines.

§4 I include specially designed tables under the subject of simples to enable you to survey the facts rapidly as to the adjuvants for treating disease by simples.

§5 I have deemed it best to consider compounded medicines, their adjuvants, and how to mix them separately in a formulary. This it is my intention to compose after the special subjects are dealt with. Disorders not confined to one member are described in this book; cosmetics are spoken of, and the knowledge set forth in previous books is assumed. God helping me to complete this volume, the formulary will be added to it. Every follower of my teachings, who wishes to use them profitably, should memorize most of this work, even though he not understand it all.

§6 It is my intention to prepare further volumes if God should prolong my life still further, and if circumstances prove propitious. [Avicenna was to complete five volumes of which this is the translation of the first volume. Adp.]

A brief summary of the contents of remaining volumes, II, III, IV, and V of *The Canon* [which have not as yet been trasnlated into English, Adp.] are:

Volume II: Simple Drugs

This volume gives a detailed material medical pharmacology and therapeutics of drugs. It has two parts.

Part One. General Principles: These deal with the temperament or constitution of drugs, and how it is determined: (1) by experiment; and (2) by deduction. Conditions of the experiment such as, its being on the human body, drug to be free of extrinsic and intrinsic alterations, the trial to be allopatric and made on simple diseases, drug to be qualitatively and quantitatively corresponding to the severity of the disease, etc., have been described. Part one also gives an account of all the actions which drugs may possess and describes the method of collection and preservation of the various herbal and other products.

Part Two. List of Drugs: It gives 797 drugs in seriatim

according to the Abjad system. The properties of each drug have been described under the following headings: general description of the drug, tests for its purity, qualities, general and special actions on each system of the body or on special diseases; specific actions; antidotal properties; alternative remedies and adjuvants.

VOLUME III: DISEASES OF INDIVIDUAL MEMBERS

In this volume, the various diseases have been discussed systematically, with their etiology, symptoms, diagnosis, prognosis and treatment with simple drugs. Special mention may be made of the following sections:

Head: brain, (intemperaments, headache in all its aspects, organic diseases of the brain, epilepsy, paralysis, etc.) eye, ear, nose, mouth, throat, and teeth. Chest: lungs, heart, breasts. Alimentary tract: stomach, intestines, liver, gall bladder and spleen. Intestines and the anus, disorders of the rectum. Urinary tract: the kidneys, bladder and urine. The male reproductive system; the female reproductive system, conception, pregnancy, and diseases of women. Muscles: joints, and feet.

VOLUME IV: GENERAL DISEASES

Part One. Fevers: general description of fevers; their periodicity; causes such as constipation, diarrhea, dietetic indiscretion; excessive activity; excessive wakefulness; fear or anger; pain, inflammation, putrefaction, humoral disturbances; etc. Diagnosis of fevers; epidemic fevers; small pox; phthisis. Prognosis. Management of symptoms such as thirst, rigors, diarrhea, vomiting, sleeplessness, pain, headache, etc. Treatment of fevers: general and specific. Subject of crisis.

Part Two. Boils and swellings. Leprosy. Minor surgery. Wounds and their general treatment. Injuries: fractures and dislocations. Ulcers. Glandular swellings.

Part Three. Poisoning with mineral, vegetable and animal products. Bites from animals and man.

Part Four. Beauty culture. Leanness and obesity. Hair, nails and skin. Treatment of offensive odors and discolorations including leucoderma. Pediculosis. Pitting from small pox, etc.

VOLUME V: THE FORMULARY

This volume gives details of special prescriptions and antidotes; their form such as pills, powders, syrups, decoctions, confections, elixirs, etc, and their method of preparation. A thorough discourse about laxatives; purgative and non-purgative powders; medicinal powders, dosages; electuaris; potions and thickened juices; jams and preserves; pills; greens and cereals; lotions; and ointments and dressings. Prescriptions for different diseases. Weights and measures.

PART ONE
THE SCOPE OF MEDICINE AND ITS PHYSICAL BASIS

Lecture 1: The Scope of Medicine and Its Topics

1.1. The Definition of Medicine

§7 Medicine (*tibb*)[1] is the science by which we learn the various states of the human body in health and when not in health, and the means by which health is likely to be lost and, when lost, is likely to be restored back to health. In other words, it is the art whereby health is conserved and the art whereby it is restored after being lost.

§8 While some divide medicine into a theoretical and a practical [applied] science, others may assume that it is only theoretical because they see it as a pure science. But, in truth, every science has both a theoretical and a practical side. Philosophy has its practical and theoretical sides as well. A division of this nature has, of course, its own special significance in each of the various branches of knowledge. While it is unnecessary for us to enter into a consideration of such differences in regard to the other branches of knowledge, in medicine, with which we are concerned here, it must, however, be understood that this division into the theoretical and practical aspects does not mean that the physician should regard medicine as being of two different varieties—the theoretical and the practical. It should rather be interpreted as having two parts: the theoretical, which deals with the basic principles of medicine and the practical, which explains how these principles are to be applied in practice.

§9 The theory of medicine, therefore, presents what is useful in thought, but does not indicate how it is to be applied in practice—the mode of operation of these principles. The theory, when mastered, gives us a certain kind of knowledge. Thus we say, for example, there are three forms of fevers and nine constitutions.

§10 The practice of medicine is not the work which the physician carries out, but is that branch of medical knowledge which, when acquired, enables one to form an opinion upon which to base the proper plan of treatment. Thus it is said, for instance, that "for inflammatory foci," the first agents to employ are infrigidants, inspissants, and repellents; then we temper these with mollificants; and finally when the process is subsiding, resolvent mollificants will accomplish the rest. But if the diseased focus contains matter which depends for its expulsion on the integrity of the principal members, such treatment is not applicable. Here the theory guides to an opinion, and the opinion is the basis of treatment. Once the purpose of each aspect of medicine is understood, you can become skilled in both even if you are never called upon to use your knowledge.

§11 Another thing is that there is no need to assert that there are *three* states of the human body—sickness, health, and a state which is neither health nor disease. The first two cover everything. Careful consideration of the subject will make it clear to the physician either that the threefold grouping is unnecessary or that the group which we reject is unnecessary. The first two states really cover everything. Careful consideration will convince the physician that the third state is dual—on the one hand an infirmity, and on the other a habit of body or a condition which cannot be called strict health although the actions and functions of the body are normal. One must not risk defining health in an arbitrary fashion and include in it a condition which does not belong to it. However, we do not propose to argue this matter out because a disputation of that kind does not really further medicine.[2]

1.2. Concerning the Subject-Matter of Medicine

§**12** Medicine deals with the states of health and disease in the human body. It is a truism of philosophy that a complete knowledge of a thing can only be obtained by elucidating its causes and antecedents, provided, of course, such causes exist. In medicine it is, therefore, necessary that causes of both health and disease should be determined.

§**13** Sometimes these causes are obvious to the senses but at other times they may defy direct observation. In such circumstances, causes and antecedents have to be carefully inferred from the signs and symptoms of the disease. Hence, a description of the signs and symptoms of disease is also necessary for our purpose. It is a dictum of the exact sciences that knowledge of a thing is attained only through a knowledge of the causes and origins of the causes—assuming there to be causes and origins. Consequently our knowledge cannot be complete without an understanding both of symptoms and of the principles of being.[3]

1.3. The Causes of Health and Disease

§**14** There are four causes—material, efficient, formal, and final. On the subject of health and disease, we have the following:

1.3.1. The Material Causes

§**15** The material (*maddi*) cause is the physical body which is the subject of health and disease. This may be immediate as the organs of body together with their vital energies and remote as the humors and remoter than these, the elements which are the basis both for structure and change (or dynamicity). Things which thus provide a basis (for health and disease) get so thoroughly altered and integrated that from an initial diversity there emerges a holistic unity with a specific structure (or the quantitative pattern of organization) and a specific type of temperament (the qualitative pattern).

1.3.2. THE EFFICIENT CAUSES

§16 The efficient (*failiya*) causes are capable of either preventing or inducing change in the human body. They may be external to the person or internal. External causes are: age, sex, occupation, residence, and climate and other agents which effect the human body by contact whether contrary to nature or not. Internal causes are sleep and wakefulness, evacuation of secretions and excretions, the changes at different periods of life in occupation, habits and customs, ethnic group and nationality.

1.3.3. THE FORMAL CAUSES

§17 The formal (*suriyah*) causes are three: temperaments (*mizajat*) (or the pattern of constitution as a whole) and the faculties or drives (*qawa*) which emerge from it and the structure (the quantitative patterns).[4]

1.3.4. THE FINAL CAUSES

§18 The final (*tamamia*) causes are the actions or functions. They can be understood only from a knowledge of both the faculties or drives (*qawa*) and the vital energies (breaths, *arwah*) that are ultimately responsible for them. These will be described presently.

1.4. OTHER FACTORS TO CONSIDER

§19 A knowledge of the above-mentioned causes gives one insight into how the body is maintained in a state of health and how it becomes ill. A full understanding of just how health is conserved or sickness removed depends on understanding the underlying causes of each of these states and of their "instruments." For example, the diet in regard to food, drink, choice of climate, regulations regarding work and rest, the use of medicines, or operative interference. Physicians treat all these points under three headings as will be referred to later: health, sickness, and a state intermediate between the two. But we say that the state which they call intermediate is not really a mean between the other two.

§20 As the aim of medicine is to preserve health and eradicate disease, there are some other factors which deserve consideration: (1) the elements; (2) the temperaments; (3) the humors or body fluids; (4) the tissues and organs—simple and composite; (5) the breaths and their natural, nervous and vital faculty or drives; (6) the functions; (7) the states of the body—health, sickness, intermediate conditions; and (8) their causes: food, drink, air, water, localities of residence, exercise, repose, age, sex, occupation, customs, race, evacuation, retention and the external accidents to which the body is exposed from without; (9) the diet in regard to food, drink, medicines; exercises directed to preserving health; and (10) the treatment for each disorder.

§21 With regard to some of these things there is nothing a physician can do, yet he should recognize what they are and what is their essential nature—whether they are really existent or not. For a knowledge of some things, he depends on the doctor of physical science; in the case of other things, knowledge is derived by inference or reasoning. One must presuppose a knowledge of the accepted principles of the respective sciences of origins in order to know whether they are worthy of credence or not; and one makes inferences from the other sciences which are logically antecedent to these. In this manner one proceeds step by step until one reaches the very beginnings of knowledge—namely pure philosophy; to wit, metaphysics.[5]

§22 Things which the medical practitioner should accept without proof and recognize as being true are: (1) the elements and their number; (2) the existence of temperament and its varieties; (3) humors, their number and location; (4) faculty or drives, their number and location; (5) vital forces, their number and location; and (6) the general law that a state cannot exist without a cause and the four causes. Things which have to be inferred and proved by reason are: (1) diseases; (2) their causes; (3) symptoms; (4) treatment; and (5) their appropriate methods of prevention. Some of these matters have to be fully explained by reason in reference to both amount (*miqdar*) and time (*waqt*).

§23 If a physician like Galen attempted a logical explanation of these hypotheses, he would be discussing the subject not as a medical practitioner, but as a philosopher, and in this way would be like a jurist trying to justify the validity of, say, consensus of opinion. Of course, this he might do, not as a jurist but as a man of knowledge. However, it is not possible either for a medical practitioner, as such, or a jurist in his own capacity, to prove such matters by logic and reason; and if he does so, it will be at his own peril.

§24 The physician must also know how to arrive at conclusions concerning: (1) the causes of illnesses and the individual signs thereof; and (2) the method (most likely to) remove the disorder and so restore health. Wherever they are obscure, he must be able to assign to them their duration, and recognize their phases.

Lecture 2: The Elements

§25 The elements are simple substances which are the primary constituents of the human body and which cannot be subdivided into further ingredients. It is by their combination and appropriate organization that the various orders of things in nature have been formed.[1]

§26 Natural philosophy speaks of four elements and no more.[2] Two of these are light and two heavy. Fire and air are light while earth and water are heavy.

§27 Earth is a simple substance whose normal location is in the center of existence. In this position it remains stationary but when away from the center it tends to return to its normal position. This is the reason for its intrinsic weight. Earth is naturally cold and dry. These qualities of the earth can be easily appreciated by our senses as long as there is no interference by extraneous agents and it obeys its particular nature. It is by means of the element of earth that the parts of our body are fixed and held together into a compacted form. This is how our outward form is maintained.[3]

§28 Water is a simple substance which in its natural state surrounds the earth and is, in its turn, surrounded by the air, subject of course, to the other elements being also present in their own natural positions. This positing is because of its relative density. The nature of water is cold and moist. It appears to our senses as long as there are no influences to counteract it. It lends itself readily to dispersion and therefore assumes any shape without permanency. It allows things to be molded and spread out and attempered in their construction because, quite unlike the earth, it easily parts with its old shape and readily accepts a new one. Being moist, shapes can be readily made with it and as easily lost and resolved. Dryness, on the other hand, permits forms to be assumed only with difficulty and they are resolved with similar difficulty. When dryness and moisture alternate, dryness is overruled by the moisture, and thus the object is easily susceptible of being molded into a form whereas if the moisture were overruled by dryness, the form and features of the body would become firm and constant. Moisture serves to protect dryness from friability. Dryness prevents moisture from dispersing.[4]

§29 Air is a simple substance which lies above water and beneath fire. This is due to its relative lightness. In nature it is hot and moist as per the rule we have given. Its effect and value in the world of creation is to rarefy and render things finer, lighter, more delicate, softer, and consequently better able to move to the higher spheres.[5]

§30 Fire[6] is a simple substance whose natural position is above all the other elements. Thus, in nature it is located in that region of the sublunary world. Hence, its absolute lightness. Fire is hot and dry in temperament. It matures, rarefies, refines, and intermingles with all things. Its penetrative power enables it to traverse the substance of the air. With this power it subsumes the coldness of the two heavy cold elements. By this power it rings the elementary properties into harmony.[7]

§31 The two heavy elements enter more into the construction of the organs and fluids of the body and contribute to its stability. The two light elements enter more into the formation of the breaths and contribute to their movement as well as to the movement of the organs—always remembering that it is the inclination that is the motor. So much for the elements.

Lecture 3: The Temperaments

3.1. A Discussion On the Temperaments

§32 Temperament[1] is the quality which results from the mutual interaction of the four contrary, primary qualities of elements. By dividing up into minute particles, the elements are able to secure an intimate contact among themselves.

§33 These elements are so minutely intermingled as each to lie in very intimate relationship to one another.

§34 Their opposite powers alternately conquer and become conquered until a state of equilibrium is reached which is uniform throughout the whole. It is this outcome that is called "the temperament."[2]

§35 Since the primary powers in the elements are four in number (namely: heat, cold, moisture, dryness), it is evident that the temperaments in bodies undergoing generation and destruction accord with these powers.

§36 A simple, rational classification is of two types: (a) Equable or balanced. Here the contrary qualities are present to exactly equal degrees of potency—neither of them being in excess or deficiency. This temperament has a quality which is exactly the mean between the two extremes. (b) Inequable or unbalanced. Here the quality of the temperament is not an exquisitely exact mean between the two contraries, but tends a little more to one than to the other. For example, to hot more than to cold; to moist more than to dry; or contrariwise.[3]

§37 It is to be noted that a temperament, as understood by medicine, is never strictly equable or strictly inequable. The physician should abide by the philosopher who is aware that the really "equable" temperament does not actually exist in the human being any more than it exists in any "member" or "organ." Moreover, the term "equable," used by doctors in their treatises does not refer to weight but to an equity of distribution. It is this distribution which is the primary consideration—whether one is referring to the body as a whole, or only to some individual member; and the average measure of the elements in it, as to quantity and quality, is that which standard human nature ought to have—both in best proportion and in equity of distribution. As a matter of fact, the mean between excess and deficiency of qualities, such as is characteristic of man, actually is very close to the theoretical ideal.[4]

3.2. The Eight Types of Equable Temperaments

§38 Equilibrium is valid concerning the bodies of humans also; that is, in comparison with others (non-humans) not possessing such equilibrium.[5] The aforementioned equability does not approach that of humans in the first case. For (humans), in this regard, there occur eight aspects: (1) Whether, with regard to the species, when compared with others, he is excluded; (2) whether, with regard to the species, when compared with others, he is included; (3) whether, with regard to the genus of the species, when compared with others, he is excluded, but included in the species; (4) whether, with regard to the individual of the genus of the species, when compared with others, he differs from (another) individual, but is included in the genus and species; (5) whether, with regard to the individual of the genus of the species, when compared to others, he differs from (another) individual, but is included in the genus and species; (6) whether, with regard to the individual, when compared with others, he differs in his states and his essence; (7) whether, with regard to the (body) organ, when compared with those of others, he differs in them; and (8) whether, with regard to the (body) organ, when compared with those of others, he differs in its states and essence.

§39 With the first group, the human being, amongst all beings, is nearest to equable temperament. The range of temperament is too wide to be included in one definition although there are certain definite limits of excess and deficiency. If it goes beyond those limits, the temperament ceases to be a human one.

With the second group the temperament is between two extreme limits of the range of temperament shown by a person throughout his life—that is, that shown at the period of his life at which his growth has reached its limit. This is not, however, only the theoretical equilibrium referred to above although it closely approximates that. This type of person is near the approximate equilibrium only as far as his temperament corresponds to the co-equation of his members or the interchanging contra-action of his hot members (like the heart); with his cold ones (like the brain); moist ones (like the liver); with dry ones (like the bones). Were all of these of equal influence, the resulting condition would be very near to one of ideal equilibrium although not so as regards each individual member except in the case of the skin itself which will be explained later. In regard to the breaths (spirits) and principal members, the temperament cannot possibly approximate this exquisite balance. It oversteps in the direction of heat and moisture. The heart and the breath are the root of life and they are both very hot, indeed to excess for life itself depends on innate heat and growth depends on innate moisture. Indeed, the heat is present in and maintained or nourished by moisture. In regard to the three principal organs, the brain is cold, but its coldness does not modify the heat of the heart and the liver. The heart is dry, or nearly so, yet its dryness does not alter the moisture of the brain or liver. Neither is the brain absolutely and entirely cold, nor the heart absolutely and entirely dry. The heart is dry compared with the other two and the brain is cold compared with the other two.[6]

The limits of the third type are more narrow than those of the first, although still quite wide. This is a special equilibrium peculiar to the race, climate, geographical position or atmosphere. Indians, in health, have a temperament different from that of the Slav and so on. There is a temperament suitable to the people of India; for the Slavs there is another. Each equilibrium is appropriate for its class/genus, but inappropriate for another. If the body of an Indian be formed with a Slavic temperament, it will become ill or perish; the same would be true if a Slavic body were formed with an Indian temperament. So it seems that the various peoples of the earth have received a temperament appropriate for the conditions of their particular climate, and in each case there is a corresponding range between two extremes.

The fourth type is one which is a mean between the two limits of the range of the climactic temperament. It is more attempered than the temperaments of the third group.

The fifth type is more narrow in range with respect to the first and third groups. It is a temperament that necessarily belongs to a particular individual as long as he is living and healthy. He, too, possesses a breadth, the two limits of which are excess and deficiency. One must realize that every individual person has a temperament entirely peculiar to himself and it is impossible for any other person to have an identical temperament or even to approximate thereto.

The sixth type, too, is in the median between the two extremes. It is the temperament which, if possessed, is the most excellent that one could desire to have.

The seventh type is the equilibrium of temperament characteristic for each of the several members of the body because each is different from the other. In the case of bone, the equable temperament has dryness more than other qualities. In the case of the brain, moistness is more obvious; in the case of the heart, heat; in the case of the nerves, coldness. There, also, there is a range between excess and deficiency consistent with equability but less than in the other types mentioned.

The eighth type is that form of equable temperament which is proper for each given member. When it has this particular temperament it is in the best state possible to it.

§40 The human being, amongst all beings, is nearest to equable temperament. In the absence of factors to the contrary, that is, the presence of seas and mountains in the vicinity, the inhabitants of the equatorial regions are the most balanced of all. It has already been proven that neither the proximity of the sun or the vertical fall of its rays at the equator would make that atmosphere so abnormal as some of the other factors which are prevalent in places like ours or in places which are still farther from the equator. Indeed, people living in the equatorial regions are more balanced than those of the other regions. This matter has already been dealt with in a separate paper on this subject. Next to the inhabitants of the equatorial region are those living within the fourth region. They are neither exposed to the overhead sun for so long as people in the second or third circle, nor in winter do they suffer from the severe cold of the fifth circle which produces immature and imperfect development. Nearest to the absolute balance is the most balanced individual of the best balanced community in the most equable part of the world.

§41 Reference has already been made indirectly to the fact that the temperamental pattern of the vital members is not as close to the balance as of some other members. It is the flesh which is nearer to the balance and next comes the skin. The skin is evenly balanced because it fails to appreciate the temperature of water prepared by mixing equal quantities of snow and boiling water. It is in some such manner that the cold of the nervous tissue in the skin is counter-balanced by the heat of the breath and the blood vessels which contain the hot blood and vital force. When the driest element—earth—and the wettest element—water—are mixed in equal parts, the skin fails to appreciate any dryness or moisture. For it must be remembered that material objects influence one another through their contrary qualities. Things of a similar quality act upon one another only if their qualities are of different degrees.

§42 Of all the various parts of the body, the skin of the hands and from the hands, the skin of the palm and from the palm, the fingers and from the fingers, the index finger and from the index finger, the skin of the terminal phalanx is the most evenly balanced. It is for this reason that the terminal phalanges of the index and other fingers are the best organs for sensory perception.[7]

§43 It is worth remembering that when a medicine is

referred to as being evenly balanced, it does not mean that its temperament is the same as of a human being, or that it is even similar to it, for it would then be like a human being. It merely means that such a medicine, after being acted upon by the innate heat [metabolized] fails to produce any material change in the normal state of the body, and that its pharmacological actions remain within the limits of normal human temperament. In other words, when this medicine is given to a normal person, it does not produce any appreciable change or imbalance in the body. When it is said that a drug is hot or cold, it does not mean that the physical quality of the drug is particularly hot or cold or that it is colder or hotter than the human body. If this were so there would follow the unwarranted inference mentioned above that an evenly constituted medicine is the one which has exactly the same temperament as the human body. It means just that such a medicine produces a greater amount of heat or cold than what was originally present in the body. A drug which, for example, is cold for the human being may be hot for the scorpion, or the medicine which is hot for the human being may be cold for the serpent. In fact it may also mean that the same medicine may be less hot for one person than for another. This is the reason why physicians are advised to change their medicine when it fails to produce the desired result.

3.3. Imbalanced Temperaments

§44 Having fully described the evenly balanced temperament, a description of the various imbalances (dyscrasias or intemperaments) may now be given. They are classified according to race, individual and organs. There are eight types, all of which agree in being contrary to the eight equable temperaments outlined above. The simple types show a deviation from the normal equipoise only in respect of one contrary. The compound types show a deviation from the normal equipoise in respect of two contraries at once.

3.3.1. The Simple Imbalances

§45 The simple imbalance of temperament or intemperaments are where there is an active contrary quality which is in excess. That is the temperament is more hot than it should be, not more moist or drier. This is called hot intemperament. Or the temperament may be more cold than it should be, not more moist or drier. This is known as cold intemperament. Where there is a passive contrary quality which is in excess the temperament may be more dry than it should be, but not more hot nor cold. This is dry intemperament. Or the temperament may be more moist than it should be, but not more hot nor cold. This is called moist intemperament. Simple imbalances do not, however, last long, as they tend to be soon converted into compound imbalances. That is, an imbalance in the direction of excessive heat promptly leads to dryness and a change in the direction of cold increases the moisture. Dryness no doubt quickly increases cold in the body, but moisture, provided it is excessive, makes it much more cold. If, however, the increase of moisture is moderately cold, it would appear only after some considerable time. From this it will be seen that heat is generally more favorable than cold for maintaining the proper balance and general health of the body.

3.3.2. The Compound Imbalances

§46 As mentioned above, these temperaments have a dominance of two qualities: hot and moist, hot and dry, cold and moist, and cold and dry. It is clear that it cannot be simultaneously hotter and colder or drier and moister.

§47 Each one of these imbalances of temperament is further sub-divisible into two forms [making sixteen imbalances]. First of all, those apart from any material substance [qualitative, formal]. Here the temperament is altered only in regard to one quality because the fluid pervading it has the same quality as that towards which the body is being changed as a whole. Yet it does not do so unless it be because of heat [in fever] or cold [extraneous cold]. Secondly, those in which some material substance is concerned (material). Here the body is only affected by the quality of the imbalance because of the increased amount of some particular body-fluid. For instance, the body is cooled by serous humor and heated by leek-green choleric humor.

§48 Examples of these sixteen varieties will be given in Volumes III and IV.

§49 Imbalance or intemperament in which some material

substance is concerned can be of two types: a member may be pervaded by the material substance entering from without or it may be pervaded by the material substance which has reached the tissues of the body and fails to get out through the orifices of the channels or from the cavities of the body. Such retention of material may be the beginning of the formation of an inflammatory mass.

§50 This completes our description of the temperamental patterns. Let the physician accept from the natural scientist that which is not clear to him.

3.4. The Temperament of the Several Organs

§51 The Almighty Creator has bestowed upon every animal and every one of its organs the most appropriate and the best adapted temperament for its various functions and passive states.[8]

§52 Since the verification of this truth is a matter for philosophers and not physicians, we may accept that the human being has been bestowed a most befitting temperament and most appropriate faculty or drives for the various active and passive states in the body. Similarly, every organ and member is endowed with the proper temperament appropriate to its own functional requirement. Some He has made more hot, others more cold, others more dry and others more moist.[9]

3.4.1. The Hot Organs

§53 The living-principle (vital force, *ruh*) and heart, which is the center of vital activity, are hottest in the body. Next is blood which, although produced in the liver, due to its contact with the heart, is hotter than the liver. The next is the liver which is really a mass of almost solidified blood. After this is the flesh which is colder than the liver due to the cold nervous tissue in it. The next is the muscle which due to its cold ligaments and tendons is not as hot as the flesh. After this comes the spleen which, due to its high content of the residue from broken up blood, is not as hot. The kidneys are less hot because they have only a little blood. Then there are the breasts, testicles and muscular coats of the arteries which in spite of being nervous in origin are warm as they contain hot blood and other vital fluids. The next in order are the veins, which are slightly warmer because of blood in them. Last is skin of the palm, which is evenly balanced.

3.4.2. The Cold Organs

§**54** The coldest thing in the body is phlegm. Then in order of coldness are hair, bones, cartilage, ligaments, serous membranes, nerves, spinal cord, brain, solid and liquid fats, and lastly the skin.[10]

3.4.3. The Moist Organs

§**55** Phlegm is the most moist. Next in order are blood, solid and liquid fats, brain, spinal cord, breast, testicles, lungs, liver, spleen, kidneys, muscles and the skin. This order has been laid down by Galen. It should be noted that the lungs are not really so moist in structure and temperament as is implied in the list. The primary temperament of an organ is always similar to that of its nutriment, while its secondary temperament is determined by its excrement. The lungs, as Galen himself stated, are nourished by the hot blood which contains an appreciable quantity of the bilious humor. If the lungs are moist it is because of the vapors from below and the catarrhal secretions from above. The liver is more moist than the lungs due to the intrinsic moisture while lungs appear to be moist because of the extrinsic moisture. As they are constantly soaked in the extrinsic moisture (secretions), this makes them even structurally moist in the end. Similar is the case with phlegm and blood. The moisture in the phlegm is of a kind which merely moistens the tissues, while the moisture in the blood is of such a type that it is integrated into the very structure of the organs. Although normally there is more moisture in the phlegm than in the blood, in the maturation of phlegm into blood, it becomes dispersed as will be fully explained later on because normal phlegm is nothing but imperfectly digested blood.

3.4.4. The Dry Organs

§56 Hair is the driest of the tissues. It is, as it were, solid residue from the evaporation of moisture from the ethereal element. Next in order are the bones, which due to dryness, are the hardest of organs. Bones are however, a little more moist than hair, because they are formed from blood and are constantly absorbing moisture from attached muscles so that its fume is dry and it dries up the humors naturally located in bones. This is the reason why they are a source of nutrition for many animals, while hair is reported to be consumed by only bats. Next in order of dryness are cartilage, ligaments tendons, membranes, arteries, veins, motor nerves, heart, sensory nerves and the skin. Motor nerves are colder and drier at the same time and are therefore in equipoise. The sensory nerves are colder but not drier in proportion and are probably very nearly in equipoise since their coldness is not very far distant from that of the motor nerves.[11]

3.5. The Effect of Age On Temperament

§57 Life is divided into four periods: the period of growth which extends to the age of thirty; the period of adulthood from thirty-five to forty years; middle age, which extends to sixty years; and old age, during which the centers become weak. This continues until death.

§58 The period of growth is divided into five stages: infancy, during which limbs have not developed sufficiently; childhood, the stage in which a child can walk, but its limbs have not become firm. This period lasts until the second dentition; youth, begins after the limbs and organs of the body have become firm and the second dentition completed. It lasts until nocturnal emissions begin to appear; adolescence lasts until the appearance of moustache and beard in boys [and menstruation in girls]; youth continues until further growth stops. The period of childhood (i.e. from infancy to adolescence) is balanced in regard to heat, but has an excess of moisture. Heat (or metabolism) in childhood and youth has been a subject of dispute amongst the earlier teachers. According to some, children have greater heat as they show more rapid growth and have more persistent and more active physical functions like appetite and digestion. Moreover, their innate heat, having been derived originally from the semen, is relatively fresher and stronger than that of the grownups.

§59 Others, however, think that heat is more powerful in adults because their blood is greater in quantity and thicker in consistency, as may be inferred from the greater amount and severity of epistaxis amongst them. Moreover, adults tend to be bilious, while children are generally phlegmatic. Adults also show more powerful movements and possess a stronger digestion, thus indicating more heat. Appetite, however, does not depend upon heat, but is due to cold, hence the proverbial "dogs appetite" which is frequently a result of the cold. The stronger digestion of adults can be inferred from the fact that they do not suffer so much from nausea, water rash, vomiting and revulsion from food as children do. Adults are more susceptible to hot diseases and bilious vomiting than to cold or moist diseases as are children. Children also bring up quite a lot of phlegm in their vomit. The rapid growth observed in children is due not so much to the greater heat as to the moisture. The excessive appetite in children also shows that they have a lesser degree of heat. Such, indeed, are the arguments given by the two schools.

§60 It is, however, interesting to note that Galen was opposed to both schools. According to him, heat and moisture are about equal in children as well as adults. In children, the heat is quantitatively more but qualitatively less than in the adults, in whom it is quantitatively less but qualitatively more. According to Galen, this difference could be understood better if we keep in view the effect of the same amount of heat on a relatively larger quantity of water and a smaller quantity of dry material like a stone. The water would absorb more heat but its heat would be of a lesser intensity. The stone, on the other hand, would absorb a smaller amount of heat but would be hotter than the water. The difference between the heat in children and adults appears to be of the same type.

§61 Children derive heat from the sperm, which is very hot. This initial innate heat is being steadily used up, but the loss is made up by the progressive growth. Even during adulthood there is no special increase or decrease in this heat. In the end, due to some decrease in the quantity and quality of the protective moisture, heat begins to decline, so that when the senility is reached, it becomes less.

§62 In this connection it should be remembered that even this reduced amount of moisture, though insufficient for growth and development, is sufficient for the protection of heat. In childhood there is always sufficient moisture to meet both requirements. During the intervening period of maturity, it is just enough for maintaining body heat. In the end it is, however, not enough for either. It would of course be difficult to believe that a quantity of the moisture which is sufficient for growth should not be sufficient for the production of heat, but when a thing cannot even maintain itself it can hardly provide something additional for growth and development. It is clear from this discussion that moisture in adults is sufficient only for maintaining the heat, but is insufficient for growth and development. As some others have said, it is not true that the development of children is solely due to the moisture. Moisture is the material for growth and the matter, of course, cannot be altered or grown without an efficient cause. In this case, efficient cause is the "self" or nature which, according to the will of Almighty God, operates through the innate heat.

§63 It would be equally wrong to say that the excessive appetite of children is due to their cold temperament. A morbid appetite due to coldness of temperament cannot result in good digestion and nutrition. Children usually have the best digestion. Growth of the body as a whole implies that more food is being assimilated than is being used up. When digestion is faulty, the cause is either gluttony—eating food voraciously or inordinately, errors of diet—taking a diet badly designed and including articles of food which are unwholesome or moist in temperament or in excess, neglect of the movement of the bowels and other emunctories whereby effete matters accumulate and become knit together in them (which is an indication for purging), or other emunctories. The lungs especially need purgation by making the respiration deeper and quicker although its power is never as great as it sometimes is in the second period of life.

§64 These observations on the temperament of children and adults are really those of Galen and have merely been included here for their general interest.

§65 Innate heat begins to decline after middle age. This is due to the dispersive effect of the atmospheric air on the moisture which is the basic material for heat. The innate heat (vital activity) gradually disperses the body moisture, and the various secretions of the body, are also constantly drying up from normal physical and emotional activity.

§66 It has been proven in natural philosophy that the faculties or drives of the body are not everlasting, hence the system gradually fails to cope with the various dispersive factors, and in the end, the faculties or drive which supplies nutrition also fails. Even if these faculty or drives had been everlasting, and even if the system could replenish the daily loss of wear and tear, the natural dissolution which is incidental to the aging process would prevent adequate replacement. When both factors cooperate in furthering the decline of the body from its original perfection, it can be readily understood why in the end the material [moisture] should decay, and with it the heat [or activity] come to an end, and this all the more so because the moisture which is being constantly received from the impaired digestion, acts as a contributory factor.

§67 Moisture, then, must come to an end and the innate heat become extinguished. This occurs sooner if another contributory factor to destruction is present like the extraneous excess of humor arising out of imperfect digestion of food. This extinguishes the innate heat by smothering it, enclosing it and by providing the contrary quality. This extraneous humor is called the cold serous humor. That is how natural or physiological death ensues. The duration of life depends on the original temperament which retains a certain degree of power to the end by fostering its intrinsic moisture. (Death from accident or disease has, however, a different origin. Whether from physiological or pathological cause, it is, of course, ultimately determined in accordance with divine decree).[12]

§68 It may be summarized that both children and the young are balanced in regard to heat, while the middle aged and the senile are relatively cold. Children, however, possess a moderate excess of moisture to fulfill the requirements of growth. The excess of moisture in children is evident from the softness of their bones and nerve tissues and also from the fact that it has not been long since they grew and developed from the semen, blood and ethereal vital force.[13] The middle-aged and the old are not only cold but dry. This can be observed from their bones being hard and the skin dry, and inferred from the long time having elapsed since they originally developed from the blood, semen and ethereal vital force. Both the children and the young adults are fiery to the same extent. There is more water and air in children than in the young. The middle-aged and particularly the old and senile show a larger amount of earth in their constitution than children and the young adults, but the young are more balanced than children. The grownups are, however, drier than children and hotter than the old and the middle-aged. On the other hand, elderly persons are drier than the young and middle-aged persons in their primary temperamental constitution. They are, however, more moist because of the abnormal moisture which makes their tissues temporarily and superficially moist.

3.6. The Effect of Gender on Temperament

§69 Observation shows that women are colder in temperament than men. This is why they are normally of a smaller build. They are, also, more moist because their greater cold leads to the excessive formation of excrements, and because they do not indulge in so much activity, their flesh is loose and lax. The denseness of male flesh renders permeation through its veins and nerves more difficult.

3.7. The Effect of Residence on Temperament

§70 People living in the northern countries are more moist and colder than people living in southerly countries.

§71 So too are those whose occupation involves work with water. If, however, the circumstances are contrary, they would be dry.

§72 The signs of various temperaments will be described when dealing with the general and special signs and symptoms of health and disease.

Lecture 4: The Humors

4.1. The Nature of the Humors and Their Types

4.1.1. The Nature of the Humors

§73 Humor (*akhlat*)[1] or body-fluid is that fluid, moist, physical substance into which our aliment is transformed. That part of the aliment which has the capacity to be transformed into body substance, either by itself or in combination with something else thereby being capable of assimilation by the members or organs, and completely integrated into the tissues, is the healthy or good humor. It is what replaces the loss which the body substance undergoes.[2]

§74 The residue from this process, the "superfluity," is called unhealthy or abnormal humor. It is the fluid which, in the absence of proper digestion or conversion, is unsuitable for assimilation and is therefore eliminated from the body.[3]

§75 Body fluids may be primary or secondary. Primary fluids are the sanguineous humor (blood), the serous humor (phlegm), the bilious humor (yellow bile) and the atrabilious humor (black bile). Secondary fluids of the body are either non-excrements or excrements. The non-excrements have not yet been subjected to any action by any of the simple organs and they are not changed until they reach the destined tissues.

They are of four types: (1) that which is located at the orifices of the minutest channels near the tissues and thus irrigating them; (2) that which permeates the tissues like a dew and is capable of being transformed into nutriment if it becomes necessary; (3) the third type forms a nutrient which which will be changed into the substance of the tissues, whether to the extent of entering into their temperament or to the extent of changing into their very essence, thereby attaining an entire likeness to the member or organ. (4) The fourth type accounts for the continuous identity of the member or organ or of the body throughout one's life. It is derived from the semen, which in its turn is derived from the humors.

§76 The non-excreted fluids have not as yet been subjected to the action of any of the simple members or organs and they are to be changed until they reach the tissues for which they are destined. The second type mentioned above—the fluid which is present in the tissues as dew drops and is capable of being utilized as a nutriment in times of dire necessity, also moistens the organs which have been dried up by excessive activity.

4.1.2. The Four Types of Humors

§77 Both the normal and abnormal humors are of the following four varieties: the sanguineous humor, the most excellent of all; the serous humour; the bilious humour; and the atrabilious humour.

4.1.2.1. The Sanguineous Humor

§78 The nature [dynamic aspect] of the sanguineous humor is hot and moist in temperament.[4] It may be normal or abnormal, conforming to its nature or not. Normal blood is red in color, sweet in taste and free from smell. Abnormal blood has two varieties: first of all, blood which has become abnormal from some intrinsic change in the temperament, such as getting hot or cold, but not because of any admixture with any foreign matter and second of all, blood which has become abnormal from admixture with some morbid or unhealthy fluid derived from within or without. This second type of abnormal blood may be caused by either an unhealthy fluid coming to it from without, penetrating it and so causing decomposition in it or by a putrescent change in a portion of itself (the rarefied product becoming bilious humour and the denser product becoming atrabilious where either one or both together may remain in the blood). Abnormal blood of the first type is named according to what which is mixed with it—whether serous humour or atrabilious or simply bilious fluid. Abnormal blood of the second type is named according to its color and wateriness—sometimes it is turbid, sometimes attenuated, sometimes very dark from much blackness, sometimes pale and its taste and bitter, salty or sour.

4.1.2.2. The Serous Humor

§79 The nature of the serous humor[5] is cold and moist in temperament. It may be normal or abnormal. Normal (sweet) serous humor can be transformed into blood at any time as it is an imperfectly matured blood. It is a kind of sweet fluid which is only slightly colder than the body, but it is much colder than the bilious and blood humors. Sweet serous humor has a variety which is abnormal. This variety is tasteless unless it is mixed with blood, when it becomes somewhat sweet. This happens frequently with sputum and catarrhal excretions.

§80 According to Galen, the normal variety of the sweet serous humour has no special place in the body, as is also the case with the bilious and atrabilious humors. The reason is that like blood, the serous humor is required by nearly every organ in the body, hence, it always circulates with the blood. There are two special reasons why it has no special place. The first reason is essential and the second is accessory.

§81 The essential function is two-fold: the serous humor has necessarily to remain in close contact with the tissues as an easily available material for emergencies, such as a temporary failure of the food supply from the stomach and liver as in starvation. This material is normally acted upon by the vegetative faculties or drives which change and digest it and are themselves maintained thereby.

§82 The transformation of lymph into blood is achieved by the innate heat. Alien heat [bacterial infection] would only putrefy the material and decompose it. This kind of relationship does not hold in the case of the two bilious fluids because neither of them turns into blood at any time as the serous humor does under the influence of innate heat. However, they resemble the serous humor in undergoing putrefaction and decomposition under the influence of alien heat [bacterial infection]. Secondly, the serous humor must be mixed with the sanguineous humor before it can reach and nourish the tissues of the lymphatic temperament. When the serous humor is present in the blood for subserving nutrition, it must be in definite proportion before it reaches the parts to be nourished, that is, the cerebrum. It is the same in the case of the two bilious humors. The accessory function is that of moistening the joints, tissues and organs concerned in movement. Otherwise the heat of the friction of the movement would produce dryness of their surfaces. This function is within the range of necessity.

§83 Abnormal phlegm has a few varieties: sticky and of an apparently abnormal consistency; immature, but of an apparently normal consistency; abnormally thin and watery; and thick and of white color. The thinner portions of the serous humor are dispersed by stagnation in the joints and passages. This is the thickest of all varieties. Another variety of the serous humor is the one which is salty and is more dry than all the other types.

§84 The salty, serous humor is warmer, drier, and lighter than any of the other types. It is salty because the oxidized earthy matters of dry temperament and bitter taste are mixed with the watery (nearly or quite insipid) "moisture," in equal [in terms of potency, not weight] proportions. If these particles are in a greater quantity than the normal, the fluid becomes bitter instead of salty. Both natural and artificially manufactured salts are made in this way.

§85 In the artificial method, alkaline, ash-like or lime is boiled in the water and then filtered out. The remaining solution is then either boiled to yield a deposit of the dissolved salt or is left to crystallize out.

§86 Attenuated serous humor may be insipid or have only a slightly salty taste. This taste comes from the mixture with an equal amount of oxidized bile which is dry and bitter. The resultant heating salty fluid is called "bilious serous humor." According to Galen, the taste of salt in the serous humor is due to either putrefaction or mixture with fluid. We would rather say that it is really the oxidized portion of the serous humor is turned into a sort of dry ash which makes it salty. Mixture with the fluid alone would not give salinity to the serous humor, unless the other factor, (i.e., the oxidized ash) is also present. It is possible that Galen meant "putrefaction and fluid" rather than "putrefaction or fluid."

§87 The serous humor becomes bitter if mixed with the atrabilious humor (which is itself bitter) or too much infrigidation tales place whereby the taste changes from sweet to bitter. The process consists in a congealing and degradation of the watery element into something dry and, therefore, earthy in character. The degree of heat is too little to ferment it and make it sour. A strong heat would completely alter it into something else.

§88 The serous humor, which is sour, has also two varieties. One is where the sourness is intrinsic in origin and the other is where it is introduced from without. In the latter case it is acrid atrabilious humor that is the extraneous factor. This will be discussed later. When the sourness is intrinsic, it is comparable with the change that takes place when the others juices go sour. In other words, it is sour because the humor has fermented and then gone sour.

§89 There is a variety of serous humor which is bitter. The astringent taste in this humor may be due either to an admixture of some astringent atrabilious or bilious itself may become so cold that it tastes astringent. This is because cold solidifies the moisture into earthy particles and in this process the heat being neither so little as to ferment it into sour serous humor nor so strong as to mature it into an assimilable form makes it astringent.

§90 Serous humor may be thick and viscid like melted glass or it may be sour or tasteless. In fact, it should not be surprising if the tasteless variety of the thick serous humor proves to be really an immature humor or if the immature humor turns out to be an altered form of the tasteless kind. This serous humor is originally cold and thin and is free from putrefaction and admixture of any kind. Its greater cold and viscosity are due to its local stagnation. It is now clear that the abnormal serous humor has four varieties in regard to taste: salty, sour, bitter and tasteless. The latter also has four varieties: watery, slimy, viscid and thick white. The immature serous humor is really a variety of the slimy.

4.1.2.3. The Bilious Humor

§91 The bilious humor is the foam of blood.[6] It is bright in color. It is light and pungent. The more red, it is, the hotter it is. It is formed in the liver and then follows one of two courses: either it circulates with the blood or it passes on to the gallbladder. The part which passes into the blood stream assists in two purposes. First of all, the portion which goes to the blood is essential for nutrition of organs like the lungs. It makes the blood light and thin for easy passage through the narrow channels of the body. The portion which goes into the gallbladder is thus prevented, from vitiating the body and providing nutrition to the gallbladder. Its subsidiary functions are the cleansing of the intestine from the thick and viscid mucus and stimulation of the musculature of the intestine and rectum for proper defecation.

§92 That is why stasis or obstruction in the bile duct may produce colic.

§93 Bilious humor becomes abnormal either from vitiation with some external factor or from some change in its composition. Of these two types, the former has two sub-varieties. One of these is the well known variety which is admixed with the serous humor and is produced in the liver. The less known variety is that which has atrabilious humor mixed in it. The variety which has the serous humor in it may be thin or thick. The latter, which is a mixture, is of a vitelline yellow color. The less known variety is the oxidized bilious bile. This is formed by oxidation of the bilious humor which instead of separating out remains in the bile. This is the worst type of bile.

§94 Bilious humor may also get mixed up with the atrabilious humor derived from outside. This kind of bile is not so bad. It is often red, but not of bright color. Both in color and appearance it resembles blood from which it could be distinguished only by its consistency. Occasionally, its color may be changed by some other factors. The bile which has become abnormal from some intrinsic change is also of two varieties. One is formed in the liver and the other in the stomach. In the liver, the burning of the thin and lighter portions of the blood produces pure bilious humor, while the burning of thicker portions produces pure atrabilious humor.

§95 Bile produced in the stomach may be either green bile or brown bile. Green bile is formed by the mixture of the dark viscid burnt out bile with the normal atrabilious bile. Brown bile is formed from the oxidation of the green bile. Oxidation destroys the moisture, and thus makes the objects white. Moist things are first darkened by heat, but later with the actual destruction of moisture, the dark color gradually turns into white. This can be observed from the action of heat on a moist piece of wood. The heat would first turn the wood into dark charcoal and then into white ash. This happens because heat makes the moist objects dark, and the dry ones white, while cold whitens the moist objects and darkens the dry ones. These remarks about the green and brown bile are, however, tentative and thus cannot be vouchsafed as facts. Brown bile is the most hot and poisonous of all varieties. It is said to be formed of the hot, vapory material, as it were.

4.1.2.4. The Atrabilious Humor

§96 Atrabilious humor is cold and dry in nature.[7] There are a natural and abnormal varieties.

§97 Normal atrabilious humor is a sediment of the normal blood. It has a taste between sweetness and bitterness. After being formed in the liver, a part goes to the blood and another to the spleen.

§98 The part which goes with the blood is essential for two purposes: the nutrition of organs such as the bones which have an appreciable quantity of the atrabilious bile in their composition, and to make the blood properly thick and heavy.

§99 The portion which is in excess of these requirements is taken up by the spleen essentially for its own nutrition but also to save the blood from being damaged. The portion which goes from the spleen into the stomach serves the purpose of making the stomach strong and firm. It also stimulates the appetite by its sour taste.

§100 This action of atrabilious humor is somewhat similar to that of the bilious humor. Just as the surplus of bile in the blood goes to the gallbladder, and the surplus from the gallbladder passes into the intestine, the excess of atrabilious humor from the blood goes to the spleen, what is left over from the spleen goes to the stomach to induce appetite. The surplus of bilious humor excites peristaltic movements and thus assists evacuation, but the surplus of atrabilious humor encourages the intake of food. So, blessed be God, the best of creators and the mightiest of rulers!

§101 The abnormal form of atrabilious humor is formed by the oxidation of material or ash formed from an oxidation of the commingled bilious humor. When there is some earthy matter mixed something moist, the earthy matter separates out either by sedimentation, as does normal atrabilious humor, or as an ash by the oxidation process, dispersion of the thinner elements leaving the heavier matter behind. This is what takes place in the humors of which the atrabilious humor which is to be excreted is the segregate.

§102 Blood is the only body fluid which yields a precipitate of this kind. Serous humor is too sticky to leave any deposit. It acts like oil. Bilious humor does not do so because it is attenuated and is deficient in earthy matters. Also, it is constantly moving. Whatever little that is formed is either oxidized or quickly eliminated by the body. Moreover, it can be separated from the blood only in minute traces.

§103 Abnormal atrabilious humor is produced in four types: The ash from oxidized bilious humor is bitter in taste. It differs from the partially oxidized bilious humor in being all ashes, rather than a small quantity of the oxidized bile being still mixed with it. If the ash from the oxidized serous humor is light and thin, its product is salty, otherwise it tastes acid or bitter. The ashes from oxidized sanguineous humor has a sweetly salty taste. If the ash from the oxidation of normal atrabilious humor is thin, its oxidized product is extremely acrid like vinegar. On being spilled, vinegar "boils" immediately, giving a foul acrid smell which even flies shun. When the normal atrabilious humor is thick, its oxidized products are bitter rather than acrimonious.

§**104** Three varieties of morbid atrabilious humor are particularly injurious: (1) oxidized bilious humor where the attenuated portion is removed—there are two types of this kind; (2) sero-atrabilious humor which is less injurious and acts at a slower rate; and (3) choleric-atrabilious humor which is more injurious and undergoes decomposition very readily. The first atrabilious humor derived from the serous humor is slow in action and not so harmful. The second is more acrid and more injurious but if treatment be begun early, it will be more amenable thereto. A third form effervesces less when poured upon the earth and penetrates the tissues less easily and is more slowly destructive. On the other hand, it is very difficult to disperse or mature or treat by any remedial measures.

§**105** According to Galen, blood is the only physiological humor and all the others are merely excremental and unnecessary to the body. This is not correct. If blood had been the only nutriment, every organ in the body would have had the same temperament and structure. Bones would not have been harder than the flesh and brain softer than the bones. If the bone is hard, it is because its blood supply contains some hard and black bile material, and if the brain is soft, it is due to soft and moist material in its blood supply.

§**106** The other humors can also be actually seen in the blood. Thus, when after the venesection blood is allowed to settle down, it develops a foam on the surface (serous humor or yellow bile). The heavy matter which settles down at the bottom is atrabilious humor (black bile). The material which remains mixed with blood, like the white of an egg, is the serous humor. There is also a watery portion which is mostly excreted in the urine. Water is, however, not of a strictly humoral nature because it is of no nutritional value. Water dilutes the food for its easier passage through the narrower channels of the body.

The humors are made of the material which is of a nutritional nature. A thing can be nutritious only if its qualities are similar to those of the body, and a thing which has a qualitative resemblance to the body can only be a compound and not a simple substance like water.

§107 It is not true that the strength of the body depends upon the presence of a large quantity of blood in the body and that weakness is due to its deficiency. Strength or weakness depends upon the amount of nutrition available in the blood and on the quantity actually assimilated by the body. Others, again, believe that whether the humors be increased or lessened in amount, the maintenance of health depends on the preservation of a certain quantitative proportion between the several humors, one to another, peculiar to the human body. This is not exactly correct. The humors must, besides that, maintain a certain constant quantity. It is not a matter of the composition of one or other humor, but of the body itself. The proportions which they bear one to another must also be preserved.

§108 A further consideration of the humors will now be omitted as this subject is not quite appropriate for physicians, but really concerns the philosophers.[8]

4.2. The Production of the Humors

§109 Digestion begins from the time of mastication as the lining of the mucous membrane of the mouth is in direct continuity with mucosa of the stomach. The food is altered by its contact with the lining of the mouth. Saliva aids the digestion further by its own innate heat or activity. This is the reason why the application of chewed wheat matures boils and sores, but not of the merely ground, moistened and cold wheat. Some say that mastication produces some vital change which is evident from the altered taste and odor of the masticated food (that is, prior to this, there is neither odor nor taste).

§110 The stomach digests food, not only by its own heat, but also by the heat of the surrounding organs, like the liver on the right and spleen on the left. It is true that the spleen is temperamentally cold, but due to its rich vascularity it also provides heat to the stomach. There is, also, in front, the omentum whose fat easily retains heat and reflects it onto the stomach. Above is the heart which warms the diaphragm and so warms the stomach.

§111 The first stage of digestion gives the essence of the digested material which, in many animals, becomes chyle with the help of mixing with the fluid it has consumed. The chyle is of the consistency of a broth, as thick as sodden barley.

§112 The part of this chyle which is thus diluted is drawn from the stomach into the intestines and then is caused to enter into the roots of the mesenteric vessels which are found all along the intestinal tract. The vessels are thin and light. Once entering these channels, the nutriment passes into the portal vein, enters the gateway of the liver, and then travels along finer and finer divisions until it comes to the capillaries (the very fine hair-like channels), which are the ultimate source of the vena cava emerging from the convexity of the liver. These channels are, however, so narrow that food can only pass through them with the help of water, which has been taken in excess of the strict requirements of the body. By being distributed over the whole liver in this way, the chyle is exposed to the digestive function of the whole organ, and the function of the liver is thus accomplished most vigorously, energetically, and speedily. The change of nutriment into blood is now complete.

§113 The various products and by-products of digestion up to this point are in healthy digestion by the blood itself; by-products include a foam which is the bilious humor and a sort of precipitate which is the atrabilious humor. In unhealthy digestion by-products include: an oxidation product where digestion is carried too far—an attenuated portion shows a morbid bilious humor, and a dense portion shows a morbid atrabilious humor; and (2) a product when digestion is not carried far enough which is the serous humor.

§114 As long as it stays in the liver, the blood which the liver forms is more attenuated than it should be because the wateriness is in excess for the reason already given. But when the blood leaves the liver, the excess of water is removed, for it is taken to the renal vessels and so provides the kidneys with the quantity and quality of the blood best suited for their nutrition. The fat of the blood nourishes the kidneys and the superfluous wateriness and a certain degree of sanguineous material passes down to the bladder and so away from the body.

§115 The good blood ascends into the veins, emerging from the convexity of the liver and enters into the main channel from where it spreads into the smaller branches until it reaches the tissues in the manner best known to God.

§116 The material cause of blood are those parts of the solid and fluid digestive material which are of equable temperament; of the bilious humor are the attenuated hot, sweet, oily and sharp by-product of digested material; of the serous humor are the dense, humid, viscid, cold by-product of the digested material; of the atrabilious humor are the very dense by-product of the digested material, very deficient in moisture and exceeding in heat. The formal causes of the humors are: of blood, exact and good digestion; of bilious humor are the digestion verging on excess; of the serous humor, imperfect digestion; and of the atrabilious humor, the precipitative tendency preventing the flow or dispersal. The efficient causes are: of blood, attempered heat; of bilious humor, attempered heat for normal bilious humor (foam), and undue heat for abnormal bilious humor whose site is the liver, for serous humor, feeble heat; for atrabilious humor are medium heat (that is, a heat of oxidation which surpasses the limits of equipoise). As to the final cause for the blood it is to nourish the body. For the bilious humor, the primary cause is nutrition or attenuation of blood while the secondary cause is cleansing the bowel wall and desire for stool. For the serous humor, the primary and secondary purposes [see §79ff]. For the atrabilious humor, the primary and secondary purposes [see §96ff], include nutrition, inspissation of blood, nourishment of the spleen, tone to the stomach, and aid to the appetite.[9]

§117 Further details regarding the efficient causes include the following.:(1) The action of heat and cold. One must not forget that the most fundamental agents in the formation of the humors are heat and cold. When the heat is equable, blood forms. When heat is in excess, bilious humor forms. When in great excess, so that oxidation occurs, atrabilious humor forms. When the cold is equable, serous humor forms. When cold is in excess so that congelation becomes dominant, atrabilious humor forms. (2) The faculty or drives. There is also a proportionate relation between the active and passive drives [which has to be considered in thinking of the formation of the humors]. (3) The temperaments. One must not get the idea that every temperament gives rise to its like and never to its opposite. A temperament often gives rise to its exact opposite (indirectly, of course. It cannot do so directly). A cold and dry temperament may give rise to visible moisture, although this would not be beneficial, but would indicate that digestion is feeble. A person with such a temperament would be thin, with supple joints, and hairless skin, cold to the touch, the surface veins narrow and he would be gentle and timid in nature. He would be like the elderly person who produces too much serous humor and is cold and dry in temperament.

§118 Excessive formation of atrabilious humor may be due to: (1) immoderate degree of heat in the liver; (2) weakness of the spleen; (3) a degree of cold sufficient to be congelative and cause marked and long-continued constriction; (4) the existence of various long-standing or often repeated diseases whereby the humors are reduced to ash.

§119 When the atrabilious humor is plentiful, it virtually lodges between the liver and the stomach with the result that the formation of blood and healthy fluids is interfered with and less blood is formed.

§120 Blood and its other humors, while in circulation, undergo a third digestion.[10]

§121 A fourth digestion also occurs when they have actually reached the tissues.

§122 The waste products of the primary digestion in the stomach are eliminated by the intestine. Those of the second digestion in the liver are mostly eliminated in the urine, and it is only a small portion which is directed towards the gallbladder and spleen. Wastes from the third or fourth digestion are eliminated partly in the sweat, ear, nasal and aural secretions and partly through the invisible pores of the body. Sometimes they are even discharged through boils and abscesses. Hair and nails have also been considered by some to be of an excretory nature. Persons with thin humors are apt to be easily debilitated by eliminants. This is particularly true in the case of those whose bodily pores naturally produce a greater dispersion and thus cause loss of vitality. As long as the chyle stays in the liver, the blood which the liver forms is more attenuated than it should be because of the wateriness being in excess (the reasons given above). When the blood leaves the liver, the excess water is removed, taken to the renal vessels and provides the kidneys with the quantity and quality of the blood best suited for their nutrition. The "fat" of the blood nourishes the kidneys and the superfluous wateriness and a certain degree of sanguineous material passes down to the bladder and so away from the body.

§**123** Lastly, it must be clearly understood that not only the causes of origin, but also the causes of movement of the humors must be taken into consideration. Exercise and heating agents set in motion the sanguineous humor, the bilious humor, and even the atrabilious humor (which is thereby strengthened). Rest sets the serous humor in motion and strengthens it. Rest also strengthens some kinds of atrabilious humor. Even imagination, emotional states and other agents cause the humors to move. Thus, if one were to gaze intently at something red, one would cause the sanguineous humor to move. That is why one must not let a person suffering from nose-bleed see things of a brilliant red color.[11]

§**124** This description of the humors is the only one pertinent to the subject of medicine. The rest is a matter for philosophy.

Lecture 5: The Members (Anatomy)

5.1. The Nature and Types of Body Members

§125 Members or organs are formed primarily from the mixing of the normal humors just as the humors are derived primarily from the mixture of the digested material and the digested material is formed primarily from the mixing of the elements.

§126 They are of two kinds: simple and compound organs. Simple organs are those in which all the visible and perceptible tissues carry the same name and definition as the whole organ, i.e., muscles, nerves etc . They are recognized by the uniformity of their structure and are thus known as elementary tissues. Compound organs are those in which the parts, irrespective of size, differ in nature as well as name from the corresponding organ as a whole, i.e., hands, feet, face, etc. Thus, a part of the face cannot be called a face and a part of the hand a hand. These organs are also called "instrumental" because they are the instruments whereby the passions and actions of the soul [mind, emotional expression] are expressed.[1]

5.2. The Simple Members (Elementary Tissues)

5.2.1. *Bones*

§127 Bones form the foundation or skeleton for the body as a whole and serve as the basis for its movement.

5.2.2. *Cartilage*

§128 Cartilage is softer than bone. It can be easily bent but is relatively harder than the other tissues. It provides a firm cushion between the bone and soft tissues so that the soft organs or members not be injured when exposed to a blow or fall or compression. Examples of this are the shoulder-blade and the bones over the precordia and the ribs or the epiglottis and xiphisternum. In the case of joints, it prevents the tissues from being torn by the hard bone. It allows for a muscle to obtain extension in places where there is no bone to give support (like the muscles of the eyelids) and gives attachment to muscles without being too hard for them (like the epiglottis).

5.2.3. *Nerves*

§129 Nerves arise from the brain or the spinal cord. They are white, soft, pliant, difficult to tear and were created to subserve sensation and movement of the limbs.

5.2.4. *Tendons*

§130 Tendons form the terminations of the muscles. They resemble the nerves in appearance. They are attached to movable organs and when the muscles contract and relax, the parts to which the tendons are attached move to and fro. They may broaden when the muscles expand and then become narrow again on their own, lengthening and shortening apart from the lengthening and shortening of the muscle. Sometimes this is through the intervention of ligaments. The upper part of the muscle is called flesh and that which leaves the flesh and passes to the joint, bringing the two close together, is called the tendon.

5.2.5. *Ligaments*

§131 Ligaments have the appearance and feel of nerves. They are of two kinds: true and false. False ligaments extend to the muscle while true ligaments to not reach as far as the muscle but simply join the two ends of the bones of a joint firmly together. The false ligament does not have the feel of ligament and is not painful when moved or rubbed. The auxiliaries of the ligaments are the structures attached to them.

5.2.6. Arteries

§**132** Arteries arise from the heart and are distributed to the body. They are hollow, elongated organs which are nerve-like in appearance but are structurally similar to the fibrous tissue. They display movements of contraction and expansion which distinguishes them from the veins. They serve the purpose of ventilating the heart and expelling the fuliginous vapor and distributing the breath [oxygen] by their means to all parts of the body.

5.2.7. Veins

§**133** Veins are like the arteries but veins arise in the liver. They do not pulsate (like the arteries). They carry blood away to all parts of the body.[2]

5.2.8. Membranes

§**134** Membranes [viscera] are made of extremely minute interwoven fibers which are extremely delicate: they are formed into thin sheets which cover the various organs. They serve these purposes: (1) to form the external covering for other structures and thereby (2) to preserve the form and outline of these structures, (3) to support the members; (4) by means of their fibers to bind together the nerves and ligaments with the members. For example, they hold the kidneys in position; (5) to give sensation to organs which are themselves insensitive because by providing a sensitive covering, they enable the member to be aware of anything happening to it. Things which are in direct contact with the membranes are felt directly but those within the organs are perceived indirectly, i.e., lungs, liver, spleen, and kidneys which are all insensitive. It is in this way that affections such as the distension from gas or swellings are perceived.[3] Distension is felt by the tension it creates when stretched and inflammation by the awareness of the weight.

5.2.9. Flesh

§135 Flesh fills up the spaces in the tissues left within the organs, thus making them firm and solid. Flesh includes muscles, fasciae, tendons, ligaments, connective-tissues and so forth all together.

5.2.10. The Faculties

§136 The body depends for life on the faculties or drives. Thus, every organ has been provided with a primary innate faculty or drive (force or power) for its nutrition. Nutrition consists of the absorption, retention and assimilation of food, its integration into the structure of tissues and excretion of its wastes. Organs may, therefore, be classified accordingly. In addition, some members have a further faculty which passes from them to another organ, while others have no such faculty or drive. Therefore it is possible to assume the following associations: (1) receiving (receptor) and also giving an faculty or drive (effector); (2) giving (effector) and not receiving an faculty or drive (receptor); (3) receiving (receptor) and not giving an faculty or drive (effector); (4) neither giving (effector) nor receiving (receptor) an faculty or drive.

5.2.10.1. Receptor-Effector of a Faculty

§137 There is little doubt regarding the existence of the first group [receiving and giving a faculty or drive]. Physicians generally agree that the brain and liver both receive their power of life (innate heat), natural heat and breath from the heart and that each of them is also the starting-point of another faculty which it sends out to other organs. But there is disagreement about the second [giving and not receiving a faculty or drive]. Thus in the relation between the brain and sensation, is sensation confined to the (literal) brain or not? In the relation between the faculty or drive of nutrition and the liver, is it integral in the liver or not?

5.2.10.2. Effector and Not a Receptor of a Faculty

§138 In regard to the heart, there is a great disagreement between the philosophers and the physicians. The great philosopher [Aristotle] held views different from physicians. He said that the heart is an organ which gives and does not receive. In other words, it is the first root of all the faculties or drives and gives the faculty or drive of nutrition, life, apprehension, and movement to the several other organs while physicians and some other philosophers contend that these faculties or drives were distributed among several organs (the faculty or drive of nutrition in the liver, of vital power in the heart, of mental faculty or drives in the brain) and that there is, therefore, no such thing as an organ giving without receiving. Although this view appears to be superficially more plausible, it is really the philosopher's [Aristotle] view which is valid.[4]

5.2.10.3. Receptor and Not an Effector of a Faculty

§139 In regard to the third association, we consider that there can be no doubt about the fact that some organs receive and do not give. Thus the flesh receives the power of sensation and life, but does not have the power of imparting this to another faculty or drive in return.

5.2.10.4. Neither Receptor Nor Effector of a Faculty

§140 Regarding the fourth, there is also a difference of opinion between the philosophers and the physicians. According to some that insensitive organs like bone and fibrous tissue could not continue to live unless these drives or powers resided in them and they, therefore, do not need to receive them, that the power provided by the digestive tract conveyed to them is adequate, and that therefore they neither furnish an faculty or drive or power for another organ nor does another organ furnish them with a drive or power.

§141 The opposite opinion is that the powers in those members do not reside in them, but are formed in the liver and heart and when they reach these members, they come to rest within them.

§142 There is no way to decide between the two views by argument but the inability to do so is no hindrance to the practice of medicine. As to the first of these views, one must realize that it does not matter whether the heart is the source of sensation and voluntary motion in the brain or not or whether the source of the nutritive faculty be in the liver or not. It is of no significance whether the brain has in itself the source of the powers of the soul or whether these powers only come by way of the heart. In any case, it is only a relation. If the liver is the starting-point of the nutritive faculty, that, too, is only in relation to other organs.

§143 In regard to the second of the two views, one must realize that it does not matter whether the faculty or drive in an organ like bone is innate in it by virtue of its temperament or whether it arose in the liver first or whether neither is true. One must, rather, realize that the faculty or drive could not be there at all were it not for the liver and that, therefore, if the path were obstructed, the bone would cease to receive the necessary nutriment and its functions would cease—exactly as holds in the case of movement when some nerve-connection with the brain is severed. There is the natural faculty in the bone as long as its temperament is maintained.

§144 The discrepancy is removed by considering some organs as principal or vital, some as auxiliary and some as neither vital nor auxiliary.

5.2.11. The Principal or Vital Members

§145 The principal (or vital) organs are those in which the primary faculty or drives of the body arise like the faculty or drives that are necessary either to the life of the individual or to the life of the race.

§146 The principal or vital organs are three in number, (1) the heart—the center of vital power or innate heat; (2) the brain—the center of the mental faculties, sensation and movement; and (3) the liver—the center of the nutritive or vegetative drives.

§147 There is a fourth faculty or drive, part of which is principal or essential and the other, auxiliary. The essential function is that of forming generative elements; the auxiliary functions are those of giving the masculine and feminine form and temperament. These functions are inseparable from the race and yet play no part in the essence of life.

5.2.12. *The Auxiliary Members*

§**148** These are of two kinds: (1) those which are auxiliary to the vital organs [adnexa] (coming into operation before the vital organs can come into play); and (2) those which are the instruments of their functions (coming into operation after the vitals organs have functioned). Thus, the lungs supply air to the heart and the arteries carry the blood. The brain is supplied with nutrition and the vital force, while the nerves carry its impulses. The liver is supplied food by the stomach (intestine), while the veins carry its final products. The testicles in the male produce and discharge semen from the preparatory tissues and ducts which connect the testes with the urethra. In women, the fallopian tubes discharge the egg into the uterus and thus serve the final purpose, the preservation of the race.[5]

5.2.13. *Classification of the Members According to Their Action*

§**149** Classification of the organs according to their action—Galen classified the organs into those which effect an action (like the heart) and those which assist in the action (like the lung) and those which do both (like the liver). For my part, I consider as "action" that particular kind of action by means of which a given member accomplishes the maintenance of the person's life or the perpetuation of the species. Therefore, the heart gives rise to the breath. Action is assisted when one organ is prepared to receive the action of the other organ thereby completing the process either of giving life to the individual or of propagating the race. Thus, the lung prepares the air. The liver carries out the first digestion to prepare for the third and fourth digestion. The more perfectly the liver functions in the second digestion, the more likely is the blood so made to be adequate to nourish the tissues. Therefore, in this respect, the liver effects an action and, in so far as the liver assists in accomplishing a further action, it is considered to be preparative for that action.

5.2.14. Classification of the Members According to Their Origins

§150 Classification of the members according to their origins—some organs develop from semen and this includes all elementary tissues except fat and flesh. These organs (other than fat and flesh) develop from both male and female sperm, while fat and flesh are formed from blood. According to the ancient philosophers, the process of generation can be compared with the processes which take place in the manufacture of cheese. Thus the male sperm is equivalent to the clotting agent of milk and the female sperm is equivalent to the coagulum of milk. The starting point of the clotting is in the rennet; so the starting-point of the clot "human being" is in the male semen.[6] Just as the beginning of the clotting is in the milk, so the beginning of the clotting of the human form lies in the female "sperm." Then, just as each of the two—the rennet and the milk—enter into the substance of the cheese which results, so each of the two—male and female sperm—enters into the "substance" of the "embryo."

§151 Galen has another point of view. He considers that each of the sperms has both a coagulative and a receptive power for coagulation. Therefore, he says that the coagulative power is stronger in the male than in the female while the receptive capacity for coagulation is stronger in the female than the male. The real truth, however, is expounded in our own works dealing with the fundamental principles of natural science.

§152 In regard to relations between the female menstrual blood and the embryo during pregnancy, the blood which is otherwise discharged from a woman at the time of menstruation becomes nutriment for the embryo in three ways. One portion is changed into the likeness of the substance of the sperm and the organs derived therefrom. This is the nutriment which enables growth to take place. Another portion is not nutriment of that kind but has the capacity to be formed into the material which fills up the interstices in the vital organs and becomes flesh and fat. A third part is waste material that is not useful for either of the above two purposes. It remains in the same situation until the time of birth and is then expelled with the infant.

§153 After the child is born, the blood formed in the liver goes to make the tissues which were previously being developed from the mother's blood. It arises, therefore, from an organ which itself was formed out of maternal blood.

§154 The infant's flesh is formed from the gross blood, congealed by heat and dryness, while fat is developed from the thin and oily blood which cold has congealed and heat dispersed.

§155 Repair of damaged organs: derived from the sperm. It should be remembered that if ever the tissues derived from semen get damaged or broken, restoration can only take place, and then only in a few of them, if the individual is spare in habit and has not passed the age of youth. These organs are: the bones, the small branches of veins; medium-sized veins and arteries because when severance occurs in such organs as bones and nerves, they will not grow again.

§156 Repair of damaged members derived from blood. On the other hand, if the organs derived from blood are damaged, they are renewed out of like substance like the flesh.

§157 Repair of damaged members derived from both blood and sperm. If the organ which is damaged arises both from blood and sperm, then, as it is not very long since the sperm was there, it will be restored (like the teeth of a child) unless the blood has in the meantime undergone a change in temperament.

§158 Here, it may also be mentioned that some organs have the same nerve to serve both sensation and movement or there are separate nerves for sensation and movement as is the case with most of the cranial and spinal nerves.

§159 Serous membranes, which cover the viscera, are derived either from the pleura or the peritoneum. The covering for the organs in the thorax which derive their covering from pleura are: the diaphragm, lungs, veins and arteries. Abdominal organs and their vessels are enclosed by the peritoneum which cover the muscles of the abdominal wall.

5.2.15. Texture of the Members

§160 All members are either fleshy in texture or fibrous (as the flesh found throughout muscles) or are devoid of fibrous texture (as the liver). Fibrous texture goes with the power of movement—voluntary in the case of contrary muscles and involuntary in the case of the uterus and veins. Compound movements such as that of deglution depend on the direction of the fibers varying—longitudinal, oblique, transverse. Thus, reception is carried out by the longitudinal fibers, expulsion by the oblique and retention by the transverse fibers. The transverse fibers also help to extrude and expel.

§161 Tubular or hollow organs which contain substances different from their walls have one or two muscular coats. Organs which possess only a single muscular coat have all the three sets of fibers intertwined with each other. Organs which possess two coats have the transverse fibers in the outer coat and the longitudinal and oblique fibers in the inner coat. This arrangement prevents the expulsive and retentive fibers from interfering with the gripping and pulling fibers although they are very close to each other.

§162 The presence of two coats serves the following purposes: (1) They give the necessary strength to the walls so that there is no risk of the proper power of movement failing at any time like in the arteries. (2) They ensure that the contents will not dissipate or escape. One coat would not be enough to retain so tenuous a substance as the breath which the arteries contain. It would make the risk of rupture or severance in injuries too great in which case death would be very likely to occur because the blood would then drain out.[7] This would be a great danger to human life. (3) Where there is a need for vigorous suction and expulsion, it is beneficial to have a separate instrument available for the performance of both actions rather than to distribute both powers over one coat. This applies in the case of the stomach and intestines. In this organ absorption and elimination rather than retention are necessary. The two muscular coats of the longitudinal and transverse fibers are necessary for the organs like the stomach and intestine which have to perform strong movements of propulsion and expulsion. (4) Where each coat of an organ subserves its own action or where each action requires its own special temperament, in the case of the stomach, there is a need of a power of sensation (which can only exist in a tissue containing nerves) and also a power to execute the movement of digestion (for which a fleshy tissue is needed). Therefore, each need is supplied by its own muscular coat—the nerve-containing tissue for the power of sensation and the fleshy coat for the power of executing the movements entailed in the work of digestion. Nature made the inner coat capable of sensation and the other coat, fleshy. The operation of sensation requires actual contact with the nervous tissue as is true in the case of the sense of touch but the movements necessary to enable digestion do not require contact of the material to be digested with the fleshy walls. Sensation of food is best secured through direct contact with the nervous layer while for digestion it is necessary that the muscular layer should be in direct contact with the food. Some tissues are temperamentally so near the blood that the nutriment does not require any substantial change before assimilation. Therefore, flesh and other tissues have no sinuses or cavities for the prolonged detention of blood as the nutriment comes in contact with the tissues and is easily assimilated.

§**163** Members such as the flesh that have a temperament near to that of blood need to undergo little change in order to subserve nutrition. Therefore, there is no need for spaces or cavities in these members to retain nutrient material pending its transformation into their own substance. In such members, the nutrient at once becomes identical with their substance.

§**164** In the case of organs and tissues which are temperamentally different from blood like bones, blood has to be suitably altered before it can incorporate in their structure. Therefore, bones have always one or more cavities to give time to the blood to enable the conversion to take place. The femur and humerus are this way. In the case of the lower jaw bone numerous spaces are seen scattered through it. In this way more nutriment can be accommodated than is necessary for the moment and the transformation into their own likeness can take place little by little.

§165 Strong organs expel their waste matters into the adjacent weaker members. Thus the heart expels waste matter to the axilla; the brain to the tissues behind the ears; the liver to the groin.[8]

5.3. The Skeleton

5.3.1. A General Description of Bones and Joints

§166 There are certain bones in the body which act like a foundation. The vertebral column is like the central beam of a boat on which the remaining framework is built. Some bones provide a covering and protection for the various parts of the body like the cranium.

§167 Some bones act as the instruments of defense and protection from friction, shocks and injury like the spinous processes of the vertebrae. Some bones fill up the cavities of joints like the sesamoid bones between the phalanges. Some are attached to the parts of the body which need support like the muscles of the tongue and the larynx.

§168 Bones which are required for the protection of the body and not for movement are solid although they may be somewhat spongy. Bones which are responsible for movement have larger cavities and a central canal to supply nutrition so as not to make the bone too soft. Indeed, bones of this type are generally harder as they have only the central canal filled with the nutrient marrow. The central canal is made larger to prevent the bone from becoming too heavy. They have also been made hard to avoid fracture during vigorous exercise.

§169 Bone marrow provides moisture to counteract the dryness produced by exercise. Another advantage of the marrow is that it fills up the spaces and thus, reduces the hollowness and makes the bone more solid. When there is need for greater strength, the bone has smaller cavities, but when there is less need for strength, its cavities are larger. Some bones have been made spongy to provide better nutrition, others to facilitate access to the odors, as in the ethmoid bone. Apertures of the skull are for proper elimination of the excrements from the brain.

§170 Joints are formed by the approximation of bones. They have several varieties. Some joints have sufficient space for movement. In some, the articular distance is so little that they can move only with difficulty. There are others in which the joint is fixed, that is, embedded, sutured or united.

§171 A joint is moveable if one bone moves in conjunction with the other as in the wrist joint. A partially mobile joint is like the joint between the scapula and thorax or between the two rear bones of the foot. An immovable joint is the one in which one of the two articulating bones are unable to move without the movement of the other like the joints of the ribs with the sternum.

§172 A fixed joint is one in which one of the articular bones has a process and the other a socket to receive it and both are joined together in such a way that there is no movement as in the case of the roots of the teeth fixed in the jaw bone.

§173 A suture joint is one in which there are sharp saw-like serrations entering into one another like those employed in the making of copper utensils. Such joints are found in the skull.

§174 A pivot joint is one in which the bone moves around the long axis, that is, the joint between the two bones of the forearm. Another type of pivot joint is the one which moves on its transverse axis like the joints of the lower vertebrae at the back. Joints between the upper vertebrae are not so mobile.

5.3.2. The Anatomy of the Cranium

§175 The function of the skull is to protect the brain. The skull is made of several bones for the following reasons. An injury or putrefaction in a part of the skull might involve only that part and not the whole skull. The various parts of the skull vary in thickness, hardness and density according to the requirements.

§176 Another reason is that the skull, in this way, is able to give passage to the various nerves and allows the escape of thick vapors excreted by the brain. There is also an advantage for the brain and other structures—the veins and arteries are able to pass through the intervening spaces while the weight of the thick membranes is dispersed by attachment to the several bones.

§177 The skull is normally spherical in shape. This gives more space to the contents than the straight borders would have provided and it minimizes the chance of their being affected by shocks from outside. The shape of the skull is however, not entirely spherical but ovoid. This is to give more space to the many nerves which arise lengthwise from the brain. The skull has prominences both in front and at the back to accommodate the nerves which arise from the front and hind parts of the brain.

§178 The skull has three "true" and two "false" sutures. One of these, which is common with the frontal bone and is curved like a bow over the forehead, is called the coronal suture.

§179 The second is a straight line which divides the skull longitudinally into two halves. It is like an arrow which in reference to the coronal suture is designated as the sagittal suture.

§180 The third suture is common to the vault and the base of the skull. It meets the sagittal suture at an angle and since it looks like the letter lambda, it is known as the lambdoid suture.

§181 The two false sutures run parallel to the centrally situated sagittal suture. They do not penetrate the bone but overlap each other like fish scales—hence, the name squamosal sutures.

§182 There are three abnormal shapes of the skull. In one, the frontal prominence is missing and there is no coronal suture. In the second, there is no prominence at the back of the skull and there is no lambdoid suture. In the third type, both elevations are missing and the skull is absolutely round with the length and breadth being equal. In this case, both the coronal and lambdoid sutures are absent.

§183 According to the great physician Galen, when length, breadth and height are equal, the sutures divide the skull into equal parts. In a normal skull, this division is such that there is only one true suture in the length and two in the breadth of the skull. In this case, there is only one suture in the length and one in the breadth. The suture which is in the breadth crosses the one in the length and runs from ear to ear.

§**184** According to the great Galen, there could be no other abnormal shape of the skull, because if the length had been shorter than the breadth, the contents of the skull like the substance of the brain, would have itself become deficient and this would be a supposition incompatible with life. Amongst the ancient physicians, Hippocrates was the first one to express a correct opinion as he, too, classified the shapes of skull into four varieties—one normal and three abnormal. It is necessary that this question should be well understood.

5.3.3. The Anatomy of Other Head Bones

§**185** The skull has five bones other than the two parietal bones. Four of these are like the side walls and the fifth is a base on which they are erected. The side bones have been made stronger than the top bones because they are more exposed to injuries. The skull bones have been made spongy for the passage of vapors and so as not to be top heavy for the brain.

§**186** The strongest of the skull bones is the occipital bone which covers the sensory organs at the back. In the front is the frontal bone. This is bounded above by the coronal suture and below by a suture which runs from the lower end of the coronal suture on one side and passes through the orbit beneath the two eyebrows. It joins the coronal suture on the other side.

§**187** On the sides of the skull there are two temporal bones which lodge the ears. They are stone-like and are termed as such. They are bounded above by the squamosal suture and below by the sutures which join the coronal suture in front and the lambdoid suture behind. The fourth wall is at the back of the skull.

§**188** It is bounded above by the lambdoid suture and below by the suture between the skull and the sphenoid bone. On both sides, it is bounded by the ends of the lambdoid suture. In the base of the skull is the sphenoid bone which carries the weight of the skull. This is made very hard for two reasons: it helps to support the weight of the skull and it can resist the damage from the putrefied excretions.

§189 On both sides of the skull there are two strong bones which enclose the nerves entering the temporal muscles. These bones are placed obliquely in the temples and are thus known as the temporal bones.

5.3.4. The Anatomy of the Bones of the Jaws and the Nose

§190 In this section, the various bones of the jaw and the nose and their sutures are described.

5.3.4.1. The Upper Jaw

§191 The upper jaw is bounded above by the suture which starts between the upper jaw and the frontal bone and passes beneath the eyebrows, ending on either side at the temples. At the side of the frontal bone is another suture which comes from the ear and passes between the jaw and the sphenoid bone. Behind the molars it turns slightly inward forming another suture which separates it from the two palatine bones. These are the four boundaries of the upper jaw.

§192 Of the sutures in the body of the upper jaw, there is one which separates the palate lengthwise. Another suture starts between the two eyebrows and ends between the two upper flat incisors. The third suture on the right side starts from the origin of the second suture and ends between the incisor and the canine teeth. The fourth suture on the left side is just like the third.

§193 Between the central and the outer sutures and the roots of the teeth there are two triangular bones with their bases separated from the root of the teeth by a suture which runs from the base of the nostrils. From here, the three sutures reach near the roots of the teeth, where in close proximity to the two triangles, are two bones which are surrounded on all sides by the bases of the two triangles, the roots of the teeth and the two side sutures. These bones are separated from each other by a central suture. Thus, each bone makes two right angles near the dividing suture, one acute angle near the roots of the teeth and another obtuse angle near the two nostrils.

§**194** One of the sutures of the upper jaw starts from the upper common suture and descends to the outer side of the eye. When it approaches the orbit, it divides into three branches. The first branch passes beneath the common suture at the upper part of the orbit and joins the eyebrows. The second branch ends beneath the orbit without entering it. The third branch ends like the second one but enters the orbit. All the sutures described above are beneath the eyebrows, but orbit the suture which touches the palate at some distance from this point. The bone which is separated by the first suture is the largest. The next in size is the bone which is separated by the second suture and then in the same order is the bone which is separated by the third suture.

5.3.4.2. The Nose

§**195** The nose has three functions: (1) It holds a large quantity of air for smell and conditions the same before passing it on to the lungs. Although most of the air goes to the lungs, an appreciable quantity is passed directly to the organ of smell for keener perception. These three purposes have been grouped together as one. (2) It helps in the proper intonation of voice and the utterance of syllables. Thus, it prevents the collection of too much air in the voice organs and during phonation, it releases the air in a regulated manner as from the holes of a flute. (3) It keeps the excretion from the brain hidden from sight and blows it off with the air as and when necessary.

§**196** The nose is formed of two triangular bones which are joined together anteriorly from the apex downward. Their bases are separated from each other at an angle below. Their posterior borders are joined to the cheek bone with a suture on either side which has already been described. At the lower margins of the nasal bones there are soft cartilages.

§**197** In the center of the nasal cavity there is another cartilage which is placed vertically in such a way that its harder part lies above and the softer one below. This cartilage is harder than the two cartilages described above. It divides the nose into two halves. When the nose receives the excretions from the brain, it directs them towards the one and not both the nostrils to ensure that the fresh air passes through for reconditioning the nervous system.

§198 There are three advantages in having the cartilages at the sides of the nose: (a) the same advantage as that of its attachment to other bones; (b) helping the nostrils to expand fully to receive a large volume of fresh air in blowing the nose and in taking deep inspirations; (c) enabling the smoke and other irritant vapors to be expelled forcefully and in an explosive manner.

§199 The nasal bones have been made thin and light, as lightness rather than strength is required, and this particularly because they do not adjoin any part which is easily diseased. The nose is also well away from the sensory organs.

5.3.4.3. The Lower Jaw

§200 There is an obvious advantage to its special shape. The lower jaw is formed from the union of two bones which are firmly joined at the chin. Both at the sides and towards its ends, the bone is flat and curved. The ends carry the processes which are thin, almost like a tooth. Each process is fixed to the articular bone with a strong ligament so that it may not dislocate in the chewing movements.

5.3.5. The Anatomy of the Teeth

§201 There are thirty two teeth in both jaws. Sometimes the four wisdom teeth may be absent. In that case, there would be only twenty eight teeth. The central incisors both above and below are flat. Next to these are the lateral incisors, one on each side, both in the upper and lower jaws. These eight teeth are used for biting. Outside the incisors there is a canine tooth both above and below. This has pointed ends and is used for cutting. Outside these teeth, both above and below, is a set of the four or five molars for grinding. This makes the total thirty two, provided all the five molars are present. When there is no wisdom tooth (i. e., the fifth molar has not erupted) there are only twenty-eight teeth. Wisdom teeth generally appear during the period of growth. Since this is between puberty and adulthood, that is, up to thirty years, they are called the wisdom teeth.

§202 Teeth have sharp roots embedded in the edge of the jaw. They are lodged in bony sockets with fibrous attachments which keep them firm. Every tooth has at least one root, but the teeth of the lower jaw have two roots. The wisdom tooth often has three roots. In the upper jaw, the crowns of the molar teeth have at least three tubercles in each tooth. Sometimes, the wisdom tooth may have four tubercles. In these teeth, the crowns are larger for fulfilling the tougher job. In the lower jaw the crowns are again larger as a counter-poise to the upper teeth. The teeth in the upper jaw have more roots to keep them firmly suspended from above, gravity acting against them. This is not so in the case of the lower jaw.

§203 None of the bones other than the teeth are sensitive. This is the opinion of Galen, and it is also confirmed by the observation that teeth have nerves reaching directly from the brain. That is why teeth can not only appreciate cold and other sensations, but are also able to differentiate between them.

5.3.6. The Function of the Spinal Column

§204 The vertebral column has four functions. It affords passage to the spinal cord which is essential to the life of animals. The purpose of the spinal cord will be described in detail under the heading of spinal cord. Here it may briefly be mentioned that: (a) if the brain supplied all the nerves, it would be too big a burden for it. (b) If all the nerves had arisen from the brain, the nerves for the hands and feet would have to travel quite a long distance and thus be exposed to greater risks of injury and damage. The nerves would also be too weak to contract and expand the heavy muscles (of the leg and the thigh). Almighty God has therefore, granted this further benefit by providing a spinal cord from the lower part of the brain. (c) The spinal cord arises from the brain like a canal from a spring so the nerves may reach both sides of the body and also go right up to the ends. (d) The source of the nerves has in this way been brought closer to the recipient organs.

§205 The spinal cord has been protected by lodgement in a canal formed of hard bone. The vertebral column also gives protection to the important organs lying in the front. That is why it has been provided with hard prominences and spines. Like the central beam of a boat, the vertebral column provides a sort of foundation for the framework of other bones. This is the reason why it has been made particularly hard. In the human being, the vertebral column has been made into a strong and stable pillar so that on flexion, side to side movements, and on standing it should maintain its proper position. The vertebral column has been built of several irregularly shaped bones which are not as big as to make movement difficult. The intervertebral joints are also neither so hard as to interfere with movement nor so loose as to make it sluggish.

5.3.6.1. The Vertebrae

§206 The vertebra is an irregular piece of bone with a central foramen for the spinal cord. On both sides it has four processes. The two processes on each side are placed one above the other. Sometimes a vertebra may have six processes with four on one side and two on the other. At times there may be even eight. These processes provide firm articulations with the processes of one vertebra entering into the corresponding depressions of the other. The processes also protect the vertebrae against shocks and injuries.

§207 Vertebrae are covered with hard, broad and long ligaments which are attached from below upwards to the full length of the vertebral column. The backs of the vertebrae have spinous processes and the sides transverse processes. The vertebrae give protection to the structures like nerves, blood vessels and muscles which are placed lengthwise. The transverse processes of the vertebrae have smooth, glistening facets for articulation with the heads of the ribs.

§208 Just as there are two smooth facets on each side of a vertebra, there are two rounded heads on each rib for articulating with the facets to form joints. Some transverse processes are bifid and look like double transverse processes. This peculiarity however, exists only in the cervical vertebrae. The advantages of this formation will be described shortly.

§209 In addition to the vertebral canal, there are foramina for the passage of nerves and blood vessels. In some vertebrae, the foramina are within the substance of the vertebrae, while in others they are intervertebral, being formed of semicircular notches on the articular margins of the two adjoining vertebrae. These foramina may be large or small and may be present both above and below the vertebra or only on one side. They are located in the sides because at the back there would be no protection for the structures passing through them and in front these structures would be liable to damage from the movements of the spine.

§210 If the vertebral column had no ligamentous attachments, it would not have the strength and firmness which it now has. The vertebral processes of the spine which are of a protective nature are always covered with ligaments and tendons. The ligaments also keep the processes moistened with exudation, and thus, on the one hand, facilitate movement and on the other protect the local muscles. The articular processes of the vertebrae, being protected by fasciae and ligaments from all sides, make strong joints. The anterior ligaments are stronger than the posterior ones because there is a greater need of forward movement than backward extension.

§211 The space behind the vertebrae is formed by the stretched fibrous tissue and is filled with viscid exudation. Although this material is very little, it does help to provide rest and stability to the vertebral column. The advantage of the vertebral column being made of several vertebrae is that its movement is free and easy. This would not be the case if it had been made of a single bone.

5.3.6.2. The Functions of the Neck

§212 The neck has been designed to accommodate the trachea, which will be described in detail at its appropriate place. The bones of the neck, especially the atlas, are placed one above the other. They are smaller in size, particularly the atlas, which is supported by other vertebrae. A thing which is supported has always to be lighter than its support, especially if it is normally expected to move.

§213 The spinal cord is thickest at its origin because of the large number of nerves arising from there. The vertebral canal here is also wider and the vertebrae thinner for the same reason. These two factors ultimately produce weakness of the vertebrae at this place. This is, however, rectified by the measures already described.

§214 The cervical vertebrae have also been made more compact than the other vertebrae. It should also be remembered that cervical vertebrae have thin bodies and shorter spinous processes to reduce the risk of injury which longer processes would have entailed. The transverse processes in these vertebrae are however big, as more movement than stability and firmness are required in this region. Moreover, these vertebrae do not have to carry as much load as the lower vertebrae. Hence, the joints of the cervical vertebrae are more loose and mobile than those of thoracic vertebrae. The weakness and laxity of the cervical spine have been compensated for by strengthening the joints with a complete cover of the muscles, blood vessels and nerves.

§215 The upper and the lower articular processes of the cervical vertebrae are as big as those of the lower vertebrae. The bases of the articular processes of the cervical vertebrae are longer and the ligaments which cover them are looser. The foramina for the emergence of nerves are formed, as already described, by a union of two vertebrae. The thinness and smaller size of the cervical vertebrae and the larger size of their vertebral canal do not leave room for any other foramina than the foramina in the transverse processes of the cervical vertebrae for transmitting the vertebral artery. The cervical vertebrae will now be described in some detail.

§216 The cervical vertebrae are seven in number. Their number, size and length are most appropriate for the body. There are eleven processes in each vertebra except the first: one spinous, two transverse, four articular processes, two pedicles and two arches making the total of eleven. In some vertebrae, these processes are quite prominent while in others they are not so distinct.

§217 Every transverse process splits into two and has a circle to complete with the semicircle of the adjoining vertebra. The first and the second cervical vertebra have some special characteristics which are not found in other vertebrae. The movements of the head to the right and the left sides are carried out in the joint between the head and the first vertebra and the forward and backward movements of the head occur between the first and the second vertebra. We shall first describe the joint between the head and the first vertebra.

§218 On the upper side of the first vertebra there are depressions over the two articular processes to receive the two articular condyles of the skull. If one of the two condyles is elevated, and the other depressed, the head gets tilted to that side. Since there is no more room in this vertebra for another joint, the next vertebra has been provided with a long hard process on the front, i. e., on the inner side to enter the vertebral foramen of the first vertebra in front of the spinal cord.

§219 The vertebral foramen of the first is in continuity with the vertebral foramen of the second vertebra, but the foramen of the latter is larger antero-posteriorly, rather than transversely to accommodate this additional structure.

§220 This process of the second vertebra is known as the odontoid process. Near this process, the spinal cord is protected from pressure and injury by a covering of the ligaments arising from both the odontoid process and the spinal cord. After passing through the first vertebra, the odontoid process disappears in the foramen magnum, forming a joint for the forward and backward bending of the head.

§221 There are two advantages of the odontoid process: first of all, it gives good protection and secondly, it prevents the thin, anterior portion of the first vertebra from dislocation. The first vertebra has no spinous process as that would have made it too heavy and exposed it to shocks and injuries. The principle is that a process which is sufficiently strong to give protection from injury is also an invitation to damage of the delicate structures. Moreover, a spinous process in this vertebra would have damaged the large number of muscles and nerves surrounding the first vertebra. There is also no real need for it, as the first vertebra is well protected by the second vertebra. That is why it also has no transverse process. Besides, in this area there is a good packing of vessels and nerves arising from the brain and these leave no room for this process.

§222 Another characteristic of this vertebra is that the nerves do not pass through the inter vertebral foramina at the sides of the vertebra but through the foramina on the top of the posterior part. If the nerves had come out near the condyles, they would be damaged by the movements of the joint. The case would be similar if they had emerged from the place where the articular processes of the second vertebra enter into the articular depressions of the first. It would not have been proper for them to arise from the anterior or the posterior parts of the first vertebra nor from its sides which have been thinned for receiving the odontoid process. Hence, there is no other way for the nerves to emerge from the spine except from behind and slightly below and to the sides of the vertebral joints. Since these foramina are rather small, the nerves which pass through them are also very thin and fine.

§223 In the case of the second vertebra, the nerves could not have emerged from above the vertebra because the movement and rotation of the first vertebra over the second would have caused damage. It was also not possible that these nerves should emerge from either above, behind or from the sides of the second vertebra because in that case both the first and the second cervical nerves would have arisen so close to each other that they would have joined together as one. Had the nerves emerged in this way, they would have become too weak and fine and thus would create the same difficulty as mentioned before. Hence, the only suitable place for the nerves to emerge is from foramina by the sides of the spinous process, where the first vertebra has also a corresponding aperture and where its body can also participate.

§224 The odontoid process of the second vertebra is firmly joined to the first with ligaments. The joints of the skull with the first and the second vertebrae are very loose and mobile as compared to the other joints of vertebral column. The reason is that in these joints there is a greater need of movement for rotating the head in all directions. In the movements of the head, the upper two vertebrae move like a single vertebra. Thus, when the head moves forward or backward, both the first and second vertebrae move together. Similarly, when the head tilts to the right or left side without any movement of the neck, both the first and the second vertebra move together as one.

This is a summary of the various special features of cervical vertebrae.

5.3.6.3. The Function and Anatomy of the Thoracic Vertebrae

§225 The ribs articulate with the thoracic vertebrae and encase the lungs. Eleven of the thoracic vertebrae have spinous as well as transverse processes, but the twelfth vertebra has no transverse process at all. The spinous processes of these vertebrae are of unequal size, being particularly large and strong near the vital organs. The transverse processes of these vertebrae are very hard and strong as compared to those of the other vertebrae because they have to join with the ribs.

§226 Thus, in the upper seven thoracic vertebrae, the spinous processes are enormous in size and the transverse processes exceptionally thick for a thorough protection of the heart. The tubercles over the transverse processes of the vertebrae up to the ninth have been made short and broad to correspond with the heads of the ribs.

§227 The upper articular processes of these vertebrae have facets for articulation with the tubercles on the under surface of the vertebrae above, so that the lower articular process of each vertebra has a tubercle to articulate with the smooth facet on the vertebra below. The spinous processes of the upper vertebrae are directed slightly downward, but the spinous process of the tenth thoracic vertebrae is strong, straight and erect.

§228 The articular surfaces of this vertebra are smooth and free from tubercles and articulate with the vertebrae both above and below. The vertebrae below the tenth have depressions on their upper surface for articulating with the processes on the lower surface of the vertebra above. The spinous processes of these vertebrae have been directed slightly upwards for a purpose which will be described later. There is no transverse process in the twelfth vertebra as the twelfth rib does not articulate with it, hence, there appears to be no need for it and the necessary protection has been given in some other beneficial manner to it.

§229 It is necessary for the lumbar vertebrae to be of larger size and stronger joints to carry the weight of the upper vertebrae, hence, they have more articular facets and processes than the other vertebrae. The first lumbar vertebra which articulates with the twelfth thoracic closely resembles it. The articular processes of the first lumbar vertebra are larger because this vertebra has a surplus of bone available from the absence of transverse processes. The articular processes in the lumbar vertebrae are so broad that they look like transverse processes.

§230 There are two reasons for this. The posterior part of the diaphragm is attached to the twelfth thoracic vertebra. Moreover, the vertebrae above the twelfth, being small, have no need of larger articular processes for additional strength as their long transverse and spinous processes are a sufficient compensation. Since the thoracic vertebrae are larger than the cervical vertebrae, the vertebral canal progressively decreases in size from above downward until the tenth thoracic vertebra comes to have a small vertebrae foramen and the remaining thoracic and lumbar vertebrae are so small that they are unable to accommodate the whole of the spinal cord. That is why they have the foramina on either side to let out the lumbar and sacral nerves.

5.3.6.4. The Anatomy of the Lumbar Vertebrae

§231 Lumbar vertebrae are five in number. They have spinous processes and broad transverse processes. Their articular processes are flat like the protective transverse processes. In collaboration with the sacrum, lumbar vertebrae form a base and a pillar for the whole spine. They also support the pubic bone and provide exit for the nerves to the legs.

5.3.6.5. The Anatomy of the Sacrum

§232 There are three vertebrae in the sacrum. These are very hard and have strong joints and broad transverse processes. Foramina for the nerves are placed rather posteriorly to avoid obstruction to the hip joint. The pieces of the sacrum are just like the lumbar vertebrae.

5.3.6.6. The Anatomy of the Coccyx

§233 The coccyx is made of three cartilaginous vertebrae which are devoid of processes. They are small, hence, the nerves pass through the intervertebral foramina as in the cervical vertebrae. There is only one nerve which emerges from the side of the third coccygeal vertebra.

5.3.6.7. A Final Description of the Functions of the Vertebral Column

§234 In the description of the various bones of the vertebral column, its advantages have been dealt with to some extent. Here it may be mentioned that the vertebrae of the spinal column jointly act as a single bone. They have the best possible shape, i.e., cylindrical to withstand hits and jolts. The spinous processes of the upper vertebrae are directed downward and those of the lower upwards.

§235 The spinous process of the tenth vertebra lies in the center. This central position is, however, not in accord with the number of the vertebrae, but with the length of the spinal column. When the spine is moved to the right or left side or backwards and forwards, it does so by inclining from the center to the opposite side.

§236 In this way, the upper or lower portion of the spine can bend sideways or forwards with the ends of the spine brought close to each other. In order to facilitate this, the vertebral column has been provided with articular facets rather than large tubercles. To bring the vertebrae in close contact with each other, the margins of the upper vertebrae are directed downward and of the lower vertebrae upwards. The surfaces of the articular tubercles in the upper vertebrae face somewhat downward, while in the lower they face upwards to facilitate movement.

5.3.7. The Anatomy of the Ribs and Their Functions

§237 The ribs encase and protect the respiratory organs and the upper part of the stomach and intestine. The thorax has not been made of a single bone lest there should be too much weight and the whole cage get involved in case of injury. The ribs are able to expand freely to meet the excessive demands of ventilation and to accommodate the stomach when distended with food or gases. They also provide the necessary space for muscles of the chest and respiration. It is obvious that the ribs encircle the chest to protect the lungs, heart and other such organs as any injury to these organs may sometimes prove fatal. Since it is necessary that the vital organs should not be easily damaged or compressed, the upper seven ribs have been joined to the sternum to give protection. The ribs which cover the digestive organs arise from the vertebrae but do not join the sternum. They progressively decrease in size from above downward. The ends of the first ribs in the upper set are nearest while those of the lower set are farthest from one another. This is to protect the liver and the spleen and to provide sufficient space for a distended stomach.

§238 The upper seven ribs which encircle the chest are called the thoracic ribs. The central ribs in this set are the largest and longest, while those at the two extremes are the smallest. The shape and the placement of the ribs are the best for affording cover and protection to the underlying organs. The ribs descend from their vertebral origin but then curve upwards to join the sternum and thus provide plenty of space.

§239 The heads of the ribs on either side articulate both with the transverse processes of the vertebrae and with the articular facets which are made half and half from each of the two adjoining vertebrae. That is why there is a ridge across the articular surface of the head for making a double joint. This is the case with all the upper seven ribs which are joined to the sternum. The last five ribs which are known as the false or floating ribs have cartilage attached at the inner ends. This is to protect the delicate membranes of the abdomen from damage by the hard ribs.

5.3.8. The Anatomy of the Sternum

§240 The sternum is not a single bone but a union of seven pieces, as already mentioned. It has been designed to facilitate the expansion of the underlying respiratory organs. It is porous and spongy and has been supplied with cartilage at the junction of the individual pieces to facilitate movement. Had this union been overly strong and immobile, it would not have been as useful as it is now. The seven pieces of the sternum articulate with the seven ribs. At the lower end of the sternum there is a flat piece of cartilaginous bone which has a curved lower border. Due to its resemblance to a dagger it is called the xiphoid cartilage. This part of the sternum covers the epigastrium and acts as a soft, intervening medium between the hard and soft tissues for the purpose mentioned several times before.

5.3.9. The Anatomy of the Clavicle

§**241** The medial end of the clavicle articulates with the notch on the side of the sternum. Behind the inner convex part of the clavicle, there is a space for the passage of blood vessels which ascend to the brain and for the nerves which descend from it. Its outer side, which is concave, articulates firmly with the scapula to strengthen the shoulder.

5.3.10. The Anatomy of the Scapula

§**242** The shoulder bone has a dual purpose. It enables the arm and the hand to remain free and not be tied up with the chest. It also gives protection from behind to the structures inside the chest. This serves a substitute purpose as in this region there are no spinous and transverse processes of the vertebrae to afford protection and no sensory organs to intimate the impending dangers. The outer border of the scapula is thin except at the upper part where it has a shallow depression for articulating with the rounded head of the humerus.

§**243** At or near this place there are two processes. The one above and behind is known as the coracoid. This process gives attachment to all the ligaments of the scapula and thus prevents the humerus from dislocating upwards. The other process of the scapula is placed medially and somewhat lower down to prevent the inward dislocation of the shoulder. The scapula is wider on the inner side. This is to provide a good cover to the thoracic organs from behind.

§**244** On the posterior surface of the scapula there is a triangular prominence with its base on the outer side and the apex on the inner to avoid irregularity in the back. If this prominence had been at a lower place, it would have unnecessarily exposed it to injury and damage. This prominence, like the spinous processes of the vertebrae, has been formed for protection. It is known as the spine of the scapula. The part of the scapula which articulates with the round head of the humerus is flat and lined with cartilage for a purpose which has been mentioned many times over.

5.3.11. The Anatomy of the Humerus

§245 The arm bone has been made cylindrical so that the risk of injury may be minimized to the maximum extent. Its smooth and convex head articulates with the cavity of the scapula and forms a loose movable joint which, not being very strong, is frequently dislocated.

§246 There are two advantages in its being loose: one is a need and the other a protection. By need we mean the necessity of free movement in this joint. Protection means that, although the joint is able to move in all directions and perform various movements, its movement is not so strong and quick as to cause damage or dislocation. On the other hand, the joint tends to remain stationary even when the whole arm is moved. That is why the shoulder unlike the other joints has not been made so very strong.

§247 The shoulder joint has four ligaments. The first of these is sheath-like and envelopes the joint completely as in some other joints of a similar kind. The second and third ligaments arise from the acromion process. Of these, one is flat and attached to the humerus and the other which is large and hard, descends with the fourth in a tunnel. Thereafter, both become flat for attachment to the humerus and merge with the aponeurotic muscle on its inner side.

§248 The humerus is somewhat concave on the inner side and convex at the outer side. This is to provide accommodation to the muscles, nerves and vessels of the arm. It enables objects to be carried under the armpit and facilitates movement of the one hand towards the other. At the lower end, the humerus has two prominences with an intervening depression. The inner prominence is thin and long. It does not take part in the joint but serves to protect the vessels and nerves. The outer prominence forms a part of the elbow joint and articulates with the depression on the head of the radius.

§249 The remaining part of this joint is formed in a manner which will be described later on. Between the two prominences there is a pulley-like surface on which the ulna moves. On both sides of it there are two articular processes which are smooth from back to front and top to bottom. The inner process is smooth at its upper part and has no obstructions. The outer prominence is longer than the inner. The process which articulates with the inner depression is however, neither smooth nor completely round but has an abrupt posterior wall. When the olecranon process of the forearm moves backwards, it is held by the vertical obstruction. The purpose of this formation will be described shortly. Hippocrates termed this joint a hinge joint.

5.3.12. The Anatomy of the Radius and Ulna

§250 The forearm has two bones which are attached to each other lengthwise. They are the radius and ulna. The bone which is in line with the thumb is thinner at its upper part and is known as the radius. The lower bone which is in line with the little finger is the ulna; it carries the weight of the radius. The purpose of the radius is to supinate and pronate the hand while the ulna flexes and extends the elbow joint. Both the bones are thin at the middle lest the forearm should become too heavy. Their ends are thick for the attachment of several ligaments and to prevent damage from the movement and friction of the wrist joint. Moreover, there is no fleshy, muscular tissue to give the necessary protection to this part. The radius has a curve which starts from the inner side and ends at the outer. The purpose of this curve is to facilitate pronation of the wrist. The advantage in the ulna being straight is that it is helpful in flexion and extension.

5.3.13. The Anatomy of the Elbow

§251 The elbow is formed by the articulation of the radius, ulna and humerus. At the upper end of the radius there is a depression which articulates with the outer prominence of the humerus and is held in position with the ligaments. When the head of the radius rotates with its articular depression, the forearm is pronated and supinated. The ulna has two processes, with an intervening concave surface which articulates with the convex pulley-like prominence at the lower end of the humerus to form the elbow joint. When the notch of the ulna moves backwards, the arm is extended. But when after gliding over the pulley (trochlea), the olecranon process of the ulna is held up by the posterior wall of the humeral depression, there is no further extension. This brings the arm and the forearm in alignment with each other.

§252 When the surface of the trochlear notch moves forward, the forearm is flexed and brought close to the arm. The lower ends of both the radius and ulna are joined together and form a common articular surface, most of which is made of the radius. That part of the bone which does not articulate is convex and smooth as a precaution against injury. Behind the articular surface of the ulna there is an abrupt prominence which is called the styloid process. The purpose of this will be described shortly.

5.3.14. The Anatomy of the Wrist

§253 The wrist is formed from a union of several bones because damage to or disease in a single bone would have affected the whole wrist. There are seven bones in the wrist. There is also another bone which is not in alignment with them. The bones of the wrist are set in two rows. There are three bones in the first row. These are towards the wrist joint and being proximal are thinner and smaller. The second row has four bones, which are adjacent to the bones of the palm and fingers and articulate with the three bones of the first row described above. The proximal ends of the wrist bones taper upwards for proper articulation, but the lower ends are flat and lack the articular depressions. The eighth bone which is out of alignment with the two rows gives protection to the ulnar nerve of the hand. The proximal ends of the first row form a wedge which articulates with the lower end of the radius and ulna for the flexion and extension of the wrist. The styloid process of the ulna enters the joint for the pronation and supination of the wrist.

5.3.15. The Anatomy of the Metacarpus

§254 The palm is formed of a set of metacarpal bones which are placed like the teeth of a comb. Under this arrangement, disease or injury of one does not affect the others. The large number of bones in the palm enables the hand to form a suitable depression for holding fluids and round objects. The bones can also come together with such a force that the hand can hold and grip the objects firmly. When the skin has been dissected away from the metacarpus, the bones appear to be so close to one another that their intervening joints are not visible. The metacarpal bones can be bent slightly to form a depression in the palm. The four metacarpal bones articulate with the phalangeal bones of the four fingers. The proximal ends of the metacarpal bones are in firm articulation with one another but fan out distally to meet the fingers. The metacarpus is concave on the palmar side for obvious reasons. At the wrist, the metacarpal bones articulate with the carpal bones through marginal processes and are held there with cartilage.

5.3.16. The Anatomy of the Fingers

§255 The fingers are used for grasping. They are fleshy but not devoid of bone like the fish and worms which are slow and sluggish in movements. The presence of bone in the fingers ensures that their movement is not slow and sluggish, like that in tremor disease. Fingers have not been made of a single bone, because in that case there would have been no flexion and extension of the phalanges as may be in case of some congenital or acquired disease.

§256 Each finger has three phalanges. If there had been more than three, the fingers would have certainly obtained a greater range of movement but they would be considerably weakened in strength. If the phalanges had been less than three, that is, each finger had only two phalanges, the fingers would have certainly become stronger, but then there would have been a lesser range of movement when they actually require greater movement and only nominal strength.

§257 The bones of the phalanges have wide bases and narrow heads, but to give proper proportion, the proximal phalanges have been made wider than the distal ones. Fingers have been rounded for protection against injury and are made solid to give proper strength for grasping, lifting and moving objects. They are concave on the inner side and convex at the outer, for the gripping, pressing and rubbing of objects. The fingers do not have any convexity or concavity on the outer or inner side. This is to ensure proper adduction.

§258 The fingers on the sides, i.e., the thumb and little finger, are convex on their outer side as there is no adjoining finger. This enables the fingers to come together for protection against injuries. On the palmar side, the fingers are fleshy to provide greater comfort and a better grip. The outer side is not fleshy, as this would have made the fingers unnecessarily heavy; as it is, they can join together to make an effective weapon (as a fist in boxing). The phalanges of the middle finger are the longest. Next in size are those of the ring finger, then of the index finger and smallest are those of the little finger. That is why on flexion, the finger tips can come in line with each other and together with the palm are able to form a concavity for the proper gripping of spherical objects.

§259 The thumb has been placed at the most appropriate position with respect to the fingers. Had it been placed elsewhere, it would not have had its present advantages. If the thumb had been placed in the middle of the palm, it would not have functioned properly, and if it had been placed beyond the little finger, it would have been impossible to bring the two hands together as in the lifting of an object. The worst position for it would be the back of the palm.

§260 The metacarpal bone of the thumb has not been placed in line with the others, as that would have reduced its present distance from the fingers and made it difficult to lift the objects with the thumb on one side and the four fingers on the other. Now we can lift even big objects in the palm with the thumb holding them from above and the ring and little fingers from below. The phalanges articulate with each other by sharp processes and articular depressions which hold a viscid secretion to keep the joints moist and thus prevent dryness from the movement. The phalangeal joints are lined with cartilage and have sesamoid bones in the joint cavities.

5.3.17. The Function of the Finger Nails

§261 The nails have four purposes: (a) they support the fingers in catching objects firmly. (b) They help to pick up even small objects. (c) They help the fingers in scratching. (d) They are used as weapons or instruments for tearing thin delicate sheaths during operations.

§262 The first three purposes are specially meant for the human beings, while the fourth is mainly for animals. Nails also have round borders for the reason already described. Nails are made of soft bone so that they do not damage the underlying structures and are not easily broken. They are continuously growing to replace the loss from undue friction.

5.3.18. The Anatomy of the Pelvis

§263 There are two hip bones, one on each side of the sacrum. They are joined together anteriorly by a strong joint and serve as a base for the support of the upper bones and carry the weight of the lower ones. The hip bone is divided into four parts. The outer part is the ilium, the one united anteriorly is the pubis. The posteromedial part is the ischium and it has the acetabulum for articulating with the convex head of the femur. In the pelvis, nature has placed delicate organs like the bladder, uterus and the spermatic cord.

5.3.19. The General Purpose of the Legs

§264 The legs have two functions: (a) They help in standing and maintaining the erect position. This function is performed by the feet. (b) They enable one to walk and move from place to place despite the unevenness of the ground; this function is performed by the leg and the thigh. When the foot is injured, standing and stability are interfered with, but there is no trouble in walking. If there is some trouble in the muscles of the thigh, it would be possible to stand up, but walking would be difficult.

5.3.20. The Anatomy of the Thigh

§265 The thigh bone is the largest bone, as it has to support the body above and carry the structures below. Its upper end is rounded and fits completely in the cavity of the ischium. The femur is convex on the outer side and concave on the inner. If the head of the femur had gone straight into the acetabulum, the gait would have become abnormal and the muscles, blood vessels and nerves would have lacked the protection now enjoyed by them. Moreover, it would not have been possible to sit in the normal way. If the head of the femur had not been directed inward, another type of deformity would have developed and the symmetrical standing and balance which is normal for both legs would be impossible. At the lower end of the femur there are two masses of bone. They are known as the condyles. Now the legs and the knee joint will be described.

5.3.21. The Tibia and Fibula

§266 Like the forearm, the leg also has two bones. The bigger and longer one is placed medially and is called the tibia. The other bone is thin and small. It articulates not with the femur but with the upper end of the tibia. This bone is called the fibula. The lower ends of both tibia and fibula are at the same level.

§267 The tibia above is convex on the lateral side. At the lower end, it has a medial convexity to give it proper shape. The tibia is to the leg what the femur is to the thigh. It has been made smaller than the femur for two reasons. A bigger bone facilitates standing and carrying the weight of the parts above, and a smaller bone facilitates movement. Since the leg has to be more mobile, the tibia has been made smaller, and because the femur has mainly to provide support, it has been made bigger and longer.

§268 Nature has provided such a medium-sized and a well proportioned leg that any increase in its size would have interfered with activity, as in those suffering from elephantiasis and varicose veins. Similarly, any decrease in the size would have produced weakness and inability to raise the legs. The fibula gives cover and support to the tibia. It also protects the vessels and nerves lying between the two bones. It further helps the tibia to form a strong ankle joint for flexion and extension.

5.3.22. The Anatomy of the Knee

§269 This is formed by the two condyles at the lower end of the femur, which articulate with the two depressions on the upper end of the tibia. The two bones are kept firmly joined together by a complicated ligament within the joint. There are also two strong ligaments, one on each side, to strengthen the knee from outside. In front of the knee joint there is the patella, which is like an eyeball to the knee joint. It is somewhat round in shape. It protects the knee joint and prevents its dislocation on sitting and in moving the leg forward as in walking. It has been placed in front because the knee is more vulnerable to injury from the front, both in sitting and standing positions.

5.3.23. The Anatomy of the Foot

§270 The foot has been designed for standing. It has been elongated on the front mainly for this purpose. On the ventral side, it has been provided with a sole to give firmness to the foot during the forward movement of the other foot, as in walking. If the sole does not obtain proper contact with the ground, the foot would not be firm and steady. The sole enables a straight and steady progression of the legs over long distances without any discomfort. It helps in climbing the stairs and serves to protect the feet from irregular and pointed objects.

§271 There are manifold advantages in having several bones in the feet. One is that feet can rest on the ground just as firmly as the hands can grip an object tightly. If the feet had been made of a single bone, the adjustment to irregular surfaces would not have been possible. There is also an overall advantage that, when a part of the foot is damaged or diseased, the remaining part of the foot escapes involvement. The foot is made of twenty-six bones. One of these is the talus, which forms the ankle joint. The other is the calcaneus which gives firm support to the heel. There is also another bone which is called the scaphoid. This is related to the sole. The cuboid is the fourth of the tarsal bones which articulates with the metatarsal bones. It has six sides and lies on the outer side of the foot to which it gives a strong support.

§272 The ankle in the human being is more complex than in the animals. The talus is most useful in the movements of the foot just as the calcaneum is for giving firmness to it. The talus is enclosed in a strong and firm socket made of the lower processes of the tibia and fibula. The scaphoid lies in front of the talus. Due to the concavity of the sole, it has been depressed on the outer side. It articulates behind with the talus, in front with the metatarsais and beneath with the calcaneum.

§273 On the outer side it articulates with the cuboid which may be the fourth bone of the tarsus or a separate bone. The calcaneum lies beneath the talus. It is hard and rounded for protection from friction and injury. It is smooth below for giving the foot a firm grip. The bone has been made big, as it has to carry the heavy weight of the body. It is of a triangular shape and tapers towards the side of the sole. The tarsal bones differ from the carpal bones in being all in a single row. Besides, they are four rather than seven.

§274 They also differ in their functions. In the hand there is a greater need of movement and gripping of an object, while in the foot, there is a greater need for firmness and stability. Hence, there are more bones in the hands and fewer in the feet. The larger the number and smaller the size of the bones, the easier would be the grip, and the larger the size of the bones and smaller the number, the greater would be the firmness.

§275 There are five metatarsal bones. Each bone articulates with the five corresponding toes because the feet require greater gripping and holding than the fingers of the hand. All toes, except the big toe, have three phalanges. The big toe has only two.

§276 The description of the bones and their anatomical relations have now been completed. The body has three hundred and forty-eight bones other than the sesamoid bones and the hyoid bone, which is shaped like the lambda of the Greek alphabet.

5.4. The Muscles

5.4.1. General Remarks Concerning the Nerves, Ligaments, Tendons and Muscles

§277 Voluntary movement occurs when the energy (impulse) from the brain reaches the muscles through the nerves. It is of course obvious that bones are directly involved in movement, but they are connected with the nerves only indirectly. Since bones are hard and the nerves soft, nature has interposed nerve-like fibrous tissue between them.

§278 At its origin from the brain or spinal cord, the nerve has been especially thickened with the fibrous tissue so that it is not damaged in passing through the foramina. As the nerve proceeds towards its destination, it gets divided into smaller and smaller branches, and in the end these become so fine that they can be easily damaged. Hence, Almighty God in His perfect wisdom, has strengthened the nerves by interposing the fibrous tissue in between the nerve fibers. The fibrous tissue envelopes the muscle along with its nerve and keeps it attached to the bone. The whole neuromuscular unit, with its interspersed fibrous tissue and the covering fascia, is the apparatus with which voluntary movement occurs. When a muscle contracts, its tendon which is made of nervous and fibrous tissue, pulls the attached organ (bone) towards itself (flexes). When the muscle expands, the tendon relaxes and produces extension.

5.4.2. The Muscles of the Face

§279 It is evident that the facial muscles should be the same in number as the facial movements. The movable parts of the face are forehead, eyelids, cheeks, lips, outer parts of the nostrils and the jaw.

5.4.3. The Anatomy of the Muscles of the Forehead

§280 The forehead is moved by a thin, flat (aponeurotic) muscle which is spread under the skin and is attached to it. It has no tendon because it has to move only the flat skin of the forehead, which could not have been moved properly by a tendon. This muscle elevates the eyebrow by its contraction and assists in the closure of the eyes by relaxation.

5.4.4. The Anatomy of the Muscles of the Eyeball

§281 There are six muscles of the eyeball. Each of the four sides has a muscle attached to it to elevate, depress, abduct or adduct the eyeball. The other two muscles are attached obliquely and rotate the eye. Behind the eyeball there is another muscle, which supports the optic nerve and functions as its ally. This muscle prevents the eyeball from bulging out and controls the optic nerve during the fixation of the eye towards an object. Its fascial covering is branched, creating the impression of its being two muscles. Some anatomists, therefore, regard it as one, some two, and others as three muscles. Whatever the number, it is a single organ.

5.4.5. The Anatomy of the Muscles of the Eyelid

§282 The lower eyelid does not need movement, as the opening and the closing of the eye is carried out by the upper lid. God employs the minimum of means, as the larger the number, the greater would be the hazard. He, therefore, develops the organs close to their origin and directs the various causes towards their objectives. This obviously is the best principle. Thus, it is the upper lid which has been chosen for movement as it is nearer to the origin of the nerve and does not require its nerve to turn backwards. Moreover, the upper lid has to open and also close the eye. For closing the eye a muscle is required to pull the lid downward. Hence, the nerve would have to bend and then turn upwards pulling the upper lid downward to meet the lower one. The nerve would also have to go either straight to the center of the lid margin or to its inner or outer ends.

§283 If it had gone to the center of the lid, then only the central portion of the eyeball would be covered. If it had gone to one side, there would be a partial closure of the eye at one end with sagging of the lid at the other, as in paralysis. In view of such difficulties, nature has provided not one but two muscles, which, arising from both the ends, close the upper lid evenly from below. For opening the eye, there is a single muscle which spreads in the upper eyelid from the center towards the sides. When it contracts, the eye gets opened. In view of the above-mentioned principles, nature has placed a muscle in between the two layers of the facial and has attached it to the cartilaginous plate (tarsal plate) of the eyelid.

5.4.6. The Anatomy of the Muscles of the Cheeks

§284 There are two types of movement in the cheeks. The first of these occurs in association with the movement of the lower jaw, and the second with the movement of the lips. In the former case, movement is produced by the muscles of the lower jaw and in the latter case by the muscles of the lips. Hence, movement at this part of the cheek is an associated movement and is carried out by the muscles of both cheeks. Being flat, it is known as the flat muscle of the cheek. It has four sets of fibers arising from four different places. One set arises from the sternum and clavicle and terminates beneath the angle of the mouth. It pulls the mouth obliquely from below. The second set of fibers arises from the outer part of the sternum and clavicle, and, after decussating obliquely with the fibers of the other side, ends at the lower margin of the lip on the opposite side. The fibers of the left lip cross those of the right lip and vice-versa.

§285 When the fibers of both sides contract, the mouth becomes narrow and purses forward as in blowing. This action is similar to that of a purse, which, on its string being pulled from both sides, closes. The third set of fibers arises from the acromion process of the scapula and is attached above the fibers already described. When these fibers contract, they pull the lip to their side. The fourth set of fibers arises from the spinous processes of the cervical vertebrae and, passing in front of the ears, joins the cheeks. These fibers pull the cheeks and lips outward. In some cases, these fibers pass near the root of the ear, but at times they are not only attached to it, but also move the ear.

5.4.7. The Anatomy of the Muscles of the Lips

§286 We have already described some muscles of the lips which are common to the cheeks and the lips. There are, however, some others which belong only to the lips. These are four muscles. Two of these arise from the upper part of the cheeks and are attached to the margin of the ears. The other two arise from lower down. These are the four muscles responsible for moving the lips so that when one contracts, the lip moves to that side and when the two contract, on both the sides, the lips move in all the four directions. Since there is no other movement of the lips, there is no need to have any other muscle except the four described above. The four muscles of the lips, and also their associated muscles, join the substance of the lips in such a way that they cannot be easily seen in the soft and fleshy tissues which have no bones.

5.4.8. The Anatomy of the Muscles of the Nostrils

§287 There are two small but strong muscles on both sides of the nostrils. They have been made small to avoid encroachment on the space required for the important muscles of the lips and cheeks, which have to be constantly moving. Movement in the lips is more important than in the nostrils. Since there are no bones in the nostrils, these muscles have been specially strengthened by being brought from the cheeks from where they also assist in opening the nostrils outward.

5.4.9. The Anatomy of the Muscles of the Lower Jaw

§288 It is the lower jaw and not the upper one which moves. In this, there are special advantages. Movement in the lower jaw, which is lighter than the upper one, is easier. It is also better that this jaw, which does not lodge any important organ, should be moved rather than the one which has an important organ, whose movement would produce discomfort.

§289 Moreover, the lower jaw unlike the upper one is not firmly united with the skull. The lower jaw does, however, produce more than three movements, that is, opening and closing the mouth and mastication. When the lower jaw is raised, the mouth is closed and when it is lowered, the mouth is opened. Mastication has a rotatory movement in which the lower jaw opens and closes the mouth and moves from right to left. For closing the mouth, it is necessary to have muscles arising from above and contracting upwards. To open the mouth they should arise from below and pull downward. The muscles of mastication are oblique.

§290 Nature has provided two muscles for closing the mouth. These are the temporal muscles. These are small in the human being as the lower jaw is small and hollow and its movements are not so strong. The lower jaw in animals, however, is large and heavy and has to perform several types of movements, i.e., crushing, biting, uprooting and cutting.

§291 The jaw muscles have been made soft because of the soft and delicate nature of the neighboring brain which is separated from the (temporal) muscles only by a single bone and is thus liable to be damaged or diseased by their involvement. Nature has, therefore, protected the brain by providing an arch over the temporal bone. When the temporal muscles contract, the jaw is elevated.

§292 They are assisted by two other muscles, which are supplied to the lower jaw from within the cheek. It is well recognized that when a heavier part is to be lifted, some special measure and additional strength is required. Hence, these muscles have been provided with tendons which, for additional strength, arise from the center of the muscle and not from its end.

§293 The muscle which opens the mouth and lowers the jaw arises from the process behind the ear (mastoid) and originally being fleshy, it later forms into a tendon to gain additional strength. It again expands into a small, fleshy muscle rather than a long, vulnerable one and is finally attached to the mandible near the chin. When this muscle contracts, the jaw retracts and is also depressed. Since this movement is aided by gravity, there is no need of having any other muscles.

§294 There are two muscles for mastication—one on each side. Each muscle is of a triangular shape with the apex at the angle of the cheek. From there, one set of fibers goes to the lower jaw and the other ends at the temporal bone. In this way they provide a base extending between them. The muscles are so firmly attached to the surrounding structures at the angles that various types of movements become possible for proper mastication.

5.4.10. The Anatomy of the Muscles of the Head

§295 Some movements of the head are confined to the head alone while others involve both the head and the other structures, including the first five cervical vertebrae. In some of the movements, the neck participates with the head. The movements of the head, whether specific to the head or jointly performed with the neck, move the head forwards or backwards and to the right or the left side. Some muscles rotate the head.

§296 There are two muscles on either side of the neck which are specifically meant for bending the head. Both arise from the sternum below and are attached above to the mastoid bone. As both ascend together, some anatomists regard them as one. One of these has two sets of fibers. One set arises from the sternum and the other from the clavicle. Some anatomists regard them as three muscles.

§297 When the muscles of one side contract, they bend the head to that side, but when the muscles of both the sides act together, the head is bent forwards. For bending the head and neck forward, there are two muscles. These are situated behind the esophagus and after arising from the first and second vertebrae are attached to the head and the neck. When the muscle nearer the esophagus contracts, only the head is bent forward, but when the muscle attached to the vertebrae also contracts, there is bending of the neck as well.

§298 There are four pairs of muscles which turn the head backwards. They are underneath the muscles as described above. These muscles arise from above the joint between the head and the neck. Some of the muscles arise from the spinous processes of the vertebrae, slightly away from the mid-line, while others arise from the transverse processes near the mid-line. There are some pairs which arise from the transverse processes of the first vertebra and are situated above the muscle arising from the spinous process of the second vertebra. Among these is the pair of muscles whose fibers arise from the transverse processes of the first vertebra and end at the spinous process of the second vertebra. This muscle keeps the head slightly bent during the rotation of the head.

§299 The fourth pair arising from above passes obliquely under the third pair and after emerging from there is attached to the transverse process of the first vertebra. Amongst the four pairs, the first two move the head backwards with or without any deviation to either side. The third pair keeps the head erect with a slightly backward deviation. The fourth pair moves the head backwards with a slight bend. When the third and fourth pairs act together. the head is moved backwards, but without any deviation.

§300 There are three pairs of muscles for the rotation of the head. These are placed deep in the neck. The muscles of the outer pair are triangular in shape with their narrow bases at the occipital bone and the apices at the sides of the neck. The lowest of the three arises from the sides of the vertebrae and is inclined more towards the transverse processes. The third pair lies midway at the sides of the vertebrae.

§301 There are two pairs of muscles which move the head towards the sides. These are adjacent to the joint between the head and the neck. One of these pairs covers the space anteriorly between the head and the second vertebra and has one muscle on the right side, and the other on the left. The second pair which lies posteriorly rests between the head and the first cervical vertebra. One of its muscles is on the right side and the other on the left side.

§302 When any one of these four muscles contracts the head is bent to the corresponding side with a slight deviation. When two of these contract, the head bends to their side without any deviation. When the two front muscles contract, the head bends forward, but when the two muscles at the back contract, the head bends backwards. When all the four act together, the head is kept in the erect position.

§303 Although these muscles are rather small, they have a good cover of other muscles and are thus well protected. The joint for the head requires two things which are contradictory to each other. Firstly, the joint should be sufficiently strong to withstand its various movements, and at the same time, it should be loose enough to permit the performance of these movements. Nature has, therefore, made this joint sufficiently loose as well as enormously strong, and it has covered it with muscles for additional strength and easier movements. So blessed be God, the best of all creators!

5.4.11. The Anatomy of the Muscles of the Larynx

§304 The larynx is a cartilaginous structure designed for the production of sound. It has three cartilages. The first cartilage can be seen in the neck beneath the chin. This is the thyroid cartilage. It is concave on the inner side and convex at the outer, thus resembling a shield. The second cartilage is placed behind the first and is attached to it. It has no special name. The third cartilage is placed in an inverted position over the other two and is attached to the one which has no name.

§305 The thyroid cartilage is in touch with the third cartilage, but without any union. There is a double articulation between the second and the third cartilage, so that there are two depressions over the latter for receiving the two elevations of the unnamed cartilage. Both are firmly joined to each other with ligamentous fibers and are known as the epiglottis and the arytenoid cartilages respectively.

§306 The expansion and the contraction of the larynx is determined by the distance between the thyroid cartilage and the cartilage which has no name. The opening and closing of the larynx is determined by the inversion, elevation and depression of the arytenoid cartilages over the thyroid cartilage. Above the thyroid cartilage there is a triangular bone, which resembles the letter lambda of the Greek alphabet and is known as the hyoid bone. This is close in front of the larynx and beneath the chin. The hyoid bone acts as a supporting and a resting place and gives origin to the muscles of the larynx.

§307 The larynx needs a muscle to join the thyroid cartilage with the cartilage which has no name and also another to separate the arytenoid cartilage from the thyroid cartilage for opening the larynx. A pair of muscles which helps to open the larynx arises from the hyoid bone and is inserted in front of the thyroid cartilage and covers it completely. When this pair contracts, the front of the arytenoid cartilages is raised and the larynx opens.

§308 The second pair of muscles, which is also included among the pharyngeal muscles, pulls the larynx downward. This pair appears to be common to both the pharynx and the larynx. It arises from behind the sternum and is attached to the thyroid cartilage. Occasionally, this pair is supported by another pair in animals. In addition to these, there are two other pairs of muscles. One pair comes from behind the arytenoids and has a fleshy attachment with them. It elevates the arytenoid cartilages and pulls them backwards from the thyroid cartilage, thus widening the larynx.

§309 The muscles which contract the larynx arise from the hyoid bone and are attached to the thyroid cartilage. They enclose the cartilage which has no name from both sides and contract the larynx. There are four other muscles for closing the larynx. Some regard these muscles as being merely two double muscles. The muscles attached to both the thyroid and the cartilage which has no name narrow the lower part of the larynx.

§310 According to some anatomists, one of the two muscles mentioned above lies on the inner side of the larynx and the other on the outer side. The one which is inside occupies the best shape and position, i.e., it is right within the larynx. When this muscle contracts, it pulls the arytenoids downward, thus narrowing the larynx.

§311 For this purpose, nature has provided another pair which, arising from the inner side of the thyroid cartilage, is attached to the arytenoid cartilage and to the roots of the cartilage which has no name. When this muscle contracts, it closes the larynx completely and in this way is in strong opposition to the muscles of the thorax and the diaphragm. The muscles on the inside of the larynx have been made smaller to prevent narrowing of the larynx. They are, however, so strong that, even with their smaller size, they can close the larynx completely and thus hold the breath.

§312 After arising from below, these muscles pass obliquely upwards and are attached to the thyroid and the cartilages which have no name. Occasionally, two other muscles are seen below the arytenoid cartilages. These act as supportive to the muscles which have already been described.

5.4.12. The Anatomy of the Muscles of the Throat

§313 The throat as a whole has two pairs of muscles which pull it downward. One of these has already been mentioned under the laryngeal muscles. The other pair, arising from the sternum, passes upwards by the side of the hyoid bone. It ends in the pharynx, which it pulls downward. There are two muscles placed near the fauces in the pharynx. These assist deglutition and are known as palatopharyngeous and saplingopharyngeous (*nufnughatan*).

5.4.13. The Anatomy of the Muscles of the Hyoid Bone

§314 Some muscles exclusively belong to the hyoid bone and some are common to the hyoid and other bones. Muscles of the hyoid bone are in three pairs. One of these arising from the lower jaw is inserted in the middle of the hyoid bone and pulls it towards the jaw. The other pair, arising from beneath the chin, passes downward under the tongue and is attached to the upper margin of the hyoid bone. This pair also pulls the hyoid bone towards the jaw. The third pair, arising from the arrow-like (styloid) process near the ear is inserted below in the horizontal part of the hyoid bone. The muscles which are common to both the hyoid bone and the other structures have already been described, and some of these will be described again.

5.4.14. The Anatomy of the Muscles of the Tongue

§315 There are nine muscles which move the tongue. The first pair arises from the styloid process and ends at the second pair at the sides of the tongue. The third pair, which moves the tongue obliquely, arises from the lower end of the hyoid bone and is inserted in the substance of the tongue. The fourth pair makes up the central mass and lies beneath the six muscles already described.

§316 The fibers of all these muscles run transversely under the muscles described above and are all attached to the jaw. There is only one muscle which belongs exclusively to the tongue. This is placed between the tongue and the hyoid bone. Each muscle can move the tongue either way, i.e., the muscle which lengthens the tongue during protrusion shrinks it, too, on retraction.

5.4.15. The Anatomy of the Muscles of the Neck

§317 There are two pairs of muscles especially meant for moving the neck. One is on the right side and the other on the left. If one muscle contracts, it bends the neck obliquely to its side, but if both muscles contract on the same side, they bend the neck to that side without any deviation. When all four contract, the neck becomes straight and erect.

5.4.16. The Anatomy of the Muscles of the Chest

§318 Some muscles of the chest produce expansion, others contraction, but there are some others which produce both expansion and contraction. The muscles which expand the chest are nine, including the diaphragm, which lies between the organs of respiration and the stomach and will be described shortly.

§319 Amongst these muscles there is a pair which lies behind the clavicles. Each muscle arises from the outer half of the scapula and is attached to the first rib and pulls the clavicle to its own side.

§320 There is another pair to expand the chest. This is a double muscle with two heads. The upper head is attached to the neck and moves it. The lower head along with another muscle is attached to the first and sixth ribs and it moves the chest.

§321 The third pair of muscles which expands the chest arises from beneath the scapula. This pair is joined by another pair which arises from the first vertebrae and goes to the scapula. Both pairs join as one pair and are attached to the smaller ribs.

§322 The fourth pair for expanding the chest arises from the seventh cervical and the first two thoracic vertebrae and is inserted to the external ribs.

§323 These are the muscles for expanding the chest. Some muscles narrow the chest indirectly by contraction, i.e., the diaphragm not in motion, while others act directly.

§324 Some muscles are inserted beneath the ends of the upper ribs. Their function is to strengthen the chest and hold the various parts together. There are some pairs of muscles on the side of the chest which are attached to the sternum and xiphoid cartilage. The rectus abdominis is amongst these muscles.

§325 There are two other pairs to assist the muscles described above. The muscles which produce both expansion and contraction of the chest are the intercostal muscles. After a thorough consideration, it has however, been found that muscles for expansion and contraction are separate and that each intercostal muscle is in reality a set of four muscles which look like a single muscle.

§326 The fact is that the intercostal muscles consist of several sets of fibers. The fibers on the inner side of the chest are oblique. These are attached near the strong posterior ends of the ribs. The outer fibers are attached near the cartilaginous ends. Thus, the two sets of fibers differ markedly from each other, the one attached to the cartilaginous end has a different shape and position from the other at the posterior side. The outer set of fibers is for expansion and the inner set for contraction of the chest.

§327 Keeping this description in view, there are eighty-eight muscles of the chest. There are two other muscles which assist the muscles of the chest. They arise from the scapular ends of the clavicles and are attached to the first ribs. They help in raising the ribs and thus producing expansion of the chest.

5.4.17. The Anatomy of the Muscles Which Move the Arms

§328 There are three muscles which move the arm at the

shoulder joint. They arise from the chest and pull the arm towards it. One of these arises from under the breast and is attached to the front of the arm. This muscle adducts the arm and pulls it somewhat downward. The second muscle arising from the upper part of the chest goes round the head of the humerus from its inner side. This also adducts the arm, but with a slight rise of the shoulder. The third muscle is thin and double and of a larger size. It arises from the chest and is attached to the lower part of the front of the arm. Its upper fibers adduct the arm with some elevation (of the shoulder), and the lower ones adduct the arm with some depression. When both fibers act together, there is a simple adduction of the arm.

§329 Two muscles arise from the ilium. These are joined together more intimately than even the double muscle ascending from the chest. One of these arises from the ilium and the smaller ribs and pulls the arm towards the ribs. The other muscle is thinner and smaller than the first. It does not arise from the iliac bone but from its aponeurosis. It comes forward to join the tendon of the other muscle which lies under the breast. It draws the arm slightly backwards.

§330 There are five muscles of the arm which arise from the scapula. The first one arises from the upper part of the scapula and fills up the space between the shoulder and the first rib and ends at the upper part of the arm. The second muscle is on the outer side. It moves the arm away from the chest with some inward deviation. Two of the five muscles arise from the upper ribs. The one which is bigger sends its fibers under the diaphragm as already described. It fills up the space between the diaphragm and the lower ribs and is inserted on the outer side of the head of the humerus. This muscle draws the arm away from the chest with a slight outward rotation. The other muscle [the third] becomes a part of the first and is directed the same way and has a similar action. It is, however, not connected with the upper part of the scapula but is inserted obliquely on the outer side of the arm which it rotates outward. The fourth muscle fills up the depression in the scapula. Its tendon is inserted on the inner side of the medial crest of the humerus which it rotates backwards.

§331 Another muscle which arises from the margin of the

ribs under the scapula has a tendon, which begins from the large muscle ascending from the ilium. Its action is to pull the head of the humerus upwards. There is one more muscle of the humerus which has two heads and thus two different actions. It arises both from the clavicle and the neck and ends at the head of the humerus, where the large muscle of the thorax is also inserted.

§332 Physicians have described an inner head of the muscle which lies obliquely out and an outer head which goes towards the back for insertion to the lower part of the outer margin of the shoulder bone. When both heads act together, the arm is elevated upwards. Some physicians have mentioned two other muscles of the arm. One of these is a small muscle which arises from the breast; the other, is in shoulder and is related to the muscles of the elbow joint.

5.4.18. The Anatomy of the Muscles of the Forearm

§333 The muscles which move the forearm are the flexors and extensors. They are attached to the humerus. There are also some muscles of the forearm which produce pronation and supination. These have no connection with muscles of the arm. Extensors of the forearm are two muscles of which one extends the forearm with some inward rotation. It arises in front from the lower end of the humerus and the ribs beneath the scapula. It ends at the inner side of the elbow.

§334 The other muscle extends the forearm with some outward rotation. It arises from behind the humerus and ends on the outer side of the elbow. When both muscles act together, they produce a straight extension of the arm. The flexors of the forearm are two muscles. The one which is larger flexes the forearm with some inward rotation. This muscle arises from the coracoid process of the scapula and passing over the inner side of the arm is inserted at the upper part of the radius.

§335 The other muscle flexes the forearm with some outward rotation. It arises from behind the humerus and divides into two halves. One goes to the front and the other behind the humerus and then both pass downward for insertion on the front of the ulna. The part which rotates the forearm outward during flexion is attached to the lower end of the ulna, and the part which turns the forearm inward is attached to the upper end of the ulna. When both parts act together, the forearm is kept straight during flexion. Sometimes there is a muscle in between the two extensor muscles. This covers the humerus but appears to be just a part of the flexors.

§**336** The supinator muscles of the forearm are also a pair. One of these muscles lies on the outer side of the forearm in between the radius and the ulna and is attached to the radius without any tendon. The second muscle is long and thin. It arises from the outer side of the head of the radius and passing through the whole length of the forearm reaches the wrist, where it is inserted along the lower end of the radius.

§**337** The pronators of the forearm are also a pair of muscles placed on the outer side of the forearm. One muscle arises from the medial side of the head of the humerus and is inserted at the lower end of the radius just before the wrist. The other muscle (pronator quadratus) is smaller and has broad fibers and a very strong tendinous attachment. This muscle arises from the ulna and is inserted on the radius near the wrist joint.

5.4.19. The Anatomy of the Muscles Which Move the Wrist

§**338** The wrist has extensor, flexor, supinator, and pronator muscles.

5.4.19.1. The Extensors

§**339** Extension of the wrist is carried out by two muscles which are so firmly joined together that they look like one. One of these arises from about the middle of the ulna and is attached to the thumb as an abductor. The other muscle arises from the radius and is attached to the first metacarpal bone by a tendon. When the two muscles act together, they extend the wrist with some pronation. If the second muscle extends the wrist, it also produces some pronation. The first muscle abducts the thumb away from the index finger. In addition to these there is another muscle which arises from the outside of the radius and the lower end of the humerus. It has two tendons, one of which is attached between the metacarpal bones of the middle and index fingers and the other to the lower end of the radius near the wrist. This muscle pronates the wrist with some extension.

5.4.19.2. The Flexors

§340 These are a pair of muscles on the outer side of the forearm. The lower of these arises from the medial side of the lower end of the humerus. It is attached below to the metacarpal bone of the little finger. The upper muscle arises from the upper part of the previous one and ends just there.

§341 In addition to these, there is another muscle which arises from the lower end of the humerus and passes downward in between the two muscles mentioned above. It has two ends which cross each other and then join up again between the index and the middle fingers. When the above-mentioned muscles act together, there is flexion. When they act obliquely, there is pronation or supination according to the direction of the movement. If the muscle which is attached to the proximal end of the metacarpal bone of the little finger acts alone, it pronates the hand. When this muscle is assisted by the muscle attached to the thumb and the one which is to be described presently, there is complete supination. Similarly, if the muscle attached to the metacarpal bone of the thumb acts alone, it pronates the hand, but if the one attached to the little finger also acts with it, there is full pronation of the hand.

5.4.20. The Anatomy of the Muscles Which Move the Fingers

§342 Some muscles of the fingers are in the palm and some in the forearm. If all had been in the palm, the hand would have become too heavy with the muscular tissue. The forearm being distant, its muscles have been provided with tendons; and in order to give additional strength, they are covered with membranes. In these muscles, the tendons are strong and round except at their attachments. They are flattened to give a firm hold during movement.

5.4.20.1. The Extensors

§343 The extensors of the fingers are placed on the outside of the forearm at its middle. They arise from the raised surface at the lower end of the humerus and send extensor tendons to all the four fingers.

5.4.20.2. The Flexors

§344 These are three muscles. Two are partly joined with each other. One of the muscles arises from about the middle of the lower end of the humerus, in between the two elevations at its outer side. It sends down two tendons: one to the ring and the other to the little finger.

§345 The second muscle of this group is really a double muscle. Part of it arises from the lower end of the humerus at the inner side of its two elevations and from the margin of the ulna. It ends in two tendons, one of which goes to the index and the other to the middle finger. Part of the second muscle, which is really the third muscle of this group, arises from the upper end of the radius and is attached to the thumb.

§346 Close to this muscle is another muscle of the wrist. It arises from about the middle of the ulna and ends in a tendon which moves the thumb away from the index finger.

§347 The muscles which close the fingers are from either the upper part of the forearm or inside of the palm. Muscles from the forearm are three and placed one over the other at the middle of the forearm. The one which is most important is hidden beneath the others and lies on the ulna. It arises from the inner side of the outer prominence at the lower end of the humerus. It splits into five tendons, one for each finger and ends at the inner (palmar) side of the fingers.

§348 The tendons which proceed to the four fingers flex the first and the third joints. The first phalanx is flexed by a ligamentous attachment from the tendon and the third is flexed by the tendon which ends there. The tendon which goes to the thumb moves its second and third joints by ligamentous attachments. The muscle which immediately covers the important muscle is relatively a smaller one. It arises from one of the two inner prominences at the lower end of the humerus. It joins the ulna and passes across the area between the outer and the inner surfaces known as the upper surface of the radius. It turns near the thumb and sends out tendons towards the middle of each finger for flexion. A branch goes to the thumb moving away from the other tendons. It arises from another place. The smaller head originates from the ends of both the radius and the ulna, and the larger head from only the ulna. Flexion of the thumb is carried out by only one muscle, as this movement is more important to the fingers, while extension and abduction are more important to the thumb. The third muscle does not flex the fingers but spreads out as a tendon in the palm for improving sensory perception and to prevent the growth of hair. It also provides a supporting cushion to the palm and strengthens the hand for various purposes. This was a description of the muscles from the forearm.

5.4.20.3. Palmar Muscles

§349 There are eighteen muscles in the palm placed in two layers, one over the other. The first is deeper, and the second superficial, which lies under the skin. In the first layer, there are seven muscles. Five of these extend the fingers and the thumb. The one which goes to the thumb arises from the first carpal bone. This muscle is small and flat and has oblique fibers. It arises from the metacarpal bone of the middle finger and ends in a tendon, which is attached to the thumb. It flexes the thumb.

§350 The seventh muscle after arising from the metacarpal bone goes to the little finger which it flexes. These are the seven muscles which contract the fingers: five raise the fingers and two lower them. The muscles of the superficial layer which lie beneath the flat muscle of the palm have been described by Galen. These are eleven, of which eight are attached to the four fingers in pairs. The muscles, which are attached on the dorsal side, pull the joints (extend the phalanges) while the muscles which are attached to the palmar side flex the fingers.

Contraction of the upper muscles also produces slight extension of the fingers.

§351 When both the dorsal and ventral muscles act together, the fingers are kept in the mid position. The other three muscles are only for the thumb. One of these is attached to its proximal phalanx while the other two are attached to the second phalanx, as already mentioned.

§352 For the extension of the fingers, there are five muscles and for the flexion, other than that of the thumb and little finger, there are two for each finger. Thus, there are five muscles for opening the fingers and for closing them other than the thumb and little finger, two for each finger. For closing all the fingers, there are four muscles, but for opening there is only one muscle.

5.4.21. The Anatomy of the Muscles Which Move the Spine

§353 Some muscles of the trunk bend the spine backwards, while others bend it forwards and in this way all the movement of the spine are performed. The muscles which bend the spine backwards are the most important muscles of the trunk. These are two, but as it will soon be evident, each is made of twenty-three small muscles because a separate set of oblique fibers arises from each vertebra, except the first cervical.

§354 When there is a moderate contraction, the spine becomes erect, but with a greater contraction, it bends backwards. When the muscles of one side contract, the trunk bends to that side. The muscles which bend the trunk forward are two pairs. One of these is at the upper part of the spine on either side of the esophagus. This muscle arises from the upper five vertebrae in some persons while in others it arises also partly from the head and the neck.

§355 The second pair arises from the eleventh and the twelfth thoracic vertebrae. It passes downward and bends the spine forward. Since it is only the middle of the spine which has to be bent forward, backward, outward and rotated, these muscles are sufficient for these requirements.

5.4.22. The Anatomy of the Muscles of the Abdomen

§356 In the abdomen, there are eight muscles which jointly serve the various purposes. They produce contraction and evacuation of the bowels, bladder and uterus, provide support to the diaphragm during distension and by covering the stomach and intestine keep the abdomen warm. Among these muscles there is a pair which extends vertically from the xiphisternum to the pubic bone (*rectus abdominis*). This is entirely muscular.

§357 There are two muscles which cross transversely in front of the membranous lining of the abdomen and behind the rectus muscle. There are two muscles which cross each other obliquely and extend on either side from the ilium to the xiphisternum and from the pubis to the ends of the ribs. Thus, each muscle arising from the right or left side crosses each other above the pubis. The upper margins of both muscles meet each other at the xiphisternum.

§358 There are two other muscles which cross obliquely from either side. Their fibers remain fleshy until their attachment to the rectus muscle where they turn into a flat fascia-like aponeurotic tendon. These two pairs are placed in front of the rectus muscle which in turn is placed over the flat (internal) oblique muscle.

5.4.23. The Anatomy of the Muscles of the Testes and Ovaries

§359 There are four muscles of the testes in the male. These muscles protect and support the testes and thus prevent them from becoming loose and lax. In the male, there are two muscles for each testis, but in the female, there is only one muscle for each ovary as they do not hand outside the abdomen as do the testes of the male.

5.4.24. The Anatomy of the Bladder Muscle

§360 There is only one muscle, which encircles the mouth of the bladder with its fibers running obliquely around it. This prevents the voidance of urine except when it is passed voluntarily. During micturition, this muscle becomes relaxed and the abdominal muscles squeeze the bladder in such a way that the urine is squirted out as if from a syringe.

5.4.25. The Anatomy of the Muscles of the Penis

§361 There are a pair of muscles which move the penis on each side. When this contracts, it dilates and expends the urethra and makes it straight for the passage of urine and semen.

§362 Another pair arises from the pubis and is obliquely attached to the root of the penis. If this contracts normally, the penis becomes erect, but when the contraction is excessive, the penis is pulled back towards the abdomen. If the muscle contracts on one side only, the penis is deviated to that side.

5.4.26. The Anatomy of the Muscles of the Anus

§363 There are four muscles of the anus. One of these encircles the anus. This is firmly attached to the surrounding tissues and is like the muscle of the mouth and lips. It constricts and squeezes the anus and forces out the fecal matter from the rectum. The second muscle is inside the anus and is placed on the top of the first. According to some, it has two heads joined together at the root of the penis. There is also an internal sphincter hidden within the anus and lying above the external sphincter. The third muscle is placed obliquely over the other muscles of the anus. This muscle is flat and serves the purpose of lifting the anus. When it becomes relaxed, the anus becomes prolapsed.

5.4.27. The Anatomy of the Muscles Which Move the Thigh

§364 The large muscles of the thigh are those which extend the thigh. Next to them are the muscles which flex the thigh. Of the two important functions of the thigh, extension is more important than flexion, because it is by extension that the human being is able to stand erect. In addition to these muscles, there are those which abduct the thigh or adduct it. Finally, there are muscles to circumduct the thigh.

§365 Of the muscles which extend the thigh, one is the largest muscle of the body. This is the muscle which covers the pubis, ischium and inner side of the thigh up to the knee. Its fibers arise from several places. Some arise from the lower side of the pubic bone and are spread over the inner side of the thigh. The fibers which arise from higher up flex the thigh, but those which arise from a still higher position flex the thigh with some inward rotation. The fibers which arise from the ischium extend the thigh.

§366 There is another muscle which covers the hip joint. It has three heads and two ends. The three heads arise from the ilium, ischium and coccyx, respectively. Two of these are fleshy and the third is membranous. The two ends of the muscle are inserted behind the head of the femur. When one contracts, the thigh is extended with rotation to that side, but when both contract there is a simple extension.

§367 There is another muscle of the thigh which arises from the outer side of the ilium and is inserted at the greater trochanter. It spreads over the inner side of the thigh for some distance.

§368 There is also another muscle which is similar to the previous one but is inserted at the lower part of the lesser trochanter, from where it proceeds behind the thigh. This muscle produces greater flexion than extension and arises from the outer side of this lower margin of the ilium. In the thigh, there is another muscle which arises from the lower margin of the ischium and spreads backwards and medially.

§369 In the flexors of the thigh there is a muscle which produces some medial rotation with the flexion. This is a long muscle which arises from two places and descends downward. A part of this muscle is inserted at the back and another part starting from the ilium is attached to the lesser trocanter. Another muscle arises from the pubis and is attached beneath the lesser trocanter. The third muscle which lies obliquely in the thigh is often regarded as a part of the longer muscle. The fourth muscle arising from the anterior spine of the ilium flexes both the thigh and the leg. The muscle which adducts the thigh has already been described under the flexors and extensors, but there is also another muscle for the same movement. This arises from the pubis and goes to the knee.

§370 There are two muscles which abduct the thigh. One of these arises from the ilium. There are two muscles which rotate the thigh. One arises from the outer surface and the other from the inner surface of the pubis. They are placed in layers and travel obliquely for insertion into the depression near the posterior part of the greater trocanter. Whichever contracts, it rotates the thigh to the same side with some slight extension.

5.4.28. The Anatomy of the Muscles Which Move the Knee Joint

§371 There are three muscles which extend the knee. These are situated in front of the thigh and are its biggest muscles. One of these is a double muscle with two heads. One head arises from the greater trochanter and the other from the front of the femur. The muscle ends in two tendons, one is fleshy and inserted on the patella and the other which is membranous is attached to the inner side of the femur.

§372 Of the remaining two muscles, one has already been described under the extensors of the thigh. The other muscle arises from the lateral prominence of the femur. Both unite to form a broad tendon which encircles the patella, gives protection to it and the underlying structures, and after attaching itself to the upper end of the tibia, extends the knee.

§373 Of the extensors of the leg, there is a muscle which arises from the symphysis pubica and runs obliquely downward and medially for attachment to the upper part of the leg. It extends the leg with some medial rotation.

§374 In some books of anatomy, one more muscle has also been described. It is placed on the lateral side of the thigh in front of the muscle described above. This muscle arises from the ischium and travels obliquely outward to reach the leg below the patella. No muscle is so oblique as this one. It extends the leg with some outward rotation. When both muscles contract, there is a simple extension.

§375 Among the flexors of the leg, there is a thin narrow muscle which arises from the pubis, the ilium and its membranous fascia. It descends obliquely on the inner side of the knee and from there turns outwardly for attachment to the tuberosity below the patella. This muscle flexes the leg towards the thigh with a slight inward rotation.

§376 In addition, there are three other muscles which occupy the inner, outer and middle positions in the thigh. The outer and the middle muscles flex the leg in a somewhat medial direction. The inner muscle flexes the leg medially. This muscle arising from the base of the ischium passes obliquely behind the thigh and on reaching the inner side of the leg beneath the patella gets attached to it. It is of a greenish color.

§377 The other two muscles also arise from the ischium and ,reaching the outer side of the patella, are attached to it. In the knee, there is also a muscle hidden in the fossa of the knee joint. This has a similar action as the central group of muscles. According to some physicians, the double muscle which arises from the fascia flexes the knee in an indirect manner. Its two heads join to form a tendon, which binds the knee joint firmly and brings its neighboring structures close together.

5.4.29. The Anatomy of the Muscles Which Move the Foot

§378 Of the muscles of the foot, some raise the foot while others lower it. Of the muscles which raise the foot, there is a large muscle which lies on the anteromedial side of the leg. It arises from the outer side of the tibia and passing downward from the leg is attached to the base of the great toe. The other muscle, arising from the upper end of the tibia and the fibula, has its tendon inserted at the root of the little toe. When it acts with the other muscle, the foot is raised.

§379 Of the muscles which lower the foot, there is a pair, which arising from the lower end of the femur and descending into the calf on the inner side, becomes fleshy and forms a large tendon known as the tendocalcaneus. This tendon is inserted in the calcaneum which it pulls obliquely from behind, upwards and outward. This tendon is responsible for keeping the foot firmly supported on the ground. It is assisted by the muscle which arises from the outside of the head of the fibula and is of a violet color. It descends downward and is inserted through its fleshy portion just above and behind the insertion of the tendo calcaneus.

§380 When any of these two muscles or tendons is damaged or diseased, the foot cannot be moved. The foot has another muscle which has two tendons. One flexes and the other abducts the big toe. Arising from the medial side of the head of the tibia, it descends between the two bones and then divides into two tendons. One tendon is attached to the ventral side of the big toe and lowers the foot, while the other emerges as a part of the other muscle which goes forward beyond the insertion of the first tendon for attachment to the first phalanx of the big toe. It extends the big toe obliquely inward.

§381 Occasionally, there is a muscle which arises from the lateral condyle of the femur and is attached to one of the two calcaneal muscles. When this muscle reaches the inner side of the leg, it forms a tendon which spreads under the foot like the corresponding muscle of the palm and has a similar purpose.

5.4.30. The Anatomy of the Muscles of the Toes

§382 There are several muscles to flex the toes. One arises from the outer side of the tibia and descending downward divides into two tendons of which one is spread out on the middle toe and the other on the fourth toe.

§383 The other muscle which is smaller of the two, arising from behind the leg, forms a tendon which divides into two to flex the index and the little toe. Each tendon again divides into two and joins the other tendon to form a single tendon, which flexes the big toe.

§384 There is a third muscle which has already been described. It arises from the outer surface of the tibia and passes downward between the two long bones. A part of it flexes the foot and another part goes to the first phalanx of the big toe. These are the only muscles which move the toes. They are all placed at the upper and posterior part of the leg.

§385 Among the muscles in the sole of the foot there are ten which had not been identified by the anatomists. Galen was the first to discover them. These muscles are attached to the five toes.

§386 There are two muscles on the sides of each toe which flex the toes. When these muscles act from the two sides, the toes become straight, but if they move from one side the toes are bent to that side. There are four muscles of which each is attached to a metatarso-phalangeal joint. There are two other muscles, one each for the big and the little toe, which produce flexion.

§387 All the muscles described above are so inter-related that if one is injured or diseased, the function of the other also gets impaired. This is why it is impossible to flex one toe without flexing the other. There are five muscles of the toes which are placed over the foot. These move the toes outward. There are five muscles in the sole, one for each toe which move the toes inward. All these muscles, including the two muscles of the big and little toes, are similar to the seven muscles of the hand.

§388 According to the above description, there are five hundred and twenty-nine muscles in the body.

5.5. The Nervous System

5.5.1. A General Description of Nerves

§389 There are direct as well as indirect advantages of the nerves. The direct advantage is that the brain receives sensation and controls movement through them. The indirect advantage is that the nerves give strength to the muscles and thus to the body as a whole. Organs like the liver, spleen and lungs are insensitive. There are, however, nerves in their membranous coverings. These enable the appreciation of disease or injury through a tension on the covering membranes or a pull on their attachments as in swelling or distension from gas.

§390 As mentioned before, nerves arise from the brain and spread out as a network of fine branches in the tissues and the superficial skin. Nerves are connected with the brain in two ways. Some arise directly from the brain and are known as nerves of the brain, while others arise indirectly, emerging from the spinal cord, which runs downward in the vertebral column.

The nerves which arise directly from the brain are responsible for movements of the head, face and internal organs, while spinal nerves supply the remaining organs. Galen has pointed out that it is one of God's great favors that He has especially protected the nerve which supplies the internal organs.

§391 Nerves which traverse a long distance are carefully supported and strengthened. Hence, the nerve to the internal organs has been covered in a sheath, which in its structure lies midway between the nervous and fibrous tissues.

§392 This sheath is found at three different places in the course of the nerve—one near the larynx, another near the posterior ends of the ribs where the nerve passes downward, and the third after it has passed through the thorax. The nerves which arise from the brain go straight to the recipient organs. Hence, they have not been especially strengthened.

§393 Sensory nerves are not so strong as the motor nerves. Motor nerves have a tortuous course and traverse a longer distance, and as they proceed onwards, they go on gradually losing the softness of the structure inherited by them from the brain. Nerves which have a soft structure are more sensitive. Hence, the nerves of the special senses originate from the softer forebrain, while the motor nerves arise from the relatively harder hindbrain.

5.5.2. The Anatomy of the Nerves of the Brain and Their Paths

§394 There are seven pairs of cranial nerves.

§395 The first pair of nerves (olfactory) originates from a nipple-like prominence, beneath the ventricle of the forebrain. These are responsible for the perception of smell.

§396 The nerves of the second pair [optic] are thick and somewhat hollow. The one which arises from the left side crosses over to the right while the other which arises from the right crosses over to the left. This crossing is however not (exactly) like that of a crucifix because the nerve from the right side goes partly to the right eye and the nerve from the left goes partly to the left eye. According to Galen, both the nerves cross (completely) without any complication. Physicians have recognized three advantages of this incomplete crossing. First, in case of disease or injury to one eye, the vital force is diverted to the other eye in full. Thus, when one eye is closed, the visual equity of the other is increased and particularly so, when one eye has gone blind. The closure of one eye also produces a dilatation of the pupil in the other eye, because the vital force from the closed eye gets diverted to the open eye. The second advantage of the crossing is that it enables the visual images from both eyes to overlap at the crossing. It is for this reason that in a squint, the vital force from the affected eye does not reach the crossing as normal and thus produces double vision. Thirdly, the crossing enables the nerves to receive a strong support from each other and bring the eyeballs closer to the brain.

§397 The third pair [occulomotor] arises from the outer side of the brain just behind the first. After passing through the orbital foramen on each side, it is distributed to the muscles of the eyeball. This nerve has been made especially thick to compensate for the softness of the structure inherited by it from the neighboring brain and to strengthen it because it has no support from any other nerve. The neighboring third nerve has itself to move a big organ like the lower jaw and has no strength to spare for others when indeed it is itself in need of some assistance.

§398 The fourth pair [trochleal] originates from the base of the brain in between the forebrain and the hindbrain. It soon joins the next pair but later on separates and divides into four branches. The first branch passes through the foramen for the common cartoid artery and descending from the neck, reaches the diaphragm where it supplies the other structures but not the diaphragm. The second branch emerges from the foramen in the temporal bone and joins with a branch of the fifth nerve to be described shortly. The third branch passes through the foramen for the second nerve and supplies the face. This does not pass through the foramen for the first nerve because it would then compress that important nerve and deprive it of its characteristic hollowness.

§399 After emerging from the foramen, this branch divides into three sub-branches. The first sub-branch supplies the outer canthus of the eye, temporal muscles, muscles of mastication, eyebrows and the upper eyelids. The second sub-branch passing through the inner canthus of the eye enters the nose to supply it with sensation. The third sub-branch, which is a short one, emerges from the small cavity of the maxillary bone and divides into three further branches. One of these is distributed inside the mouth to the teeth. The part which goes to the molar teeth can be felt and easily identified, but the part which goes to other teeth ends in the gums and cannot be distinguished. The second branch goes to the external tissues of this area, i. e. , the skin over the cheeks, the side of the nose and the upper lip. This was a sub-division of the third branch of the third nerve. The fourth branch of the third nerve emerges from the foramen in the upper jaw and is distributed to the outer side of the tongue for the taste sensation. A branch of this nerve supplies the gums of the lower teeth and the lower lip. The branch which goes to the tongue is thinner than the one which goes to the eye, so that the harder tongue may be counter balanced by a finer nerve, and the softer eye by a thicker nerve.

§400 The fifth pair [trigaminus], as mentioned earlier, arises from the base of the brain right behind the origin of the third pair. Soon after leaving the third pair, it goes to the palate to provide sensation. These nerves are smaller and harder than the third one because they have to be distributed to the palate, which has a membranous covering much harder than the surface of the tongue.

§401 The sixth pair of nevers [alidocens] arises in the hind part of the brain and is connected to the fifth pair as though they were one at first. Then they separate. A part of the nerve spreads inside the ear cavity. This part arises from the hind brain and conveys hearing. The second part is shorter than the first. It enters the foramen in the temporal bone and travels a complicated and irregular route, which makes it thicker. After emerging from the foramen, it joins the branches of the third nerve. A greater part of this nerve supplies the cheek, the flat muscle of the cheek and the temporal muscles.

§402 The seventh pair [pharynx], after arising from the hind brain, is so firmly tied to the fifth nerve with the membranous fascia that both the nerves appear as one. After travelling for some distance, it leaves the fifth nerve and emerges from the foramen at the lower end of the lambdoid suture as three branches. The first branch supplies the pharyngeal muscles and is spread into the root of the tongue where it assists the seventh nerve to strengthen movements of the tongue. The second branch goes to the shoulder and supplies its muscles and neighboring structures. A greater part of this branch is distributed below to the flat muscle of the scapula as a large thick nerve suspended from above. The third branch is the largest. It descends to the viscera from the carotid foramen and is tied there to the carotid artery.

5.5.3. The Anatomy of the Cervical Nerves and Their Paths

§403 There are eight pairs of cervical nerves arising from the spinal cord.

§404 The first pair emerges from the foramina above the first vertebra and supplies the muscles of the head. These nerves have been made short and fine because of their site.

§405 The second pair emerges from the foramina between the first and the second vertebrae as mentioned in the description of the bones. Most of the branches go to the head and give sensation to it. Part of it goes obliquely towards the upper vertebra and then curves forward to the external ear. It supplies a wider area to compensate for the smaller size of the first pair. The remaining part of the nerve controls the movement of the flat muscle at the back of the neck.

§406 The third pair, after emerging from the foramina between the second and third vertebrae, divide into two branches. One branch is distributed to the various groups of muscular fibers and especially to those between the head and the neck. From there it ascends to the spinous process of the second vertebra, which it surrounds at the root and then reaching the top, becomes attached to the membranous fascia arising from there. It then goes on to the ear in animals, but not in man, to move the ear muscles. The second branch starting from the front reaches the flat muscle of the cheek where it is joined with the blood vessels and the muscles of the area for additional strength. Occasionally, this branch goes to the muscles of the ear and temporal muscles, but more often it goes only to the muscles of the cheek.

§407 The fourth pair emerges from the foramina on the sides of the third and fourth vertebrae. Each nerve also divides like the third pair into anterior and posterior branches. The anterior branch is smaller and joins nerves of the fifth pair. Occasionally, it gives off a branch, as fine as a spider's web. It passes near the carotid artery and by coursing along the mediastinum arrives near the spinous processes of these vertebrae. From there it gives off a branch which reaches the muscles of the head and the neck. In animals, it turns back to supply the muscles of the ear and the cheek. Some physicians have described it as also going to the spinal column.

§408 The fifth pair arises from the lateral foramina between the fourth and the fifth vertebrae and each nerve divides into an anterior and a posterior branch. The anterior branch is smaller and supplies muscles of the cheek, muscles which bend the head and those which are common to the head and the neck. The other branch divides into two sub-branches, one of which passes between the two main branches and supplies the upper part of the shoulder bone. A part of this joins nerves of the sixth and the seventh pairs. The other sub-branch joins the fifth, sixth and seventh nerves and spreads over the middle of the diaphragm.

§409 The sixth and seventh pairs emerge from the foramina between the last cervical and the first thoracic vertebrae. The branches of all these pairs join each other. Most of the branches of the sixth pair supply the upper part of the shoulder. Some of its branches together with the fourth and a few branches of the fifth go to the diaphragm. Most of the branches of the seventh pair supply the arm, although one branch, after supplying the muscles of the head, neck and back, reaches the diaphragm. After uniting with the branches of the other nerves, the eighth pair reaches as far as the of the arm and forearm, but none of its branches goes to the diaphragm. The sixth pair supplies the shoulder and does not go beyond it. The seventh pair supplies the arm and ends there, but the branches of the eighth pair supply both the arm and the forearm. This pair originates from the spinal cord at the level of the first thoracic vertebra.

§410 The diaphragm is supplied by the nerves already described. The nerves which originate from lower down do not go to the diaphragm because the branches received from above give a better distribution. Moreover, an important function of those nerves is also to supply the mediastinal pleura in the upper part of the chest.

§411 If the nerves from the lower part of the spinal cord had gone to the diaphragm, they would not have taken the straight route. Nature did not supply the diaphragm with nerves coming directly from the brain because these nerves would have had to travel a considerable distance. The nerves to the diaphragm arrive at its middle. Their distribution from the sides would have been unsuitable, because the nerves would not have then taken the straight course.

§412 In the muscles, movement starts from the end and proceeds towards the center. This is also the case with the diaphragm; hence, it is essential for the nerves to the diaphragm to end at the periphery rather than start from there. Since it is essential for the nerves to be distributed from the center, the diaphragm had to be lifted up from its center. The diaphragm is protected by a covering of fascia derived from the mediastinum. As the diaphragm has to perform a very important function, it has been supplied with several nerves. Had it been supplied with a single nerve, injury to it would have caused a complete loss of function.

5.5.4. The Anatomy of the Thoracic Nerves

§413 The first pair of thoracic nerves emerges from the foramina between the first and second thoracic vertebrae. Each nerve divides into two branches. The larger branch supplies the muscles of the ribs and the spinal column, and the smaller one crosses over the upper ribs to reach the eighth pair for attachment. It then comes to the arm for supplying the forearm and the palm.

§414 The second pair emerges from near the same type of foramina and divides into two branches. One branch goes to the outer side of the arm to give it sensation. The second branch, along with the branches of the other thoracic nerves, supplies the muscles of the shoulder joint and gives out branches to the muscles of the vertebral column. The branches which emerge from the upper thoracic vertebrae supply not only muscles of the vertebral column, but also the intercostal muscles and the external muscles of the chest.

§415 The thoracic nerves, which emerge from the vertebrae attached to the smaller ribs supply the intercostal and the abdominal muscles. Arteries and veins also run parallel to the branches of these nerves and reach the spinal cord through the foramina of the corresponding nerves.

5.5.5. The Anatomy of the Lumbar Nerves

§416 Muscles of the vertebral column and the abdomen are supplied by the lumbar nerves in such a way that one branch supplies the superficial vertebral muscles and the other is distributed to the abdominal muscles and the deep muscles of the vertebral column. The three upper lumbar nerves join the nerve from the brain but not the other lumbar nerves. The lower lumbar nerves join with a branch of the third pair and a branch of the first sacral nerve to form a large nerve trunk for the legs. The two branches which have thus joined do not go beyond the hip but terminate in the muscles of this area. The larger branch goes to the leg and supplies the calf muscles. The nerves of the lower limb, unlike the nerves of the upper limb, go deeper into the thigh. This is because the femur articulates with the ischium in a different way from that of the humerus with the scapula. Moreover, the nerves for the leg arise differently from those of the arm and are thus disposed in a different manner. Also, the nerves which emerge from the sides of the pubic bone are unable to descend to the leg from the posterior or medial aspect of the thigh because of a large number of vessels and muscles being there; hence, this nerve has been made to traverse deeper in the thigh. After supplying the testicles and the pubic bone, it passes downward to supply the muscles around the knee.

5.5.6. The Anatomy of the Nerves of the Sacrum and Coccyx

§417 The first pair of the nerves from the sacrum joins with the last pair of the lumbar nerves, as described above. The remaining pairs of the sacral nerves and the coccygeal nerves emerge from the sides of the coccyx. They supply muscles of the penis, bladder, uterus and its adenexae, structures under the pubic bone and the muscles which arise from the sacrum.

5.6. The Arteries

5.6.1. A General Description of the Arteries

§**418** Pulsating vessels are known as the arteries. All arteries except one have two coats. Every artery has an inner coat which is directly affected by the pulsation and the powerful movement of the vital force which is responsible for the various functions of the body. Moreover, the artery has to be sufficiently strong to carry the vital force and to protect it. Arteries arise from the upper part of the left cavity of the heart as the right cavity is closely connected with the liver and is thus concerned with the collection and disposal of the nutritional material.

5.6.2. The Anatomy of the Venous Artery

§**419** Two vessels arise from the left side of the heart. One artery goes to the lungs and supplies them with the blood and an element of fresh air for nutrition. The heart in this case merely affords passage to the nutritive material but does not change it. The part of the heart from where this artery arises is very thin; there are also some pulmonary veins entering the heart at this very place. Contrary to the other arteries, the venous artery has only a single coat. The reason for this is: (a) this artery has to be soft and flexible; (b) its contraction and relaxation has to be easy; (c) the passage of the light, mature blood to the lungs must be easy because unlike the blood in the vena cava, this does not require further maturation from the heart—indeed, the blood which goes to the lungs from the heart, being suitable for the nutrition of the heart, should be quite suitable also for the nutrition of the lungs; and (d) this artery is in the vicinity of a very soft and delicate organ which is incapable of causing any injury to it.

§**420** Thus, there is no need for the venous artery to be as thick as the arteries which supply the harder tissues. The arterial vein which will be described later has been made thicker, although it, too, goes to the substance of the lungs, but to their posterior part on the other hand, the venous artery comes out of their anterior part. If the venous artery in regard to its strength, hardness, softness and flexibility, is compared to the arterial vein, it would be readily seen that the venous artery requires softness and flexibility and not the strength and hardness which are required by the latter for its contraction and relaxation and for the free circulation of blood. The second artery which comes out of the left side of the heart is the biggest in the body. It has been given the name of aorta by Aristotle. Soon after its origin from the heart, it gives off two branches: one, which is longer, goes around the heart and is distributed to its substance; the other supplies the muscle of the right heart. The aorta itself divides into two branches of which the lower one is the larger and the upper one smaller. The reason for the lower branch being larger is that it has to supply the organs which are larger in size and number. The largest of these organs is near the heart. At its origin, the aorta has three tough membranes directed from within outward. If there had been only one or two membranes, it would be necessary to have them thicker, but that would have produced sluggishness. If there had been four membranes instead of the normal three, they would have been so thin as to be functionally useless. If the membranes had been thicker than the normal, the lumen would have been narrowed. The venous artery has two membranes directed from within outward. Here, only two are sufficient as they do not have to be but soft and delicate for the easier exchange of air and blood in the lungs.

5.6.3. The Anatomy of the Ascending Aorta

§**421** This divides into two branches. The larger branch goes upwards towards the manubrium sterni and from there turns to the right and reaches close to the soft fleshy muscles. Here, it divides into three branches. Two of these are the carotid arteries which together with the internal jugular veins ascend on either side of the neck and give out various branches which will be described at their appropriate places. The third branch sends out smaller branches to the muscles attached to the sternum, first rib, upper six cervical vertebrae, clavicle, and the border of the scapula. It then goes to the arm and supplies the muscles there. The smaller branch of the ascending aorta goes towards the axilla and divides there in the same manner as the third branch of the larger division of the aorta does.

5.6.4. The Anatomy of the Carotid Artery

§**422** At the upper part of the neck, each carotid artery divides into an anterior and a posterior branch. The anterior branch again divides into two. The one which is deeper goes to the tongue and deep muscles of the lower jaw, and the other which is superficial, crosses in front of the ear and reaches the temporal muscles. From there, it gives off several branches to the top of the skull. These anastomose with similar branches from the opposite side. The posterior branch also divides into a larger branch and a smaller one. The smaller branch is distributed mostly to the muscles around the joints of the skull, while some of the other branches reach the base of the skull and enter through the foramen near the lambdoid suture. The larger branch higher up enters the foramen in the temporal bone. All these branches interlace with each other and form a fine network of branches which cannot be easily separated. This network is spread all over the right and the left side, and in front and behind and finally collects into two vessels which, after piercing the meninges, enter the brain and supply branches to the pia-arachnoid, the ventricles of the brain and their membrane. The finer branches of these vessels anastomose at their narrower ends with similar branches of the veins descending towards them.

§**423** The upward and the downward directions of the blood vessels are determined by the requirements of blood supply to the brain. The recipient brain has been given the best shape with its sides inclining downward. This provision is also helpful to the vital force, though being light and diffusible, it does not really require any such assistance. On the other hand, the blood which carries the vital force tends to gravitate downward when the natural tendency of the vital force is to rise upwards and reach the brain unhindered for activity on the required basis. The arterial network has been spread over the hind brain in order that the blood and the vital force may both circulate in it freely and thus get adequately matured for steady assimilation by the brain. This arterial network has been spread out between the brain and the thick fibrous membrane.

5.6.5. The Anatomy of the Descending Aorta

§**424** This runs vertically downward up to the level of the fifth thoracic vertebra opposite the apex of the heart. Here it is supported by a soft mulberry-shaped glandular tissue which lies between the aorta and the esophagus and vertebral column. Later on, the aorta shifts over to the right side and moves away from the esophagus. At its passage through the diaphragm, the aorta is fixed and surrounded by fascia to avoid constriction. In front of the fifth vertebra, the aorta shifts to the side and descends close to the vertebral column until it reaches the sacrum. While coursing through the chest, it gives off several branches, one to each rib and a small branch to the lungs and trachea. As it traverses the chest, it gives out a branch in front of each vertebra. These branches, passing between the ribs, reach the spinal cord. At the diaphragm, it gives out a branch on either side. Below the diaphragm, it sends out branches to the stomach, liver and spleen. The branch to the liver sends a sub-branch to the gallbladder. A branch is also sent to the small intestine and colon. Lower down it gives out three branches to the kidney. Of these, the smaller one supplies the capsule and substance of the kidney for their life and heat (activity); the other two absorb water from the blood. Sometimes these branches also carry impure blood from the stomach and intestine. Two branches are sent to the testes. The one which goes to the left testis is often a branch from the artery to the left kidney. Sometimes this branch may arise directly from the main vessel (aorta) from where the artery to the kidney arises. Further down, the aorta gives out two more branches for distribution around the rectum. A branch is also sent to the spinal cord through the intervertebral foramen and the same branch is sent to the hip and the bladder.

§425 In females, in addition to the branches described above, a small pair which will be described later goes to the vulva. The other branches are common to both the male and the female and finally anastomose with the veins. When the descending aorta with its accompanying veins reaches the last vertebra, it bifurcates like the Greek letter lambda into two branches, each of which goes to the sacrum and finally enters the thigh. Their further course will be described later. Before reaching the thigh, however, it gives a sub-branch, which supplies the bladder and uterus and anastomoses with the arterial branch of the opposite side. During pregnancy, these branches are quite prominent, but after childbirth they dry up, leaving behind a root which gives out a branch to supply the muscles attached to the sacrum. The branch which goes to the bladder gives off a sub-branch to supply the penis. In the female, this branch gives out two smaller branches for supplying the uterus. The artery which goes to the thigh is divided into two branches, one medial and the other lateral. The one which is lateral is inclined somewhat medially and gives out a few branches to supply the neighboring muscles.

§426 As the femoral artery descends downward, it gives out two further branches—one larger and the other smaller. The larger branch goes as far as the big toe and the first toe. The other branch remains hidden under the calf muscles and sends further branches to supply them. These course under cover of the accompanying veins which will be described later. The arteries which generally travel over the veins are the fetal artery from the liver to the umbilicus, branches of the pulmonary artery, arteries to the vertebral column up to the fifth vertebra, arteries which reach up to the suprasternal notch, axillary artery, carotid arteries and their thin branches which form the choroid plexus, arteries which supply the diaphragm, artery to the scapula and its branches, arteries which supply the liver, stomach, spleen, intestine, peritoneum and the artery which goes to the sacrum. In all these cases, the principle is that the less important structure should bear the weight of the more important one. In the superficial organs, the arteries, however, course under the veins for protection. There are two advantages in keeping the veins near the arteries: first of all, arteries provide a firm membranous attachment to the veins and secure a good covering for themselves and secondly, arteries and veins are able to interchange moisture with each other. All this was a description of the arteries.

5.7. The Veins

5.7.1. A General Description of the Veins

§427 Non-pulsating vessels are called veins. All veins emerge from the liver. Of the two main vessels, one arises from the concave side of the liver. Its chief function is to carry the nutritive material from the intestine to the liver. This vein is known as the portal vein. The other vein emerges from the convex side of the liver and carries nutrition for the other organs. It is known as the vena cava.

5.7.2. The Anatomy of the Portal Vein

§428 The portal vein has five branches which form a network of the vessels, extending from the concave side to almost near the convex side. One branch goes to the gallbladder. These branches look like the roots of a tree reentering the earth. As it enters the liver on the concave side, the vein receives eight tributaries. Two of these are smaller and six somewhat larger. One of the smaller branches draws nutritive material from the body of the pancreas. The other runs along the lower border of the stomach and receives branches from the pylorus. It draws nutritional matter from the stomach and carries it to the liver. One of the six major branches is spread over the outer surface of the stomach and gives nutrition to it.

§429 The inner surface of the stomach receives nutrition from the food which is in direct contact with it. The second branch goes to the spleen to supply nutrition, but before it reaches the spleen, it gives off a few branches to the pancreas supplying a relatively purer blood for its nutrition. After the vein has entered the spleen, it gives off a branch which turns backwards to supply nutrition to the left side of the stomach. When the branch to the spleen reaches at about the middle of this organ, it divides into two branches. The upper one provides nutrition to the upper part of the spleen, and the lower divides into smaller branches which are distributed to the fundus of the stomach. One of these supplies nutrition to the left and the outer side of the stomach, and the other enters the mouth of the stomach (cardiac end) and as already described, pours the sour black bile excretion of the spleen to stimulate appetite.

§430 The other branch to the spleen also divides into two branches: one provides nutrition to the lower half of the spleen and the other goes to supply the omentum. The third branch goes to the left side and reaches the rectum where it divides into a surrounding network of vessels which absorb nutriment from the fecal residue. The fourth branch divides into thin, hair-like branches. Some of these are spread over the right side of the stomach opposite to the branches which arising from the spleen are spread over the left side. Some of the branches are spread over the right half of the omentum opposite to those spread over the left half and received from the lower part of the spleen. The fifth branch forms a network around the colon to absorb nutritional material for transportation to the liver. The greater part of the sixth branch spreads over the jejunum, while the remainder goes to the ilium, which is next above the cecum. It absorbs nutritive material from there and brings it to the liver through the portal vein.

5.7.3. The Anatomy of the Vena Cava and its Branches

§431 The root of the vena cava is spread into the liver as fine, hair-like branches, which anastomose with similar branches of the portal vein to receive nutritive material. The branches of the vena cava enter the liver from its convex side, whereas those of the portal vein enter from the concave side. After emerging from the convex side of the liver, the vena cava divides into two branches. One goes downward, while the other ascends upwards. The latter passes through the diaphragm and gives two branches for its nutrition. On reaching the pericardium, the vena cava gives it fine, hair-like branches for nutrition. It again divides into two branches. The larger one enters the right heart. This is the biggest vessel of the heart. All other vessels supply aerated blood to the heart, while this provides nutrition. It is therefore obvious that the food material being denser than the air, it should be carried by a bigger vessel.

§432 At its place of entry into the heart, the vena cava has three tough membranes (valves), with their margins directed inward so that the heart may draw its nutritive material from the vein during diastole and prevent it from going back during systole. These membranes are the hardest in the body. Near the heart, the vena cava gives out three vessels of which one comes out of the heart and goes to the lungs. This branch first inclines towards the left side of the heart and then passing near the origin of the arteries goes into the right ventricle and finally reaches the lungs.

§433 Like the other arteries, it has two coats and is, therefore, called the arterial vein. It has two coats because it has to transmit a thin type of blood, which is quite suitable for the thin structure of the lungs and also because this blood having left the heart only recently did not have sufficient time for complete maturation, which has now to take place in this type of vessel. The second branch goes round the heart and enters its substance to provide nutrition. The entry takes place close to the place where the vena cava enters the right auricle of the heart. The third branch in the human being usually goes to the left and then after reaching the fifth vertebra is distributed to the lower eight ribs, their muscles and other connected structures.

§434 After giving out the three branches mentioned above, the vena cava ascends upwards and passing by the side of the heart gives out hair-like, fine branches to the mediastinal membrane, pericardium and the supportive glandular tissue. Near the clavicle, it gives out two more branches which obliquely travel away from it. Each of these gives out two more branches. One goes by the side of the sternum and ends at the xiphoid cartilage; on its way, it gives out further branches which anastomose with the blood vessels in the muscles of the ribs and some branches supply the external muscles of the chest.

§435 On reaching the xiphoid cartilage, they let out a few more branches which are spread out into the muscles of the scapula. A few branches are sent to the rectus of the abdomen and a terminal branch goes downward to anastomose with the branches of the sacral vein which will be described later. The other branch is a pair with each blood vessel giving out five branches. The first branch goes to the chest and supplies nutrition to the upper four ribs. The second branch supplies nutrition to the shoulder muscles. The third branch supplies nutrition to the deep muscles of the neck. The fourth branch enters the foramina of the upper six cervical vertebrae and reaches the head. The fifth, which is the largest branch, goes to the axilla and divides into four sub-branches; the first spreads into the sternal muscles which move the shoulder, the second goes into the axillary glands and fascia. The third passes from the side of the chest to reach the hypochondrium and the fourth, which is the largest of these, further divides into three branches. Of these, one goes to the deep muscles of the scapula, the other supplies the big muscle of the axilla and the third, which is the largest, passes down from the upper arm to the hand. This is known as the axillary vein. After its division into the above mentioned branches, the remaining part of the vein goes to the neck, where it immediately divides into two further branches. One of these is the external jugular vein.

§436 The external jugular vein divides into two branches near the clavicle. The first branch immediately becomes superficial and turns to the side. The second branch comes forward and descends immediately downward. It then ascends upwards and appears above the clavicle. It goes round the clavicle and ascends upwards to unite with the first branch to become the external jugular vein. Before the two join together to form the external jugular, the vein gives out two more branches. The first branch travels horizontally to join the branch from the opposite side in the supra-sternal notch between the two clavicles. The second branch travels obliquely outward in the neck and does not join its opposite number. It gives off branches which are so minute that they cannot be easily seen. The second pair has many branches, but only three are sufficiently thick and prominent. One of these goes towards the scapula and is known as the scapular vein which gives out the cephalic vein. Two branches of the scapular vein reach the shoulder. One of these is distributed there and the other ends at the upper part of the arm. The scapular vein finally reaches the hand and is distributed there.

§437 The external jugular, soon after its emergence, branches into two. One branch goes deep and subdivides into two. One of these goes deeper and divides into several branches of which the smaller ones go to the upper jaw and the bigger ones to the lower jaw. Some of the other smaller and bigger branches are spread as a network around the tongue and its superficial muscle. The second branch of the external jugular is distributed to the ear and the head. The internal jugular vein ascends upwards by the side of the esophagus and gives off a few branches which join the branches of the external jugular and are distributed to the esophagus, trachea and deep muscles of this area. The terminal part of the internal jugular vein near the lambdoidal suture gives out several branches which are distributed to the structures around the first and the second cervical vertebrae.

§438 A thin vein comes out of the internal jugular vein near the junction of the head and the neck. It gives a few branches to the membranous lining of the skull. They pierce the thin membranes of the brain and spread out into branches which go side by side with the arterial branches and help to bind them across the irregular surfaces of the thick membrane over the brain. After this, the vein reaches a spacious place (sinus) under the occiput where the blood arrives from various sides. This place lies in between the two parts of the brain and arriving near the middle ventricle of the brain, widens to receive the blood from the veins of both sides. At about the middle of the brain, they reach the front and anastomose with the arterial branches that have ascended to this part of the brain. Afterwards, they form a network, which is known as the choroid plexus.

5.7.4. The Anatomy of the Veins of the Arms

§439 The cephalic vein in the arm gives off a few branches to the skin and its superficial structures. At the level of the elbow joint, it divides into three branches. The first branch is known as the accessory cephalic. Its branches spread over the outer side of the radius and after passing over the convex side of the ulna are finally distributed to the lower and outer part of the wrist. The second branch appears at the outer side of the forearm at the level of the elbow joint. It joins with a branch of the axillary vein to form the median cubital vein. The third branch goes deeper into the tissues to unite with a branch of the auxiliary vein. The axillary vein gives off a branch which goes deeper into the upper arm and spreads into the neighboring muscles. It also gives out a branch which goes to the wrist.

§440 When the axillary vein reaches the elbow, it divides into two branches. One branch goes deep into the arm and joins with the deep branch of the cephalic vein. These two branches travel together for some distance and then separate. One of these goes inward and downward until it reaches the little, the ring and the half of the middle finger. A branch from this vein turns upwards and is distributed to the various tissues between the bones of the hand. The second main branch of the axillary vein divides into four branches. The first branch goes to the lower part of the forearm and ends near the wrist. The second, like the first, spreads out with more branches. The third branch is distributed in the same way, but in the middle of the forearm. The fourth branch is the largest of all. It is quite superficial and gives out a branch which joins the cephalic vein and thus forms the basilic vein.

§441 The basilic vein and the median vein join the deep hidden cubital vein. The medial cubital vein starts from the medial side of the forearm and reaches the radius. It deviates laterally and bifurcates like /\—the Greek letter lambda. The upper branch goes towards the radius. It reaches the wrist and spreads over the back of the thumb and is distributed between the thumb and the index finger. The lower branch goes towards the ulna and divides into three branches. One of these is distributed between the index and the middle fingers. It also joins with a branch of the upper one and is distributed between the thumb and the index finger. All these branches join together to form a single vein. The second branch lies between the middle and the ring fingers. The third branch spreads between the ring and the little fingers. Thus, all the three branches fan out towards the fingers.

5.7.5. The Anatomy of the Inferior Vena Cava

§442 The superior vena cava which has already been described is relatively smaller than the inferior vena cava. The inferior vena cava arises from the liver. Before reaching the vertebral column to receive support, it gives out delicate, hair-like branches to the capsule and the substance of the right kidney for nutrition. A bigger branch is sent to the left kidney. This divides into minute, hair-like branches for the capsule and substance of the left kidney. The inferior vena cava also sends out two larger branches to the kidney for the purification of blood. The kidneys separate out the water containing waste products and receive their own nutrition from the blood. Sometimes, the left renal vein sends a branch to the left testis in both the male and the female in the way described under the heading of arteries. It should not, however, be mistaken that the females have no testes.

§443 It should also be understood clearly that the testes receive their veins directly from the veins of the kidneys. The vein for the left testis comes from the vein to the left kidney, but some branches come out from both veins of the kidneys. The vein to the right testis is generally a separate one but sometimes, though rarely, it is from the right renal vein. There is also a passage between the kidneys and the testes in which the semen matures and changes its color from red to white. It has an extremely convoluted and circuitous course. Some veins reach the testes from the spinal column as described in the section on the arteries. After giving out the renal veins and the other branches, the inferior vena cava descends in front of the vertebral column and gives out branches, one to each vertebra for supplying the vertebral and neighboring muscles. Some branches are spread across the ilium and terminate in the muscles of the abdomen. Afterwards, it gives off some more branches which enter through the vertebrae and reach the spinal cord. It finally divides into two veins at the level of the last lumbar vertebra. These veins are at first close to each other, but later on gradually diverge to enter the thigh.

§444 Before entering the thigh, each vein gives out ten

branches. The first branch is spread into the muscles of the back. The second divides into minute, hair-like branches which are distributed under the peritoneum. The third spreads into the muscles attached to the sacrum. The fourth supplies the muscles of the rectum and the sacrum. The fifth branch in the female supplies the vagina and its neighboring structures. It also gives out a branch for the bladder, which divides into a branch for the fundus and a branch for the neck of the bladder. In the male, this branch is bigger and goes to the penis. The sixth branch is distributed to the muscles over the pubic bone. The seventh branch spreads into the rectus muscle of the abdomen and anastomoses with the veins from the chest; both spread over the hypochondrium as already described. In the female, the main vessel gives out further branches. Some of these go to the uterus and some branches ascend to reach the mammary glands. It is these veins which establish a relationship between the mammary glands and the uterus. The eighth branch is distributed to the external genitalia of both the male and the female. The ninth branch goes into the deeper muscles of the thigh. The tenth branch runs along the ureter and goes to the outer part of the iliac bone and anastomoses with the terminal branches of the veins which come from the mammary gland.

§445 A large branch goes to the muscles of the testis and divides into several branches which reach the thigh. One of these goes in front, while another goes to the deep muscles of the thigh. The remaining branches go into the various other deep muscles of the thigh. When the femoral vein reaches the knee, it divides into three veins. The outer vein passes across the fibula and reaches near the ankle. The middle vein descends below the knee joint and gives off two branches to the deep muscles of the calf. One of these disappears in these muscles while the other descends downward between the tibia and fibula and arrive near the ankle. Where it anastomoses with the outer vein described above. The third branch which is medial proceeds towards the calf from where it turns towards the convex side of the tibia and the ankle. This runs medially and in front it becomes the saphenous vein and divides into four branches. Two of these branches are on the outer side. They descend along the side of the fibula and reach the foot. The other two branches are on the inner side: one of these goes in front of the foot and is distributed to the upper part of the little toe, and the other branch joins with the outer branch and goes to the deeper structures. All the veins have been described in detail.

§446 An essential description of the simple organs has also been given. The anatomy of the compound organs will be described when their diseases and treatment are discussed. Now the discussion of the faculty or drives follows.

Lecture 6: General Physiology

6.1. A General Description of the Types of Faculties or Drives

§447 Faculties or drives (or psycho-physical forces) are to be distinguished from functions. The difference is that faculties or drives originate functions. However, as each function depends on its own special faculty or drive, they can be treated together.[1]

§448 There are three kinds of faculties or drives in the body and also three types of functions arising from them: vital (*haywaniyya*), natural or vegetative (*tabiyya*), and sensitive or animal (*nafsaniyah*).[2]

§449 Many philosophers and all physicians who follow Galen consider that each faculty or drive has its own principal organ which forms its storehouse and from which its functions emerge. In this view the rational faculty or drive resides in the brain and its functions proceed from the brain.

§450 The natural or vegetative faculty or drive is of two kinds: (1) One is concerned with the preservation of the individual and is responsible for his nutrition and growth. This is located in the liver and its functions emerge from there. (2) The other is the reproductive faculty or drive which pertains to the generation and preservation of the race and is responsible for sexual functions like the formation of germinal fluid and its fertilization of the ovum into the specific form ordained by the Almighty Creator. This faculty or drive is located in the generative organs and its functions proceed from them.

§451 The animal, faculty or drive consists of perception and motivation. Perception contains five external and five internal senses. The vital faculty or drive preserves the integrity of the breath. It allows the breath able to receive these impressions. Having reached the brain makes it capable of imparting life and then spreads in every direction.

§452 Aristotle, the great philosopher regards the heart as the real source of all the faculties or drives, the principal organs being employed (by the heart) for expressing various functions. Similar is the case with the brain which is the center of all sensation but needs the eyes to see and the ears to hear. It is in this sense that the brain is the center of these functions. But physicians still maintain the opinion that the brain is the chief seat of sentient life, and that each sense has its own distinct member whereby it manifests function. As regards the verification of this truth, physicians should better leave this question properly to the philosophers and physicists and accept these as formulated principles. So long as one looks at the problem more as a physician than a philosopher, it is immaterial whether all systems are centered in the heart or each has its own corresponding center. Knowledge on these matters is of course essential for philosophers, and it would be considered a piece of ignorance if they did not understand them.

6.2. The Natural or Vegetative Faculty or Drive

§453 The natural or vegetative faculty or drive consists of dominant or directing and subservient or obedient faculties or drives. There are two dominant, natural or vegetative faculties or drives. The first is concerned with the preservation of the life of the individual—the nutritive and augmentative power of growth. The second is concerned with the preservation of the race—the generative and formative or plastic natural faculty or drive.[3]

6.3. The Faculties or Drives Pertaining to the Preservation of the Life of the Individual

§454 Nutrition alters the food in such a way that it becomes temperamentally akin to the body, and is thus rendered suitable for the repair of daily wear and tear of the tissues. The faculty or drive of growth develops the organs in their appropriate spatial relationships and integrates the nutritive material according to the requirements of the individual growth.

Nutrition serves the natural faculty or drive of growth by providing the necessary nutriment. Sometimes the quantity of nutriment may be sufficient only for the day to day needs of repair, but at times it may be more or less than the daily requirements. Growth is, however, possible only when the quantity of nutriment is in excess of the actual requirements. But this would not always produce growth. Thus, after the completion of normal growth, there may be increase of weight, that is, after the recovery from some wasting disease, but this would not constitute growth. Growth is an increase of size within the limits of the normal physical proportions and it can only occur before the completion of full development. Similarly, during the period of growth there may be loss of weight but no reduction in the dimensions of the body, unless of course, this be the result of some special disease.

§455 Nutrition consists of three special functions: (1) Absorption or apposition of the altered material, namely, the blood or a humor which is potentially like the tissue to be nourished. If this process is defective, as may happen in disease, there is “atrophy,” which is a defect of nutrition. (2) Assimilation or agglutination—a later stage. Here the nutriment apposed to the tissue is now fully united up to it and made a part of it. This may be lacking owing to disease and then what happens is called “fleshy dropsy.” (3) Formation or true assimilation—a stage still further where that which has been made into a part of a member becomes absolutely like it in all respects, in essence and color.

§456 That is, the formative process, though essentially the same throughout the organism, acts differently than organs of the body according to the requirements of their special structures and appearances. Thus, every organ has its own natural faculty or drive according to its temperament which enables it to acquire its own distinctive color and pattern by making suitable changes in its nutritive material. This fails in such conditions as leprosy and vitilego in which case the first two functions are achieved, but not the third.

§457 These three functions are the work of the transformative power. This is really a single faculty or drive although it is distributed among the respective members. For in every organ this faculty or drive corresponds to its temperament, and so transforms the digestive material into the likeness of that organ. In each case it differs from that which transforms the digestive material into the likeness of the various other organs or tissues. So we may say the transformative faculty of the liver ramifies throughout the whole body.

6.4. The Faculties or Drives Pertaining to the Preservation of the Race

§458 The generative faculty or drive is twofold: (1) reproductive—this serves the race and is responsible for the formation of male and female "sperm" (the reproductive units); (2) the formative power (that is, the male element), which separates from one another the various faculties in the sperm and rearranges them in such a way that each organ (and tissue) receives the temperament appropriate to it. That is, to the nerve, its distinctive temperament and to the bone, its distinctive temperament. The one "sperm," apparently homogeneous, opens out in all these directions. This is called the primary transformative faculty.

§459 Inherent in the informative or plastic faculty or drive in the female element is the plastic process which, as ordained by the beloved and exalted Creator, gives shape and appearance to the various organs and develops them complete with cavities and foramina in their appropriate spatial relationships and also produces the proper degree of smoothness, roughness, etc.[5]

6.5. The Faculties or Drives Subservient to the Natural Drive

§460 With the vegetative life or the natural faculties or drives, the real secondary faculties or drives are the various processes which assist nutrition which are fourfold: attraction,[6] retention (or maturation, *masikah*), digestion [ferment actions of the body], and elimination.

§461 The attraction or receptive process draws suitable or apparently suitable material inside the body for nutrition. It is served by longitudinal fibers. The liver attracts the chyle from the stomach by sucking, as it were, the purer parts through the mesenteric veins.

§462 The retentive process retains the food while the alterative (transformative) faculty or drive is engaged in preparing sound nutritive substances from it. It generally acts through the oblique but sometimes also through the transverse fibers.

§463 The digestive process is that which alters the material attracted and held by the two above drives. It transmutes the material from its former state until it works up into a temperament such as enables it to become efficient nutrient material. This process is "digestion" in the strict sense. At the same time, it produces a change in the superfluities so that they can be easily discharged from the organ containing them. This process is called "maturation" (that is, the liquefaction of the waste products for proper elimination). Through it three things happen: (1) the texture of the superfluities becomes attenuated when it is inspissation that hinders expulsion; (2) the texture of the superfluities becomes thickened when it is attenuation that prevents their discharge; (3) the superfluities are entirely broken up if it be viscidity that hinders expulsion. It is a mistake to use the terms "digestion" and "maturation" as synonymous.

§464 The eliminative process is concerned with the elimination of the non-nutritive excremental matters left over from the digestion of food, the nutritive material taken in excess of nutritional requirements and the material which, having served its purpose, is no longer required like water which is eliminated in the urine. The waste matter is expelled through the natural channels of excretion, that is, the urinary tract for the excretion of urine and large intestine for the elimination of feces. When, however, these routes are not available, waste matter is diverted either from a superior to an inferior organ or from a hard organ to a soft one. The principle of nature is that when excrements are tending to eliminate through the normal channels, the system helps rather than hinders their elimination, that is, black bile is eliminated through vomiting.

§465 Interrelation between the faculties or drives and the qualities. The four physical faculties or drives are served by the four primary qualities—heat, cold, dryness and moisture. Heat is the underlying factor in all the subservient faculty or drives.

§466 The action of cold serves all four faculties or drives but only indirectly except in so far as it is the contrary of all the faculties or drives. All the faculties or drives act by virtue of movement which is shown not only as attraction and expulsion, but even in the transformative process (digestion proper); for the latter consists in the separation of gross and aggregated particles from one another, and in the condensation together of the finer and separated particles. The movements of dispersion and aggregation are simultaneous. Movement is also concerned indirectly in the retentive faculty or drive because the transverse muscular fibers come into play. Coldness enfeebles, stupefies, and mortifies, and hinders this faculty or drive in all its functions; yet indirectly it helps it by fixing the fibers in the position referred to. Therefore it is not directly concerned with the faculties or drives. It simply causes their instruments to be in a state which will help to maintain their functions.

§467 Cold helps expulsion by: (1) increasing the density of gases; (2) by keeping the particles of the digested material as coarse; (3) and by its astringent action upon the transverse muscular fibers. This action being preparatory, may be regarded as an indirect help. In short, cold helps the faculties or drives indirectly. If it had been concerned directly, there would have been no movement at all and the real purpose would have been completely defeated.

§468 The action of dryness is directly instrumental in the functions of two faculties or drives—transformation and retention. It is secondary and auxiliary in the case of the other two—attraction and expulsion. This is because dryness delays the movement of the breath enabling it to take on with it those faculties or drives which it has encountered with a vehement impact. It also prevents the moisture present in the substance of the breath or its instrument from flowing away. Dryness helps the retentive drive because it favors muscular contraction (that is, upon the contents of the organ). The transformative drive needs moisture (and not dryness). The action of moisture, on the other hand, hinders strong and free movement by unduly relaxing the fibers. Dryness serves the retentive process by increasing the contractility of the fibers. This is, however, of little use to digestion.

§469 Comparative relations between the qualities and the drives. If one compares the degree of active [heat, cold] and passive [dry, wet] quality needed for the various drives, one finds that the retentive drive needs more dryness than heat. This is because more time is required for a movement to come to rest than is needed to start the transverse fibers to move in contraction.

§470 Heat is necessary for movement and it takes only a short time to produce its effect so that the remainder of the time is occupied in holding the material and coming to a state of rest. This explains why the temperament of children tends to moistness for their digestive power is weaker.

§471 The attractive drive needs more heat than dryness because the main feature of attraction is movement and movement needs heat. The organs concerned must move rather than be at rest and contracted which requires dryness. This drive, however, does not require much movement although at times violent activity becomes necessary. (1) Attraction is brought about by an attractive faculty or drive—as when a magnet attracts iron; (2) by heat as when oil is drawn up in a lamp. Some physicists say that the last-named is really an example of filling up of a vacuum. Heat increase the power of attraction exerted by the attractive drive.

§472 The expulsive process requires less dryness than the attractive and retentive process because there is not the need of the muscular contraction requisite for retention nor for the apposition necessary for attraction nor a need to maintain contraction upon an object until the next stage of the process is reached. Nor is there a need for rest, but, on the contrary, there is a need of movement and also a small amount of inspissation, just enough to insure that degree of compression and expulsion which is necessary to make the contracted viscous an instrument. Lastly, whereas the retentive faculty requires a long period of time and the attractive power only a short period—namely that necessary to bring one thing in contact with another—so there is less need of dryness.

§473 The digestive drive requires more heat than the other three. It does not need dryness but moisture for by moisture the nutrients are rendered fluid and so become able to enter the pores and become molded into the conformation of the channels to be traversed. But one must not suppose that because moisture aids digestion, children (whose temperament is moist) can digest hard or indigestible foods. This can be done in youth, but here the reason is not to be found in their moisture. It is because at that period of life, their nature is similar to that of the foods in question. Foods of a hard nature are not appropriate for the temperament of children (which is soft) and therefore their transformative drive cannot cope with such food. Their retentive drive cannot hold it and their expulsive drive rapidly expels it. In the case of young people, on the other hand, such hard food is quite suitable for nourishment.

§474 The attractive drive has a quite short duration of muscular contraction and a marked amount of longitudinal movement achieved; the retentive drive has a long, continued duration of muscular contraction and a moderate amount of longitudinal movement achieved; the alternative drive has a continued duration of muscular contraction and no amount of longitudinal movement achieved; the expulsive drive has a momentary duration of muscular contraction and a considerable, but super added from without, amount of longitudinal movement achieved.[7]

§475 Therefore the various drives make use of these four qualities in diverse ways and to different extents.[8]

6.6. The Vital Faculty or Drive

§476 The power which the organs receive before they can acquire the capacity for the drives of sensation and movement and for accomplishing the various functions of life is called the vital drive. Closely related to this subject is that of the breath and therefore also of the emotions of fear and anger because they coincide with the expansion and contraction of the breath.[9]

§477 This brief description needs to be further amplified by saying that while the dense structure—organs and their various tissues—are formed of the heavier portions of the humors of the corresponding temperament, the "breath" or vital force is formed of the light and vapory part of the humors of corresponding temperament.

§478 The liver is concerned with the production of the former (the heavier portions of the humors), while the heart serves as the center of the production for the latter (the light and vapory parts of the humors). As soon as the breath and the appropriate temperament meet, the vital power comes into being and thus all the members are rendered capable of receiving all the other drives of the soul—sensation and otherwise. The drives of sensation do not appear in the breath and organs until this vital power has come into being and so even should the drives of sensation in a given organ be lost, life will remain in the part until the vital power has forsaken it. Does one not find in practice how a limb is devoid of sensation from paralysis (whether as a result of a temperament which renders it incapable of receiving sensation or showing movement, or because of some obstruction to the current from the brain and nerves into the limb) yet continues to live? And does one not find that a limb which has lost the vital power loses also sensation and movement, dies, and undergoes putrescence and decomposes? That shows that the power which renders an organ living is still there even in the paralyzed member so that sensation and movement would return again if the obstruction could be removed. In fact, the intact possession of this vital power makes the limb always ready to receive the attributes in question. That which obstructs these attributes does not interfere with the power of receiving vital breath; the member itself is not dead.

§479 Also, it is not the nutritive drive that prepares a member for receiving sensation and motion. It is not the nutritive drive that is fundamental for the life of an organ. One cannot say that an organ perishes as soon as the nutritive drive is gone. The statements just made about a paralyzed limb apply equally to the nutritive drive. For sometimes the nutritive drive ceases in a member and still the member continues to live. Sometimes the nutritive drive is unimpaired and nevertheless the member tends towards death. Then again, if it be the nutritive drive which provides the power of sensation and movement, should not plants also share in these powers?

§480 Therefore it is clear that there is something else preparing the organs for these powers, something akin in temperament to itself—and this something is the vital drive. This is that drive which appears in the breath at the very moment at which the breath develops out of the rarefied particles of the humors. As the philosopher Aristotle says—from the moment the breath receives its first beginning and all the other drives flow out from it. Not that the activities of these drives are directly derived from the breath any more than the sensation proceeds from the animal breath in the brain until the sense-impression has passed the crystalline lens or the tongue or the other sense-organs. It is when the particular portion of the breath reaches the appropriate parts of the brain that it becomes impressed with the temperament of the brain and thereby becomes adapted for the operations of the faculties proceeding from and reposing in it. The same applies in the case of the liver and reproductive organs.

§481 Physicians, however, believe that unless the vital force on reaching the brain acquires an altogether new temperament, it would not be able to function as a source of sensation and movement. This is so with the liver, too. In other words just as the vital force is primarily differentiated in the heart into the vital faculty or drive, in other organs it is differentiated into their appropriate faculties or drives.[10] Thus, according to them, the various individual functions are differentiated by their own respective 'soul,' rather than by a common one as the philosophers believe.

§482 The primary differentiation of the vital force into the vital faculty or drive occurs as an end product with its own vital energy and its own faculty or drive. But the physicians believe that the appearance of this faculty or drive does not necessarily lead to the differentiation of the other faculties or drives unless the vital force acquires a new appropriate disposition for each of these faculties or drives.

§483 If the primary temperament helps the breath to receive the primary drive, then the vital powers, the breath and the drives are its perfection. The primary vital drive is not sufficient by itself to enable the breath to respond to the other drives, but needs an appropriate temperament first. The physicians also claim that this drive, besides paving the way for "life," itself initiates the movement of the attenuated spiritual substance (the breath, that is) towards the various organs and is the agent which brings about the contraction and expansion of respiration and pulse. When it assists life, it is "passion." When it assists the activity and functions of mind and pulse, it is "action."

§484 The vital drive resembles the natural or vegetative faculty or drive in that its actions are beyond the scope of the will. It resembles the animal (sensitive) drive in carrying out contrary actions in that it expands or dilates and contracts at one and the same time effecting two contrary movements at once.

§485 When the ancient philosophers use the word "soul" (*nafs*), they refer to the earthly or corporeal soul, the perfection of the corporeal body, which is its instrument. It is the source of all those drives upon which the movements and various bodily operations depend. The natural drive in medicine thus corresponds to the animal drive in philosophy. The soul is not understood in this sense but is the power which originates understanding and voluntary movement. In philosophy, the natural drive means every drive from which any bodily function proceeds. But this is not the animal drive of medicine but a natural drive of a higher order than that named natural in medicine. So if natural drive is defined as that which is concerned in nutrition, whether for the preservation of the individual or of the race, then another and third term would be required to represent this other drive. Anger, fear, and similar emotions are passions of this same drive and admittedly arise from the senses, the judgment and the apprehensive drives.[11]

Lecture 7: The Breath: Its Origin, Forms, Sources and Relation to Being

7.1. General Remarks

§**486** God created the left side of the heart and made it hollow in order that it should serve both as a storehouse of the breath and as the seat of manufacture of the breath. He also created the breath to enable the drives of the "soul' to be conveyed into the corresponding members. In the first place the breath was to be the rallying-point for the faculties of the soul and in the second place it was to be an emanation into the various members and tissues of the body (whereby these could manifest the functions of those drives).

§**487** Now He produced the breath out of the finer particles of the humors and out of heat and dryness (fire) and at the same time produced the tissues themselves (the visible body) out of the coarser and cold and dry (earthy) particles of these humors. In other words, the breath is related to the attenuated particles as the body is related to the coarser particles of the same humors. Just as the humors are intermingled to produce a temperamental "form," whereby the members of the body are enabled to receive a physical appearance, impossible were they separate, so the attenuated portions of the humors, being intermingled into a temperamental form, enable the breath to receive the powers of the soul—impossible were the humors separate.

§488 The beginning of the breath is as a divine emanation from potentiality to actuality proceeding without intermission or stint until the form (preparation, state) is completed and perfected. Each member, though derived from the self-same substance of the humors, nevertheless has its own particular temperament—for the proportional qualities of the (denser portions of the) humors and the form of their commixture are peculiar to each member. Similarly, although derived from the same attenuated portions of the humors, nevertheless each of the three breaths (natural, animal and vital) has its own particular temperament, because the proportional quantities of the more attenuated portions of the humors and the manner of their commixture are peculiar to each breath.

§489 Although the body consists of several organs, there is one from which they all originally arose. As to what this organ actually was, there are various opinions. The fact remains that one organ necessarily came to light before other organs could arise out of it. Exactly the same is true in the case of the breaths. There is one single breath which accounts for the origin of the others. This breath, according to the most important philosophers, arises in the heart, passes thence into the principal centers of the body, lingering in them long enough to enable them to impart to it their respective temperamental properties. Lingering in the cerebrum it receives a temperament whereby it is capable of receiving the drives of sensation and movement; in the liver, it receives the drive of nutrition and growth (vegetative drives); in the generative glands it acquires a temperament which prepares it for receiving the drive of generation (reproduction).

§490 The foundation or beginning of all these drives is traceable to the heart as is agreed upon even by those philosophers who think that the source of visual, auditory and gustatory power lies in the brain.

§491 Some philosophers consider that the breath is made able to receive these drives and so be perfected in other organs than those named. Thus, visual power results from the union of the temperament of the breath with the moist temperament of the crystalline lens, that the auditory power results from the union thereof with the temperament of the auditory nerve; that gustatory power is produced by the mediation of the moist temperament afforded by the soft spongy sub-lingual glands.

§492 Others reject this view and consider that the earth carries the faculty or drives from the brain and receives nothing from the temperament of the member to which it travels, as nothing is necessary to perfect it. The member itself is an instrument well adapted for the action of the vegetative drive and contributes nothing of its own essence.[1]

7.2. The Nature of the Breath and Its Purpose

§493 Life and every perfection and every goods for which creatures are destined, comes from nothing but the primal Truth—the source of all good and from the strong desire ever proceeding therefrom

§494 Nevertheless, the recipient thereof requires a specific capacity for reception of the good. A creature cannot receive indifferently. For instance, wool cannot be wool (lit., half the "form" of wool) and at the same time have the character of a sword. Water cannot be water (lit., have the "form" of water) and at the same time receive the "form" of human nature.

§495 All corporeal bodies may receive life, except the four first principles, and whatever is of like nature to them. For these are non-living bodies, and are also of negligible bulk. In fact their bulk is infinitesimal compared with the planets, and still more strikingly so compared with some of the fixed stars. Indeed it can be shown that these first principles in their totality have not as much bulk as a point compared with the body of Saturn; how mulch less then are they when compared with the higher bodies?

§496 Those who realize the Truth know the reason why these elementary bodies do not receive the "form" of life. Even the simplest of living beings is quite different from them; and the celestial bodies, adapted as they are to a very wonderful kind of corporeal life, are very different from them also. The first-principles are entirely beyond the possibility of life.[1]

§497 It is the mingling of substances in the compound bodies which accounts for their ability to receive life. The commingling of the components so modifies their contrarieties (see §20) as to produce an ensemble (i.e., the temperament, see §27), in which all the various seeming contraries [nothing is really absolutely contrary to anything else—a typical Sufi concept] are blended harmoniously. The more harmonious the blending, the more adapted is the resultant compound for being the vehicle, not merely of life, but of a very particular kind of life. Perfect equilibrium and perfect balance renders possible the manifestation of the perfection of rational life which celestial beings possess. And it is just this kind of character which is to be found in the case of the human breath!

§498 The breath, then, is that which emerges from a mixture of first principles, and approaches towards the likeness of celestial beings. It is a luminous substance. It is a ray of light.

§499 This accounts for the fact that the mind rejoices when it looks towards the light, and is depressed when exposed to darkness. Light is in harmony with the breath. Darkness is in discord with it.

7.3. The Common Emotions in Relation to the Vital Breath: Their First Causes: Potentiality and Disposition

§500 Sages and those physicians who agree with them, are satisfied that joy and sadness, fear and anger, are passions peculiarly; related to the breath of the heart. Each of these emotions is maintained or discontinued: (1) by the agent [in the scholastic sense]; (2) by the persistence or cessation of the disposition exhibited by the substance of the patient.

§501 Sages perceive a subtle distinction between potentiality and disposition.[2]

7.3.1. Joy and the Causes of Delight and Sadness

§502 Joy is a form of delight. A thing is delightful when it is the perfection of its corresponding faculty or drive. For instance, the perception of a sweet or sapid taste or a pleasant fragrance; the overruling of a feeling of anger by a good judgment; the realization of some useful outcome of the reasoning or imaginative drive.

§503 There is a certain power accruing from every perfected delight. It is the perfection of the given power which produces joy.[3]

§504 Some people have expressed the opinion that delight is really nothing but the departure of abnormal disposition, and that there cannot possibly be delight where there is no possibility of going beyond the natural disposition. This view has arisen because there are some forms of power which cannot bring delight until some abnormal disposition has first been eliminated. Nevertheless this opinion is wrong; it takes a thing which is an accident for a thing per se—a fallacy of reasoning which is mentioned in "the definitions."

§505 Delight[4] implies attaining a goal, and the one who apprehends it can only be aware of the delight because he is aware of the change. For instance: (1) in the case of touch, it is evident that the quality of tangibility can only provide delight as long as the tactile organ continues to be in the opposite phase. Once the polarity has reached equilibrium, the character of the organ will have become "setup" and cannot provide further change. From this time there ceases to be any sensation of pleasure. (2) In the case of the hectic patient who does not suffer from heat subjectively however high the body temperature may be, a patient with an acute fever may feel hotter than the other even though his temperature be not so high. This is because in the hectic case, heat is already resident in tissues of the corresponding constitution; in acute fevers, it is as if the heat flew past, afraid of the manner in which it may find the elements mingled in the tissues. Doctors rightly consider the state of the members of a hectic case as "bad, though balanced," and in the other case regard the quality as "unbalanced and therefore bad."

§506 It is clear then that pleasure ceases as soon as one is accustomed to the completed sense perception because one can now no longer be aware of the entry of sense perceptions. The reason why pleasure is experienced at the departure of an abnormal disposition is that one is now sensitive to the slightest change in the now normal disposition. It is possible that this sensitiveness to change in the natural disposition may appear synchronously with the departure of the abnormal disposition.

§507 People are then apt to think the latter was the cause of the former when it is not so. The real explanation lies in the attainment of perfect perception. It is this that is the intrinsic basis of delight.[5]

§508 In other words, the disposition towards delight depends on the constitution of the participating breaths, and on the degree to which the disposition is favorable to their presence always provided that the substance of the breath is not diminished, and the disposition likely to be favorable is not an abnormal one.

§509 The effect of quantity of breath—should a breath with a tendency towards delight be abundant, its action will be correspondingly powerful, the greater its vigor, and the greater is the amount of it which will persist at the place of its origin—that is, in its "matrix." Consequently, under these circumstances it will radiate out in greater measure to the various members and produce that particular state of expansion which spells joy and pleasure. For, if the breath in question were only moderate in amount, the substrate concerned would hold it greedily, and not allow it to expand as freely as otherwise would be the case.

§510 The effect of the quality of the breath—the more noble the character possessed by it and the more noble its substance, the more luminous does it become, and the more like celestial substance will it be.[6]

§511 Such, then, are the various points about the tendency towards pleasure and joy. As regards sorrow and grief, it is just a question of the converse. Once the general sources of delight and pleasure are thoroughly grasped, the sources of joy become intelligible, since joy is a form of delight.

§512 By way of summary, it may be said that when the breath residing in the heart is plentiful (as it is when there is plenty of that material from which it is rapidly and constantly being generated); when it is balanced in temperament; when it has a luminous, beautiful and bright substance then there is a strong tendency to joy.

§513 When the breath is scanty (as occurs in convalescents, in long-standing illnesses, and in elderly persons); when it is not balanced in character (as in morbid states); and when it is: (a) very dense and coarse in substance (as in melancholy and elderly people), it cannot arouse joy; (b) very delicate in substance (as in convalescents and in women), it will not allow of expansion; and (c) confused (as in melancholy people). In all these cases there is a very strong tendency to depression, sadness and grief.[7]

7.3.2. The External Causes of Delight and Sadness

§514 When all the conditions required for a given act are present, the slightest agent will now suffice to effect the act. Thus, when sulphur is used for kindling, it is because sulphur is set afire by a moderate amount of heat, whereas wood cannot be made to burn without twice as much. So, when the mind has a breath whose tendency to receive the impress of gladdening agents is complete, a slight agent will suffice to evoke gladness.

§515 The action of wine on emotions and on breath—this is shown in the instance of those who drink excellent wine, for in such persons gladness increases to such a pitch that onlookers wonder how they can be jovial without reason. Such a thing, of course, cannot be. No impression is possible without an impresser.

§516 But the fact is that when wine is taken in moderation, it gives rise to a large amount of breath, whose character is balanced, and whose luminosity is strong and brilliant. Hence wine disposes greatly to gladness, and the person is subject to quite trivial exciting agents. The breath now takes up the impression of agents belonging to the present time more easily than it does those which relate to the future; it responds to agents conducive to delight rather than those conducive to a sense of beauty. It also takes up an impression from agents which are prone to evoke conjecture rather than from those which are concerned with real understanding. The explanation of this is that normally the power of the mind brings about an act in the brain such as will expel the breath (when it is in the phase of having a mild degree of moisture); the brain thus becomes able to obey the motions of the thought and the exercise of the faculty of understanding. In inebriety, however, there is a very great inclination towards excess of moisture (which is incompatible with obedience to the understanding), owing to admixture with ascending and overflowing vapors, which render it too humid. This moisture prevents it from obeying the intellectual faculty and the tendencies of the thought, except in respect of very material and corporeal topics. It cannot serve in respect of very delicate spiritual matters. Whether stable or agitated, moisture cannot take part in the formation or presentation of spiritual affairs; it can only respond to corporeal ones.

§517 The stages in inebriety: the following are the various steps of degradation of the mind, not arranged chronologically: First, recognition of truth is impaired, and the operation of the mind is imperfect. The intellectual power falls in proportion. The substrate continues to attract breath until the temperament of one has reached up to that of the other after which the flow of breath of course comes to an end.

§518 The power of the mind—which is in the "heart"— has a greater affinity for joy during the state of drunkenness; the gladdening things that come to it do not reach it by the usual route between the senses and fantasy (or even the cogitative faculty or drive), because the sensitive drives have come into dominance. The repletion of the breath with moisture has altered its vigor. The senses now dominate the inner breath, and are more powerful than the understanding. The understanding (as, for instance, for geometry and other exact sciences), meeting as it does a breath which is so wanton towards it, unreadily submits to the senses. Things being so, no wonder that the conception of future, of beauty, of rational affairs, has become blurred in the intoxicated person's mind; the sense perception of sweet, glad, and delectable things prevails, and the sense of the present is very strong. It is the very strength of this tendency that accounts for the fact that quite a slight agent will evoke gladness and mirth. Onlookers think that such persons are jovial without reason. But this cannot be so. As a matter of fact, some causative agents of joy and gladness are powerful, while others are weak; some are known and obvious, others are not known and occult. Many of the latter are not known, not because they occur only rarely do they occur regularly. The fact is that we notice things less particularly the more often we encounter them.

§519 It is now necessary to detail the powerful and obvious sources of joy and gladness. Instances of sources of joy are the following: (1) gazing upon the daylight, among cheerful people. The evidence of this is that being in the dark makes them sad; (2) having intercourse with those of like beliefs. The evidence of this is that solitude makes such people sad. Gladdening influences are things such as: (3) obtaining that which is wished for; (4) satisfying an intention without meeting opposition; (5) preferring to do something peaceful, (6) confidence; (7) the memory of past and future joys and hopes; (8) thinking about ambitious things; (9) mutual argumentation with kindred minds; (10) relief from pain; (11) contact with curious (interesting, unusual, remarkable, new) things; (12) uplifting of the mind; (13) meeting friends and friendly surroundings; (14) overcoming deception in small matters; and many similar things to be found mentioned in books of rhetoric and morals.[8]

§520 All these vary in different races according to their affections, habits and ages. None of them is invariably absent. If two agents usually having a gladdening effect occur together the effect is not so much the greater. All that happens is that the disposition is more drawn to one than the other. The effect of one only overrules that of the other if the agent in question be very powerful, or, if it be weak, only if it be very persistently at work (see §1041). This accounts for delight being able to persist during the state of inebriation, and for the fact that melancholy persons with confused breaths keep sad after agencies producing a sense of desolation and sadness—such as the following: (1) reflecting that one's homeland is distant; (2) pondering over many injuries already past and done with; (3) hate and rancor; (4) bad health; (5) difficult circumstances of life; (6) thinking terrible things are going to happen in the future; (7) thinking of the necessity for death, which natural judgment ignores because of the obvious fact-—that we must die; (8) thinking about something that it is disturbing to meditate upon; (9) being away from an agreeable occupation; (10) having thoughts that distract from one's occupation; (11) distraction from that which is desired for and wished for; (12) many other similar things, and others which are beyond comprehension. Things of this sort easily sadden a mind which is disposed to become sad. Moreover, in melancholy persons the vividness of the imagination of depressing things itself causes (them to appear, because the thing whose image is represented to the mind is already there in actuality. Hence depression persists.

§521 Vividness of imagination goes with dryness of the breath, the movement of which the will has power to correct. We find that the understanding is drawn away from rational actions by the senses and by the fantasies whenever the character of the breath is perverted; for the breath moves characteristically towards that direction in which a lack of congenial disposition arises, as when the quality of the breath is very bad, and when it is confused.

7.3.3. How Each Emotion Tends to Generate its Own Type of Breath

§522 It is not to be thought that every agent tending towards joy or depression necessarily depends only on the quantity or quality of the substance of the breath. Other agencies are concerned. For instance, the emotions of the mind have to be considered. These tend to one or other of the aforesaid, true though it be that they act through the agency of factors internal in the breath itself (namely, quantity, quality) They do this by modifying the temperamental substrate or by rectifying the breath or by increasing its quantity Thus, they dispose towards joy. On the other hand, an agent of the opposite sign will tend to induce depression. These are the immediate and remote, external factors.

§**523** The internal factors are traceable to one single source, because every act of contrary type, if it be repeated often, comes to be more efficient in imparting an effect Every increment of power carries with it so much more tendency to the accomplishment of the effect. This is sufficiently plain from a purely logical point of view. A body which is very heating tends to impart heat rapidly; and similarly—in the case of cold, rare and dense bodies. The same holds good in the case of the internal potencies. This is how it is that a strong character is formed by repeated practice and repeated experience of emotion. It is in this way that moral character is acquired. Perhaps the reason underlying this is that when an emotion appears, it often makes the substance of the breath become conducive; and what is suitable for one thing is unsuitable for its opposite. The more often it is repeated, the less does the tendency to the opposite become, for that which is conducive to the opposite, is expelled little by little. This is saying the same thing as logic says. It would be tedious to prove it by syllogism by an acceptable and convincing argument from known premises. It emerges from the aforesaid that a reiteration of being glad disposes the breath to a state of gladness; a reiteration of being sad disposes it to depression.

§**524** Natural enquiry shows the source of increase of gladness to depend on: (1) a strengthening of the natural faculty: (2) a rarefaction of the breath—the latter is due to the expansion following gladness: (2) the strengthening of the natural drive is contributed to by three factors, each of which is itself a source of gladness; (a) the temperament of the breath; (b) overproduction of the breath beyond that which is lost by dispersal; (c) prevention of excessive dispersal of breath. Rarefaction of the breath is followed by two things: (i) a tendency towards movement and expansion—this is related to the fineness (rarefaction) of its substance; and (ii) an attraction to itself of its own particular nutriment.

§**525** This is due to the movement of expansion towards a

place away from the movement of the nutriment. This particular attraction is really the natural corporeal tendency to avoid emptiness. In its essence, it is the same with any movement which in itself brings it to pass that the latter things shall take the place of the former. It is the outcome of this law that very distant waters are drawn towards their primary source, and that winds follow the course they do.

§526 Two things follow great depression: (1) weakening of natural power; and (2) concentration of the breath. The explanation of this is that violent condensation and aggregation of the breath obliterates the natural heat and results in coldness. Two opposites follow upon this, as has already been intimated.

§527 It is therefore evident that intense gladness disposes the breath to gladness, sadness to depression; that associated depressants do not make an impression on gladness unless they are vigorous; whereas weak stimulants may and do impress themselves thereon. It is, of course, the other way about in the case of depressants.

7.3.4. The Distinction Between Weakness of the Heart and Cowardice, Sadness and Their Opposites

§528 Weakness of the heart and sadness, which some people call "contraction of the chest or heart," are similar and yet different. The same thing may be said about their opposites (vigor and gladness of heart), which some people call "enlargement of the chest or heart.[9] The difference between them is difficult to identify because so commonly one passes into the other. Most people think the two former are passive dispositions; others think they are active. But there is an obvious difference between the extremes of each: (1) Not every weak heart is associated with depression nor is depression always accompanied by a weak heart. A vigorous heart is not necessarily accompanied by joy; and conversely. (2) The basis is different in each. Weakness of the heart is a disposition assumed in respect of things evoking dread, because it is incapable of tolerating them. Depression has to do with saddening things and the heart does not tolerate them much. Fear concerns the body; depression concerns the mind. (3) There is a difference in regard to the mental effect. Weakness of the heart impels to flight; depression impels one to stand still for the purpose of either resisting or repelling. This is the opposite action to flight. Weakness of the heart inhibits the powers of motion; depression stimulates them. Consequently there are two emotions associated with weakness of the heart: (a) that of a threatening injury; and (b) that of the desire to prolong movement. In the case of depression (oppression of the chest) there are: (i) a sense of threatening injury; (ii) no desire to flee. In the event of there being a decision to flee, it is because of some contingent circumstance rather than because of an intention to give ground. It is as likely that attack and struggle will be decided upon in place of flight. (4) They differ as to the after effects on the body. Weakness of the heart and escape from danger are followed by loss of natural heat, by cold. Depression, after the particular cause has passed away, is followed by kindling of the natural heat. (5) They differ in regard to the disposing causes. Too fine and too cold a complexioned breath tends to weakness of the heart; coarseness and hot temperament of the breath tend to depression.[10]

7.3.5. The Relations Between the Various Blood States and the Several Emotions

§**529** The part played by imagination in emotions—the persistence of an imagination which s disposed towards taking vengeance for a thing is related to persistence of anger although there is not sufficient propulsive power to execute the vengeance. The anger is neither marked enough nor mild enough. For it must be understood that when anger ceases quickly, the hurtful image does not persist in the imagination, but is quickly destroyed; so rancor becomes impossible.

§**530** In like manner, too much tendency to secure vengeance is countered by two factors: rancor and hate. The one is due to the mind being wholly impelled to vengeance, but prevented from continually reflecting upon the hurtful conditions by remembering the things which follow upon having hate fixed in the memory. The mind naturally hesitates to face impending hurts. Externals tend to draw away from internals and vice versa.

§531 It must also be remembered that when there is too much tendency to vengeance in a fearless person, the impression results as if the imagination had already become possessed of the thing desired for. In aiming at the realization of a power, and hastening towards it, the imagination of such a person takes it as actually handled. The image is impressed on the imagination as if actually present; then the image of the thing in which the purposed action will end is added to the imagination, and the desire for it ceases to be maintained; the image is abolished, and therefore does not linger in the memory. That is how it is that rancor is not there.

§532 When the noxa is big, as where a sultan or very high dignitary (usually looked on with fear) is concerned, then the urgent anxiety to gain vengeance, coupled with the fear, together prevent the image of the desire from staying in the mind. The result is that the picture of the desire and of the noxa are both abolished from the imagination, whereas the image of the fear is so much the more dominant to the mind that it evokes a desire to flee and not attack. Here again, the image of rancor cannot persist in the mind. In the case of persons under puberty, or weakly persons, it is so easy to take vengeance on them, and there is so little fear entertained of them that the vengeful mind pictures the vengeance as if already accomplished. Excessive ease in securing vengeance makes it pictured as if already in one's hand. The imagination acts not according to what is in the matter at issue, but according to that which it pictures to itself. So, when ease of fulfillment arouses the thought that vengeance is attained, the weak-minded person takes it as actually attained. So the love for it vanishes and is entirely obliterated from the mind.

§533 Moreover, that the imagination moves according to that which is represented to it and not according to the outcome of things, is shown by the fact that men dislike honey when it is served up like bilious matter; and they dislike laudable sapid foods should their color be made like repugnant substances: or even when they are served in the appearance of repugnant objects even though such things are not believed to exist at all.

§534 Similarly with this: when a given likeness to the above named thing is portrayed (either because of the intensity of the impulse of the desire, or because of the worthlessness of realizing the desire as though it had actually been attained) it has the same effect as if it had been realized; therefore there is no rancor.

§535 From what has been said in the preceding chapter, it is evident that the last-named kind of temperament is that which is most disposed towards rancor.

7.3.6. How the Appropriate Medicines Stimulate And Strengthen the Breath

§536 We can now understand how the appropriate medicines can stimulate. Wine, for instance, restores the breath by nourishing it; pearl and silk (which counteracts disagreeable things) supply the breath with brilliance and luminosity. Embolic myrobalan, amber, and coral concentrate the breath or prevent it from dissipating rapidly; doronicum modifies the temperament of the breath by giving it heat; camphor and rosewater do so by imparting cold; sweet aromatics strengthen the breath by endowing its substance with agreeable and sweet fragrance; bugloss and lapis lazuli act by separating off black bile and fumosity. Changes are produced by adding or removing a drug; i.e., coral may be joined with amber and bugloss.

§537 In some cases, gladness is the outcome of the intrinsic property of the drug. This is so in the case of *sunbul*. In other cases, the intrinsic property of the drug produces its effect indirectly by acting upon one or other of the primary causes of gladness. Thus, musk and amber act on the breath by way of their aromaticity. The juice of matian gives rise to gladness by virtue of an intrinsic property. But when used in a case where the temperament of the breath is hot, the stimulant action is effected by way of infrigidation. When the temperament of the breath is cold, doronicum acts as stimulant both by virtue of its intrinsic property and by imparting warmth to the breath.

§538 In dealing with all these drugs, then, it is necessary to know whether the properties are general or specific. When the property is general there is no need to make any modifications in employing it for weakness or depression of the heart. An instance of such an agent is afforded by aromaticity. On the other hand, where the property is specific, it requires modification. For instance, the juice or syrup of matianus is cold, and will stimulate one kind of temperament but not another. If it be desired to use matianus to make a person of cold temperament glad, it is necessary to counteract its coldness by a calefacient; and it would be more efficient to choose a calefacient which itself is intrinsically a stimulant. For instance, musk or amber is mixed with syrup of matian, because they supply both warmth and stimulating power.

§539 Aromaticity and sweetness are potencies which, though opposite, are yet attracted towards qualities which are agreeable to the substance of the breath. They supply the taste and fragrance which the natural and vital power respectively desire to receive.

§540 Where two drugs are of equal power, the sweeter and more aromatic of the two will prove a more efficient adjuvant, because these properties are more attractive to the members (especially the liver). Should nutrient properties be present as well, the breath is more rapidly nourished; and being medicinal in character, it acts more rapidly on the breath.

§541 These indications guide as to which drugs to use to obtain a more rapid effects.

§542 The essence of aromaticity lies in its rarefaction; the essence of sweetness lies in its concentration and earthiness. This explains why aromatics are so much better adapted to feed the breath, while sweet substances are better fitted to nourish the body. Consequently aromaticity is more efficient for the heart than sweetness, while it is the other way round in the case of the liver. The heart is the matrix of generation of the nutriment of the breaths, whereas the liver is the matrix of generation of the nutriment of the body. That is why it needs less aromaticity and more sweetness to nourish it than does the heart. All the same, aromaticity is required by the liver, because that organ is the matrix of the natural breath—not a matrix of generation of the breath, only a substrate for the breath to reside in (according to those acquainted with the truth; not according to those who merely speculate).

§543 The natural breath has a desire for aromaticity and is invigorated and refreshed by such. It is easy to-see that the natural faculties will also be invigorated in consequence.

7.3.7. What "Property" Means and How It Differs from "Nature"

§544 Strictly speaking, the specific "property" of a thing is the same as its "nature." The one term would really be defined by the same word as the other. The specific property is the source of movement or rest in whatever thing it occurs.

§545 Nevertheless, there is a difference between the two concepts in the same way as the particular differs from the universal. It is not true, as the laity think, that the two terms belong to opposite things. The truth is that the first principles behind all generable and corruptible substances are primary, active or kinetic energies and occur either simply in fire, air, water, and earth, or linked to a composite temperament.

§546 There are two views about this: (1) that the disposition appears synchronously with the production of physical form; (2) that the disposition is inherent in matter from the outset. Once matter assumes a given physical form, it can only assume some other form by dispersing the first form. That is, matter relapses to the natural power of the disposition.

§547 Whichever view is correct, it is true that from such a physical form (whose constituents have become so to say blended) there emerges a power which could not have appeared in the several separate constituents. For instance, the attractive power of iron in a magnet is not in any of its component powers. It arises out of the divine emanation which pervades all things and makes latent energies kinetic. This happens in one of two ways: (1) by means of something primarily inherent in matter; or (2) by means of the temperament which itself disposes it to receive the given power, and is yet itself neither power nor physical form.

§548 We now have the answer to the questions, what is "specific property?" What is "nature?" If one asks, "Why does fire burn?," one must needs answer, "because the thing burning has a combustible nature." If one asks, "Why does a magnet attract iron?," it can only be said, "It has an attractive power by nature." To say that fire burns because of heat is no better than saying a magnet attracts iron because of having the power and nature to attract iron; we may say the nature of the energy called "heat" is to burn up in fire, and call this "combustible nature," "combustible power," but there is no name for the other. The giving of a name has not imparted complete knowledge about the matter; to know the name does not remove the real lack of knowledge about a difficult phenomenon.

§549 But people are not usually satisfied by the preceding answer because they want to believe that every property arises out of the "heat," "cold," "dryness," or "moisture" of a body by virtue of heaviness or lightness or movement or of any of the things which are obviously really dependent upon the components. When they find that actions are not to be attributed to any of the aforesaid, and that the real reason for an act is not apparent, they come to the conclusion that every one of the first beginnings is inscrutable. That is not true. Actions proceed either from natural, vital, intellectual or accidental (contingent) properties.

§550 We may pass over as untrue the other theories held about magnetic force that it attracts iron because of: (1) heat; (2) cold; (3) a spirit residing in the magnet itself; (4) sending out hook-shaped bodies; (5) likeness between the nature of the magnet and the nature of the iron; or (6) a vacuum in the iron. The fallacy in all these ideas is easily seen when we reflect on how a green twig acquires nutritive properties from its constitution, which is the same sort of thing as the reception of magnetic properties from a constitution in the iron. What is not understood is why the magnetic power is so much greater in iron than in any other thing; yet this ignorance is no greater than that which exists in reference to other matters.

§551 This ignorance is in two directions: (1) we do not know the initial factors which go to produce this attractive power. Neither do we know them in regard to any other force; (2) we do not know why this body is more disposed to take on magnetic power than any other body. But neither do we know more in regard to other phenomena. We are in exactly the same case concerning colors, fragrance, powers of the mind, and such like matters. Of course we can say that all such phenomena arise out of the active principles originally blessed by God, and we can allow that the basis of the disposition which comes from the particular constitution is due to a rearrangement of matter. But though we may guess that it is the proportions of ingredients which account for the existence of a temperament, it is quite another thing to be definite about the absolute proportions of this commixture, and we shall be ignorant of this as long as we live in this world. So it is evident that our ignorance of the real causes of the power in the magnet is not as remarkable as our ignorance of the real causes which dispose the corporeal or mental body to redness or yellowness.

§552 The fact is that we take little interest in the common things of life; the mind neglects to study them; so often is it true that the rare things are the ones to excite admiration and be inquired after and their causes speculated about.

§553 In conclusion, "specific property" is the "nature" met with in compound substances after a characteristic temperament (and its correspondingly special and characteristic state) has been initiated in them out of the supreme and limitless influence. This is the real truth about specific property. In spite of this being so, it is common for people to say that specific property differs from "nature" in that the former appears in complex bodies after a special act has occurred to make its nature manifest. On the other hand, the "nature" of a thing is said to be the power by which simple bodies are operated. This is as far as the laity and feeble searchers-after-truth can see. If fire is a difficult thing to make, and is carried from distant places, surely the laity might wonder at the specific properties of this more than of other things, and look more closely into the causes of its specific property than they do into those of other phenomena that appear to be more remarkable. To think how fire removes visible forms, cannot be touched, rises upward, makes the things over which it can prevail, ascend, can be generated from a small quantity in large amounts within an hour, destroys whatever it meets and transmutes it into its own essence, is not lessened by however much is taken from it. Surely these facts are more wonderful than the attraction of iron by a magnet, or than other specific properties. But, being so common, seen so much everyday, these things evoke no admiration. There is no interest displayed in seeking their explanation. The action of the magnet seems extraordinary and receives universal wonder, and everyone is interested in inquiring into its nature and origin.

LECTURE 8: PSYCHOLOGY

8.1. THE ANIMAL FACULTY OR DRIVE

§554 The animal faculty or drive consists of perception and motivation. The perceptive process operates externally through the external senses and internally through the interior senses. Each of these have five faculties or drives. When perception operates externally, it is termed sensation. According to some, there are five varieties of sensation, but according to others there are eight. The five varieties are the vision, hearing, smelling, tasting and touching.[1]

§555 When sensation is differentiated into eight varieties, the sensation of touch is sub-divided into four (pain, temperature, smoothness or roughness, softness or hardness) even though these may all be perceived from a common sensorium, that is, taste and touch from the tongue and touch and vision from the eyes. The validity of these conclusions should be left to the philosophers for necessary consideration.

§556 When perception operates internally, it is deemed as the mental faculty or drive consisting of the following five varieties.[2]

§557 The interior senses. There are five groups of interior faculties or drives: common sense or the composite drive, imagination, apprehensive or instinct, the retentive or memory and the ratiocinative. According to the physicians, this (the composite and imaginative) is a single process, but according to the philosophers, it is of two kinds: (1) receptive perceptibility which receives all sensation, composes them into percepts and enables proper sensory appreciation; and (2) imagination, which comes into action after the stoppage of perception and is concerned with the storage and retention of percepts.

§558 The composite or common sense. This is the drive which receives all forms and images perceived by the external senses and combines them into one common mental image.[3]

§559 Imagination (fantasy). This preserves the percepts of the composite sense after they have been so conjoined and holds them after the sense impressions have subsided. Common sense is the recipient and imagination is the preserver. The proof of this belongs to the philosopher. The main place of the activities of these two faculties is the anterior part of the brain.[4] The difference from common sense is that common sense only deals with objects when they are present.

§560 The imaginative or cogitative faculty or drive. The faculty or drive which medicine calls cogitative is taken in two senses in philosophy. It is regarded sometimes as "imaginative sense" [*mutakhayyalah*: animal] and sometimes as "cogitative" [*mutafakkirah*: human]. In the view of the philosopher, the imaginative sense is where the apprehensive sense or instinct comes into play and the cogitative sense is where reason controls or decides that a given action is advantageous. There is also the difference that the imagination deals with sense form percepts whereas the cogitation uses the percepts which have been stored in the imagination and then proceeds to combine and analyze them and construct quite different images, for example, a flying man or an emerald mountain. The imagination does not present to a person anything but what it has already received through the sense-organs.[5]

§561 The apprehensive or instinctive sense. This faculty or drive is the instrument of the power called instinct in animals. With it, for instance, an animal knows that a wolf is an enemy and a child distinguishes its nurse as a friend from whom he need not flee. Such a decision is not formed by the reasoning powers but is another type of apprehension. Friendship and enmity are not perceived by the senses nor do the senses comprehend them. They are not perceived by reason either. The human being employs the same faculty or drive on very many occasions exactly as does an irrational animal.

§562 In regard to the apprehensive faculty or drive vs. imagination, apprehension executes a judgment while imagination only stores sense-perceptions.

§563 In comparing the apprehensive faculty or drive and the cogitative, apprehension relates to one single act while cogitation does not make a judgment but opens the way to a series of discursive processes and decisions. The cogitative sense is concerned with the synthesis and analysis of sense impressions whereas the apprehensive sense makes a judgment on the super sensuous ideas in the particular sense percepts. The cogitative sense is concerned with forms perceived by the senses; the apprehensive sense deals with derivatives therefore ("supra sensuous forms").

§564 Some writers however call the apprehensive sense "cogitative" as a matter of convenience saying that the terms are unimportant as long as one understands the things themselves and the primary differences between them.[6]

§565 The apprehensive sense need not be considered much by the physician because disorders in it are always consequent on disorders in the prior senses of imagination and memory as we shall show later on. It is only necessary to consider those faculties or drives the disturbances of whose functions bring on disease. It is enough to know that the lesions in one which are interfering with the other arise in the temperamental state of the member or in depravity of its constitution because on this knowledge depends the selection of the remedy and how to guard against the disease. Not to know about the state of a faculty or drive which is affected only indirectly is of less moment compared with accurate knowledge about a drive which is affected directly.

§566 The retentive faculty or drive: memory: the power of memory is as it were a treasury or repository for those suprasensuous ideas discovered by the apprehensive faculty or drive just as the imagination is the treasury or repository for the sense impressions of forms and sensible images (formed by common sense). The place of this faculty or drive is in the posterior region of the brain.[7]

§567 There is still one more faculty or drive distinguishable in them and, namely, the ratiocinative or understanding. Physicians do not concern themselves with this any more than they do with the cogitative drive and for the same reason. They only study the operations of the four other faculties or drives.[8]

8.2. The Power of Movement

§568 Movement. This power is that which contracts and relaxes the muscles whereby the organs and joints are moved, extended or flexed. This power reaches the limbs by way of the nerves and there are as may forms of power as there are of movement. Each muscle has its own peculiar purpose and it obeys the decree of the composite sense.[9]

8.3. Bodily Functions

§569 Some functions are performed by a single faculty or drive, that is, digestion. Other functions are performed with the collaboration of two faculties or drives, that is, the appetite for food depends upon the combined receptivity and sensitivity of the stomach. The drive of attraction is achieved by a contraction of the longitudinal fibers which draw the object inward and extracts from the humors that which is required. The faculty or drive of sensation enables the organ to be aware of the acridity of the atrabilious humor for this it is which excites appetite. In saying that this one function is achieved by two faculties or drives together, one relies on the fact that something noxious befalling the drive of sensation destroys that desire which is called hunger and appetite. Even the need of nutriment does not account for desire.

§570 The faculty or drive of swallowing is also carried out by two processes, that is, reflex attraction and voluntary propulsion. The reflex attraction is due to the movement of longitudinal fibers in the esophagus and upper part of the stomach, while voluntary propulsion is due to the contraction of ordinary muscle fibers concerned in swallowing. In the absence of either factor, swallowing becomes difficult if not impossible, that is, in the absence of true appetite swallowing becomes difficult. In fact, when there is aversion to food, the receptive process fails to propel it towards the stomach in sheer disgust.

§571 The progress of transmission of nutriment is secured by the action of two processes: one of these is the propulsion of food by the expelling part and the other is reception by the part which receives it next.

§572 The elimination of waste matters (like defecation) is also affected in a similar manner. Sometimes both sensitive and vegetative faculties initiate the function simultaneously.

§573 In some cases, an faculty or drive may be associated with a quality. Thus cold holds material and also arrests the flow of humor (or intestinal contents) either absolutely by repressing its formation or relatively by driving it back. Cold restrains by: (a) congealing the material (rendering its particles closely aggregated); or (b) narrowing the powers. Incidentally it has a third action; (c) that of obliterating innate heat (which is concerned with the drive of attraction).

§574 On the other hand, heat acts in quite the opposite way. Whether the absorption is by heat or capillary action, it is always the thinner portion which is taken up first, and the denser portion absorbed later. The physical faculty or drive absorbs only those portions of the food which are specially required for assimilation and those which have been suitably converted into an assimilable form. This suitable and specific material is generally of a thick consistency.[10]

Part Two
The Classification of Diseases: Their Causes

Lecture 9: A Discussion of the Cause of Disease and Symptoms

9.1. General Remarks

§575 Cause, as a medical term, refers to a factor or factors which precede and initiate some new state in the human body or maintains a fixity of such a state.[1]

§576 Disease is an abnormal state of the body which primarily and independently produces a disturbance in the normal functions of the body. It may be an abnormality of temperament or form (structure).[2]

§577 Symptom is a manifestation of some abnormal state in the body. It may be harmful as the colic pain or harmless as the flushing of cheeks in peri pneumonia.[3]

§578 An example of a cause is decay or putrescence while the corresponding malady may be fever and the corresponding symptom, thirst or headache. Another example of a cause is fullness of lacrymal sacs from developmental error; its corresponding malady may be obstruction of uvea with a corresponding symptom of loss of vision. A third example might be a cause of acrid flux resulting in a corresponding malady of ulcer in the lung and a corresponding symptom of flushed cheeks or curved nails.

9.1.1. The Difference Between Symptoms and Signs

§579 A symptom may not only be a symptom but also a sign. A symptom refers to that which relates to its own intrinsic character or in relation to that to which it belongs. A sign is that which guides the physician to a knowledge of the real essential nature of the disease.[4]

9.1.2. One Disorder May Originate a Second

§580 As an example, colic produces syncope or paralysis or spasms and convulsions.[5]

9.1.3. A Symptom May Be the Cause of a Disorder

§581 Thus, violent pain causes the suffering of colic and syncope is the effect of the pain. The violent pain of an inflammatory mass is due to the flow of matter to that spot.[6]

9.1.4. A Symptom May Also Be a Disease

§582 A headache may be an effect of fever, but may also last so long as to amount to a "disease."[7]

9.1.5. One and the Same Thing May Be at Once Disease, Symptom and Cause

§583 Considered in relation to the present, a fever may be a disease; considered in relation to the past, a fever is cause; considered in relation to the future, a fever is a symptom. Examples: the fever of consumption is the sign of ulceration of the lung. Considered in itself, it is the disease. Considered in its effect, it is the cause of gastric weakness. Again, a headache which fever gives rise to (in those cases where fever causes headache, especially meningeal disease) may remain behind (after the subsidence of the fever) and be itself the disease. To particularize the malady itself sets up inflammation of the meninges and this sets up a headache.

9.2. The Various States of the Human Body and Types of Illness

§584 According to Galen, there are three states of the human body: (1) Health. This is a state in which the temperament and form of the body are such that all its functions are performed wholly and in a balanced manner. (2) Disease. This is a state opposite to health. (3) Intermediate state. According to Galen, this is neither health nor disease.

§585 There are three varieties: (1) Neither perfect health nor definite disease such as old age, convalescence, infancy. (2) Health and disease being present in one and the same organ or in two different organs. In the former case, the temperament may be normal but the form abnormal or the shape may be normal but not the size or position. The abnormality may be in the active qualities but not in the passive ones. (3) Health and disease may alternate with each other like a person may remain healthy during winter but become ill in summer.

§586 Disease may be simple or complex. Simple diseases are those which have a single abnormality of either temperament or structure. Complex diseases are those in which two or more abnormalities combine to form a single disease.

9.2.1. Simple Disorders

§587 Disorders of temperament primarily and independently affect only the simple organs. When a compound organ is affected with these, it is due to the involvement of the simple organs composing it. Hence, diseases of temperament are referred to as affecting every kind of simple organ, but not a compound organ. There are sixteen kinds of disorders of temperament.

§588 Disorders of the configuration affect the compound organs which in reality are comprised of the simple organs and are the instruments of special functions.

§589 There is a loss of continuity in diseases which directly and independently involve both simple and compound organs. This may be as a dislocation of a joint without any injury to the composing structures or with damage to simple tissues such as nerves and blood vessels. It may be summarized that simple diseases are of three kinds: disorders of temperament, deformities, and/or diseases involving loss of continuity. A disease is thus always described as belonging to one or other of these varieties.

The sixteen varieties of abnormal temperaments have already been described.

9.2.2. The Disorders of Configuration

§590 Deformities (of structure) are four which involve errors of development (malformations; errors in shape; errors in number; and displacements).[8]

9.2.2.1. Abnormalities of Development

§591 Abnormalities of development may involve shape, ducts, cavities or surfaces of the organs.

9.2.2.2. Abnormalities in Shape

§592 There may be an increase as in elephantiasis, unduly large penis (priapism); or macroglossia like the disease which befell Nicomachus whose body became so huge that he could not be moved. Or, there may be a decrease such as shortness of tongue so that it cannot reach the other parts of the mouth (tongue-tie), atrophied and wasted members, or general decline.[9]

9.2.2.3. Abnormalities in Number

§593 There may be an increase in normal organs: additional teeth; supernumerary fingers. There may be an increase which is entirely abnormal: warts, calculus, enlarged glands. There may be a decrease in normal organs: congenital absence of a finger, accidental loss of a finger through amputation (accidental or surgical), dilatation of the pupil or dilatation of the blood vessels, i.e., varicose veins.

9.2.2.4. Displacements

§594 These may be as displacement from the proper

anatomical position, replaceable such as the hernia of the intestine; tremor (which occurs through a quite unnatural to and fro involuntary movement), or not replaceable such as the fixation of a joint in a new position as in gout where joints are hardened (ankylosed). There may be displacement from the normal position in regard to neighboring anatomical structures. This results in their being too near together or too far from one another. In such a case, one part cannot move towards another as it should. For instance, adjoining fingers cannot touch one another or one part cannot be moved away from another, either at all, or only with very great difficulty. For instance, in the case of joints flabby because of paralysis or in the case of the eyelids. There may be a difficulty in opening the hands or in opening or raising the eyelids.

9.3. Injuries (Loss of Continuity)

§595 Loss of continuity occurs in the organs (and tissues) as mentioned here.

§596 (1) The skin (and the flesh beneath it): as excoriation, scarification, wounds. If pus is not formed or discharged, it is called a wound; if a discharge of pus is present, it is called an "ulcer." The presence of pus is due (a) to effete matters ("superfluities") being discharged at that spot; for the reason that it is weak. (b) The tissue is not able to digest all the nutriment which is brought to it, the excess being changed into pus. (2) Bone. A fracture into two parts, large or small; or longitudinally in the form of a fissure. (3) Cartilage. The fracture may be in any of these three ways. (4) Nerve. Transverse section from incised wounds; longitudinal, and over a short distance, as "scission." Longitudinal and also extensive—in a contusion. (5) Muscle. If near the ends, or in the tendon: attrition. If transverse: severance, or incision. If longitudinal, but small in extent, with the formation of a deep hollow, it is called cavitation. If multiple, with the appearance of several swellings and hollowings, it is attrition with contusion. If the loss of continuity is in the belly of the muscles, it is called attrition or incision, or contusion, whatever the direction of the injury be. (6) Arteries and veins. When these undergo injury or loss of continuity, they are "opened." If the injury is transverse, it is an incision; if longitudinal, it is called fission. They may be punctured (perforation). There may be a partial loss of continuity, whereby the blood escapes into the surrounding tissue spaces until their pressure arrests its further progress; this is called an aneurism. (7) Membranes (including the diaphragm): disruption. Note that not every member can undergo loss of continuity with impunity. For instance, in the case of the heart, death ensues.

§597 If one of two parts of a composite member be separated from the other, such that there is no actual injury to either, it is called a dislocation. A nerve may be twisted out of place and this is also called a dislocation or contortion.

§598 Any break of continuity occurs where there are foramina. It may widen them. When it occurs in a place where there are no foramina such may come into existence.

§599 Any break of continuity, whether it be in the form of an ulcer or the like, will heal quickly if the temperament of the member be good. But if the temperament be not good, healing may be delayed for a long time. Healing is especially delayed in persons with dropsy or cachezia or suffering from lepra.

§600 If wounds are tightly bandaged, they may end in a very deep ulcer. Ulcers appearing in summer may last on into winter and exhaust the patient's strength.

9.3.1. Complex Diseases

§601 By the term "complex diseases" we mean not that several diseases are conjoined—but that a number of morbid states concur and out of them there emerges one single disease. Frequently the morbid material which produces boils and abscesses is kept in check by the healthy fluids of the body. When these fluids are lost physiologically as in lactation, or pathologically as in hemorrhage from wounds, the system tries to eliminate the morbid matter towards the skin as in boils and abscesses.

§602 The following kinds of morbid state go together to make up an inflammatory mass: (a) a disorder of temperament, this being associated with matter; (b) a perversion of form; (c) unhealthy configuration—one never meets with an inflammatory deposit without there being disfigurement, change of size, and there is often displacement as well; and (d) loss of continuity. This is the necessary accompaniment of the discharge of superfluities into the tissue-spaces, penetrating as they do into them all, and separating one from the other in order to make space for themselves.

9.3.1.1. The Site

§**603** Swellings occur in soft members and sometimes also in bone in which case the cavities in the bone widen and the exudate accumulates in them. It is not surprising that a tissue which can accommodate nutrients should also accommodate waste material if these should by change penetrate into it or should form in it.

9.3.1.2. Causation

§**604** (1) The primary cause may not be evident, the corporeal change showing that material has been removed from one tissue to another (at a lower level). This is called a "catarrh." (2) The material cause from which boils and other inflammatory swellings arise may be immersed within other humors, without being deprived of its own harmful qualities.

§**605** Good humors may be discharged either by natural processes (as for instance in the case of women at the times of parturition and lactation), or by unnatural processes (as when good blood is lost through a wound). The bad humors, however, remain and continue to be harmful. Nature then expels them. If the discharge is by the skin, pustules form.

9.3.1.3. The Classification of Swellings.

§**606** Swellings may be classified according to the different kinds of matter of which they are made up, namely, according to the six kinds of material cause—the four humors, wateriness, and gas.

§**607** There are both hot and cold inflammatory swellings, but the fact of their being hot does not mean that they are derived from bilious humor or blood. Any material intrinsically of a hot nature, or any material which has become hot because of putrefaction, can give rise to a hot inflammatory mass.[10]

§608 Physicians as a matter of course call inflammations due to disturbance of the blood humor as "phlegmonous" and those of the bilious humor as "erysipelas." When both of the humors are involved a double name is given like phlegmonous erysipelatodes or erysipelas phlegmonodes according to the predominant humor. When there is pus, the inflammation is called an abscess. There is an inflammation of the glands in the axilla, the neck, behind the ears and in the groins which is of a very grave type. This is known as "bubo" which will be described separately.

§609 There are four stages in the development of a hot swelling (inflammation): (1) onset—the humor makes its way to the surface and increases in size until the cavity is so distended as to be evident; (2) growth or rise—when the size and tension increase; (3) acme—when the inflammation having reached its maximum is stationary; (4) decline—state of softening from digestion of the contents and resolution or maturation into pus or other kind of matter or a conversion into a hard or indurated mass.

§610 Swellings other than those of the hot type are produced by black bile, phlegm, fluid or gas. They may be composed of atrabilious humor including induration (generally autumnal), cancer (generally autumnal), and glandular (scrofulous); other nodules and nodosites.[11] They may be composed of serous humor as in lax or soft glands and winter swellings. Another type is composed of watery fluid like dropsy, hydrocephalus, hydrocele and the like. Or the swellings may be composed of gases as in tumefaction, puffiness,[12] or distension.

§611 The glandular form is either quite loose within the tissues among which it lies and is therefore easily moved to and fro by the finger; or there is adhesion, simply to the skin (as in strumous swellings). The other two kinds of swelling are intermingled with, and inter fused with, the substance of the tissues among which they lie.

9.3.1.4. The Difference Between Cancerous Swellings and Induration

§612 Induration is a slumbering silent mass which destroys the sensation (so that the part is numb), and is painless and stationary. It may produce weakness of the part. A cancerous swelling progressively increases in size, is destructive, and spreads roots which insinuate themselves amongst the tissue-elements. It does not necessarily destroy sensation unless it has existed for a long time and then it kills the tissues and destroys sensation in that particular part. It would seem that indurations and cancerous swellings differ less as to substance than in the inseparable accidental qualities [induration may be what is now called "scirrhus"].[13]

§613 Hard swellings which arise from the atrabilious humor are usually hard from the outset. They are often autumnal and become indurations especially if there be sanguineous humor present. The same sort of change may take place in the swellings arising out of serous humor.

9.3.1.4.1. Swellings arising out of serous humor

§614 These are of two types: (1) diffuse or (2) circumscribed (nodular). The difference lies in the fact that the latter form is discrete among the surrounding tissues whereas the other form is intermingled with them and is, therefore, not discrete, but diffuse. Swellings formed of serous humor often arise in winter (the raining or stormy season). Even if they are hot, they are white in color.

9.3.1.4.2. The Difference Between Soft Glands and Ganglia

§615 Ganglia are more adherent to the surrounding tissues. They feel nodular to the touch. They always slip back to the original position after manipulation, but they may be dispersed by certain strong medicines without compression and then disappear permanently. They are often produced by toil. The application of a very heavy weight such as lead may disperse them.

§616 Swellings arising out of serous humor vary in consistency according to the density of the contained fluid. They may be soft, thin, lax, or hard, or resemble the atrabilious type of swelling or resemble the gaseous form. Tenuous serous humor flows down along the course of the nerve-fibers and so reaches the muscles beneath the epiglottis and larynx.

9.3.1.4.3. Watery Swellings

§617 These include dropsy, hydrocele, hydrocephalus and allied conditions [cysts].

9.3.1.4.4. Gaseous Swellings

§618 These are two different kinds: (1) tumefaction, and (2) inflation. These differ both in essence and in mode of commixture. In tumefaction, the gas is intimately mixed with the substance of the tissue. In inflation it is aggregated, tense, tumescent, and discrete from the substance of the tissue. The former feels soft; the latter feels more or less resistant.

9.3.1.4.5. Papular Swellings

§619 These show the same subdivision as inflammatory swellings in general. They are formed of: (a) blood or sanguineous humor (true pustules); (b) purely of bilious humor: miliaria, sudamina, certain forms of eczema; (c) both serous and atrabilious humor—morbilli, myrmecia, clavus, scabies, warts, and the like; (d) watery fluid—full, vesicles; (e) gaseous material—emphysema.

§620 The points of distinction which apply in regard to the kinds of pustules will be adequately dealt with in the fourth book, should God be willing for its accomplishment.

9.3.2. Disfigurements

§621 In a discussion of the various disease entities it is customary to include certain conditions which strictly speaking are not diseases. These generally pertain to beauty i.e., affections of hair, complexion, odor, and the form of the body.

§622 These are baldness with a local or a general loss of hair, shortness, scantiness, splitting, undue fineness, undue thickness, excessive curliness, excessive straightness, greyness, discoloration of hair.

§623 Changes in complexion may be due to imbalance of temperament, which may be humoral like the accumulation of bile as in jaundice or non-humoral like the chalky pallor from the simple excess of cold or yellow complexion from the simple excess of heat; or due to extraneous agents and environmental effects like the scorching sun, extreme cold and much exposure to wind, abnormal pigmentation—as in unnatural colors in the skin, moles, freckles and general unnatural pigmentation of the body, or scars and pock marks;

§624 Disfigurements may be associated with bad odors such as fetor of the mouth or objectionable odor of the whole body or portions of it.[14]

§625 Disfigurements may be like extreme emaciation, excessive bulk, undue thinness, or fatness.

9.3.3. The Stages of a Disease

§626 Most diseases have four stages: onset, increment, acme, and decline. What is not covered by them is included in the state of health. The onset is that period of time during which the disease is becoming manifested, and its characteristics are beginning to develop. There is no evident change in degree.[15] The increment is the period during which the degree of illness is hourly becoming more and more decided. The acme is that period during which all the characteristics of the illness have become manifest and remain so. The decline shows the signs of illness abating; and the further this period advances, the more nearly is there freedom from the symptoms of the diseases.

§627 These stages may be applied both to the illness as a whole, and in regard to each of its component attacks or paroxysms. In regard to the whole course of the disease, they are called "general"; in regard to each of the attacks which occur in its course, they will be called "special" or "particular" or "individual" phases.

9.3.4. Concluding Remarks About Disease

§628 Diseases are named (1) according to the member affected (i.e., pleurisy, pneumonia, sciatica, podagra, nephritis, arthritis, ophthalmia, etc.); (2) according to the chief symptom (epilepsy, spasm, tremor, paralysis, palpitation, cephalalgia, otalgia, cardialgia, odontalgia, neuralgia, etc.); (3) from the originating humor (i.e., atrabilious disorder); (4) from resemblances to animals which the disease produces (i.e., leontiasis, elephantiasis, satyrism); (5) from the first historical example of the disease; (6) according to the substance and essential nature of the disease (i.e., fever; inflammatory swelling).

§629 Galen classified diseases as external—those which can be observed by the senses and internal—those which are not so obvious but can be recognized from the symptoms like gastric pain, pleuritic pain or those whose recognition is difficult like diseases of the liver and the bronchial passages, or those which have to be inferred like affections of the urinary tract.

§630 Diseases may occur in single members or in more than one. In the latter case there are the following possible relations: (i) Association by natural connections such as stomach and brain which are associated through nerves; the uterus and breast which are connected by the veins. (ii) One member is the channel for the other. Thus, the groin is the natural channel for inflammation to travel into the leg. The weaker of two of so related members will take up the excrementitious matters from the stronger such as the axillary region from the heart. (iii) Simple contiguity such as the neck and the brain. (iv) One member initiates the function of another. For instance, the diaphragm is concerned in the drawing of air into the lungs. (v) One member is the servant of another; Thus, the nerves serve the brain. (vi) Some third member is associated with two related organs. Thus, the brain is related to the kidney, and both these organs are related to the liver. (vii) Vicious circles. Disorders of the brain affects the activity of the stomach and impairs the digestion. Consequently, the stomach supplies morbid vapors and imperfectly digested aliment to the brain, so increasing the disorder of the brain. Hence from the original illness, the malady spreads and continues and runs in a circuit.

§631 There are the following six degrees, ranging from health to disease: (1) Blameless health. (2) Not absolute health. (3) A state neither of health nor disease as people assert. (4)

Potential illness where the body is on the verge of illness. (5) Slight ill-health. (6) Declared disease.

§632 Diseases are curable or incurable. A curable disease is one which offers no resistance to treatment. An incurable disease is one in which there is some impediment to complete cure so that whatever the doctor applies, the desired effect is not reached. For instance, headache which is due to "rheumatism." A disease is more likely to be curable when the temperament, the age, and the season are in proper relation. If not, there must be a serious causal agent at work. One can only hope to cure or disperse the diseases of one season during the contrary season.

§633 Disease is regarded as curable when there is nothing to hinder its efficient treatment. It is deemed incurable when it is associated with factors likely to interfere with an effective treatment like headache which is due to rheumatism. A disease is more likely to be mild and curable if the age, temperament and the season are favorable. In fact, only a very strong and potent cause can produce the disease in such a case.

§634 Some diseases turn into new ones, and so themselves disappear. This is very satisfactory. One disease becomes the medicine for curing another. Thus, quartain malaria often cures epilepsy, also podagra, varices and arthralgias.

§635 A spasmodic disease may be cured by scabies, pruritus, and furunculosis. A certain type of diarrhea is cured by inflammation of the eyes. Lienteria cures pleurisy. Bleeding piles removes atrabilious disorders including sciatica, renal and uterine pain. But the passage from one disease to another may be a serious matter. For instance, when an empyema spreads into the substance of the lung; when meningitis becomes lethargia.

§636 A disease may be transmitted from one person to another by: (1) transmission by infection: (a) from one house to an adjoining one—here belong lepra, scabies, variola, pestilential fever, septic inflammatory swellings and ulcers; (b) from a house in the wind-track to another; (c) when one person gazes closely at another (as ophthalmia); (d) fancy as when a person's teeth chatter because he thinks of something sour; (e) diseases such as phthisis, impetigo, leprosy; (2) hereditary transmissions as vitilego alba, premature baldness, gout, phthisis, lepra; (3) racial transmission; and (4) endemic transmission as with the sweating sickness of Anglia, elephantiasis in Alexandria, aurigo in Apulia, endemic goiter, and many the like.

§637 Do not forget that weakness of members and a frail body may supervene upon intemperaments.[16]

Lecture 10: The Causes of Illness (Etiology)

10.1. A General Discussion of Causes

§638 There are three groups of causes of those states[1] of the body which have been referred to as: health, disease and the intermediate state. These groups are (1) pre-disposing, primitive or extra-corporeal causes. These befall the body from without (trauma, heat, cold). (2) Antecedent causes include those things which befall the body from within (repletion, starvation).

§639 The primitive causes are extra-corporeal from external agents such as blows, exposure to very hot air, use of hot or cold foods; or from the mind which is here considered as distinct from the body. Here belong the causes of states of anger, fear, and the like.[2]

§640 Resemblances—the primitive causes resemble the antecedent in that there is a certain intermediate condition between each and the three states of the body named above. Primitive causes sometimes resemble the conjoined in that there is no intermediate condition between them and the three states of the body. The antecedent and conjoined causes resemble one another in both being corporeal or humoral; that is, either temperamental or compositional.

§641 Differences—the antecedent differ from the primitive causes in being corporeal and in requiring an intermediary between them and the bodily state. Such an intermediary is not necessary in the case of the primitive causes. The conjoined causes differ from the primitive in being corporeal, but without an intermediary between them and the bodily state. An intermediary may occur, but is not essential in the case of the primitive causes. The antecedent differ from the conjoined causes in that with the former the state does not become immediately manifest, but only after a number of other intermediate causes have come into operation, these being near to the state than are the antecedent causes.[3]

§642 Essential causes are such as pepper which warms; opium which cools. Accidental causes are such as cold water which warms because it closes the pores of the skin and therefore the heat is retained; hot water which cools because it opens the pores and liberates the heat; scammony which cools by expelling the calefacient humor.[5]

§643 It does not follow that a causal agent will alter the body even if it reaches it. Before the agent can act, one of three conditions must be fulfilled. (1) The agent must be powerful enough; (2) the preparatory power of the body must be adequate; (3) there must be an appropriate time factor.

§644 The agent must be exposed to the causative agent long enough for the latter to act. The states of the causes vary in their results. One single causal agent may give rise to quite different diseases in different persons, or at different times.

§645 It may be reasserted that the various factors responsible for the maintenance of health or disease may be essential or subsidiary. The essential causes are those which are acting on the body throughout the life. These are: (1) atmospheric air, (2) food and drink, (3) physical rest and activity, (4) psychological activity, (5) sleep and wakefulness, (6) elimination and retention.

10.2. The Unavoidable Causes of Disease

10.2.1. The Effects of the Atmospheric Air and Its Influence Within the Body

§646 Air is an elementary constituent of our physical body and its vital forces. Through its constant supply, the vital force is kept actively conditioned. It is the agent which modifies the breath, not simply as element, but by virtue of its constructive and attempering nature.

§647 The vital force in our language is as described earlier, and not what is termed “breath” (*nafas*) by the philosophers. That is, the term “breath” is not synonymous with what philosophers and theologians call “spirit” (*ruh*).

§648 There are two processes whereby the breath reaches its attempered state from the air—namely depuration and ventilation. Ventilation is the means whereby the temperament of the breath is modified in respect of the undue warmth which is usually the effect of condensation and imprisonment of the breath. (By temperament we mean that relative temperament which has been defined.) Air is carried in the body both through the lungs and the innate openings of the vessels (capillaries) and distributed through the arteries.

§649 The air which surrounds the body is relatively colder than the temperament arising from the imprisonment or condensation of the breath. When the outer air enters the breath, it drives it on and mingles with it, and so prevents its transformation into the astringent fire element; for such a transformation would render the temperament of the breath faulty and unfitted for receiving the impressions of the sensitive soul (that is, for maintaining life) and would interfere with the dispersal of the moist vapor of the substance of the breath.

§650 Purification is a process which maintains the vital force in its normal temperament by a judicious elimination of the hot vapor during expiration. This hot vapor is to the vital force what waste matters are to the body. Thus, air conditions the vital force by cooling it during inspiration and purifying it during expiration. (In this way the temperament of the breath is maintained).

§651 When the air is first drawn in, it necessarily cools the breath, but after the air attains the quality of the breath, through continued contact with its heat, it ceases to be an adjuvant, and is superfluous. Therefore, new air is needed and when breathed in, supplies the place of the other. The old air must be expired in order to give place for the new, and at the same time remove with it the superfluities of the substance of the breath.[6]

§652 As long as the air is attempered and pure and has no substances admixed which would be contrary to the temperament of the breath, health will come and remain. Otherwise the contrary occurs.

§653 The air is liable to natural as well as non-natural changes and may even undergo preternatural changes. The natural changes are those of the seasons. At every season the air changes to a new temperament.

10.3. Natural Mutations

10.3.1. The Influence of the Seasons on the Atmosphere

§654 Physicians[7] have defined the seasons differently from astronomers. According to astronomers, the four seasons are the four periods during which the sun, starting from the vernal equinox travels a quarter of the zodiac in each season, beginning with the spring. According to physicians, the spring in the temperate zone is neither so cold as to make warm clothing necessary nor hot enough to require cooling measures. This is the season when trees begin to leaf. It starts with the sun at the vernal equinox and lasts until it reaches the middle of Taurus [early June].

§655 In temperate countries the season directly opposite to the spring is the autumn. In other countries, the spring may begin a little earlier and the autumn somewhat later. Summer lasts throughout the hot weather while winter continues all through the cold. From the medical point of view, both spring and autumn last for a shorter time in the year. Summer and winter vary in length according to the geographical position of the country. In brief, spring is the flowering season when fruits begin to form. Spring is the season of the year between (or about, or slightly before, or slightly after) the vernal equinox and that at which the sun has reached the middle of Taurus. Autumn is the opposite portion of the year in our latitude. The intervening periods between these seasons are the summer and the winter.[8]

§656 The influence of spring is equable in temperament. As it is generally believed, spring is not hot and moist, but the proof of this rests with the physicists. Physicians should, however, regard this season as being properly balanced.

§657 The influence of summer is hot because the sun lies directly overhead, and therefore, due to its relatively shorter distance from the earth, its rays are stronger. From the overhead position, the sun's rays fall either vertically downward or in very acute angles, thus concentrating the heat on the ground below. The fact is that when a beam of light strikes the earth cylinderically or conically, a portion of the sun rays falls axially on the point of contact on the earth and another portion falls circumferencially at the periphery. Due to the concentration of rays, there is more heat at the center than at the periphery.

§658 Therefore, during summer, northern countries like ours which are nearer to the axial center of the conical rays are exposed to greater heat for a longer time even though the sun is at a longer distance from the earth. During winter we are, however, near the periphery of this cone and are thus exposed to lesser heat. The variations of distance between the sun and the earth have been fully discussed in astronomy, which is a branch of mathematics and thus of natural philosophy.

§659 The question as to whether it is the greater intensity of light which is responsible for the greater heat is a question of physics which is also a branch of philosophy.

§660 The summer, in addition to being hot is also dry, as the excess of heat produces evaporation of moisture and makes the ethereal elements of air almost like fire; moreover, in this season there is also less rain and humidity.

§661 The influence of winter is opposite to the above and is thus cold and moist.

§662 The influence of autumn is such that the heat becomes less, while cold has not yet fully developed. In other words, during this season we are midway between the center and periphery of the conical rays. Autumn is more balanced in respect of heat and cold but not so in respect of moisture and dryness. This is understandable because dryness which had come from the summer continues in the autumn without the addition of any moisture.

§663 Moisture has a natural tendency to cool, but it is difficult for the dryness to become moist. The process of drying by heat is different from the production of moisture from cold. Even a small quantity of heat is sufficient to dry the moisture, but a little cold would not be able to produce any moisture. On the other hand, in an appropriate material, a small amount of heat could produce more moisture than a corresponding degree of cold. This is because a small amount of heat merely separates the water vapor but does not evaporate it. Mild cold however, is unable to condense the moisture.

§664 Persistence of the winter moisture into the spring is not like the continuation of summer dryness into the autumn. During the spring, the heat is able to reduce the moisture more easily than the winter cold could reduce the dryness of the autumn. Moistening and dessication would thus appear to be not just contraries of each other, but two separate processes depending upon the presence or absence of moisture. Dessication in this sense means the destruction of moisture, but moistening does not mean the destruction of dryness; it only means an acquisition of moisture.

§665 When we speak of the air as being moist or dry, we do not mean that the nature or the temperament of the air has become moist or dry. If this happens at all, it is only to a minor degree. What we do mean is that the moist air contains plenty of water vapor or it has become so dense that it begins to resemble water vapor. Thus, dry air is the one from which either the water has completely disappeared or the air has become so rarefied that it comes to resemble the elemental heat or the air has clouds of dry dust particles.

§666 It would be seen from the above that the moisture left by the winter is dispersed during the spring by the relatively greater heat of the overhead sun. On the other hand, the cold in autumn is insufficient for moistening the dryness brought from the summer. This is supported by the observation that a moist thing dries up quicker by heat than a dry thing becomes moist by the same amount of cold.

§667 Another important point is that moisture is unable to withstand heat or cold for long without a steady reinforcement. But dryness needs no such help. The atmospheric air, as well as the various objects exposed to it, is unable to retain the moisture for long without a corresponding reinforcement. This is because there is always enough heat in the atmosphere (to produce evaporation). If the air is said to be cold, it is because it feels cold to the body. Our neighboring countries are never so cold as to hinder evaporation. The sun and the stars have always sufficient warmth to promote evaporation there.

§668 Due to the absence of further reinforcement, the continued evaporation of moisture, however, produces dryness in the atmosphere. During the spring, evaporation is more active but there is little formation of the water vapor. Vapor forms in the presence of two factors: a mild degree of atmospheric heat and a sufficient degree of latent heat in the earth which raises the moisture towards the surface.

§669 During the winter, the inside of the earth is extremely hot, as proved in the books on natural philosophy. The outside air has also a mild degree of heat. A combination of these factors—evaporation and condensation, with the direct tendency of cold to condense air—produces water vapor.

§670 In spring there is more loss by dispersal than by evaporation. The reason is (1) there is little heat and that is dispersed widely in the atmosphere; (2) much heat is shut up in the bowels of the earth. Therefore rarefied vapors are continually being breathed out towards the earth's surface.[9]

§671 During the winter the amount of heat concealed within the earth is very great—as is proved in treatises on natural science—whereas there is only a negligible amount of heat in the atmosphere. So there are two factors which together contribute to moisten the air—sublimation and condensation. This is the more so because the substance of the air in winter is so cold that it becomes more dense and adaptable for evaporation.

§672 In short, it is clear that just as the spring is balanced in respect of moisture and dryness, so also it is balanced in heat and cold. It cannot, however, be denied that the earlier part of the spring is moist to some extent. But this imbalance is not so marked as is the dryness of the autumn. It would not be wrong to say that the autumn is not balanced properly in regard to heat and cold. At about midday, heat is nearly the same as during the summer, because the dry air of the autumn has a greater capacity to retain heat. This capacity has of course been acquired by it from the preceding summer. The mornings and nights of the autumn are also disproportionately cooler because during this season the sun is farther from our heads.

§673 The light and rarefied air in this season is also more readily affected by the cold. Comparatively, the spring is more balanced because the factors which make the air hot or cold during the autumn are no more operative in this season and, therefore, there is not much difference in the night and day temperature.

§674 A question at this stage may arise as to why nights in the autumn are cooler than they are in the spring, when the air in the autumn should in fact be hotter due to its thinness in this season. The reasons for this are that: (1) The thin air, like the rarefied water is easily affected by both heat and cold—the water which has previously been heated up would freeze earlier than that which had not been so treated. In the former case, the water having become rarefied would accept the cold readily. (2) During the spring, the body does not feel the cold so much as it does during the autumn because the temperature in this season is rising from the cold of the previous winter. (3) The autumn is disposing towards the winter while the spring is drifting away from it.

§675 The human body is not as sensitive to the cold of spring as it is to that of autumn because in spring the body passes from a coldness to which it is already acclimatized to an increasing warmth. In autumn the reverse is the case because after being relaxed by the summer heat, the body is suddenly hit by cold. This is in spite of the fact that autumn approaches winter whereas spring recedes from it.

§676 Change of seasons has to do with the kind of diseases peculiar to each climate. Consequently the prudent physician will carefully study his own climate (atmospheric conditions day by day and month by month) and country in order to better treat the disease and maintain his patient's health by an appropriate mode of life and in order to better choose the diet measures appropriate to that climate and country.

§677 Sometimes one day of a season is like one day in another season and sometimes it is not. Some days in winter are spring-like. Some spring days are summer-like. Some days in autumn are not and cold during the course of a single day.

10.3.2 The Influence of Seasonal Changes on the Body

§678 When a season is harmonious[10] for a person of healthy temperament, it is appropriate for him, but not so if the person is of unhealthy temperament. But if deviation from equipoise be marked, then the season will be harmonious or not correspondingly, but the person may become debilitated. When a season is appropriate for a person of unhealthy temperament, the contrary holds.[11]

§679 If two consecutive seasons turn abnormal and develop opposite types of qualities, they would counteract each other's abnormality, provided they are neither too severe nor too prolonged. Thus, if the winter becomes like that of the south and the ensuing spring like that of the north, the effects of winter will be counteracted by the spring. Similarly, if the winter had been extremely dry and the following spring turns out to be moist, it would remove the excessive dryness of the winter. Moisture does not harm unless it becomes unduly excessive or lasts for a very long time.

§680 An abnormal variation in the course of one season is not so likely to produce an epidemic as its persistence through several seasons. Such variations, however, produce epidemics only when they are not like those described above like the variation of one season counteracting the ill-effects of the other season.

§681 Among the temperaments of the atmosphere one that is hot and moist is more favorable to putrefactive processes.

§682 Atmospheric changes are common in some regions, especially in the depths of the valleys; they are only rare on hills and high mountains.

§683 It is better when seasons are normal in character; it is better that summer should be hot and the winter cold; so with each season. If seasons are not normal in character, serious maladies will arise.[12]

§684 If all the seasons in one year are of uniform quality (for instance, wet, dry, hot, cold, all through the year) it is a bad year; there will be many diseases in conformity with the quality of the year. The subsequent seasons will be fortunate. If a single season can arouse much illness of corresponding type, how much the more will not a whole year arouse?

§685 A person of phlegmatic temperament is liable to develop epilepsy, paralysis, apoplexy, trismus, convulsions and the like in a cold season.

§686 A person of choleric temperament may develop delirium, mania, acute fevers, acute inflammatory swellings in a hot season. How much the worse would it not be if the character of that season persisted throughout a whole year?

§687 With a premature winter, winterly diseases come on early. With a premature summer, summer diseases arise early. The diseases of the corresponding season will change accordingly.

§688 An unduly prolonged season predisposes to many illnesses, especially in the case of summer and autumn.

§689 Note that the effects of the changing seasons are not due to the season itself, but to the quality which is changed along with them, for this exerts a marked effect upon the states of the body. A change from heat to cold in the course of a single day produces a change in the body accordingly.

§690 A rainy autumn followed by a temperate winter (not without some cold and yet not too cold, considering the geographical region) is more healthy. A rainy spring followed by a moderately rainy summer would be more likely to be healthy

.

10.3.3. The Properties of Healthy Air

§691 Fresh air is free from pollution with smoke and vapor and it is available in the open rather than in enclosed or covered places. Open air is the best but when the outside air becomes polluted,[13] the inside air is rather preferable. The best air is that which is pure, clean and free from contamination with vapors from lakes, trenches, bamboo fields, saline affected areas and vegetable fields, specially of cabbages and herb rockets. It should not be polluted with the overgrowth of trees especially walnuts and figs.

§**692** Once a putrefactive process has begun in the air, it is more likely to continue if the air is free and exposed than when it is enclosed and concealed. Except for that it is better that air be free and exposed.

§**693** It is also essential that the air should be open to the fresh breeze and not enclosed. Fresh air comes from the plains and high mountains. It is not confined in pits and depressions hence it is quickly warmed by the rising sun and cools after the sunset. Air would not be fresh if it is enclosed within recently painted or plastered walls. Fresh air also does not produce any choking or discomfort.

§**694** We have already learned that some changes in the air are normal, some abnormal and harmful, while others are neither normal nor particularly harmful. Abnormal changes in the air, whether harmful or otherwise, may or may not be periodical. It is best that a season remain in its own quality rather than be subject to frequent variations which produce disease.[14]

10.3.3.1. The Influence of the Changes in the Quality of the Atmosphere; The Diseases Incident to the Several Seasons and Kinds of Weather

§**695** Hot air produces dispersion of the body fluids and has a relaxing effect on the organs. A moderate degree of heat produces a rosy complexion by drawing the blood towards the surface. But intense heat would produce pallor by destroying the blood brought to the surface. Hot air induces sweating, diminishes the quantity of urine, impairs the digestion and increases thirst.

§**696** Cold air makes the body firm, strengthens the digestion and increases the quantity of urine by imprisoning the humors in the body and by reducing the evaporation from sweating. Cold also reduces the quantity of feces by producing spasm of the rectum and anal sphincter and thus prolongs stagnation.

§697 Moist air softens the skin and increases moisture in the body.

§698 Dry air makes the body thin and the skin dry.

§699 Fog causes anxiety and disturbs the humors. Fog however is not the same thing as dense air. The latter is uniformly dense while fog is mixed with coarse particles. That is why it is difficult to see the smaller stars in a fog and when seen they appear to be rather trembling. The fog is cloudy due to the admixture of excessive smoke and vapors. A further discussion on the subject of fog will be taken up again when dealing with the abnormal variations of air.

§700 Every season has its own characteristic diseases provided it remains in its own quality. The diseases which appear at the beginning or at the end of a season are the same as those characteristic of the season.

10.3.3.2. The Changes Which Spring Produces in the Body

§701 Normal spring is the best season as its temperament corresponds to the temperament of the vital force and the blood. The spring, as mentioned earlier, is evenly balanced but has slightly more moisture. Since it draws the blood towards the skin, it makes the complexion rosy. In this season, the heat being mild does not destroy the blood as the heat of the summer does.

§702 During the spring, chronic diseases are activated by the movement of humors that had been lying dormant. It is for this reason that depressed melancholics become agitated in this season. Those with an excess of humors suffer from diseases caused by the liquefaction and agitation of humors. When the spring becomes prolonged, there is considerable reduction in the incidence of summer diseases.

§703 The diseases of the spring may cause bleeding from the bowels, epistaxis, agitated forms of melancholia resulting from the excess of black bile, inflammation, carbuncles, fatal forms of throat involvement and other boils and abscesses, rupture of the vessels, haemoptysis and troublesome cough are characteristic maladies of this season. In the spring, which is like the winter, diseases which had already been there, particularly phthisis, become worse.

§704 Since the spring activates phlegmatic secretions it produces apoplexy, paralysis, and joint pains. During the spring, factors such as vigorous physical or mental activity and excessive consumption of hot seasoned dishes assist in the production of more diseases.

§705 Diseases of the spring can be prevented by venesection, purgation and the restriction of diet and wine. If wine is taken, it should be well diluted with water.

§706 In relation to the periods of life, the spring is specially wholesome for children and adolescents.

10.3.3.3. The Changes Which Summer Produces in the Body

§707 The summer[15] disperses humors and vital forces and thus enfeebles the faculty or drives and their functions. Blood tends to decrease in quantity while the bile increases. Towards the end of summer, there is a predominance of black bile as the thinner parts of humors get dispersed, leaving the heavier parts behind. Old and debilitated persons look stronger and healthier during the summer.

§708 Summer turns the complexion yellow as the blood brought to the surface is destroyed by the excessive heat.

§709 In summer disease generally has a shorter course. This is because, if the general vitality is good, it helps elimination by the dispersal of matured humors, but when the vitality is low, the summer heat with its relaxing effect debilitates further and thus hastens death. A hot and dry summer shortens the course of disease while a moist summer tends to prolong it. Moisture makes the ulcers chronic and diseases like ascites, diarrhea and looseness of the bowels are more frequent.[16]

§710 Diseases particularly associated with the hot season include increased incidence of disease in this season is also due to the migration of humors from the upper parts to the parts below. When there is heat, diseases such as tertian fever, continuous fever, wasting fever, painful affections of the eye and ear and general debility are more frequent. In the absence of regular breezes, erysipelas and other inflammatory conditions of this type are increasingly liable to occur. The summer which is mild, almost like the spring with less heat and dryness, is beneficial to the fever patients. They feel less dry and sweat more during the crisis.

§711 Heat and moisture favor sweating because heat liquifies the morbid matters and moisture opens up the pores by relaxation. A southerly type of summer which is hot and moist predisposes to the epidemics of measles, smallpox, etc. A northerly summer which is cold and dry is generally healthy, but diseases caused by chill from exposure are relatively more frequent. This is due to the cold squeezing out matters already liquefied by the internal and external heat. The diseases produced by chill are the various catarrhal conditions. A northerly type of summer which is particularly dry benefits phlegmatic men and women. Those of a bilious temperament are apt to suffer from a dry type of conjunctivitis and chronic fevers. The dominance of the atrabilious humor in a dry summer is due to the burning of bile which is readily available in this season.[17]

10.3.3.4. The Changes Which Autumn Produces in the Body

§712 The greater incidence of disease in this season is due to: (1) The hot sun during the day and cold in the night which produces wide fluctuations of temperature. (2) Excessive consumption of fruit which causes derangement of the humors: (a) abundance of fruits in the diet, (b) bad articles of diet, (c) dispersion of attenuated matter leaving dense particles behind and these then undergo oxidation. (3) The fermenting humors pass to the skin in the summer and the natural drives can be brought to bear on them so as to disperse and expel them, but in autumn the cold atmosphere causes the humors to be thrown back into the interior parts where they accumulate and are (as it were) imprisoned. (3) The vigor of the body is impaired from the effects of the preceding summer continuing into this season.

§713 There is less blood in the body because this season is qualitatively opposed to the temperament of blood. Consequently it cannot help blood to form and that which the summer has already dispersed is not replaced. On the other hand, the bilious humor becomes relatively increased during the summer and predominates during autumn. The atrabilious humor is more abundant at the end of summer because of the oxidation of the humors during summer and this produces ash-like residues which tend to sediment under the influence of the autumnal cold.

§714 The diseases of autumn. (1) Fevers: (a) composite; (b) quartan (due to the abundance of atrabilious humor and the agents already described (associated effects—enlargement of the spleen); (c) oliguria (the urine only passes drop by drop owing to the temperament of the blood being diverse—between heat and coldness); (d) lientery (because the cold drives the rarefied portions of the humors into the interior parts of the body); and (e) simple hectic fever (this is more severe during this season because it is desiccant in character.[18] (2) Diseases of the skin include impetigo, excoriating scabies, canker, and pustules (especially if the autumn be dry and the preceding summer was hot). (3) Diseases of the throat include acute choleric angina. (4) Diseases of the lungs—autumn is harmful for persons suffering from phthisis and chronic pulmonary infections. If a person had such a disease latent in him at the onset of autumn, he would show the signs of it at the end of the season. (5) Diseases of the brain include apoplexy; mental disease is common because the bilious humor is unhealthy and atrabilious humors are admixed with it. (6) Diseases of the intestine include the bowels which tend to become loose as the cold diverts the thin humors towards them. Irritative swellings of the glands and sciatica occur in this season just as phlegmatic swellings appear in the spring. (7) Pains in the joints, sciatica; pains in the back and hips (due to the stagnation and subsequent imprisonment of the insoluble parts of the humors which summer brought into circulation). (8) Worms, which multiply because digestion is deficient and there is lack of expulsive action.

§715 Autumn is, so to speak, the foster-mother for the disorders left by the summer-time. Autumn is more healthy if the weather be very damp and rainy, and is more unhealthy if the weather be dry.

§716 In relation to periods of life, the first part of autumn is to some extent beneficial to old people but the last part is very injurious to them (because there is cold and because there is the residue of the oxidation of humors of summer-time).

10.3.3.5. The Changes Which Winter Produces in the Body

§717 The winter is particularly beneficial to the digestion because: (1) due to cold, the vital force is enclosed in the body and thus becomes stronger and less prone to dispersion; (2) there is less fruit consumed during the winter; (3) the type of food is more natural; (4) there is less movement and activity after the meals; and (5) there is a greater tendency to remain in warm places.

§718 The winter is the most effective season for reducing the bilious humor. This is due to the cold and shorter days of this season. As winter tends to stagnate the morbid matters, there is a greater need for liquefying and resolving agents.

§719 Diseases of wintertime. The diseases of wintertime are generally phlegmatic. In this season, phlegm is increased so much that during emesis it comes out freely. The inflammatory swellings of this season are generally of a pale white color. Catarrhal conditions are more frequent due to the change of weather early in winter. Later on, pleurisy, pneumonia, hoarseness, pharyngitis and other affections of the throat appear. When the winter is fully established, pain in the chest, sides, back, and loins, and nervous disorders such as chronic headache and, occasionally, even apoplexy begin to develop from the excessive accumulation of phlegmatic excrements. Winter is more troublesome for the old and the debilitated, but it benefits the young and healthy persons. During this season, the urine is passed more freely and often shows a lot of sediment.

§720 In regard to relation to periods of life, winter is inimical to old persons and to those akin to them in nature. Middle aged persons are likely to be in health in this season.

10.3.3.6. The Influences of Seasonal Cycles

§721 If a southerly winter is followed by a northerly spring, which, in its turn, is followed by an extremely hot summer with excessive rains—provided the spring had kept up the morbid humors in the body—the autumn would produce a high rate of mortality amongst the children and increase the incidence of dysentery, intestinal ulcers and prolonged tertian type of fevers.

§722 If the winter is extremely rainy, women due for confinement in the spring will be liable to miscarriage and if pregnancy at all continues to term, the offspring may be weak, diseased or still-born. Amongst the elderly, conjunctivitis, dysentery and frequent colds and catarrh are common. Old persons are also liable to develop various types of catarrhal affections in the brain, which by blocking the passage of the vital force with the accumulated material may produce sudden death.

§723 If a rainy and southerly type of spring succeeds a northerly winter, acute fevers, diarrhea, dysentery and catarrhal diseases are frequent. The reason is that phlegm congealed by the winter is activated by the heat and it blocks the cavities, especially in phlegmatic persons, as most of the women are.

§724 If the summer become rainy about the time when the Dog-Star appears or when there are cold northerly winds, these diseases would disappear. This kind of season is the worst for women and children. Those who do not succumb to it develop quartan fever and in consequence ascites, painful spleen, and weakness of the liver from the incineration of the body humors. This type of season is not, however, so harmful for the elderly as is the cold one. If the summer is dry and northerly and is followed by a southerly rainy autumn, the succeeding winter would produce headache, cough, hoarseness and predisposition to phthisis from its catarrhal tendency.

§725 When a southerly type of dry summer is followed by a northerly rainy autumn, the winter as mentioned above would produce frequent headache, catarrh, cough and hoarseness. If a southerly summer is followed by a northerly autumn, it would produce many catarrhal affections of the respiratory and gastrointestinal tracts. If both the summer and the autumn are moist and southerly, the succeeding winter would produce similar type of catarrhal affections.

§726 In winter, the excess of humors and the closure of pores would produce putrefactive disorders. A winter which follows a season of this type produces a large number of diseases from the accumulation of morbid and putrefied matters. When, however, this season is dry and northerly, the following winter would benefit phlegmatic individuals and women, but others would tend to suffer from dry conjunctivitis, chronic catarrh, acute fevers and melancholia. In an extremely cold winter which is also rainy, burning of micturition is a common complaint.

§727 A summer which is unduly hot and dry produces inflammation of the throat which may be mild or grave, diffuse or localized, and which may rupture internally or externally. Dysuria and mild attacks of measles and smallpox are also common. Such a summer also produces various affections of the eye, putrefaction of the blood, anxiety, amenorrhea and hemoptysis. A dry spring which follows a dry winter is often unhealthy. Just as trees and vegetations are affected by epidemics, so are the animals which subsist on them. Since man eats both (i.e., meat as well as fruits and vegetables) he, too, is likely to be affected.

§728 A cold and rainy winter produces burning of the urine.

§729 A very hot and dry summer produces the following disorders in the following season: anginas (pernicious and non-malignant), anginas which produce a discharge (these may burst externally or internally), anginas which do not produce a discharge, cariola, morbilli (both these last two are favorable), eye-infections, mental depression, difficult micturition, retention of the menses, retention of the expectoration, and hemoptysis.

§730 If a dry spring follows a dry winter, this is bad. The trees and herbage are liable to decay and they are injurious to the animals which feed on them and, in turn, to the human beings which feed on the animals.[19]

10.4. Incidental Mutations

10.4.1. Climate

§731 We shall now proceed to describe some other changes in the atmosphere which are not necessarily pathogenic. These changes may arise from celestial or terrestrial causes. Some of these have already been mentioned while describing the influence of seasons.

§732 Celestial factors.[20] The changes dependent on celestial bodies such as the stars. If many luminous stars rise in one region of the sky and the sun approaches towards that region, the people living directly or nearly directly under the sun's rays are exposed to greater heat. But if the rays are oblique, the heating effect is lessened. The effect of a vertical position of the rays on the head is not nearly so great unless they continue vertical for some time and are direct.

§733 Terrestrial factors. These depend upon: (1) latitude, (2) altitude, (3) presence or absence of mountains in the neighborhood, (4) vicinity of the seas and oceans, (5) direction and nature of the winds, and (6) nature of the soil. These will now be described in some detail.

§734 The influence of latitude on climate in a country with the Tropic of Cancer to the north and the Tropic of Capricorn to the south, is that the summer is hotter than in the countries north of Tropic of Cancer or south of Tropic of Capricorn. It is true that the equatorial zone is not subject to extreme variations. The only special factor on the equator is that of the sun's being overhead (at the zenith) but this alone is not so effective as the continuation of this position for a sufficiently long time. It is for this reason that there is more heat at the time of the afternoon prayer than at noon.

§735 For the same reason, the sun at the end of Cancer or at the beginning of Leo (mid-August) is hotter than it is at the point of maximum declination. Similarly, when the sun passes through Cancer to a place of lesser declination, it becomes hotter than it would be if it had not yet reached the Cancer but had stayed on at the same degree of declination. In the equatorial regions, the sun lies vertically overhead but only for a few days. Afterwards, the suns rays become rapidly oblique. The reason is that the speed of declination increases much more rapidly towards the equinoxes than towards the solstices. In fact, the position of the sun at the solstices does not change much even in the course of three or four days. Hence, countries whose latitude approaches complete declination are hotter than others and next to these are those which are fifteen degrees to either side of the equator. Over the equator, heat is not as intense as it is at the Tropic of Cancer. The countries which are farther north are cooler than those at the equator. The laws mentioned above pertain to the effect of latitude on the climate of a country presuming of course that there is no change in any of the other factors.

§736 The influence of the altitude of a country, whether high or low, varies with the contour of the earth. Lowlands are hotter and highlands cooler. Where we live (the Middle East), the atmosphere near the earth is hotter than on the highlands. This is due to the sun's rays being more powerful near the earth than on the highland. This has been fully explained in the books on natural philosophy. When the rays fall on the lowland, the heat being enclosed in a basin gets increased.

§737 The influence of mountains on the climate of a neighboring country—the effect of height is the same as already described under the influence of altitude. Mountains also influence the air by their site and location. The high mountains influence in two ways: they reflect the rays or block the sun and they serve as wind screens or help in the formation of winds. The former effect can be observed in places which have mountains on the north. Due to the reflection of rays, such places become hot even though they may be in the north. The same would be true if they have mountains on the west and the east is open.

§738 If the mountains are on the east, the place would not be so hot, as it would be exposed to the sun only in the afternoon, when the sun is on the decline and the intensity of its rays is gradually waning. If the mountains are on the west, the place would be steadily exposed to the rising sun.

§739 Windscreens. With regard to the screening influence of the mountains, it may be noted that a mountain on the north would protect the place from the cold northerly winds but will expose it to the warm southerly winds. The velocity of the wind is much greater in the valleys than in open deserts because when the wind blows through a narrow passage, it gathers more speed and keeps on blowing. This has already been well explained in the books on natural philosophy. Water and other liquids behave in a similar way. The ideal position of a town in relation to the mountains is to be open on the north and the east and protected from the south and the west.

§740 The influence of the sea on maritime countries. The sea air is generally more humid. If the sea is to the north, it would have a cooling effect as the winds from the north would be passing over the cold waters. If the sea, however, is to the south, the air being charged with vapor becomes dense. This is particularly so if there are also mountains on the north to block its passage. The air becomes more humid if the sea is in the eastern side instead of the western side. The reason is that on the eastern side, waters are exposed to the rising sun; hence, there is more evaporation, but in the western side they are relatively unaffected. It may be summarized that there is more humidity in the neighborhood of the sea, but if there are constant or even intermittent breezes and no mountainous obstructions, the air will be free from putrefaction.

§741 On the other hand, when there is no breeze because of mountainous obstructions, the air tends to putrefy and it also putrefies the humors. So the best type of winds are those which blow from the north and to a lesser extent are those which blow from the east or the west. The worst type of winds are those which blow from the south.

§742 The influence of winds. The direction of the wind may influence in a general way or produce special effects in various localities. South winds are generally hot and moist. They are hot because they come from regions which being relatively nearer the sun are hot. They are moist because on our southern side there are oceans, which, being exposed to the extremely hot sun, produce considerable evaporation and thus greater humidity. North winds are cold as they pass over snow covered lands and mountains. They are also dry because there is less moisture in it due to the relative lack of evaporation in the north, where the winds pass over solid ice and flat plateaus instead of liquid waters and oceans.

§743 Easterly winds are well balanced in regard to heat and cold, but compared to the west winds, are more dry. The reason is that there is less evaporation in the northern countries of the west; and our country (Persia) is situated in the northern part of the east.

§744 Westerly winds are likely to be moist as they pass over the seas, but they are not so humid as the east winds because they move in the direction opposite to that of the sun. It is worth remembering here that the east winds blow in the morning and the west winds in the evening. The west winds are, therefore, relatively cooler than the east winds. Both are however, milder than the north and the south winds. The general characteristics of the winds mentioned above may be altered by some interfering factors, i.e., south winds usually become cold when the snow-capped mountains are in the south. Similarly, the north winds may become hotter than the south winds if they pass over the hot plains.

§745 Poisonous winds are of two kinds: those which pass over hot deserts and those which are like a sort of smoke producing a strange, fearful atmosphere like the flames of fires. When the atmosphere becomes hot, the heavier particles become illuminated and fall down towards the earth in a burning state leaving the lighter ones behind.

§746 Wind storms originate in the upper strata of the atmosphere according to philosophers, and, although they receive suspended particles from below, their movement, direction and formation into winds is determined in the higher regions of the atmosphere. That is how the formation of winds is generally explained, but its proof is to be found in physics, which is a branch of philosophy. A further reference to this subject will be made again, while discussing the influence of residence.

§747 The soil. Places differ according to the nature of soil. The soil may be pure, rocky, stony, sandy, marshy or with an excess of salt. There may be an excess of niter or other heavy chemicals. All these factors influence the water and the air of a locality.[21]

10.4.2. The Impressions Produced by Other Changes in the Atmosphere

10.4.2.1. The Effect of Unfavorable Changes in the Air Which are Contrary to Its Ordinary Nature

§748 A change in the nature of air does not mean an increase or decrease in its qualities, but it only means that its composition has become morbid and deranged.[22] A change of this kind is known as an epidemic. Epidemic is a specific putrefaction of air similar to the one which occurs in covered and stagnant waters.

§749 By air, we do not mean the air as an element but the atmospheric air which surrounds us. This air is not the elemental air even if it is supposed to have any existence. None of the primary elements is capable of undergoing putrefactive change. They only change either in their quality or character into the form of another element, i.e., water may change into air (steam).[23] Here by air, it is meant the atmospheric air which surrounds us. This air is composed of: (1) elemental air as an element of fire, (2) moisture as water vapor, and (3) earthy matter derived from smoke and dust. If the atmospheric air is termed air, it is merely in the sense in which stagnant sea water or stagnant lake water is called water.

§750 Although water is indeed the main constituent, it is not the pure elemental water but water admixed with mineral matter and possessing some degree of heat.

§751 Hence, the atmospheric air, like the stagnant sea water, is liable to putrefaction. Its epidemiological and putrefactive changes, which are more common towards the end of the summer and in the autumn, will be described later.

§752 Change in primary qualities—a qualitative change in the air implies that the air has become unduly hot or cold. This change may at times be so great that both vegetable and animal life are destroyed. These changes may be due to an increase or decrease in the original quality—for instance, a hot weather may become terribly hot. The original quality may change into its contrary, for example the hot weather may become extremely cold.

§753 The effect on the human body—these changes produce various diseases, i.e., a putrefactive change may produce putrefaction of the bodily humors. This happens first in the humor of the heat (blood) as it is more accessible to the air than the other humors.

§754 Hot atmosphere. The hot air relaxes the joints and disperses the secretions from the body. It produces thirst, impairs the digestion, causes dispersion of the vital force and enfeebles the faculty or drives by dissipating the innate heat which is an index of the system and a vehicle of its functions. It turns the rosy complexion into yellow by destroying the blood and making the bile predominant. It also makes the heart more hot and the humors more fluid and mobile. It tends to putrefy the humors and divert them towards the weaker organs. This type of air is not good for the healthy. It may, however, benefit those suffering from ascites, paralysis, the cold type of spasmodic affections, cold catarrhs, moist spasms, and facial paralysis.

§755 Cold atmosphere. The cold air helps to conserve the vital heat, provided it is not so severe as to produce shrinkage (suppression) of all vital activity. In that case, it may prove fatal. If air is not too cold, it reduces the flow of humors and thus helps to keep them in the body. It produces catarrh, weakens the nerves and damages the lungs. If cold is not very severe, it aids the digestion and helps to increase appetite and thus strengthen the inner faculty or drives. It may, however, be summarized that the cold air is more suitable for health than the hot air. Cold air is, however, injurious to the various nervous functions. It tends to occlude the pores and constrict the viscera.

§756 Moist atmosphere. Moist air benefits most people. It improves the color and complexion of the skin and makes it soft and keeps the pores open. It predisposes to putrefactive disorders.

§757 Dry atmosphere. The effects of dry air are contrary to those of the moist air.[24]

10.4.2.2. The Influence of the Winds on the Body

§758 A description of the winds has already been given under the heading of changes in the atmosphere. The subject of winds is now dealt with here comprehensively from a different point of view.

§759 The north winds. They strengthen the various faculty or drives and harden the body. They prevent the flow of visible excretions, close the pores, strengthen digestion, produce constipation and increase the quantity of urine. They also purify the air from any prevailing putrefactive and epidemic condition. When a south wind precedes a north wind, the material liquefied by the south wind is compressed by the subsequent north wind. Sometimes, the compression may be to such an extent that some of the orifices actually bulge out from the body. For the same reason head colds and chest troubles are quite frequent. Diseases which are commonly associated with the north winds are neuritic pains in the chest, diseases of the bladder and uterus, dysuria, cough, and spells of shivering.

§760 The south winds. They are relaxing to the body. They open the pores, excite the humors and direct them outwardly. They produce dullness of the mind, putrefaction in wounds and induce relapses of diseases. They are also debilitating and thus produce ulcers, gout, headache, drowsiness and itching. They further cause putrefactive fevers, but no sore throats.

§761 The east winds. When they blow during the late hours of the night or early hours of the morning, the air is thinned and balanced by the (rising) sun reducing the humidity, thus making it hot, dry, and rarefied. When, however, these winds blow in the afternoon or during the early hours of the night, they are of an opposite quality. Generally speaking, the east winds are more beneficial than the west winds.

§762 The west winds. When the west winds blow during the late hours of the night and early hours of the day, they are dense and heavy because the air then has not been acted upon by the sun. When, however, they blow during the late hours of the day and early hours of the night, they are of the opposite character.

10.4.2.3. The Influence of Places of Residence on the Human Body

§763 The influence of climate has already been referred to under the section dealing with seasonal changes. A concise description of it is again given here from a different point of view.

§764 The characteristics upon which the effect of habitable regions on people depends—it has been established earlier that the influence of climate is exercised through factors such as: (1) altitude (whether high or low-lying); (2) type of adjoining country (mountainous, maritime, open or sheltered); (3) nature of soil (clay, mud, mineral, damp, marshy); (4) adequacy or scarcity of water (stagnant or flowing); and (5) local factors (trees, mines, cemeteries, and dead animals in the vicinity).

§765 As we have also pointed out, the temperament of the air is revealed by the latitude of a territory, its elevation or lowness, the proximity of mountains and seas, prevailing winds, and kind of soil. In short, whenever the air becomes quickly cold after sunset and quickly warms after sunrise, it is attenuated. If the opposite is the case, the nature of the atmosphere is the contrary. The most harmful of all kinds of air is that which contracts the heart, hinders inspiration and makes breathing difficult. We will now discuss each kind of locality in turn.

§766 Hot countries. In these countries, complexion tends to become dark, the hair black and curly, and the digestion weak. The increased dispersion of fluids from the body leads to an earlier onset of senility. This is particularly evident in Abyssinian where people tend to become old even at the age of thirty and, due to excessive loss of vitality, are inclined to be timid. People living under these climactic conditions are generally of a soft and feeble constitution.

§767 Cold countries. Residents of cold countries are usually strong, brave and courageous. Their digestion is good. If, however, the climate is damp, they tend to become fat and obese with inconspicuous veins and joints and with soft and delicate skins.

§768 Damp wet countries. Residents of damp countries are distinctly obese and have a soft and smooth complexion. They are easily tired by exercise and are liable to suffer from prolonged fevers, diarrhea, menorrhagia and profuse bleeding of the piles. Diseases such as ulcers, fistulae, putrefactive disorders, stomatitis, and epilepsy are common. Here the summer is very hot and the winter very cold. People who live in dry climates develop a dry temperament. The skin becomes dry and dusky as a result of the great dryness and roughness of the atmosphere. The brain soon becomes dry in temperament.

§769 Rocky and exposed places. In these countries, both the winter and the summer are generally severe. The inhabitants have a dry temperament. Their skin is thin and cracks easily. Their brain also tends to be dry.

§770 High altitude. High altitude produces people who are brave, strong, and have a long life.[25]

§771 Mountains and snow-clad places. These places are generally damp and stuffy. Their inhabitants are gloomy and pessimistic. In such places, water never becomes cold, especially when it is stagnant in the lakes or has an excess of saltpeter [potassium nitrite]. The atmosphere in these places is always abnormal and hence, the water bad.

§772 Low-lying countries. The climate is generally hot in the summer and cold in the winter in these places. The body is hard and sturdy with an abundance of hair. People are strong and possess large prominent joints. They have a dry temperament, sleep little, and lack moral character. Possessed of physical strength, they are proud and tyrannous, and display great valor on the battlefield. They are often skillful but are generally temperamental.

§773 Maritime regions. People in these localities resemble those of colder countries. Such places are generally breezy during the snow, but after the snow has melted, they become hot and damp from the screening influence of mountains. [Maritime places are beneficial for nerve cases.] The summer and the winter are both mild because of the moisture from the sea. The breezes from the sea are, however, much more humid.[26]

§774 Northerly countries. Persons who live in the north resemble in character those who live in cold countries with cold seasons. Diseases of "expression" (§711) and those due to confinement of the humors in the interior parts are liable to occur. Digestion is usually good. Such persons are long-lived.

§775 Repletion with, and the lack of dispersion of, the humors predisposes to epistaxis and the rupture of varicose veins. Ulcers readily heal owing to the vigor of the body and the purity of the blood. External conditions are also favorable to healing because there is nothing to relax or moisten the tissues. The fact that the innate heat is plentiful in such people prevents epilepsy from occurring, but if fits should occur they will be correspondingly severe, for it would have to be a very powerful agent to bring on such fits at all in these regions. The great degree of heat in the heart makes such persons leonine (wolfish) in disposition.

§776 The effect on the female sex. Menstruation is defective owing to constriction of the channels and the absence of the stimulus to menstrual flow and to relaxation of the channels. Some assert that this makes the women sterile; that their wombs do not open. But this is contrary to experience; at any rate as regards the Turks. My opinion of the stimulus to flow and to dilate the channels. Abortion, it is said, is rare among women in these climates and this fact further supports the opinion that their vitality is great. However, parturition is not easy because the organs in question remain hard and will not open easily. If abortion should occur, it must be ascribed to the cold. The milk will be scanty and thick, because the cold prevents the blood from flowing easily enough to the breasts.

§777 When the vitality is impaired, people in these regions (especially nursing women) are liable to develop puerperal tetanus and wasting diseases, because the difficult labor makes them strain so much and consequently risk tearing the veins in the chest, and the nerve and muscle-fibers. The former leads to pulmonary ulcers; and the latter to spasmodic affections. Another effect of the excessive straining during parturition is ventral hernia.

§778 As regards the age of puberty in these countries, hydrocele arises, but disappears as the person grows older. Female slaves are liable to develop ascites and hydrouterus but these also pass away as they grow old. Ophthalmia is rare but is severe when it does occur.

§779 Residence in southerly countries. The climactic features of these countries are similar to those of the summer. Water is usually saline and contains sulphur. Tendency to accumulate moist humors in the head is a specific characteristic of the southerly habitat. Hence, people frequently suffer from diarrhea due to the inevitable discharge of catarrhal secretions from the head into the stomach. The limbs and other organs are generally weak and flabby. People are often mentally dull and have poor appetite. Due to weakness of the brain, they are easily affected by alcohol. Since wounds tend to remain moist and relaxed, healing is slow.

§780 The effect on the female sex. Women bleed profusely during menses and conceive with difficulty. Miscarriages are common, but this is mostly due to greater frequency of disease than to any other cause.

§781 The effect on the male sex. Men often suffer from dysentery, piles and catarrhal ophthalmia, but these disappear quickly. The middle aged persons of over fifty develop paralysis due to congestion in the brain caused by catarrh and suffer from asthma, epilepsy and other spasmodic conditions.

§782 The inhabitants tend to develop fevers characterized both by heat and cold and prolonged fevers which generally appear during winter and have nocturnal paroxysms. Temperature is, however, seldom high due to the frequent occurrence of diarrhea which disperses the lighter elements of the humors.

§783 Residence in easterly countries. Towns which are open to the east receive pure fresh air as they are exposed to the sun which purifies it. They also receive gentle breezes which travel with the sun.

§784 Residence in westerly countries. Towns exposed to the west and shielded from in the east are protected from the sun for a longer time. They are exposed to the sun for only a short time and that, too, when the sun is going away from rather than coming towards them. Hence, it fails to make the air thin and dry and leaves the atmosphere dense and humid. If there is any breeze, it is from the west and that, too, only in the evening. Residents in such places are subject to the same effect as in the moderately hot, dense and humid countries. But for the greater density of air, these places should have the same characteristics as the spring. In spite of this, these places are not as healthy as those places open to the east, as the air there is in fact never like that of the spring. It is, however, true that places in the west have a relatively better climate than some of the other localities. A particularly undesirable feature of these places is their sudden exposure to the hot midday sun after the colder nights. Due to excessive humidity, the inhabitants are prone to develop hoarseness of voice, specially during autumn, when the catarrhal conditions are most common.

§785 How should one choose a place of residence and what type of house should be selected? In selecting a place for residence one should consider the nature of the soil, the altitude of the place, whether it is exposed or sheltered, bare or covered with trees or woodlands or forests; if its water supply is exposed or covered, i.e., low lying or exposed to breezes or being at some considerable depth; if the prevailing winds are fresh and cool, whether they are salubrious or not, fresh (cold) and bracing, or dry and sultry (having blown over wide tracts of land), or moist; whether it is cold and healthy; the nature of the surrounding country with respect to the presence or absence of seas, lakes, mountains; whether it is rich in minerals or not; whether the ground air is pure and healthy, or impure and unhealthy, making the natives prone to illness; what sort of illnesses prevail; the general health of the inhabitants, regarding their strength, appetite, digestion and dietetic habits; the construction of a house, whether it should be large and roomy, or with narrow entrances, good ventilation and wide chimneys. Do the doors and windows face east and north? One must be specially careful to arrange to have the easterly winds able to enter the house and to see that the rays of the sun can enter all day because the sun's rays make the air pure.[27]

§786 There should also be plenty of sweet, pure, and clean water nearby and that, too, should be in the running state rather than stagnant in deep and covered wells. It should be cool during winter and warm in summer.

§787 Consider the amount of light, the temperature (hot, warm, cold), rainfall, and average humidity of the atmosphere.

§788 Having discussed fully the influence of air and residence, other factors which influence the body will now be described.

10.4.2.4. The Unavoidable Physical Causes Because Physiological

§789 The effect of exercise on the human body varies according to its degree—mild or severe, the amount of rest taken, and the movement of the associated humors.[28]

§790 All forms of exercise, whether moderate or excessive, slow or vigorous, increase the innate heat. It makes little difference whether the exercise is vigorous or weak and associated with much rest or not, because it makes the body very hot; but even if exercise should entail a loss of innate heat, it does so only to a small amount. The dissipation of heat is only gradual, whereas the amount of heat produced is greater than the loss. If there be much of both exercise and repose, the effect is to cool the body because the natural heat is now greatly dispersed and consequently the body becomes dry. If the exercise entail the handling of certain material, that material usually adds to the effect of the exercise, although often there is a lessened effect. As an example, if the exercise were in the course of performing the art of the fuller, an increase in coldness and moisture would result. If the exercise were in the course of the performance of the art of the spelter, there would be more heat and dryness.

§791 Rest always has a cooling effect because the envigorating, life-giving heat passes away and the innate heat is confined. It also has a choking and moistening effect because of the lack of dispersal of waste matters.

10.5. The Conditions Associated with Sleep and Wakefulness

§792 Sleep closely resembles rest, while wakefulness is akin to exercise and activity. Since both have their own special characteristics, they need separate consideration.[29]

§793 Sleep strengthens the natural faculties or drives [digestion of food and elaboration of the digestive products into good blood], by enclosing the innate heat within the body and relaxing the faculty or drives of sensation [which are asleep]. It does so because it makes the channels of the breath [mind] moist and relaxed.

§794 Sleep removes all types of lassitude (see §1716) and it restrains strong evacuations. If then followed by appropriate exercise, the power of running is increased unless effete matters accumulate which only the skin can remove.

§795 Sleep sometimes helps to expel these effete matters in that it imprisons the innate heat and procures the dissemination of the nutrients throughout the body and the expulsion of the effete matters which are under the skin as well as of those which are deep in the interior parts of the body. These innermost matters push on those which are in front of them in successive waves until they finally reach the subcutaneous tissues and are thereby discharged from the skin. The same action is achieved by wakefulness to a still greater degree, but in this case the effete matter is removed by dissipation, whereas sleep removes it by inducing sweating.

§796 Sleep induces sweating—it does this by a process of overcoming the effete matter and not by a process of continuous dispersal of attenuated matter. When a person sweats heavily during sleep, without obvious cause, nutrients accumulate in excess of the bodily requirements. When sleep encounters matter adapted for digestion and maturation, it turns it into the nature of blood and warms it and in consequence innate heat is engendered and travels through and warms the whole body. If there are hot bilious humors and the period of sleep is prolonged, there is abnormal production of heat. Sleeping on an empty stomach produces more dispersion than coldness in the body. During sleep, the indigestible foods, being partially digested, tend to produce coldness. Wakefulness has quite the opposite effect. When the wakefulness is unduly prolonged, it produces disturbance of the brain such as dryness, weakness and impairment of the intellectual faculties or drives.

§797 Wakefulness is, however, however, the contrary way in all these respects. Excessive wakefulness, by oxidizing the humors, produces hot types of diseases. Excess of sleep, on the other, hand dulls the nervous and mental faculty or drives and makes the head heavy. Due to lack of dispersion, cold type of diseases also follow.

§798 Wakefulness increases the desire for food and stimulates the appetite by dispersing the wastes. It, however, impairs the digestion by dissipating the faculties or drives.[30]

§799 A restless and disturbed sleep (insomnia), being in a state between wakefulness and sleep, is bad for all the bodily states.

§800 Undue somnolence entails an imprisonment of the innate heat and makes the body become cold exteriorly. This is why so many blankets are needed to keep the limbs warm during sleep, which are not required in the waking state. That is why the whole body has to be covered up.

§801 A detailed description of the various factors concerning sleep and their significance will be discussed in my succeeding books.

10.6. The Influence of Psychological (Emotional) Factors

§802 Mental changes (*al-awarid al-nafsaniyah*) and the associated "motions" of the breath are either interior or exterior, sudden or gradual.

§803 Where there is coldness inwardly it moves outward with the breath. Therefore if the breath were suddenly dispersed, the coldness becomes excessive, and both exterior and interior cooling occur which may be followed by syncope or even death. When there is coldness exteriorly, and heat interiorly, the coldness moves inward with the breath.[31]

§804 Great confinement of the breath, with both exterior and interior cooling, results in severe syncope or even death. The outward movement of the vital force or expansion of the breath may be sudden and forcible, as in anger, or gradual as in delight and joy. Similarly, the inward movement or contraction may be sudden, as in acute fear and terror or gradual as in sorrow or gloom. When the movement is sudden, there is a severe shrinkage or dispersal of the vital force, but when it is slow or gradual, there is only a mild contraction or expansion of the vital force.[32]

§805 Confinement and dispersal of breath only occur suddenly; languishing of breath only develops by degrees. By "languishing" I mean a slow, progressive confinement or coarctation of the breath. When I say "the nature declines," I refer to a gentle, gradual, step by step dispersal of the vitality. If two motions of the mind occur simultaneously, the breath may move in two directions (contraction within itself, and enlarging) at once. This happens (1) when there is fear, dread, and anxiety about the future. (2) When anger and gloom occur simultaneously. The two opposite movements may produce a sense of shame, because there is first the confinement of the breath in the interior parts, and after that the power of reason returns, and resolution appears, allowing the contracted breath to expand again, and bring heat to the surface. The skin now becomes red.

§806 The influence on the body of mental disturbances of a different category. The state of the mind of the parents affects the body of the offspring, as for instance, fantasies. As a rule, it is some natural object which impresses the body. For instance, some image of a boy pictured by both parents at the time of conception may be realized in the infant when born or the infant's breath may have a "color" very like the color seen (mentally) by the mother while the seminal fluid was flowing into her at coitus or by the father during the the time of this flow. Many persons are reluctant to believe such things and suppose they can understand the states of the body without having realized the fundamental state. The physician who seeks wisdom does not deny these and allied things.[33]

§807 Other instances of the influence of fantasy on the bodily state are: (1) A movement of the mind which is intent on considering red things induces a corresponding state of readiness for a movement of the sanguineous humor. (2) Energetic character: eating acrid things; hardening of the teeth. (3) Introspective character: dwelling on aches and pains in the limbs. (4) Timid character: fearing lest some imagined event should happen: change of temperament corresponding (fear of catching a certain complaint: actually developing the disease. (5) Hopeful disposition: rejoicing in the thought of something one would like to realize—change of temperament corresponding.

10.7. Dietetics: The Influence of Food and Drink

§808 Food and drink influence the body in regard to (a) quality; (b) material composition; and (c) "substance" as a whole. It is essential to define each of these three terms exactly.

§809 Influence in regard to quality. Heating and cooling food and drink respectively make the body hot by virtue of their own heat; cold by virtue of their own coldness; and yet these qualities do not become an integral part of the body.

§810 The influence in regard to material composition—the food and drink in this case change from their own nature so as to receive the "form" of one or other of the human members (tissues); and the matter of which the food is composed receives the "form" of the member without losing its own dominant primary quality right through the whole process of digestion to the end of assimilation. Thus, the temperament of lettuce is colder than that of the human body, and yet lettuce becomes blood and is thus capable of being converted into tissue. The temperament of garlic is hotter than that of the human body and it also becomes blood.

§811 The influence in regard to substance as a whole. This is an action according to what food is in itself, as apart from its four primary qualities and apart from whether it becomes like the tissues or not or apart from whether the body becomes like to it or not.

§812 Matter does not enter into action by virtue of its quality of action, but action ensues by virtue of its matter when the matter is changed by a transforming drive in the body, from the substance it originally possesses and first renews whatever has been used up in the body and then increases the innate heat in the blood. Then the effect of the primary qualities which remain in the food after that comes into play.

§813 The action occurs by virtue of the substance when the "form" of its "species"—resulting from its temperament (for the elementary components are intermingled, and one single thing emerges therefrom)—is made ready for receiving the species; a certain "form" is now super-added over and above the form possessed by the primary qualities.

§814 But this "form" is neither (1) the primary qualities of the matter, nor (2) the temperament proceeding from those primary qualities.

§815 This "form" is the perfection which the pattern of the ailment receives according to its capacity, and its capacity is the outcome of its temperament. For example, the attractive faculty of the magnet; the nature inherent in the various species of plants and animals (the nature emerging from the temperament).

§816 Nor is this "form" (3) any of the simple temperaments by themselves, for it is not hotness, moistness, dryness, or coldness, either alone or in combination. It is, in truth, something comparable with color, odor, or intellect, soul or some other "form" imperceptible by the senses.

§817 The "form" which arises after the temperament has formed may be perfected by passive action. In this case the "form" = "passive property." But it may also exhibit active perfection. In this case "form" = "active property" (active principle). This active property may be exerted upon a human being or it may not.

§818 Any property may produce an effect on the human body which is either desirable (useful, harmonious) or undesirable (inharmonious). Such an effect is not entirely derived from its temperament.

§819 It is also derived from the substance as a whole (that is, the "specific form"), and not from any of the primary qualities or from a temperamental intermingling of the qualities. For instance, the action of peony in annulling epileptic seizures is desirable. The action of aconite in destroying human "substance" is an instance of undesirable action.

§820 A substance which is eaten or is introduced hypodermically (that is, by inunction) is "hot" or "cold." we mean not only that it is so virtually (not actually), but that it is virtually hotter or colder than are our bodies.

§821 "Power" or "potentiality," is a term with two kinds of meaning. It may be used in reference to the action of the innate heat of the body upon it.

§822 As soon as the potentiality encounters the action of the innate heat, it submits to that and so becomes act. Or, the word potentiality may also be considered in reference to its utility or advantage to the body. Thus we say that sulphur is hot in potentiality ("virtually hot").

§823 When we say that a thing is hot or cold, we may mean that one of the four imponderables is dominant in its temperament and we do not refer to the effect which it has on our bodies.

§824 We may say that a certain medicine has such and such a potentiality, thereby meaning its utility or otherwise to the body. Thus a scribe who has stopped writing still has the potentiality for writing. So we say that aconite has a destructive potentiality. In the one case, there is no act until after the body has become evidently changed. In the other, the action occurs at once, from the mere presence of the agent (viper poison) or some time later, after it has undergone some certain change in quality (aconite). Between these two potentialities there is a third—that of poisonous medicaments.

§825 There are four orders of medicines—whether eaten, taken in the fluid state, or given by inunction: (1) The first degree drugs are those whose action is not ordinarily felt by the body, i.e., the heat or cold produced by them is not appreciated unless the drug is taken repeatedly or in a larger quantity. (2) The second degree drugs are a little more potent but unless taken repeatedly or in larger doses they do not disturb the normal functioning of the body and even when they do so it is only indirectly. (3) The third degree drugs directly impair the normal functioning of the body but not to the extent of causing disease or death. (4) The fourth degree drugs are those which cause death or damage to the body. These are the poisonous medicines which act on account of their quality. The poisons of course kill by their very nature and are thus specific.[34]

§826 The fate of medicines taken into the body are either:[35] (1) changed by the body in a passive or active change; or (2) they are not changed by the body at all, but rather produce a harmful and active change in the body like poison. In regard to (1), the body is (a) neither changed nor restored to health (passive actions), or (b) the body itself is changed (active action). With (a),medicine that is pure nutriment changes into the body or the medicine is called attempered medicine because it changes, but not into the likeness of the body. Where there is an active action (1), the body itself is changed by the medicine. With medicinal food, the change in medicine produces a change into the likeness of the body, while with pure medicine, the medicine is not changed into the likeness of the body, or (2) the change in the body continues until the life of the patient is destroyed. This is through venomous medicine.

§827 In saying a medicine is not changed by our body we do not mean that it does not induce a formation of heat in the body by affecting the innate heat because, as a matter of fact, most poisons only act on the body in that way, thereby producing warmth. We mean that its "form" is not changed, and that, as a result, its power continues to influence the body until the latter has destroyed the "form." For instance, if the nature of the medicine be hot, its nature reinforces its property of dispersing the breath. Examples include viper venom and aconite. Again, if the medicine be cold, its nature reinforces its property by congealing or enfeebling the breath. An example would be scorpion venom and hyoscyamus (or hellebore).

§828 Anything that is nutritious will eventually change the temperament of the body and in a natural manner. It warms the body because when it becomes blood, that is, the natural effect and the body becomes warmer. Lettuce and gourds warm in this way. So in saying "warm," we do not mean "warm" the form" but "warm that which arises out of its own intrinsic quality"—the species remaining.

§829 Medicines which are food are altered by the body first in quality and later in substance. This change in quality may be in respect of heat so that the medicine warms (e.g., garlic); or it may be in respect of cold so that the body becomes cold (e.g., lettuce). Afterwards, when the digestion and conversion into good blood has been completed, the medicines produces warmth to the same extent to which it has added to the volume of the blood thereby increasing the substance of the innate heat. How could it do otherwise than furnish heat when it has itself been made hot and its coldness thereby abstracted?

§830 But even after the medicine has been changed in substance there still remains some of its innate quality (some hot, some cold). There is some of the coldness of the lettuce left in the blood which has been made from the lettuce and there is some of the heat of the garlic left in the blood which the garlic has given rise to. This holds good for a certain period of time.

§831 Some nutrient medicines are medicinal in quality rather than nutrient and others are nutrient rather than medicinal. Some of the latter are more like the "substance" of blood in nature (such as wine, egg-yolk, and meat-juice), and others are less so (such as bread, and meat) and others are entirely different to the substance of the blood (medicinal foods).

§832 Food changes the state of the body both in quality and quantity. Changes in quality have been discussed.

§833 Changes in quantity are in two directions. Either (1) the nutriment increases in the body until there is an aversion to food, obstructions therefore arise and putrescence results; or (2) it diminishes in amount until the body wastes away and the tissues dry up.

§834 An increase in amount of nutriment is always cooling in effect unless decomposition supervenes in it so giving rise to warmth. This warmth, due to putrescent changes, is extraneous; for changes in the superfluous nutriment are the means by which extraneous heat, as opposed to innate heat, enters the body.[36]

§835 Food may be light, heavy, or of medium quality.[37] Light food produces thin blood, the heavier food thick blood, and a medium in this regard is the food which produces a medium type of blood. Food may be rich or poor in quality. Examples are:

Rich and light: wine, meat juice, cooked eggs or partly cooked eggs.

Poor and heavy food which forms only a small quantity of thick blood: cheese, part fried meat and eggplant.

Poor and light: honey diluted with rose water, vegetables of a medium quality, apples and pomegranates.

Rich and heavy: boiled eggs and beef.

All these may be further defined according to the nature of resulting chyme, as wholesome and unwholesome.

Light, rich, and wholesome: egg yolks, alcohol, and raw meat juice.

Light, rich, and unwholesome: lungs, pigeon, and young pheasants.

Light, poor, and wholesome: lettuce and apples.

Light, poor, and unwholesome: radish, mustard, and most vegetables.

Heavy, rich, and wholesome: boiled eggs and meat of one-year-old lamb.

Heavy, rich, and unwholesome: beef, horse flesh and duck.

Heavy, poor, and unwholesome: dried meat.

Heavy, poor, and wholesome: lean beef.

10.8. Various Kinds of Drinking Water

§836 Water[38] is the only one of the elements which has the special property of entering into the composition of food and drink—not that it is itself nutriment (although it will by itself prolong life for some time), but rather that it enables the chyme to penetrate into the human body and permeate and purify its substance.

§837 We do not wish to imply that water does not nourish at all, but we mean that it is not, as nutriment is, potential blood, giving rise ultimately to body tissue. As an elementary substance, it is not changed in state in such a way as to become able to receive the "form" of blood or of tissue. This can only occur with a true compound.

§838 Water is really a "substance" which helps to make

chyme fluid and attenuated so that it can flow easily into the blood-vessels and out of the excretory channels. Nutrition cannot be effective without it. It is the handmaid of nutrition.

§839 The various kinds of water differ (1) not merely in the substance of aquosity, but (2) in admixed matters, and (3) their own individual dominant primary qualities.

§840 The best type of water comes from the springs located on a soil which is pure and free from contamination and not from the springs over rocky ground. Although the rocky soil does not putrefy as easily as the pure earthy soil, its water is not as good as that obtained from a pure soil. The water from the springs of a pure soil is, however, not always the best unless it is running and is exposed both to the sun and the air.

§841 Since exposure spoils the water of stagnant springs, it is better that these springs should be deep and well covered. The water which is running over ordinary soil is better and purer than the one which runs over rocky ground. This is because ordinary soil filters the impurities better than the rocky ground. The soil should of course be really pure and not nitrous or marshy. The other characteristics of a good water are that it runs deep, its flow is rapid and its quantity so large that anything mixed with it would become relatively insignificant. Its direction of flow should be towards the sun, i.e., eastwards and particularly towards the summer east.

§842 It is also better that the water should be collected at some considerable distance from the source. The next best is the water which runs northward. Water which runs southward or westwards is of little value, specially when it is exposed to the south winds. The water which is ordinarily wholesome further improves by running from a height. The best type of water has the qualities mentioned here: (1) it has a characteristic sweet taste; (2) it is easily mixed with wine; (3) it is light in weight; (4) it becomes hot or cold easily when rarefied; (5) it cools in winter and warms up in summer; (6) it is free from any other taste; (7) it is odorless; (8) it passes down the stomach with ease (i.e., does not cause irritation or heaviness); and (9) it does not have an unduly high or low boiling point

§843 An excellent method of assessing the quality of water is by weighing it. The water which is lighter in weight is generally superior. Thus, we may test it by weighing the unknown water against an equal volume of some known water = the water which is superior would be lighter, soaking equal quantities of cotton wool in equal volumes of the waters being tested. After a thorough drying, the pieces of cotton wool are weighed against each other. The one which is lighter would be the better of the two waters.[39]

§844 Water can be purified by distillation, filtration, and decantation. If these methods are not workable, it may be boiled. Boiled water causes less distension and passes through the system quickly. The belief that there is no advantage in boiling and that the evaporation of the lighter portions from it makes it more dense is misconceived. Water is an element with particles of a uniform nature and density. It is not a compound. It becomes dense when it is extremely cold or when there is some mineral matter thoroughly mixed with it. The mineral particles are often so minute that they are unable to overcome the resistance and thus settle down at the bottom.

§845 Boiling reduces the density of water by first reducing its cold and then, by expansion, makes it light and rarefied. The result is that particles of mineral matter, which had been there due to the relatively greater density of water, now settle down as a deposit thus, leaving behind pure water of a more or less elemental nature. The water obtained by evaporation does not differ from ordinary water. It is actually like any other water. Thus, water becomes light by a reduction of the density due to cold and by the sedimentation of admixed particles. The proof of this is that when dense water is allowed to stand even for a long time, it does not leave any appreciable deposit and remains clear and transparent. But on boiling, deposit occurs due to the rarefaction of water. A similar phenomenon can also be observed when water from a big channel like that of the Oxus River (Amu Darya) is collected in a pit at some distance from the source. The water, though, originally dense and muddy is so clarified by sedimentation that it fails to yield any further deposit.[40]

§846 Some have highly praised water of the Nile for it flows a longer distance from the source. It flows on pure soil. It flows in a northerly direction, which makes it lighter; and it has considerable depth, which is however a common feature of most rivers.

§847 If impure water is daily made to stand in a new vessel, it will regularly leave some fresh deposit. Its suspended particles however do not settle down properly unless the water is allowed to stand for a considerably long time and even then it would not be purified completely. The reason is that mineral particles separate easily from liquids which are thin, light and free from viscosity or oiliness. In the liquids which are dense, sedimentation is more difficult unless they have been made thin by boiling. Next to boiling is the method of agitation in which the water is shaken or churned.

10.8.1. Commendable Waters

§848 Rain water is the best, especially when it is collected during summer and particularly after thunder. In stormy weather, it becomes dense and impure (from admixture).

§849 Rain water, even though purest, is easily vitiated. This is because it is very thin and is thus liable to prompt vitiation from both the atmosphere and the ground. When it becomes vitiated, it sets up putrefactive changes in the humors. Rain water is injurious to the throat and chest.

§850 It has been suggested that the actual reason for its putrefactive tendency is that it is formed by the evaporation of all kinds of waters from the ground, including those which are putrefied. If this had been the case, the rain water would have become impure and dangerous, but this is decidedly not so. The real reason why it putrefies so easily is that it is extremely light and thin and it is well established that anything which is of a light nature is always prone to be easily affected by extraneous influences. If rain water is promptly boiled, its tendency for putrefaction is greatly minimized. If one has to drink rain water, something sour should be taken as the necessary corrective.

§851 The worst kind is the well and water from a canal because it is usually stagnant and thus has a prolonged contact with the mineral matter. It is also somewhat putrefied as it does not spring out of its own force, but collects by seepage with gravity. The water which is carried through lead pipes is most harmful. It becomes contaminated with lead and thus produces ulceration of the intestine. Well water, by being frequently lifted is constantly replaced by the seepage of fresh water; hence, it does not stagnate for a long time.

§852 Snow water and water from melted ice are coarse in texture. When pure and free from admixture with deleterious substances, such water is good and healthy; it is also useful for cooling water, either by placing such water in it or by adding it to the water. There is little difference in the visible character of these two kinds of water but they are denser in texture than other kinds of water. This kind of water is harmful for persons suffering from neuritis. Boiling renders such water wholesome. If ice water be made of bad water or if the snow has attracted some bad property from the places upon which it has fallen, it would be better to use water free of such injurious admixture?[41]

10.8.2. Non Commendable Waters

§853 On the other hand, marshy water which moves about in the sodden pores of the soil is not so active as to rise to the surface. When it does so, it is only feebly and passively from the sheer size of its larger collection. These waters generally come from dirty and polluted soils. Well water, on the other hand, is cleansed by contact with that which separates out from it and by the gases which bubble up out of it, thereby keeping it in constant movement. Well water does not remain in a confined state long and does not linger in the channels and openings of the earth.

§854 Water in reed marshes, particularly after its exposure to the air, becomes heavy and unhealthy. During the winter, cooled by the snow, it produces phlegm [serous humor] and in the summer, rendered hot by exposure to the sun, it produces bilious humor. There are three reasons why they cause disease: (1) their inspissated character, (2) admixture with earthy matter, (3) dispersion of their subtile particles.

§855 The following are the diseases liable to develop after drinking stagnant water: Diseases of the spleen (these result in heaping up of the viscera and stretching of the peritoneum—the belly being hard and tense); wasting of the arms, legs and neck—for the nutrition fails because of the state of the spleen despite the excessive appetite and thirst; constipation; vomiting becomes difficult to induce; dropsy, from retention of the water; inflammatory deposits in the lung and spleen; dysenteric ailments with the result that the hands and feet become dry and the liver becomes enfeebled and nutrition is impaired; quartan fevers (in summer); piles, varices, and lax swellings of inflammatory nature; and insanity (especially in winter).

§856 The effect of stagnant water on women is that conception and parturition are both difficult. The offspring will be male and will be liable to develop inflammatory masses and then waste away. Moles are liable to occur because impregnation is often faulty; the offspring is found to have rupture. Varicose veins and ulcers of the leg heal with difficulty. The appetite increases and there is constipation leading to intestinal ulceration. Quartans are common.

§857 The effect of stagnant water on old persons is that ardent fevers occur as accords with dryness of their nature and of the stomach.

§858 All stagnant waters, from whatever source, are injurious to the stomach.

§859 Channel water is similar to stagnant water but is more healthy because it does not linger so long in one spot. If it is not actually flowing, this is because of some heaviness in it. In many of these waters (including water in aqueducts, water in irrigation channels) there is a certain stypticity and they quickly warm the interior organs. Therefore they are not utilizable in cases of fever or for persons in whom the bilious humor is predominant. They are more applicable for cases of disease where the treatment is to foster retention and maturation.

§860 Waters which contain metallic substances are generally injurious. Some may however be of considerable value, i.e., water with iron strengthens the internal organs, prevents stomach trouble and stimulates the appetite. They resolve the spleen and are beneficial for those who cannot cohabit properly. Waters containing salts of ammonia are aperient and carminative. They may be either swallowed as a drink or given as an enema or used in a sitz-bath. These waters will be described in detail later on. Waters containing alum suppress excessive menstruation and haemoptysis and the bleeding of piles but they make persons who are liable to develop fevers still more liable to develop them.

§861 Waters in which leeches live are injurious.

§862 Salt water makes the body dry up and become wasted. Its abstersive power makes it first a laxative and afterwards constipating because it is dry in nature. It decomposes the blood and so gives rise to pruritus and scabies.

§863 Acetous water, added to rain water which has to be consumed, arrests putrefactive changes in the water and provides immunity from such ill-effects.

§864 Milky water gives rise to calculus and obstructions. Therefore one should make use of diuretics after it. In fact, one should take diuretics after drinking any coarse and heavy waters because they linger in the bowel. Fatty and sweet things (like theriaca) are also corrective for such water. The fact that milky water brings on constipation makes it of value for some persons.

§865 Water which is only moderately cold is more healthy than all others because it stimulates the appetite and strengthens the stomach. Nevertheless it weakens the nerves and is harmful for cases of inflammatory disease in the interior organs.

§866 Tepid water incites nausea. Warm water (a little warmer than tepid water) taken on an empty stomach is cleansing both to the stomach and intestines, but it has a weakening effect on the stomach if taken often.

§867 Hot water is beneficial for the following conditions: (1) head: cold headache, inflammation of the eye, parotitis, quinsies, dry gums, postauricular inflammations; (2) mental conditions: epilepsy and melancholia; (3) chest: asthma, solutions of continuity in the thorax, ulcers of the diaphragm; (4) general: rheumatic pains, dieresis, and relief for painful micturition; (5) female conditions: it brings on menstruation. Hot water interferes with digestion and makes the food swim about in the stomach. It does not quench thirst. It may lead to dropsy, hectic fever and emaciation. Very hot water is of great value in colic as it disperses flatulence.

§868 Aerated waters are useful for certain intemperaments. When various kinds of water, good and bad, are mixed, their effect varies according to which proves dominant.

§869 The correction of impure water is referred to under "regimen for travelers."

§870 Other matters related to water and its properties and modes of action will be discussed in Book 2, God permitting.

10.9. The Effect of Retention (Repletion)/ Evacuation (Depletion)

10.9.1. Retention (Repletion)

§871 The following are the causes of retention of waste matters: (1) weak expulsive drive; and (2) unduly strong retentive drive. The latter occurs in: (a) weakness of the digestive power so that aliments remain too long in the stomach, the natural retentive drive holding them back until they are sufficiently digested; (b) narrowness of the channels; and (c) their obstruction; (d) coarseness or viscidity of the waste matter. The former holds in the case of (a) a superabundance of waste matter so that the expulsive drive cannot deal with it; and (b) insufficient informing sense for defecation, this act being aided by voluntary effort. The result may be that the effete matter is compensatorily removed to other parts of the body by the action of the vegetative drives. Thus, jaundice follows [gall-stone] colic; the colic depends on the retention, the jaundice is the compensatory evacuation. Again, at the crisis of a fever, there may be retention of urine and feces, and a critical evacuation occurs elsewhere.

§872 Diseases due to the retention of waste matters are: (1) Compositional such as constipation, diarrhea, or laxity of the bowels, *spasmus humidus* and the like; inflammatory process; furuncles; (2) Intemperaments such as septic conditions; imprisonment of the innate heat, or mutation of this into igneity. There may be so marked a coarctation that the innate heat is extinguished altogether, and coldness of the body supervenes with the transference of too much moisture to the surface of the body; and (3) General conditions: tearing or rupture of locular spaces and crypts.

§873 When repletion (as from great plenty during fertile years) develops after a long period of inanition (as from times of great famine in barren years), it is one of the most effective causes of such illnesses.

10.9.2. Evacuation (Depletion)

§874 The causes of the evacuation (depletion)[42] of matters which are normally retained include: (1) Vigorous expulsive drive. (2) Defective retentive drive. (3) Unfavorable quality of the matter which is (a) too heavy, because superabundant; (b) too distending owing to flatulent action; (c) corrosive and acrid in quality; and (d) attenuated of texture, making it too mobile and too easily expelled, and: (4) Widening of the excretory channels. This occurs in the case of the seminal flow.[43] It also occurs if they are torn longitudinally or transversely, or because their orifices become too patent (in epistaxis) from either extraneous or interior causes.

§875 The possible effects of evacuation of this type are: (1) The temperament becomes cold because the matter is lost which would otherwise increase that which maintains the innate heat. (2) The temperament becomes hot if the evacuated material is cold in temperament like serous humor or mucus. (3) The temperament becomes equable to blood if there is undue accumulation of the heating bilious humor so that the heat becomes superabundant. (4) The temperament becomes dry. This is always intrinsic in origin. (5) The temperament becomes moist in a matter analogous to that mentioned in regard to accidental increase in body heat, namely, either the evacuation of desiccant body fluid has not been too great or the innate heat is too scanty with the result that the aliment is not adequately digested and serous humor becomes relatively increased. But a moist temperament of this kind is unfavorable to the maintenance of the innate heat and foreign heat will not serve as a substitute for innate heat because of the difference of its nature.

§876 The effect of excessive evacuations on the members of the body include: (1) coldness and dryness of their substance and nature ensue, even though they receive extraneous heat and moisture beyond their need; and (2) diseases from obstruction of the vessels due to undue dryness and narrowing of the veins. Convulsions and tetanic spasms may therefore arise.

§877 When retention and evacuation are equally matched, and occur at the proper times, they are beneficial, and maintain health.[44]

10.10. The Diseases Caused by Faculties or Drives

§878 The influences on the human body from without act in these ways: (1) By penetration into the body three things may happen: (a) attenuated matter in the pores enters the body by its own penetrative power; (b) the tissues themselves draw it in through the pores; or (c) one of these factors assists the other. (2) The primary quality of the agent itself is able to produce a change in the body. There are three aspects of such a quality: (a) it may be actual, i.e., an epitheme of cooling character; a plaster which is calefacient; or (b) it may be potential—here the innate heat stirs up the power into actuality; (c) a specific property. (3) Things acting in both ways: (a) producing a harmful effect both externally and internally; and (b) harmful when applied externally, but not when taken internally, and vice versa.

§879 An example of an agent which affects the body when applied externally, but is harmless when taken by the mouth is onions applied as a plaster causing ulceration. As food, they are harmless.

§880 Another example of an agent of a contrary kind would be white lead. This is a virulent poison when swallowed, but is harmless when applied as an ointment.

§881 In explanation of this: (1) When a substance like onions is taken as food, the alternative drive breaks it up and changes its temperament into a weaker one until it is too weak to exert a harmful influence. Therefore, there is no internal ulceration. (2) When taken as food, such a substance is usually mixed with other foods. (3) Its power is broken by being submerged in the other moist substances present in the alimentary canal. (4) A substance applied externally can be kept in one spot, but when it is within the stomach, it is kept moving about. (5) A substance applied externally is usually applied very tightly and closely, whereas within the body it is only just in contiguity without any adhesion. (6) When a substance is taken internally, its own natural power determines the quick accomplishment of digestion and quickly expels the excess left after the bulk has been converted into good blood.

§882 The reason why the action of white lead is different is that white lead is of a gross nature and is made of coarse particles. Hence it cannot penetrate into the channels of the body from without, and even if it did enter the skin it would not reach as far as the channels of the breath or the principal organs. Taken in by the mouth the matter is different, for then its poisonous nature is at once brought out by the influence of the innate heat upon it. Such an interaction could not take place externally.

§883 We shall refer to these considerations again in the Book of Simples (Volume II).

10.11. Balneology

10.11.1. Baths. Friction. Exposure to the Sun

§884 This section[45] will also include a description of sand baths and oil baths and the effect of sprinkling the face with cold water. According to some, the best kind of baths are those which are housed in old spacious buildings with plentiful supply of fresh air and sweet water. There should also be proper arrangements for regulating the temperature according to individual requirements. Baths are constructed in such a way that the first room remains cold and moist, the second hot and moist, the third hot and dry. No consideration need be paid to the assertion that water has no moistening effect on the body whether used externally or internally.

§885 The natural action of the bath is that hot air warms the body and water adds to the moisture. Sometimes, baths may have some unusual effects on the body which may be direct or indirect. Thus, the hot atmosphere of the bath house produces cold from the excessive dissipation of innate heat (vitality) and dryness from the undue dispersion of natural secretions (through sweating). Some moisture may accrue, but this is only of a temporary kind.

§886 Changes and later effects of the bath are either accidental or essential.

§887 Cold air bath disperses the innate heat greatly and so dries the substance of the tissues. It disperses the natural fluids very greatly although it increases the extraneous fluids.

§888 If water is too hot, it produces "goose flesh," and by constricting the pores it prevents moisture from entering the body and there is not much dispersal of the innate heat. But the water sometimes adds to the warmth of the body and sometimes cools it. To have the former effect the water must be very hot.

§889 Sub-tepid bath cools and moistens the body. As the water cools down, the air of the bathroom becomes less warm and the effect of the cooling in both directions to which the body is now exposed is to contract the abdominal viscera.[46]

§890 The frequent use of such a bath will have a refrigerant effect. This is because (1) water is fundamentally cold in nature and even the warming of it will not ensure continuance of the "accidental" (scholastic significance) heat, the natural quality remaining and this natural coldness enters the body and makes it cold. (2) Whether hot or cold water is still wet and wets the body (interiorly) so imparting much moisture, it binds the innate heat even to the degree of extinction [as water quenches fire]. Consequently the body becomes cold.

§891 Such a bath may have a warming effect if (1) the aliment previously taken has not yet been digested; (2) there is a cold humor present in the body which is not yet completely matured. The bath will help the digestion of the aliment and the maturation of the humor.

§892 If the skin be dry at the time of the bath, dropsy or relaxed conditions would be benefited. If the skin be moist to commence with the bath will have a moistening effect.

§893 Dryness results if the person stay a long time in the bath. This is partly because of the loss of water by sweating and the dispersal of the breath so induced. A short stay in the bath will produce a moistening effect if the skin be wiped dry before sweating begins.

§894 To enter a bath fasting will make the body very dry and make the person thin and debilitated. To enter the bath after a heavy meal, on the other hand, will make a person gain weight by drawing the humors towards the subcutaneous tissues. Moreover it removes the obstructions by transferring the undigested aliment from the stomach to the tissues. To go to the bath at the moment when the first digestion has ended and before a sense of hunger returns is beneficial and produces a medium degree of weight.

§895 If the bath is taken for a moistening effect, a person suffering from hectic fever should be entirely immersed in water unless he is too enfeebled or his strength will not allow it. The air of the room should be temperate—neither hot nor cold, but gently moist. The water of the bath should be thrown freely about in order to disseminate the water vapor through the air and so fill the air with moisture. The duration of the bath should not be long. The patient should be lifted out of the water and rubbed down gently making no exertion himself. He should be laid on a couch in the bathroom and there be anointed with oil (to increase the moisture of the skin and retain in the pores the aquosity which has already gained entry into the skin thus fixing it within the skin) using cool perfumed oil. He should then lie in the tepidarium (the disrobing room) for an hour until his respiration subsides to the customary rate. After that he is anointed, robed and taken into a room where he may receive a small draught compounded of humectants like barley water and milk.

§896 Disadvantages—such patients should not stay too long in the bath as there is a risk of syncope because it renders the heart "hot" (and therefore disperses the "breath") and sets the bilious humor in motion. It produces nausea and other ill-effects. It causes morbidic matters to gravitate into the debilitated organs. It has a relaxing effect and is injurious for the nerves. It disperses the innate heat. It removes the appetite for solid food. It weakens the power of sexual intercourse.

§897 The action of baths by virtue of mineral constituents in the water—waters of this kind occur in nature or may be reproduced artificially. They are all strongly resolvent and attenuant. They make the tissues flabby and prevent humors from passing into abscesses. They are beneficial for the guinea worm and "Indian vein." Aluminous waters benefit cases of hemoptysis, melaena, menorrhage, procidentia ani or uteri, repeated causeless miscarriage, cachexias, undue sweating, causeless vomiting. They have a cooling and drying effect. Bitter waters have a heating and drying effect. Bituminous waters occasion fullness of the head. The person must therefore not immerse his head in the bath or stay too long in it. They render the temperament warmer especially that of the uterus, bladder, and colon. They are all harmful and heavy. Chalky waters have a cooling and drying effect. Copper-containing waters are beneficial for the mouth, tonsils and uvula, for relaxed ocular tissues, for humid affections of the ears. Ferruginous waters are beneficial for the stomach and spleen. Medicinal baths are prepared with laurel leaves, stavesacre, juniper berry. Nitrous baths and saline baths are beneficial for the head and chest when humors are constantly flowing into them. These baths are good for wateriness of the stomach, dropsy, swellings left after diseases and collections of phlegm. Aerated waters, ferruginous and saline waters are beneficial for diseases depending on coldness and moisture, for pains in the joints, for podagra. They benefit relaxed persons, asthma, renal disease, carbuncles, ulcers. They are very beneficial in cases of fracture. Sulphur baths soothe and warm the nerves and relieve pain, lassitude and convulsions. They cleanse the surface of the skin from furuncles and old bad ulcers and purplse marks. They benefit pannus, vitilego, and lepra. They disperse morbidic matters descending into the joints, the spleen and the liver. They are beneficial for the womb when unduly hard. They reduce the tone of the stomach and banish the appetite.

§898 Persons desiring to use thermal baths should bathe quietly, gently, and allow the waters to play gently over the relaxed body, laving, not splashing and in this way the interior organs are benefited.

10.11.2. The Influence of Sun, Sand, Oil, and Shower Baths

§899 Immersion in hot sand; oil baths, spraying of water over the face; standing, running, walking rapidly, or jumping in the heat of the burning sun—all these are powerful agents for removing superfluities, and for producing sweating, dispersion flatulence, lax swellings, and dropsies. They are beneficial for asthma, and for orthopnoea. They invigorate the brain (whose temperament is cold) and relieve inveterate "cold" headache. If the seat of the bath is dry and the floor is left wet, the bath will benefit cases of sciatica, lumbar pain, and uterine obstruction. It has a cleansing effect on the womb.

§900 One must not remain too long in the sun or else the body will become dry, thick and hard as the sun acts like a cautery upon the pores of the skin and obstructs the outflow of the insensible perspiration. The sun burns the skin more if one stands still in it than if one moves about and so it inhibits the dissipation of the sensible perspiration still more.

§901 Sea sand baths have a strong absorptive action on superficial swellings. Sand baths may be taken by sitting in the sand or by covering the body with it. Sand may also be sprinkled over the body. Sand baths relieve pain and prove beneficial in moist diseases. In short, sand baths have an extremely drying effect on the body.

§902 Taking an olive oil bath is refreshing for the fatigued. It is beneficial in chronic and "cold" type of fevers as well as in cases associated with general body aches and joint pains. Oil baths are also good in convulsions and other spasmodic conditions and in the retention or suppression of urine. Olive oil should be warmed outside the bath room. The oil in which fox or lizard excrement is boiled becomes very effective in the treatment of sciatica and arthralgia.[47]

§903 Shower baths, douching, spraying, and sprinkling of water over the face act as a stimulant to the faculty or drives weakened by dyspnea, syncope or heat of the fever. The addition of rose water or vinegar to the water would make it more effective. It may stimulate the appetite but is generally harmful to those suffering from catarrh and headache.[48]

10.12. The Agents Which Alter the Several Qualities of the Body

10.12.1. The Things Which Produce Heat (Calefacients)

§904 (1) Outward heat in various forms: summer heat, artificial heat, baths of moderate temperature (the heating effect is produced by both air and water), and heating (calefacient) plasters or local applications. (2) Heat produced by movement. Exercise, but not in excess; gymnastic exercise which is not too vigorous or beyond the right measure and duration; moderate friction; light massage with the hands on the limbs; dry cupping (wet cupping is infrigidant because it removes heat from the body). (3) Heat introduced by the mouth. Adequate supply of nutriment, hot aliments, hot or heating medicines (such as via oxidation with the body). (4) Heat arising from emotional states: anger, gloom in a degree less than would cause infrigidation; moderated joy. Also sleep and wakefulness in moderate degree.

§905 Heat derived from putrefaction. This is neither the innate heat nor derived from combustion. The warming from the innate heat is less in degree than that from combustion. It can occur apart from putrefaction and prior to a septic state. In the case of putrefaction the heat from the foreign source lingers in the body after the agent giving rise to it has left the body. This heat unites with the moisture of the humors and alters their temperament (in respect of moisture) in such a manner that it will no longer respond to the temperament of the natural breath. The difference between digestion and putrefaction is that in the case of digestion the heat and moisture which are present in matter are altered; that is, instead of being accordant with the original temperament, they are now accordant with another different one. In oxidation, moist substance is separated from dry by sublimation and evaporation, the dryness going into the residue. In the process of simple calefaction (heating), the humors simply become warmer without losing their natural breath. (6) The state of the body. When there is sclerosis of the surface, the body tends to become hot because the breath (that is, the steam) is held in or imprisoned. When there is rarefaction within the body, it becomes warm because the "breath" then expands throughout the body.[49]

§906 Galen had grouped all the above mentioned causes under the following five headings: (1) moderate exercise and activity, (2) external application of moderate heat, (3) hot foods and drinks, (4) hard skin (with constricted skin pores), and (5) putrefaction.

10.12.2. The Things Which Produce Cold (Refrigerants)

§907 The causes of cold are: (1) Artificial cold. This is a refrigerant in act, as it is cold itself. (2) Potential refrigerant. Thus when the body is hot at the time of exposure to the agent, its heat becomes dissipated like thermal waters. (3) Calefacients which are excessive. These include very hot air, thermal waters, hot plasters and fementations (which disperse the innate heat by relaxing the body); or moderate as in staying too long in the bath, or agents one time hot, but becoming cold later. (4) Excessive exercise. This disperses the innate heat unduly. Excessive repose aggregates and strangles the innate heat, thereby having an infrigidant effect. (5) Certain bodily states. Great rarefaction relaxes the body and disperses the innate heat; extreme spissitude strangles the innate heat; excessive retention (has the same action); undue evacuation from the body which destroys the material basis of the innate heat and disperses the breath and allows the effete matters to become obstructions. (6) Mental states. Great gloom, too much fear, too much joy, great delight. (7) Aliment. Excess of food and drink, cold aliments, too little food, refrigerant medicines. (8) Mechanical causes. Tight bandaging of limbs for some time which prevents the innate heat reaching them. (9) Crudity, the opposite of putrefaction.

§908 Galen grouped all the above mentioned causes under the following six headings: (1) excessive activity, (2) excessive repose, (3) applications which are either cold or not so hot as to cause excessive dispersion (diaphoresis), (4) cooling things, (5) marked reduction of food, and (6) marked excess of food.

10.12.3. The Things Which Produce Moisture (Humectants)

§909 The causes of moisture are: (1) external—baths, especially if taken after a meal; (2) diet—food taken to excess, humectant articles of food, humectant medicines; (3) retention of that which should be evacuated; (4) evacuation of desiccant humor; (5) repose and sleep; (6) joy in moderation; (7) infrigidants (these cause the humors to be retained); and (8) calefacients (a slight degree of warmth causes the humors to move).

10.12.4. Things Which Produce Dryness (Desiccants)

§910 The causes of dryness are: (1) External—cold congeals the humors and prevents the tissues from attracting nutritive material, it also constricts the channels of the body and so causes them to be blocked; in consequence nutrient material cannot reach it. (2) Great heat which disperses moisture. Therefore, too frequent hot baths have this effect. (3) Bathing in styptic waters which has a desiccant effect. (4) Diet—insufficient food, dry aliments, desiccant medicines. (5) Violent evacuations; coitus; (6) Exercise. (7) Wakefulness. (8) Frequent emotional disturbance.

10.13. The Agents Causing Deformity

§911 These may be due to: (1) congenital causes, i.e., a defect of the original formative faculty or drive inherent in the germinal fluid; (2) causes operating at the time of birth; (3) causes operating during infancy; (4) external causes, i.e., trauma; (5) efforts at walking before the limbs are sufficiently strong and firm; (6) various diseases such as leprosy, tuberculosis, paralysis, spasms and contractures; (7) excessive wasting or obesity; (8) inflammatory conditions; (9) diseases of the configuration; and (10) excessive formation of scars and keloids.

10.14. The Agents Causing Obstruction of the Channels

§912 Agents causing obstruction of the channels include: (1) Blockage of excretory channels with some abnormal material which may be abnormal in respect of composition, i. e., a calculus, size, i. e., a large accumulation of feces or quality and consistency, i. e., some unduly thick viscid or clotted material. The obstructing substance may be fixed or migratory. (2) Narrowing of channels. This may be due to scars from ulceration, polypoid growths, pressure from inflammatory processes, dryness of channels due to astringents, spasms from excessive cold, strong retentive faculty or drive, and tight bandaging. (3) Obstructions are generally common during winter due to the frequency of retentions and the constricting effect of cold. (4) feebleness of the retentive faculty or drive. (5) Excessive force of the expulsive faculty or drive, to which also belongs the forcible holding of breath. (6) Use of cleansing and relaxing medicines and those hot and moist medicines which narrow the channels.

10.15. The Agents Which Open Up the Channels

§913 Channels become dilated either from lack of retentive power or from an excessive action of the expulsive faculty. For example, holding the breath. Medicines which are relaxing, hot, moist, aperient and detergent. In short, all agents contrary to the above group, Agents Causing Obstruction of the Channels.

10.16. The Agents Producing Harshness of the Body

§914 (1) Sharp and mildly irritant chemicals, i. e., vinegar and acrid secretions. (2) Resolvents of irritative type, i. e., coral and acrid secretions. (3) Drying substances, which, like astringents may occasionally produce roughness. (4) Cold, which increases density. (5) Lodgment of dust particles. A medicinal agent may render the body harsh by its sharpness (acidity) like vinegar and acetous waste matters or by dispersion (like halcyonium = coral) and acrid waste matters or by styptic action (which produces roughness because it is dry an example being bitter substances). Infrigidants have this effect by inspissation. Terrene substances sprinkled over a limb like a dusting-powder may exert such an effect.

10.13. Causes

10.17.1. The Causes of Smoothness

§915 The causes of smoothness include applications which are gelatinous or some light substances which could remove irregularities by resolving and liquefying. Mollificants are fatty or glutinous substance that act by virtue of their viscidity. They are agents which mildly disperse the humors by attenuating them, cause them to flow while at the same time they carry off the dense particles of matter in the apertures on the surface of the member.

10.17.2. The Causes of Displacements and Dislocations

§916 The causes of displacements and dislocations include (1) forcible extension, (2) a sudden violent movement aided by the throwing of the whole weight of the body upon the member (such as luxation of the foot), and (3) relaxing and moistening factors which produce hernia, leprosy and sciatica. This happens in tearing, in corrosion, or septic change or destruction of the substance of a ligament or nerve as in elephantiasis or sciatica.

10.17.3. The Causes Which Prevent Proper Apposition and Closeness

§917 Here belong grossness, viscosity, looseness of joints, dryness of humor in a joint, spasm, ulcers which are only partially healed, calculus, thickening (from inflammation or edema), scars, spasms, paralysis, ankylosis from deposition of some dried matter (calcification), and congenital causes (malformations).

10.17.4. The Causes Which Prevent Parts From Expanding

§918 Here belongs: (1) congenital factors, (2) coarseness, (3) spasm, (4) cicatrisation after healing of ulcers.

10.17.5. The Causes of Abnormal Movements

§919 The causes of abnormal movements include: (1) dryness caused by the debility producing tremors, i.e., senile tremors; (2) dryness causing spasms, i.e., hiccup; (3) poisons which produce spasms or impair the passage of faculty or drive (nervous impulses); (4) toxic matter and poisons which being cold produce rigors or irritate the nerves, (inward) shrinkage and reduction of the innate heat, causing shivering from cold in the exterior of the body; and (5) gas which should have normally been dispersed and eliminated as in twitchings and the gas seeking dispersion as in palpitation of the heart.

§920 When this type of morbid matter is weak and ethereal it produces yawning. When it is active but otherwise stationary, it produces gaseous fatigue. The morbid matter, which is migratory, produces a different type of fatigue which will be described later. If, however, the matter is sufficiently powerful, it produces shivering or rigors. When the matter has localized in a group of muscles, jactitation is produced.

10.17.6. The Causes of Increase in the Size and Number of Bones

§921 The causes of the increase in the size and number of bones includes: (1) excess of humoral matter, (2) increase in the natural capacity of absorption and assimilation, and (3) increase in the power of absorption induced by the application of hot liniments and plasters. This will, however, increase only the size but not the number.

10.17.7. The Causes of Numerical Decrease

§922 The causes of numerical decrease include: (1) congenital,[50] as deficiency of the formative material and inherent defect or abnormality in growth; (2) external factors, such as cuts, contusions or gangrene from frost bite; and (3) internal factors such as decomposition or putrefaction.

10.17.8. The Causes of Loss of Continuity (Injuries)

10.17.8.1. The Internal Causes

§923 The causes of loss of continuity include: pathological body fluids, having a consuming, burning, moistening, relaxing, drying or cleaving action; fluids which pierce and force themselves into tissues and stretch them apart; gaseous matters also may force their way into and stretch tissues. In each of these cases the effect produced depends on: (1) the force of movement, (2) the abundance of the fluid or gas, and (3) the greatness of the expulsive power. Similar in action to these are: vociferation, leaping exercises; and the opening of abscesses.

§924 The above mentioned causes operate through either excessive activity or quantity. Thus, strong expulsive movements (as in the intestine or uterus) may produce rupture of vessels just as violent movements like jumping and shrieking produce congestion.

10.17.8.2. The External Causes

§925 The external causes of loss of continuity may be: (1) traction, which produces tears; (2) cuts from sharp weapons, which produce incised wounds; (3) burns from hot objects such as fire; (4) stings and bites of insects and animals; (5) blows from blunt weapons, especially over distended cavities; and (6) blows from piercing objects, i.e., puncture wounds.

10.17.8.2.1. The Agents Producing Ulceration

§926 An ulcer is formed either by the rupture of a matured swelling (abscess), a wound getting septic, or an abscess eroding the surrounding structures.

10.17.8.2.2. The Causes of Inflammatory Swellings

§927 Some of the causes of swellings may be due to abnormalities of humors, while others are due to abnormalities of structure. Thus, any of the six types of matter (four humors, water, and gas) may produce fullness (or congestion) in the organ affected while abnormalities of the structure may be the result of: (1) excessive excretory activity; (2) weakness or functional inefficiency; or (3) a special predisposition due to: (i) the functional peculiarity of an organ, i.e., skin, (ii) weakness and looseness of the structure, i.e., upper cervical glands, axillary glands and glands in the groin, (iii) afferent channels being wider and efferent ones narrower, (iv) lower relative position of the outlet of an organ, (v) smallness of the size, leading to a stasis of the nutriment, (vi) failure to assimilate the nutriment efficiently due to some calamity, (vii) collection of morbid humors due to injury, (viii) lack of exercise leading to the accumulation of morbid humors which are normally dispersed, and (ix) excess of heat in the tissues whether innate as in muscles, or acquired as from pain of exertion, or from using hot things.

§928 In fractures, the swelling may be due to one of the causes mentioned earlier or it may be due to a contusion, laceration or traction caused by treatment. As bones and teeth grow from nutriment, they tend to swell up from the inflammatory material.

10.18. A General Discussion of the Causes of Pain

§929 Pain is one of the unnatural states which afflicts the animal body.[51] Hence, a general description of pain will now be given. Pain is sensation produced by something contrary to the course of nature and this sensation is set up by one of two circumstances: either a very sudden change of the temperament (or the bad effect of a contrary temperament) or a solution of continuity.

§930 By "the bad effect of a contrary temperament," we mean the appearance of a quality which is contrary to the original temperament or that the temperament has become hotter or colder than the body to such an extent that it causes pain. Hence, pain is a feeling of imbalance in a temperament. A persistent abnormality of temperament does not produce pain, as it gets so integrated in the tissues so that it becomes natural to the person and is thus not felt by him. Hence, a condition which is of an integral nature and not just a departure from an established state will not give any pain. A state which has already been there would not be perceived unless some change makes it abnormal.

§931 It is for this reason that patients with phthisis do not feel the temperature so much as those suffering from paroxysmal and tertian fevers, although the heat in the fever of phthisis is much more than in the paroxysmal fevers. In phthisis, the heat is so integrated in the tissues that it tends to remain there as an abnormal feature, while in paroxysmal fevers, the heat is due merely to a temporary effect of the hot humor which is not integrated in the tissues. When the offending humor returns to normal, the superimposed heat completely disappears.

§932 It would, of course, be different if the paroxysmal fever turns into phthisis. In this connection, it should also be remembered that when a temperamental abnormality involves some organ, it does so gradually. When some temporary abnormality is allowed to continue for a long time, it assumes the form of a habit, so that in the end it fails to be appreciated by the body. Thus, a sudden hot water bath during winter time would be extremely unpleasant because that would be relatively incongruous to the cold (temperature) of the body, and the bath is enjoyed only after the cold has gradually given place to warmth.

§933 When, however, the bath is continued for some time, the body becomes so warm that the same hot water begins to feel so cold that if it is quickly poured over the body it would produce a "goose skin." Having learned this, it is important to bear in mind that every temperamental incongruity does not necessarily produce pain.

§934 The imbalances of heat and cold act as direct stimuli, while dryness acts indirectly, and the moisture never produces any pain. This is because the former two qualities are of an active nature, while the latter two are just passive and unable to influence other objects, except by making them more responsive. Dryness produces pain indirectly by causing a loss of continuity from the constriction.

§935 According to Galen, loss of continuity is the only real cause of pain. If heat produces pain, it is through a loss of continuity (from the dispersion of tissue particles). Cold acts similarly by shrinking and retracting the particles, and thus dislocating them from the original position. Galen has also mentioned in his writings that all painful sensory impressions arise either from a loss of continuity or an aggregation or dispersion of what could produce loss of continuity.

§936 Thus, looking at a black object produces unpleasant visual impressions by the forceful contraction and aggregation of visual particles, and the sight of a white object is painful because of the marked expansion and dispersion of these particles. Similarly, bitter, salt, and sour things are painful due to the active dispersion produced by them, while pungent things are distasteful due to the production of active contraction associated with dispersion as described above. Smell and hearing also act in a similar manner. Loud noises set up powerful waves in the air which strike against the ear (drum) causing dispersion.

§937 According to this author, change of temperament is itself a direct cause of pain whether this be with or without loss of continuity. It is, however, not for medicine to ascertain the truth in such matters. This is a proper subject of discussion for natural philosophy. The following brief statement may however be offered from the medical point of view: (1) Loss of continuity may be in a part of the organ but the pain is felt uniformly all over it. The feeling of pain over the area which has no loss of continuity cannot be attributed to this cause, but to the change of temperament. (2) Cold produces pain not only over the part to which it is applied, but also over the adjoining area which has become shrunken and retracted. In other words, pain is felt over the whole organ although the loss of continuity has only been in the adjoining part and not over the part to which the cold had actually been applied. (3) Pain is undoubtedly a sudden perception of a contrary object or quality.

§938 The contrary nature of the stimulus is the fundamental factor behind pain. Hence, only things which are capable of acting suddenly in a contrary manner, and whose contrary quality can be felt, act as the stimuli for pain. When cold can be severe enough to change the temperament and become painful, are we not going to accept it as the cause of pain just because there has been no loss of continuity? It is thus clear that a sudden change in the temperament is just as much a cause of pain as is the loss of continuity.

§939 Pain increases the heat, and heat by producing congestion increases the pain from tension. Occasionally, the disappearance of pain may be followed by a sensation akin to pain. This is not really pain but a perception of the state of resolution. Ill-informed physicians tend to treat it as real pain and thus cause unnecessary harm to the patient.

10.19. The Types of Pain

§940 The common types of pain are:[52]

§941 Boring pain: the cause of this pain is the retention of gross matter or of gas between the tunics of a hard and gross member (like the colon) and so continually goading it and tearing its parts asunder, boring into the interstices like a gimlet.

§942 Compressing pain: this is produced by fluid or gas when it is confined in too small a space in a member and so compresses or squeezes the tissues.

§943 Corrosive pain: this proceeds from the presence of material between the muscle-fibers and their sheaths, stretching it until it breaks not only the continuity of the membrane, but also that of the muscle therewith.

§944 Dull pain: the cause is threefold: (1) the temperament may be too cold; (2) occlusion of the pores so that the breath (of the sensitive drives) which should come to the member cannot do so; (3) over fullness of the (locular spaces or) cavities.

§945 Fatigue-pain: this is produced by (1) undue toil—laborious toil; (2) a humor which produces tension (in intensive lassitude); (3) a gaseous substance which produces inflative lassitude; (4) a humor of biting properties (ulcerative lassitude). These pains may arise out of various composite states as has already been state in the appropriate places. Lassitude as a result of several combined states is called in flammatory lassitude which is a composite of intensive and ulcerative lassitude (see tensive lassitude).

§946 Heavy pain: in this case there is an inflammatory process in an insensitive member such as the lung, the kidney or spleen. The weight of the inflammatory deposit drags on the tissues and surrounding sentient fascia and on its point of attachment. As the member is dragged on, the fascia and its point of attachment experience the sensation. The cause of the pain may be that a sentient member has had its sensation destroyed by the disease so that the weight is felt but actual pain cannot be felt any longer (i. e., cancer at the mouth of the stomach).

§947 Incisive pain: this proceeds from a humor of sour quality.

§948 Irritant pain: this is produced by a certain type of change in the humors (harshness, roughness).

§949 Itching pain: this is produced when a humor is acrid, sharp, or salty.

§950 Pricking pain: the agent producing this is material similar to that which causes boring pain. It is retained in an organ of similar type (to that which is the seat of boring pain) for a time and then ruptures it.

§951 Stabbing pain: this is the result of transverse stretching in membranes as if their continuity were being separated by a humor. It may be an equal or an inequal sensation. In the former case all the members of the body are uniformly affected. In the latter case, there are four possibilities: (1) Inequality in hardness or softness between the tissue with which the membrane is covered and the membrane itself. An example would be the clavicle or costal pleura. In a case of inflammatory process traveling from the pleura towards the upper parts of the chest; the pain is felt in the collar-bone. (2) Inequality of movement of the component parts (for example, the diaphragm and the pleura or peritoneum over it). (3) inequality of nature between the parts and the member. And (4) Unequal distribution of nocument among the parts and the member affected in that it affects one and not another.

§952 Tearing pain: tearing pain proceeds from the interposition of humor or gas between bone and periosteum or from cold which strongly constricts the periosteum.

§953 Tension pain: this is produced by a humor or gas stretching the nerve-fibers or muscle fibers asunder.

§954 Throbbing pain: the cause is a hot inflammatory process. A cold inflammatory process, of whatever type, is either hard or soft, but sets up no pain unless it changes into a hot inflammation. Throbbing pain arises in a hot inflammatory process if the adjoining member is sentient and has pulsating arteries around it. A member which is healthy does not sense their movement because they are deeply situated, but their pulsation sets up pain as soon as an inflammation arises in the member.

10.19.1. The Agents Which Alleviate Pain

§955 (1) Resolvents: Some contrary to the cause of pain—which removes the cause such as anethum, or linseed, made into a poultice and applied over the painful place. (2) Narcotics: Any agent which counteracts the acrimony of the humors or soothes, induces sleep or dulls or soothes the sensitive faculties and lessens their activity, such as inebriants, milk, oil, aqua dulcis and so forth. (3) Analgesics. These produce cold and thus insensitivity of the affected organs. The most efficient agents for this purpose are those of the first group.

10.19.2. The Effects of Pain on the Body

§956 (1) Dissipation of the faculty or drives. (2) Interference with functions of the organs, i.e., respiration is inhibited or becomes intermittent, rapid or irregular. (3) The affected organ first becomes hot and later on with the persistence of pain, becomes cold. This is due to the dispersion of vital force and decrease of innate heat.

10.19.3. The Causes of Pleasure

§957 There are two sets of causes which produce pleasure, (1) sudden restoration of the temperament to normal and (2) sudden restoration of the (structural) continuity. If these changes are not sudden, they would not be perceived and thus produce no pleasure. Pleasure is a perception of harmony. Perception depends upon the ability of a sensory organ to be affected, pain and pleasure being determined by the nature of stimulus. If the stimulus is suitable (and harmonious) it gives pleasure, but when it is incongruous, it produces pain. Since touch is the crudest of all sensations, it tends to retain the harmonious as well as disharmonious impressions for a longer time. Hence, persons of dense and thick disposition react much more to impressions from the touch than from any other faculty or drive and thus derive greater pain and pleasure from it.

10.19.4. How Movement Brings on Pain

§958 Exercise and movement may produce pain by stretching the nerves or by causing (invisible) contusions and lacerations in the muscles.

10.19.5. How Depraved Humors Evoke Pain

§959 Depraved humors which cause pain do so either by their quality, that is, irritating pain or headaches from acrid humors, or excessive quantity which stretches the fibers. Pain may also be due to a combination of these factors.

10.19.6. How Gaseous Substances Produce Pain

§960 Gas produces pain by causing tension. Thus, it occurs: (1) inside hollow organs like the stomach, as an abdominal distension; (2) within the coats of organs, as intestinal colic; (3) between muscle fibers and under membranes, i.e., periosteum; (4) around muscles or in between the flesh and the skin (i.e., in the subcutaneous tissues); and (5) around the tissues as is commonly the case with muscles attached to the chest. The dispersal or persistence of gas depends upon its quantity and consistency and on the structural pattern of the organ being solid or spongy.

10.20. The Agents Which Cause Retention and Evacuation

§961 In this connection, a reference may be made to the description already given. The reader may turn back and carefully reread what has already been said on the point.

10.20.1. The Causes of Over-Repletion

§962 The causes of over-repletion (plethora)[53] may be external or internal. (1) External: (a) A diet (fluids as well as solids) which give rise.to much moisture beyond the needs of the body; matter accumulates in the body and interferes with the action of the emunctories. (b) Taking baths frequently, especially after meals. (c) Rest: ceasing to take exercise; ceasing to secure the usual evacuations. These prevent the resolution of material in the body. (d) Improprieties in eating and drinking; depraved regimen. (2) Internal: (a) lack of digestive power so that the aliments are not completely utilized. (b) Feebleness of expulsive faculty. (c) Undue vigor of retentive faculty so that the humors are caused to linger in the body. (d) Narrowing of the excretory channels.

10.20.2. The Causes of Weakness of Organs

§963 Weakness may affect (1) the body of the member itself; (2) the breath, which conveys power to it; (3) the faculty of the member. The following produce weakness in the member itself: (a) A persisting intemperament especially a cold one. For even though the member receive some heat, the cold intemperament produces an effect like stupor in it, because it breaks up the temperament of the breath—just as happens when a person stays too long in the bath, and especially when such a procedure brings on syncope. A dry intemperament has an inspissating effect, and acts by preventing the faculties from functioning in the member. A moist intemperament relaxes and obstructs. (b) One or other of the composite diseases. (c) The most important of all (in the human being) is neither nocument, nor malady, nor pain. It is an attenuation of texture in the peripheral nerve-fibers of the member, for both vegetative and voluntary actions depend for their achievement on these fibers in all their ramifications. The retentive power, which is necessary to secure efficient digestion, depends on the condition of these fibers in the stomach.

§964 Weakness of the breath itself. This will occur if it be of bad temperament. There may also be dissipation of the breath, after an evacuation corresponding. It is also weakened by an abnormal mode of depletion.

§965 Weakness of faculty. This depends on the number of actions and the number of times they are repeated. The breath is dispersed at the same time. Moreover, loss of breath accompanies every agent which produces asthenia.

§966 The causes of asthenia may be classified in another way so as to include the remote causes with them—the causes of causes. We then consider (a) causes of intemperament; (2) causes arising from decomposition changes in the air, in water, and in the aliment; (c) causes which cause the breath to escape, or become confused, or, as it were, shaken up. Nothing disturbs the breath or causes it to escape as effectively as does a bad smell such as the fetor from putrid water or the presence of poisonous vapors in the air or in the body. [Under such circumstances, the instinctive action is immediately to "hold the breath."]

§967 Evacuations as a cause of weakness. For instance, loss of blood; diarrhea, especially of thin attenuated fluid; the sudden withdrawal of copious dropsical effusions by paracentesis; the opening of a large abscess with sudden withdrawal of much pus—whether the opening is by nature or by surgical interference; excessive sweating; severe exercise.

§968 Severe pain disperses the breath and may alter its temperament. The chief kind of pain likely to have this effect is that from distension, or incisive pain—especially in the pit of the stomach. Any pain in the region of the heart will disperse the breath.

§969 Fevers should also be included among the causes of asthenia. They act either by dispersing the breath, or by loss of blood, or through producing a change of temperament.

§970 Widening of the pores often aids in producing asthenia. Long continued semi-starvation has the same effect.

§971 Weakness in one member or in a part of a member may cause weakness of the whole body as is seen in the case of defective function of the cardiac orifice of the stomach, which produces general weakness of the body. Or, if a person suffers severely from some cardiac or cerebral trouble, shortness of breath rapidly supervenes on very slight provocation.

§972 Further, a cause of weakness may be that one has endured many illnesses.

§973 When one member is weaker than another from birth or when it is by nature weaker in itself (for example, the lung or brain), then it is receptive for matters which the stronger members reject or discard or eliminate. The brain would suffer in this way were it not for its position whereby nothing comes to it which it cannot tolerate. Even its virtues cannot persist there.[54]

Part Three
The Classification of Diseases: Their Symptoms

Lecture 11: The Signs and Symptoms (Diagnosis): General Remarks

11.1. Introduction

§974 Signs and symptoms indicate the present, past and future states of the three states of the body (health, illness, neutrality). According to Galen, knowledge of the present state is of advantage only to the patient as it helps him to follow the proper course of management. Knowledge of the past state is useful only to the physician inasmuch as its disclosure by him to the patient brings him a greater respect for his professional advice. Knowledge of the future state is useful to both. It gives an opportunity to the patient to be forewarned to adopt necessary preventive measures and it enhances the reputation of the physician by correctly forecasting the future developments.[1]

§975 The signs belonging to the first category are called "demonstrative." Those of the second category are "commemorative." Those of the third are named "prognostic."

§976 The signs of health include: (1) those which denote an equable temperament (these are referred to in §1053); and (2) those which denote equability of the composite: (i) substantial (creaturely form, position, quantity, number); (ii) accidental (comeliness, beauty); and (iii) final (fulfilling functions and fulfilled function).

§977 Every organ is healthy whose functions are adequately performed. The functional efficiency of the principal organs may be assessed by observing, in the case of the brain, voluntary movements, sensory activity and mental functions; in the case of the heart, the condition of the pulse and respiration; and in the case of the liver, stools and urine. If the stools and urine are of a meat juice color, there is likely to be inefficiency of the liver.

§978 Some signs of disease are pathognomonic of disease. Thus, rapid pulse-rate in fever itself indicates fever. Other signs indicate the position of the disease. Thus a hard pulse denotes diaphragmatic pleurisy. Undulant pulse denotes inflammation in the substance of the lung. Other signs indicate the cause of the disease. For instance, the signs of plethora or of depraved states in their various forms.

§979 Sometimes the signs and symptoms may continue throughout the illness, i.e., persistence of acute fever, piercing pain, dyspnea, dry cough and serrete pulse—essential to pleurisy. In some cases, the signs and symptoms may however appear only at a particular stage of the illness or the signs may appear towards the end of an illness, like the signs of crisis, signs indicating maturation or lack of maturation and signs portending death. These symptoms are often associated rather with acute illnesses.

§980 Sometimes other symptoms concern the state of the members. Some of them are discernible by the special senses—color, hardness, softness, heat, cold and the like. Others are discernible by all senses together—the form of the member, its position (posture, attitude), its size, its movements, or stillness. Some symptoms point to an interior state as when tremor of the lower lip reveals nausea. Changes in measure and number reveal internal states. For instance, shortness of fingers denotes small liver.

§981 Sometimes morbid states are discernible by the special senses. Thus a black or yellow color of the excrement reveals a morbid state. Black or yellow jaundice of the whole body reveals an obstruction in the biliary passages.

§982 Sometimes states are manifested to the sense of hearing—eructations reveal gastrectasis and defective digestive power.

§983 Sometimes odors and tastes also enable one to become cognizant of morbid states.

§984 Sometimes other visible evidences: curved nails denote ulceration in the bronchi, phthisis, and "hectic."

§985 Signs and symptoms based on rest and movement are of special importance (gestures, postures, attitudes). The states of the body are revealed by its movements or absence of movement: (1) motionlessness of the body as a whole: in apoplexy, epilepsy (coma), syncope, palsy; or (2) unusual movements: shivering, tremor, twitching, sneezing, yawning, stretching, cough, trembling, spasms (especially note in which member this begins).

§986 Some of these unusual movements are: (1) physiological (hiccup); (2) while others are symptomatic (convulsion or spasm, tremor); (3) and some are voluntary (tossing about in bed and turning from side to side); (4) others are partly voluntary, partly involuntary (cough, micturition, defecation). In some of these the voluntary is overruled by the involuntary (cough), while in others the voluntary overrules the involuntary (micturition and defecation, occurring too slowly owing to interference by the will); and (5) involuntary movements: some of these are evident to the senses (shivering), others are not (quivering, jactitation).

§987 These movements vary: (1) in regard to their nature: thus, cough is intrinsically more energetic and powerful than quivering; and (2) in extent—thus the act of sneezing entails the use of more muscles than the act of coughing does. Coughing is accomplished simply by the movements of the chest, sneezing entails movements of the head as well as of the chest; in degree of associated mental anxiety. Dry hiccup is associated with a greater degree of mental anxiety than the movement of coughing although the latter is more vigorous, being reinforced by the natural instinctive drive. In some cases the movement is aided by an essential primary instrument. Thus, defecation is aided by the abdominal muscles. In other cases the aid is extraneous. Thus, the natural act of coughing may be aided by the atmosphere; in origin: these movements vary: (1) according to the member—cough, nausea; (2) according to the instinctive drives involved—jactitation originates in the vegetative drives while the act of coughing originates in the sensitive drives; (3) according to the humor concerned—thus cough proceeds from an excretion while twitching from a gaseous agent. These are all evidences of conditions in the members and are chiefly external in character. Some of them reveal internal conditions as, for instance, redness of the cheeks is a sign of pulmonary inflammation.

§988 There are also internal evidences of external conditions and to discern these a perfect anatomical knowledge is necessary.

11.2. The Signs of Internal Disease

§989 It is necessary for the diagnosis of internal disease that one should have knowledge of the anatomy of various organs. Thus, one must know about: (1) The essential structure of each member, whether fleshy or not; what its normal form is. One must know (i) whether the swelling, for instance, is according to the proper form of the member or not; (ii) whether it is proportioned or not; (iii) whether it is possible for anything to be retained within the given member or not; (iv) whether that which is within (for example *jejunum*) can escape; (v) whether there can be retention in and also escape from the member; (vi) what the material is which can be retained in it or discharged from it. (2) Its site: from this one judges whether pain or swelling is actually in the part or at some distance from it. (3) Its relations: by this knowledge one judges whether pain is arising per se or reflexly from the surroundings or whether the matter is an inflammatory mass arose in it or has entered into it from neighboring parts. If it be a "superfluity which escapes, is this the matter itself or is the affected member merely the channel by which the matter finds egress from the body? (4) How to decide wither the discharge could have come from the supposedly affected member or not. (5) The normal function of a member—from interference with function one recognizes the diseased state.

§990 This is the purpose of the study of anatomy. A knowledge of anatomy is also necessary to enable the doctor to control diseases involving the interior organs.

§991 The study of the significance of the symptoms of internal diseases should follow the following six headings: (1) Interference with function. The functions have already been described in regard to their qualities and degrees. The indications here are primary and constant; (2) Discharges: the indications here are constant, but not primary. They (1 and 2) are constant in that they are always associated with morbid states. They are not primary because they denote maturation or interference with maturation. Those that are neither primary nor constant are: (3) pain; (4) swelling; (5) altered position; and (6) special symptoms.

11.2.1. Interference with Function

§992 When a function does not proceed normally, it shows that the agent at work is attacking the instinctive drive itself and the loss of function is secondary to disease of the organ subserving that function. There are three ways in which function is interfered with: (1) impairment such as failing eyesight, near sight, digestion impaired in rate or degree; (2) alteration—as when the eye sees that which is not there or perceives incorrectly; when the stomach digests food wrongly and causes it to decompose; (3) destruction—as when there is entire loss of vision; or entire loss of digestive power.

11.2.2. Significance of Discharges and Retentions

§993 The significance of discharges and retentions include: (1) Retention of that which is normally discharged (e.g., retention of urine or feces); (2) Abnormal discharge: (i) from the substance of a member (a) itself diagnostic (for example, when a piece of cartilaginous tissue is coughed up, this is a proof of deep ulceration in the air-passages); (b) diagnostic by reason of its dimensions or amount (passage of flakes in dysentery—if they are large flakes, the ulcer is in the large intestine; if fine, the ulceration is in the small intestine); (c) color of the discharge (if urinary sediment is red, it shows the disease is in the fleshy organs such as the kidney; if white it shows the disease is in a muscular organ like the bladder); (ii) Not from the substance of a member: (a) entirely unnatural (thus healthy humors or blood should not be discharged at all); (b) abnormal in quality (thus depraved blood may be discharged physiologically, or not); (c) abnormal in substance (calculus); (d) abnormal in quantity (polyuria, oliguria, excess of fecal discharge, paucity of feces which is either abnormal in quality like black feces, black urine or discharge by unsuitable or unnatural channels: i.e., passage of faces by the mouth in cases of strangulated hernia).

11.2.3. The Significance of Pain

§994 The significance of pain includes: (a) its site—if right-sided, examine the liver; if left-sided, the spleen; and (b) its type, which reveals its cause (see §434 and the doctrine of causes). Severe pain indicates inflammation in a non-essential member, or in a member which has lost sensation, but has become greatly distended by foreign matter. Incisive pain shows that the diseased material is sharp, acid or acrid.

11.2.4. The Significance in Regard to Inflammations

§995 The significance in regard to inflammations include: (1) as to essence—erysipelatous inflammation denotes bilious humor; scirrhus (induration) denotes atrabilious humor; (2) as to position—whether on (liver or spleen) the right side or the left; and (3) as to shape—a moon-shaped swelling in the right hypochondrium points to the liver; an elongated swelling refers one to the overlying muscles (rectus and adnexa).

11.2.5. The Significance of Site and Relations

§996 The significance of site and relations includes: the site may be self-evident. The relations vary in significance according to the morbidic agent. Thus a lesion in the fingers may result from injury to the brachial plexus in the neck.

11.2.6. The Significance of Special Symptoms

§997 The significance of special symptom include: wasting; black tongue; and burning fever.[2]

11.3. The Distinction Between the Disease in Itself and Its Secondary Effects

§998 Diseases may affect a member primarily or only secondarily. Thus, a disease of the stomach may become associated with one in the head. It is necessary to distinguish between the two conditions as being respectively primary and secondary. To do this, note which arises first, and then note which of the two morbid conditions persists. The former is judged to be primary; the one which develops later is considered to be secondary. Conversely, the disease is secondary which comes after the first, and ceases when the first is relieved.

§999 Errors may arise, however, because a primary disease may escape the senses (being painless) at first, and its effect may not become manifest until after the secondary disease has appeared and so one is liable to regard the secondary ones as primary, and overlook the real root of the disease.

§1000 To guard against this mistake, the physician must know the anatomical interrelations of the members, and also the several affections which each member may show. Some of these are evident to our senses, others are not. He must also avoid giving a definite diagnosis of the root of the disease until he has had time to consider the possibility of some of the states being secondary or not.

§1001 Therefore the physician will diligently question the patient in order to discover signs indicative of the various affections which can possibly occur secondarily in the neighboring or related organs. If these are not painful (tender), the patient is unaware of them, and the various signs and symptoms may be only distantly related in his mind. He cannot know the relation between remote symptoms and the real root of the disease. The wisdom of the physician alone can determine this.

§**1002** It is easier if one recalls the various points to memory under the heading of hindrances to function. If these are prior in time, the malady is secondary.

§**1003** Some affections of members are usually secondary to others. Thus, an affection of the head is usually secondary to one or other of the morbid states of the stomach. The converse is only very rarely true. All the signs of the primary and secondary temperaments will be set forth in a general way now, leaving the signs of each special organ to its appropriate place. The visible signs of a composite disease are detected by the senses, but the internal symptoms of the body as a whole cannot be described in a general way except with difficulty—with the exception of the signs of plethora, of obstructions in passages, of inflammatory masses, and of loss of continuity. It is best to describe all these together when we describe them under their specific organs.

11.4. The Diagnostic Signs of the Temperaments

§**1004** The signs from which the variety of the temperament is discernible can be arranged under ten groups: (1) the feel of the patient; (2) the state of the muscles, flesh and fat; (3) the hair; (4) the color of the body; (5) the form of the members; (6) the rapidity with which members respond to heat and cold; (7) signs derived from sleep and wakefulness; (8) signs derived from the state of the functions; (9) signs derived from the expulsive drive and from the quality of discharges; and (10) signs derived from the states of the mind during action and passion.

11.4.1. The Feel of the Patient

§**1005** One notes whether the feel of the patient corresponds to health in temperate climes and temperate atmosphere by means of touch. If it corresponds, the temperament is equable. If the physician is himself healthy in temperament and finds the patient cold or hot, softer or harder or rougher than normal, and this is not to be explained by the state of the atmosphere or of a previous cold water bath or some other contingency rendering the body soft or rough, though normal he then knows the finding is due to an intemperament.

§**1006** The state of the fingernails should be noticed. Softness or dryness of the nails not due to an extraneous agent, informs one of the state of the temperament. These qualities are not in themselves a sufficient criterion. There must be signs of balance between heat and cold. For (a) heat, by its resolving it effect, would modify hardness and roughness of feel, and make the patient seem to be attempered and his nature seem soft and moist. Or, (b) cold—i.e. the opposite—by reason of the great congelation and inspissation it induces, would make the softness of feel in an attempered person seem hard, and give the impression that his nature was dry. For instance, take snow and the sun. Snow congeals and causes coagulation; the sun causes aggregation of particles. Many persons with a cold temperament are soft to the feel, and also spare in habit owing to the presence of much immaturity in them.

11.4.2. The State of the Muscles, Flesh and Fat

§**1007** Plentiful muscular development denotes moist temperament, and warm temperament if the muscles are firm. Scanty muscular development with very little fat shows that the temperament is dry. Oiliness and fat always denote cold temperament, and the muscles are then also flabby.

§**1008** If at the same time there is constriction of the veins and lack of blood, and if there is weakness from lack of food (because there is too little blood to enable it to furnish the requirements of the tissues), this shows that this temperament is inborn and habitual. But if these other signs are absent, it shows the temperament to be an acquired one.

§**1009** Lessening of the amount of oil and fat in the subcutaneous tissues always indicates a hot temperament, because the substance of oil and fat is the oiliness of the blood, and that is derived from colds Hence these things are less plentiful in the liver-region, and more plentiful over the intestines. There is not more oil and fat over the heart than over the liver, except as to matter; it is not temperament or "form" which accounts for this; it is simply that the "nature" of the heart depends for its maintenance on the presence of such-like "matter."

§1010 Congelation of oil and fat over the body is greater or less according as the heat is more or less in degree.

§1011 If the body is fleshy, and the amount of fat and oil not great, the temperament is hot and moist.

§1012 If the body is very muscular, and there is much oil, but little fat, this denotes excessively humid temperament. If extremely fleshy, this denotes superfluity of moisture and cold. It is evidence that the body has become cold and moist.

§1013 The more spare the body is in habit, the more likely is it to be cold and dry; or (less likely) hot and dry; or, dry, for such a body is attempered as to heat and cold. Or, hot, because such a body is attempered as to moisture and dryness.

11.4.3. The Hair

§1014 The points to note are: (a) rate of growth; (b) amount; (c) fineness or coarseness of texture; (d) straightness or curliness; (e) color.

11.4.3.1. Rate of Hair Growth

§1015 Rate of growth: slow growth, or absence of growth, without evidence of lack of blood denotes extremely humid temperament. More rapid growth denotes a less humid temperament, rather tending to dryness. (Heat and coldness of temperament are shown by other signs given above than the hair.)

11.4.3.2. Amount of Hair

§1016 Amount: if the temperament is both hot and dry, the hair grows much more rapidly, and each hair is numerous and coarse. Abundance of hair means heat, while coarseness indicates much fumosity. Therefore, the hair is more plentiful in adolescent persons than in puberty, as the humors of the latter are vaporose, not fumose. The opposite characters denote the respective contraries.

11.4.3.3. Form of the Hair

§**1017** Form of the hair: curly hair denotes hot and dry temperament. It may be that there is tortuosity of the minute channels and pores, and this cannot change even if the temperament changes. But the two primary causes would change if the temperament changed. Straight hair denotes cold and temperament.

11.4.3.4. Color of the Hair

§**1018** Black hair indicates hot temperament. In such cases oxidative processes are in excess of the mean. Brown hair indicates cold temperament. Tawny and red hair indicates equable temperament. There is an excess of unburned heat so that the hair always grows red. Therefore, there is a proneness to anger (a form of heat). Very fair hair indicates a cold and very moist temperament while grey hair indicates a cold and very dry one. Note how plants lose their dark or green color when dried and become grey or white. In the human being, this change is produced towards the close of drying or desiccant diseases.[3]

§**1019** The cause of grey hair: Aristotle stated that hair turns grey because it takes on the color of the serous humor.[4] Galen ascribed it to a mustiness accompanying the nutriment supplied to the hair which retards its movement and penetration into the pores (of the hair) (i.e. hair-sac). As a matter of fact, there is little difference between the two views, because the whiteness of the serous humor is physically due to the same cause as the whiteness of the mustiness. The subject really belongs to physics.

§**1020** Observation also shows that atmosphere and geographical situation affects the hair. One would not expect to find the hair red (which denotes equable temperament) in a black person even though his temperament were equable; nor would one expect to find black hair (which denotes hot temperament) in a Slav, even though his temperament were hot.

11.4.3.5. Relation of Character of the Hair to Age

§1021 In puberty the hair is as in northern countries; in youth, as in southerly countries; after the age of fifty it is between the two. Abundance of the hair at puberty reveals the future temperament. As the person grows, it precedes the formation of atrabilious humor, and in the elderly person it shows that atrabilious humor is actually present.

11.4.4. The Color of the Body

§1022 Pallor indicates a cold temperament and the accompanying feature is lack of blood. Yellowish color indicates a hot temperament which is accompanied by lack of blood, and increase of bilious humor. Ruddiness indicates a hot temperament with abundance of blood, sanguine or bilious temperament. Sub-ruddiness indicates a hot temperament with dominance of bilious humor. Occasionally it denotes lack of blood, provided there is no bilious humor present in the blood as is the case in convalescence. A dark brown body indicates an extremely cold temperament. This is because sanguineous humor is dominant and there is deficient coagulability of the blood and it darkens and alters the color of the skin at the same time. A brown colored body indicates a hot temperament. A body the color of eggplant indicates a cold and dry temperament. The heat is such as follows upon pure atrabilious humor. A chalky body indicates a cold temperament where the serous humor is in excess. A leaden colored body indicates a cold and moist temperament. The atrabilious humor is only slightly in excess. This is because there is a trace of green in the whiteness. The latter depends on the serous humor and moistness of temperament. The greenness depends on congelative change in the blood because this tends to a blackness which, mingled with serous humor, produces a greenish tint. A grey and white body indicates a cold temperament. An ivory white body indicates a cold temperament where serous humor is in excess and the choleric humor is scanty.[5]

11.4.4.1. The Color of the Eyes

§1023 It is not easy, but it is possible, to assess the temperament of the brain from the color of the eyes.

11.4.4.2. Changes of Color

§**1024** A change to yellow (yellowish-white): suspect disorder of the liver; change to yellowish-black: suspect disorder of the spleen; change to yellowish-green: suspect piles (this does not always hold good (marginal reading). These suggestions only apply for the moment when the change of color takes place.

11.4.4.3. The Color of the Tongue

§**1025** It is not easy to assess the temperament of the stomach, intestines and veins from the color of the tongue, any more than it is to assess the temperament of the brain from the color of the eyes. There may be two different colors simultaneously in two members as a consequence of a disease. Thus, the tongue may become white and the countenance dusky. This occurs in jaundice when this is due to an intense acridity of the bilious humor.

11.4.5. The Form of the Members

11.4.5.1. Hot Temperament

§**1026** Indication from members as to hot temperament include: big broad chest; large limbs; no narrowing or shortening of the hands or feet; conspicuous full veins; big strong pulse; the muscles round the joints large (for growth and the form of composite structures requires heat).

11.4.5.2. Cold Temperament

§**1027** Indication from members as to cold temperament include: the contraries of all the above. The natural drives and the formative drive are impaired by cold, so that the natural-functions are not perfectly carried out.

11.4.5.3. Dry Temperament

§**1028** Indication from the members as to dry temperament include: roughness, curvature of form; joints conspicuous. Adam's apple prominent. Nasal cartilage conspicuous; nose of medium size.

11.4.5.4. Moist Temperament

§**1029** Indication from the members as to moist temperament include: the contraries.[6]

11.4.6. The Rapidity With Which Organs Respond to Heat and Cold

§**1030** If a member becomes "hot" rapidly and easily, it shows that it is hot in temperament, because change in the direction of its own temperament is more readily undergone than in the opposite direction. Similarly, if the organ behaves in the contrary way, it will be of cold temperament.

§**1031** Some assert that it is otherwise, because we know they say that a thing only reacts to its contrary and not to its like. But if that were the case, it would follow that a thing would react more strongly to its like. But the reply to this is that two things are only really alike when one does not interact with the other; we then know that their respective qualities are of like "species" and "nature."

§**1032** Of two things A and B, if B is less hot than A, we cannot speak of its being "like A." As long as one of the two is hotter, they cannot be called "alike." One is cold compared with the other. So an interaction (on the part of the body) is possible. B would be cold compared with A, not hot. B, too, may react with something else which is colder than itself [say C] besides reacting with "cold" [say D]. C or D may enhance the intrinsic quality of B according as they are stronger than B or not. It is easier for it to change towards that which enhances this quality of B or neutralizes the opposite quality of B on condition that the new causative agent harmonizes with A and B and neutralizes the temperamental nature.

§**1033** Therefore it is clear that when the nature is of hot temperament heat will not show any action on it until the influence of the contrary cold has first been removed, and this is achieved by preventing the malefaction (which tends to be produced by a hot temperament) from becoming greater. The result is that if both events occur simultaneously, and the inhibiting agent is destroyed, they will mutually help one another in producing heat, and the two qualities will thus reach an acme.

§1034 When the body is exposed to foreign heat, however, the balance of temperament is likely to be destroyed. The innate heat of the body is all-important for resisting this. We depend on our innate heat for the neutralization of "hot" poisons, and for their expulsion and for the dissolution of their substance.

§1035 Innate heat, therefore, is the instrument of human nature for combating the injurious action of extraneous or foreign heat. By its means, the breath gets rid of it, expels it, disperses it, and oxidizes its material basis. Further, it combats the injurious action of foreign "cold," expelling it "by contrary." Coldness has not this power. It is only the contrary to coldness i.e. foreign heat—which can combat or repress it. Coldness cannot combat extraneous "cold." Innate heat does.

§1036 Innate heat is that which protects the natural humors from being overruled by foreign calorific agents. If the innate heat is strong, the natural drives are able to work through it, upon the humors, and so effect digestion and maturation, and so maintain them within the confines of the healthy state. The humors move according to its ministration. Extraneous or foreign "heat" cannot interfere with this movement, and so they do not undergo putrefactive decomposition. If the ingrate agent is feeble, the natural drives are harassed in the regulation of the humors. For the instrument the intermediary between the natural drives and the humors is enfeebled. Stagnation sets in and foreign heat now finds the humors no longer opposed to its action. It overcomes them. It utilizes them in its own way, and imparts a foreign movement to them; and the result is what is known as "putrefaction."

§1037 Therefore, it is clear that the innate heat is the instrument of all the faculties, whereas coldness can only help them secondarily. That is why one speaks of "innate heat," but not of "innate cold;" and why that which is proportionate to heat is not comparable with cold.[7]

11.4.7. The Signs Derived from Sleep and Wakefulness

§1038 The sensitive drives make use of these things frequently, in a manner corresponding to the primary qualities. Thus we say that in the wakeful state the body is the instrument of the soul.

§1039 If there is equipoise between sleep and wakefulness, it means that the temperament (especially of the brain) is equable. If sleep dominates, it denotes a cold and moist temperament (of the brain), whereas if wakefulness dominates, it shows a dry and hot temperament (especially in the brain).[8]

11.4.8. The Signs Derived from the State of the Functions

§1040 Functions[9] may be weakened, exalted, depraved, obstructed in their action, or abolished.

§1041 Equable temperament: the activities of the body proceed fully and perfectly and naturally

§1042 Hot temperament: there is over-activity, exaggerated activity; rapid growth of stature; increased rate of growth of hair; early eruption of the teeth.

1043 Cold temperament: the activities lessen and become sluggish and delayed, but a hot temperament may cause weak and sluggish activity only if a deviation from the natural course is associated with weakness.

§1044 Many natural functions may slow down or lessen owing to heat. Thus, in the case of sleep, sometimes there is insomnia or lack of sleep from the effect of the heat of a hot temperament. Similarly some of the natural states may be intensified by cold. Thus, again, in the case of sleep, though this is not strictly the outcome of natural functions, but only an effect conditional upon some causal agent, because the necessity for sleep for life and health is not absolute. It enables the breath to separate off from its impeding factors the fatigue-substances. There is need for a recumbent posture after a meal. One cannot achieve two (contrary) things at the same time. Hence the need for sleep is simply some impotency. It is not included in "natural necessity." And if its exclusion be "natural" in the sense that it is inevitable, this is only because the word "natural" is here used for "the inevitable." One word is being made stand for two things. But the most accurate application of the term is to "equable temperament," for it is this upon which equability of functions and their final completion depends. To use the term in regard to the four qualities—heat, coldness dryness, moisture is only hypothetical.

§**1045** Among the "strong" ("jalal") actions which denote a hot temperament are: a powerful voice; a harsh or coarse voice; a rapid way of talking; constantly talking; anger; rapid gestures; and blinking of the eyelids. Before deducing a hot temperament from these, one must make sure there is no local cause for them, and that they are not confined to one particular member.

11.4.9. The Signs Derived from the Expulsive Drive and from the Quality of Discharges

§**1046** The temperament is hot if the waste matters are retained and if the feces, urine, sweat, etc., are strong in odor, acrid, of normal color, and show the normal degree of oxidation and maceration in the case of matters which normally undergo such changes. If the signs are contrary, the temperament is cold.[10]

11.4.10. The Signs Derived from the States of the Mind During Action and Passion

§**1047** Cold temperaments show the opposites to those given for hot temperaments; moist, the opposites to those given for dry. This and most of the above refers to the congenital or innate temperament. Now we refer to acquired temperaments ("intemperaments").[11]

11.5. Evidences of the Four Primary Intemperaments

§**1048** The signs of a morbid state to which there is a tendency to an acquired hot temperament is indicated when inflammatory conditions become febrile and there is a loss of vigor of a cold acquired temperament or intemperament when fevers are related to the serous humor and rheumatism develops, and of a moist or dry intemperament when there is lassitude.

§**1049** Evidence of the functional power indicates deficient energy with a hot intemperament, deficient digestive power with a cold intemperament, difficult digestion with a moist or dry intemperament. Subjective sensations indicate a bitter taste in the mouth, excessive thirst, and a sense of burning at the cardiac orifice with hot intemperament; a lack of desire for fluids with a cold intemperament; mucoid salivation and sleepiness with a moist intemperament and insomnia and wakefulness with a dry intemperament.

§**1050** Physical signs of a hot intemperament are indicated by a pulse extremely quick and frequent while approaching the weak type met with in lassitude; a cold intemperament is indicated by flaccid joints; a moist intemperament is indicated by diarrhea and swollen eyelids; a dry intemperament is indicated by rough skin and spare habit which is acquired and not inborn.

§**1051** In regard to foods and medicines with a hot intemperament, calefacients are all harmful while infrigidants benefit; with a cold intemperament infrigidants are all harmful while calefacients benefit; with a moist intemperament, moist articles of diet are harmful; with a dry intemperament, dry regime is harmful while humectants benefit (hot water, rarefied oils are beneficial to the dry temperament and are avidly taken up).

§**1052** In relation to weather, a hot intemperament is worse in the summer and a cold intemperament is worse in the winter. A dry intemperament is bad in the autumn.

11.6. The Signs of a Harmonious Temperament: Symmetry, Beauty of Form, and Good Conformation

§**1053** In addition to the signs of normal temperament

already given, there are: (a) To the feel, the body imparts sensations mean between hotness, coldness, dryness, moisture, softness, hardness. (b) In color, the body shows a balance between whiteness and redness. (c) In build, the body is neither bulky nor spare although on the whole inclined to be bulky. (d) The veins of the skin are neither prominent nor submerged; they are separated and spread. (e) The hair is neither profuse nor sparse, thick nor thin, curly nor straight, black nor white. During puberty they tend to a tawny shade rather than black, in youth they tend to blackness. Full hair where hair should be. (f) The person is equally inclined for sleep and for wakefulness.[12] (g) The person has agreeable dreams arousing hopefulness, with fragrant perfumes and alluring voices, visions and agreeable companionship. (h) Mental faculties include: vigor of imagination, intellectual power, and memory. Emotions are balanced between excess and deficiency, for example, between courage and timidity, between anger and patience, between sternness and clemency, between vacillation and perseverance. (i) Perfection in all functions.[13]

§1054 A person with such a temperament will have a happy expression, will be lovable and contented, moderate in desire for food and drink, possessing a good gastric digestion, good hermetic alley venous digestion, and good alternative and assimilative flower all through the tissues. The waste matters will be moderate in amount and will be discharged through the proper channels.

11.7. The Indications Afforded by Congenital Abnormalities: Asymmetry, Misproportion, Unshapeliness, and Ugliness

§1055 In brief, there is non-uniformity of temperament among the members; or, perchance, the principal members depart from equability and come to be of contrary temperament, one deviating towards one, another to its contrary. If the components of the body are out of proportion, it is unfortunate both for talent and reasoning power. Thus, (1) a tall person with a large abdomen and short face and round head, and short fingers; (2) a person of small stature, with small head, much flesh in the face and forehead, and even in the neck and feet—the face like the full moon, the jaws rounded and massive. Similarly, (3) if the head and forehead were round but the face very round (long, marginal reading), and the neck very thick, and if the eyes are sluggish in movement. Such persons would be the very last of people to be classed as in good health.

11.8. The Signs of Plethora

§**1056** Humoral changes may be quantitative or qualitative. Regarding plethora there are these same two aspects. Plethora in regard to cavities, tubes and juice canals (quantitative) and plethora in regard to power or strength (vitality; qualitative),

11.8.1. Quantitative Plethora

§**1057** In quantitative plethora (plethora of the channels of the body), humors and vital force are of normal quality but so excessive in quantity that the vessels become distended. In these cases exertion is apt to cause rupture of blood vessels with the humors blocking the "passages" thus causing choking of throat, epilepsy and apoplexy. This type of plethora needs treatment by venesection.

11.8.2. Qualitative Plethora

§**1058** In the case of qualitative plethora (plethora of strength of instinctive drives), the error is not in quantity of humors but in unhealthiness of quality whereby the instinctive drives are embarrassed and they become inefficient for the processes of digestion and maturation. A person who is in this state is in danger of putrefactive disorders.

11.8.3. Plethora in General

§**1059** Speaking in general of the signs of plethora of the first type are either objective or subjective. Objective: red face; full of veins; tightness of skin; sluggish movements or gestures; full pulse, high-colored urine; dense urine; scanty appetite. Subjective: sense of weight in the limbs, weak vision; dreams in which there is a sense of weight—as when one dreams one is unable to move or is carrying a heavy weight or cannot give utterance to words. This kind of dream may be compared with that associated with attenuation of humors or where the humors are moderate in amount for here one dreams one is flying through the air or moving at a great speed.[14]

11.8.4. The Signs of Plethora with the Faculties or Drives

§**1060** The signs of plethora in respect of the instinctive drives are heaviness, sluggishness, loss of appetite (these are also present in the preceding type), disinclination for exertion, and sense of burdensomeness.

§**1061** If the plethora of the instinctive drive is unaccompanied by plethora of humors, the veins are not as distended and the skin is not as tense or the pulse as full and large or the urine as gross (dense) or as red in color. There is no lassitude except after undue movement and exercise and activity. The dreams consist of sensations of itching, stinging, burning, and of fetid odors. However, in the case of plethora of the instinctive drives, illness ensues before all its signs are manifest.

11.8.5. Additional Remarks

§**1062** The age of the patient gives a clue to the kind of humor likely to be dominant. Excess of sanguineous humor is shown by signs akin to those of plethora and some of the signs given are accounted for by simple plethora. When the atrabilious humor is in excess, the blood is dusky and heavier than normal. Atrabilious humor is seldom in excess in pale and slight persons.[15]

11.9. The Signs of the Dominant Humor

11.9.1. Blood

§**1063** The signs of predominance of blood[16] resemble those of quantitative plethora and are characterized by feelings of heaviness in the body, especially behind the eyes, over the head and across the temples. Stretching and yawning is frequent. There is a tendency to excessive sleep and the mind gets dull.

Such persons are easily tired and often complain of a sweet taste in the mouth and usually have a red tongue. They are also predisposed to frequent appearance of boils over the body and ulcers on the tongue. Bleeding from the gums, nostrils and piles is frequent. Occasionally, the excess of blood can be recognized from the temperament of the person, his age, residence, previous habits and treatments and the characteristic dreams of seeing excessive blood or red things i.e., sight of a large quantity of blood being lost or someone being soaked in blood or some other such vision.

11.9.2. Phlegm

§1064 The signs of phlegm are excessive pallor, flabbiness of the body, cold and moist skin, excessive salivation and viscidity of the saliva. There is diminution of thirst, especially in the elderly, and particularly so when the phlegm is sour. A weak digestion with acid eructations, pale urine, excessive sleepiness, flabbiness of the muscles, mental torpor and softness of the pulse with slow rate and speed are characteristics of this condition. Age, occupation, residence, previous history and treatment are also helpful in identifying the predominance of phlegm. Dreams of water, canals, cold, ice, rain and thundering hail storms denote phlegm.

11.9.3. Yellow Bile (Choler)

§1065 Yellow color of the eyes and complexion, bitter taste in the mouth, rough and dry tongue and dryness of the nostrils are typical signs of yellow bile. Cool breezes are generally comforting. Excessive thirst, rapidity of pulse, lack of appetite are signs. Nausea with bilious vomiting of green or yellowish color, irritative diarrhea and often tingling of the skin are signs which point to the predominance of yellow bile. Temperament, age, occupation, residence, climate, previous habits and past treatments also help in the diagnosis. Characteristic dreams are of flames of fire and flags of yellow color. Additional signs of the yellow bile are that things seem yellow and there is burning and irritation after hot baths and on exposure to the sun.

11.9.4. Black Bile (Melancholy)

§**1066** The characteristic signs of this condition are dry and dark skin, thick and dark blood, presence of anxiety, burning in the epigastrium, false appetite, turbid urine of a blue, dark or red color, dark complexion and excessive hair. If the complexion is pale and the hair scanty, there is seldom any excess of black bile. Patches of pigmentation, chronic indolent ulcers and diseases of the spleen also indicate excess of black bile. Age, temperament, habits, residence, occupation and history of previous treatments are also helpful in the diagnosis. Dreams are usually full of anxiety and often of dark places, dark trenches and dark fearful objects.

11.10. The Signs of Stasis or Obstructions

§**1067** Obstruction is due to the retention of some normal secretion with feelings of tension and other vague signs of plethora. The obstruction of a duct which is normally free and has a regular flow of some excretion produces a feeling of heaviness, i.e., stasis or congestion in the liver, due to the blockage of the out-going hepatic veins which produce abnormal accumulation of the material arriving from the intestine. This causes a feeling of weight and heaviness which is sometimes even more than what may be experienced in inflammation. Inflammation is differentiated from obstruction by the presence of fever and relative lack of heaviness and weight.

§**1068** The blockage of a channel, which has a very little discharge, seldom causes heaviness; it is only the rupture of some blood vessel which produces this symptom. Obstruction of blood vessels produces pallor as in such cases the blood fails to reach the surface.[17]

11.11. The Signs of Gaseous Distension

§**1069** There is pain and tenderness in the affected part from a loss of continuity and abnormal movements are frequently noted. There are also some characteristic sounds and a distinctive feel. The diagnosis of gas can be made from the following.

11.11.1. Pain

§1070 Gas produces tension, but instead of heaviness it actually feels light and tends to move from place to place. There is pain when the gas has produced loss of continuity in a sensitive organ. It does not produce pain in the bones and glandular tissues. When occasionally it is of a larger quantity it may produce painless fractures. If pain does occur it is generally due to the damage of some neighboring structure caught in between the broken ends of a bone.

11.11.2. Movement

§1071 Palpitation (of the heart) and twitchings (of muscles) indicate dispersion of gas by the affected organ.

11.11.3. Sound

§1072 This may be heard directly as in flatulence or indirectly by palpation as in the case of gas over the splenic region. Sound may also be studied by percussion as in the differentiation of tympanities from ascites.

11.11.4. Feel

§1073 Distension from gas (tympanities) can be differentiated from other swellings by the amount of its pressure required to overcome the tension. Gas does not produce any thrill like the collections of fluid and it also lacks the characteristic feel of a liquid material.

11.11.5. Distinctions

§1074 The difference between inflation and gaseous distension is not in substance but in form. The form or shape of the distended area is different when standing or lying down and manipulation will alter its position.

11.12. The Signs of Solid Swellings

§1075 The presence of external tumors is easily demonstrated to the sense of sight. Deeply placed inflammatory swellings are revealed by accompanying fever as well as by a sense of heaviness if the affected member be devoid of sensation or of stabbing pain as well as heaviness if the member be sentient. Interference or hindrance to function and movement of a part affords a further sign of the presence of a tumor. A certain degree of intumescence of the overlying part is a very important sign of an inflammatory mass if sensation has access to it. Cold swellings are not accompanied by pain.

§1076 It is difficult to describe the signs of tumors in a general manner. Even if one could do so it would be at the expense of wearisome words. That is why it is simpler to defer details to the special chapters. It will suffice for the present to say that wherever heaviness and not pain are perceived and the signs of dominance of the serous humor are present, this leaves no doubt about the swelling being of pituitous nature. If there are signs of dominance of the atrabilious humor, and the swelling is hard to the touch, it will be an atrabilious mass because induration is pre-eminent among the signs of this form of swelling.

§1077 Inflammatory swellings in nerves are extremely painful and fever is intense, there is an accelerated rhythm in stretching, causing the pain, and there is delirium. Swellings in any of the inward parts of the body cause the abdominal wall to become wasted. If they are inflammatory and undergo suppuration and track outward, they cause extremely severe pain with fever; the tongue becomes very rough and there is great wakefulness; the symptoms become more and more severe—notably the sense of heaviness and weight and stiffness in the affected part. Induration and tension become evident. Sudden emaciation of the body with hollowness of the eyes may develop.

§1078 But when the process of suppuration has attained maturity, fever is high, pain lessens, the pulse softens, throbbing subsides and itching replaces the pain. If there was much redness and induration, the redness lessens, and the induration is less noticeable. Pressure on neighboring organs lessen and all the causes of pain subside along with the great sense of heaviness. When finally the abscess bursts there is a rigor produced by the acridity of the sanious matter; fever increases again because of the movement and discharge of the pus; and the pulse becomes empty, unequal, weak, infrequent, small, broad and slow. There is loss of appetite; often the extremities grow warm.

§**1079** The following signs after the bursting of an abscess are good: subsiding fever, easy breathing, return of strength, quick evacuation of pus through its proper channels.

§**1080** Sometimes, however, with deep abscesses, pus passes from one member to another and this transference is sometimes beneficial, sometimes detrimental. It is beneficial when it passes from a principal organ to a subordinate one; as for instance, when it passes from the brain to the tissues behind the ears and from the liver to the groins. It is detrimental if it passes from an ignoble organ to a noble one or to a weaker or less resistant organ as for instance when pleurisy involves the heart or lung.

§**1081** In the internal organs the inflammation may spread upwards or downward in a characteristic manner. If the spread is downward, there is a feeling of heaviness and tension across the lower abdomen and if it is upwards breathing becomes difficult and irregular and there is a sense of constriction in the chest with a sensation of burning and irritation rising upwards. Also there may be heaviness near the collar bone, headache and occasionally pain in the arm and the wrist. The spread of inflammation to the brain is a dangerous complication unless it localizes in the glands behind the ears. In these cases, as also in the inflammatory conditions of the abdomen, the occurrence of epistaxis is a favorable sign. A more comprehensive description of the abdominal inflammation will be given when the subject of inflammation is dealt with in the volume on diseases of the internal organs.

11.13. The Signs of Loss of Continuity

§**1082** Loss of continuity in the external organs is easily recognized by inspection and palpation. In the internal organs the signs are: (a) pain of a throbbing, stabbing, or tearing nature, especially when there is no fever; (b) elimination of some humor, i.e., the expectoration of blood, or the discharge of this humor into a cavity or discharge of pus from some pre-existing inflammation or matured abscess. If the discharge is not from a matured inflammation it would relieve the heaviness and fever but would be otherwise followed by an aggravation of pain; (c) a complete or partial displacement of an organ, i.e., hernia or an intestinal obstruction.

§1083 Prognosis: As you are aware, both loss of continuity and the presence of (inflammatory swellings) are more grave when they occur in very sensitive fibromuscular members. In fact, such loss of continuity may prove fatal from syncope or spasm. The syncope is due to the violence of the pain; the spasms are due to the irritation of the nerves in which the parts are so rich. Next in severity comes loss of continuity near joints, because restoration can only be slow considering the undue mobility of the parts, and the fact that spaces are opened up in and round the joints, and matters readily flow into these spaces.

§1084 Pulse and urine also provide general indications of the various states of the body. These are described in the next chapter.

Lecture 12: The Signs and Symptoms (Diagnosis): The Pulse

12.1. A General Description of the Pulse

§**1085** The pulse is a movement[1] in the heart and arteries (the receptacles of the breath) which takes the form of alternate expansion and contraction, whereby the breath becomes subjected to the influence of the air inspired.[2]

§**1086** The subject of the pulse may be considered (1) general or, (2) with regard to each of the several diseases. We defer the latter until a later period when we speak of the diseases themselves. At this stage we discuss the subject generally.

12.1.1. Description

§**1087** Every beat of the pulse comprises two movements and two pauses. Thus, expansion, pause, contraction, pause. One movement can not pass at once into another in an opposite direction. There must be a boundary or "limit of an act," as is expounded in the work on natural science.

§**1088** Many doctors consider that it is impossible to perceive the movement of contraction. Others are able to perceive it—as "strength"—if the pulse is strong as "degree of expansion" in a large pulse, as "great resistance" in a hard pulse, and, in a slow pulse, by the long period of time occupied by the movement.

§**1089** Galen also says, "For many years I was doubtful about clearly discerning the movement of contraction by touch and I shelved the question until such time as I should learn enough to fill the gap in my knowledge. After that, the doors of the pulse were opened to me. Whoever should study these things as I did will perceive that which I perceived [as it were, a brilliant light shining suddenly out from behind total darkness. Whoever allows these words to be true and not fabulous will benefit very greatly; despair will not touch him or frighten him from the pursuit of his study, even though he makes no progress for many years. Nevertheless there are conditions in which this movement cannot be perceived.

12.2.2. Reasons for Feeling the Pulse at the Wrist

§**1090** The reason for feeling the pulse at the wrist include the following: (1) it is readily accessible; there is little flesh over it; (2) the patient is not distressed by exposing this part.[3] (3) The artery runs in a straight course (which is no small help towards accuracy of diagnosis: Galen). (4) The distance from the heart is not great.

12.2.3. Technique for Feeling the Pulse

§**1091** If the palm be turned upwards the pulse will appear wider, less high and less long, especially in thin persons. If the hand be palm down, the pulse seems higher, longer and narrower.[4]

12.2.4. Emotional State of the Patient

§**1092** The pulse should be felt at a time when the patient is not in a state of excitement or anger, or affected by exertion, or under the influence of the emotions, or in a state of satiety (which renders the pulse heavy), or hungry; nor must it be a time when usual habits are neglected or new ones are being formed.

12.2. Ten Features of the Pulse

§1093 We say that there are ten features in the pulse from which we are able to discern the states of the body. Some group them under only nine headings: (1) amount of diastole; estimated in terms of length, breadth, and thickness; (2) quality of impact (literally, knocking at) imparted to the finger of the observer at each beat; (3) duration of time occupied in each movement; (4) consistency of the artery (resistance to the touch); (5) emptiness or fullness of the vessel between the beats (modern: compressibility); and (6) the feel—whether hot or cold. The remaining features concern several beats: (7) duration of time occupied by the pauses; (8) equality or inequality of force in successive beats; (9) regularity or irregularity, orderliness or disorderliness, presence of intermissions; (10) meter, rhythm, harmony, measure, and accent.[5]

12.3. Details

12.3.1. Amount of Expansion

§1094 The kind of pulse in terms of the three dimensions: length, breadth and thickness. There are nine variations in regard to one dimension alone, and these are called "simple," and there are nine compound varieties.[6]

12.3.1.1. Simple Pulses

§1095 The simple pulses are: the long, the short and the mean; the broad, the slender and the mean; the deep, the elevated and the mean.

§1096 The long pulse is one which is longer than normal. This is the type appropriate to a person of equable temperament or else approximating to this. The difference between the natural and the equable has been already made plain.

§1097 The short pulse is contrary to the preceding.

§1098 The mean pulse between these two extremes completes the first group of three. The remaining six can be understood along the same lines.[7]

12.3.1.2. Compound Pulses

§1099 As regards the compound pulses, some have received distinctive names and some have not. A pulse which is increased both in length and breadth as well as in depth is called "large." When all these dimensions show diminution, it is a "small" pulse. The moderate pulse is the mean between the two.[8]

12.3.2. Quality of Impact

§**1100** The varieties are three: strong—this resists the finger during expansion; weak—the opposite character; and the intermediate.[9]

12.3.3. Duration of Cycle

§**1101** There are three variants: rapid or short or swift—where the movement is completed in a short space of time; slow or sluggish or long—the contrary; and the intermediate or moderately quick pulse.

12.3.4. Consistency of Artery

§**1102** There are three variants: soft or easily compressible; hard, firm or incompressible; and one of moderate compressibility.

12.3.5. Fullness or Emptiness

§**1103** The full (high) pulse seems to be over full of humor and gives the impression that it needs liberating. The empty (low) pulse is contrary in character. There is an intermediate between the two.[10]

12.3.6. The Feel of the Pulse

§**1104** Hot, cold or intermediate.

12.3.7. The Duration of the Pause

§**1105** Hurried ("dense"), where the period between the two successive beats is short; sluggish ("rare"), where the period is prolonged. And there is a mean. This period of time is recognized from the contraction-period, but if contraction cannot be perceived it is estimated from the period between two expansions. In this case it is reckoned from the times of the two extremes.

12.3.8. Equality or Inequality (Rhythm or Balance)

§1106 This is reckoned according as the successive pulses are similar or dissimilar, there being a difference of size (large or small), strength (strong or weak), swiftness (rapid or slow; prompt or sluggish), hardness or softness, until it happens that the second expansion of the first pulse is overtaken by the first of the next (due to excess of innate heat), or is weaker than the next (excess of weakness).

§1107 If desired, one could expand this discourse and consider the equality or inequality in regard to the three variants in the other features of the pulse already named. But it is sufficient to consider them only in regard to strength.

§1108 Regular ("equal") pulse in the strict sense is one which is regular in all these respects; if it is regular only in one feature, it is so specified. Thus, we speak of a pulse as a regular ("equal") in strength or regular in speed. In the same way a pulse is irregular either in all respects or only in one.[11]

12.3.9. Orderliness or Disorderliness

§1109 Orderliness or disorderliness. There are two forms: the pulse may be irregularly orderly or irregularly disorderly. The orderly pulse maintains orderly succession. This occurs in one of two modes. The orderliness is absolute where there is every feature maintained; or cyclical where there are two or more irregularitics which keep on repeating in cycles, as if there were two cycles simultaneously or superposed, so that the original order reappears.

§1110 In this way, it becomes evident that the tenth feature belongs here, in a certain sense; so that those who restrict the features to nine instead of ten are justified.

§1111 For one must now see the musical character of the pulse. For in the art of music, sounds are juxtaposed in orderly relations of loudness and softness which keep on repeating at regular intervals; rates of utterance vary—some sounds coming close to one another, and others being further apart; the attack may be abrupt or gentle, sharp or dull. The notes may be sound-ed clearly or be indefinite; they may be strong or weak; the volume may be "full" or "thin." The rhythm of the sequence of the sounds may be regular or irregular.

§**1112** In feeling the pulse, all these features are also to be met with. The intervals between the beats or the successions may be harmonious or inharmonious. So, too, the irregularities may be orderly or disorderly. It is orderly when there is a proper relation of strength and weakness. It is disorderly if there is not. All this belongs to the question of order and regularity.

§**1113** According to Galen, pulse could be felt in only one of the following rhythms of music: 1:3, 1:2, 1:1.5, 1:1, and 1:1.25 [double time, three-four time, common time, four-five time, five-six time, and so on. For those who have a sensitive touch and a seen sense of rhythm with a training in the musical art, such minute of observation could be correlated in the mind. I am surprised to think how many of such relations could be perceived by the sense of touch, and yet I am confident that it can be done if one is habituated to the use of it, and can apportion metre and beats of time. On the other hand, since these variations all belong to inequality and disorderliness it is not necessary to define them particularly.[12]

12.3.10. Meter

§**1114** Even if the preceding details cannot be perceived, at least the relation between period of expansion and period of pause can be appreciated, as well as the relation between the total duration of beat and the total duration of pause. Under this heading, then, we place: first total period of pulse: next total period; period of expansion: period of pause; period of expansion plus period of pause: period of contraction plus period of pause; period of expansion: period of contraction. A relation of period of expansion: period of contraction; or period of first pause: period of second pause, is not important.

§**1115** Meter (rhythm, "beat," accent) is good (eurhythm) or bad (arhythm) according to the musical analogy. There are three kinds of arhythm: (1) pararhythm, where the beat is altered only slightly, and temporarily. An example where the adult has a metre which is only natural in youth, where a child shows a rhythm proper to an adult; (2) heterorhythm. This is a change greater in degree. Example where a youth has a metre proper to an old man; (3) etrhythm. Here the change is to something altogether different, as where the metre does not conform to the human type at all. A great change of metre denotes great change of bodily state.[13]

12.4. The Regular and Irregular Pulse

§1116 Some say that irregularity (dissimilarity) of the pulse applies to a succession of beats or to any individual beat. But when the irregularity is in the individual beat the various components are diverse, whether in the various places where one applies one's fingers, or only at one particular point of application.

§1117 When the irregularity is in regard to several pulsations there may be a regular succession of events. This begins with one pulsation and there is a change to a greater or lesser, following on regularly step by step until a maximum or minimum is reached, after which there is a break, and the original cycle is resumed. Or, the beats continue at the same level for a time and there is then an intermission and the original cycle is resumed.

§1118 The whole cycle may show only one irregularity or it may show two or more. In this case, it is as if there were two cycles distinct from one another, and yet keeping to one order, so that the whole seems to be just one single cycle.

§1119 The irregularity may consist in the occurrence of a paused when one expects a beat, or in the occurrence of a beat in they middle of a pause.

§1120 When the irregularity refers to several components of one single pulsation, this may be in regard to relative position or to movement. And as there are six components there will be corresponding irregularities: (1) expansion swift or sluggish (2) premature or delayed expansion; (3) strength or weakness; (4) largeness or smallness. All of this may be orderly and regular or may vary by exaggeration or by deficiency in two components or in three or in four. This may all be worked out for oneself.

§1121 Irregularity of the pulse in one sections is shown as an intermitting or as a recurrent or as a continuous pulse.

12.4.1. The Intermitting Pulse

§1122 With the intermitting pulse (a smaller beat occurs after one or more great pulsations.[14] Sometimes even the smaller beat is wanting. Inter-current pulse: this is the opposite. When we are expecting an interval of rest, a supernumerary pulsation occurs. These two pulses denote impairment of the cardiac power, the degree being greater in the intermittent than in the recurrent. One component is separated from the next only by a short interval and a pause is interposed in another, so that the two extremes of the pulsation vary in swifts.

12.4.2. The Recurrent Pulse

§1123 With the recurrent pulse[15] a large pulse becomes small in one component and then becomes slowly large again. In this case there may be two kinds of pulse passing into one another, so that, for instance, one pulse, by its irregularity, comes to appear like two, or two pulses come to appear like one. Opinions about this differ.

12.4.3. The Continuous Pulse

§1124 The continuous pulse[16] is one in which the expansion is continual and unbroken. There is a steady increase from slowness to swiftness, and from swiftness to slowness; from equality to inequality; from largeness to smaller, and so on. There is no break in the change, for it is continuing the whole time. Sometimes there is more irregularity in regard to some of the components and sometimes there is less.

12.5. The Types of Irregular Pulse Which Have Distinctive Names

§1125 Gazelle: [syn. goat leap pulse; modern "jerking"; "pulsus bisferiens"]: the expansion is interrupted and occupies a longer time than usual and remains at a certain height and is succeeded by at swift increase to the full height.[17]

§**1126** Undulatory ["bounding" (modern; like "rolling waves"]: the irregularity is in respect of largeness and smallness of artery, of degree of rise, and of breadth, and in the position of the beginning of the beat (whether too soon or too late), and also in softness. It is not very small; it has a certain breadth recalling the movement of waves, which follow upon one another in orderly fashion and yet vary in the extent of upward rise and downward fall and in swiftness and slowness.[18]

§**1127** Vermicular [modern "creeping"]: this resembles the preceding, but is small, soft, feeble, and very hurried. The closeness of the beats causes it to be mistaken for a swiftly or rapid pulse.[19]

§**1128** Formicant pulse: this is the smallest, most feeble and hurried of all the pulses. [It is not a quick pulse, though apparently swift. (Aeg.)] It differs from the vermicular loci pulse in the great ease with which upward rise, anteposition of beat or post position is perceived. Irregularity of breadth is not discernible. It is a weak form of vermicular pulse; and allied in character to the "hectic" pulse.]

§**1129** Serrate pulse: this [modern "harsh"] pulse resembles the undulatory in the inequality of the various components of the beat upward rise, breadth, anteposition and post position. It differs, however, in appearing harder, and in its components, being of unequal hardness. This pulse is quick, hurried, hard. The irregularity is in respect of the side of expansion, of hardness and of softness.

§**1130** Mousetail: there is progressive inequality of the components—from decrease-to increase, from increase to decrease. This may apply to several beats or only to one beat or only to a part of a beat. The inequality is in respect of volume, or of slowness (changing to swiftness), or of weakness (changing to strength).[20]

§**1131** Recurrent [modern "flickering" pulse]: this passes from minuteness to a certain volume, and then fails progressively until it reaches its former minuteness. It is like two myuri placed together end to end.[21]

§1132 Dicrotic: doctors are divided in opinion about this pulse. Some regard it as a single beat in which antecession and post position are unequal; others regard it as a double pulse, one beat following the next too quickly to give time for the second to produce full expansion. However, the presence of two beats does not make two distinct pulses. A pulse which makes a partial expansion and then resumes it would not be dual. It would only be dual if the artery were to fill first, then pause, then contract, and again refill; but otherwise it would virtually be a jerking pulse.[22]

§1133 Fading or falling: here there is a pause in the middle of the pulsation, as there is in the gazelle pulse. But in the gazelle pulse the second beat begins before the first is finished; in the falling pulse the first beat is completed before the second begins.

§1134 The spasmodic thrilling and twisted pulse: the latter is compared with a twisted thread; there is here an irregularity between the precession and the later parts of the pulsations both in position and in breadth.[23]

§1135 The chord-like pulse: this feels like a twisted cord (or sinew), and is similar to the thrilling pulse. But in the chord-like pulses the expansion is less conspicuous; the departure from regularity of position of rise is less evident; but tension is evident; the twisting is sometimes only in regard to one portion of the pulsation. The two kinds of pulse are really equally common, and equally liable to occur in "dry" diseases. All the above are simple pulses.

§1136 The varieties of compound pulse (that is, where there is more than one form of inequality or irregularity at once) am almost innumerable. In any case they have received no specific names.[24]

12.6. The Pulse Designated as "Natural"

§1137 Each of the above-named varieties (of pulse) necessitates a distinction into "increased" and "diminished." And that which is "natural" among them is the "equable" pulse, except in the case of the strong sort, because here the "natural" pulse is excessive as to strength. But in other cases, the increase is in natural proportion to the increase in force, so that, for example, as it becomes greater, it is "natural" for it also to be forcible.

§1138 As for the sorts (of pulse) in which there is no possibility of increase and diminution, in such- cases the "natural" pulse is the one which is even (equable), regular (orderly), and of good rhythm (weight).[25]

12.7. The Factors Concerned in the Production of the Pulse

§1139 The factors concerned in the production of the pulse are: (1) essential and integral in the constitution of the pulse. These are called "contentive" factors; or (2) non-essential: comprising two groups: (i) inseparable that is, if they were altered, the type of the pulse would be altered; (ii) separable; that is, a change may be produced in them without affecting the type of the pulse.

§1140 There are three contentive factors: (1) large pulse where the vital power of the heart produces the expansion; (2) the elasticity of' the artery; (3) the resistance, or urge.[26]

12.7.1. The List of Non-Essential Factors

§1141 The list of non-essential factors include: (1) natural (i.e. pertaining to the nature): age (manhood, youth); temperature of air (hot seasons; hot localities): temperament (hot temperament). (2) Non-natural: exposure to very hot atmosphere; use of hot baths; vigorous exercise or gymnastics; influence of food and wine; influence of calefacient medicines. (3) Preternatural: emotional states; secretiveness (hiding anger, concealing the fact of having taken a heating medicine in spite of the physicians enquiry); cunning persons who easily conceal matters relative; habits of the patient; hot intemperaments; decompositions occurring in the fluids (in the stomach or tissues).

12.7.2. The Effect of the Contentive Factors Upon the Pulse

12.7.2.1. Large Pulse

§**1142** If the arterial wall is at the same time yielding, and the vital power is strong and the resistance excessive, the pulse will be large. The resistance is the chief factor in the production of a large pulse, for should the power fail, the pulse will naturally weaken and if the arterial wall were also hard, and the resistance lowered, the pulse would be even smaller.

12.7.2.2. Elasticity of the Artery

§**1143** An unyielding artery will also make the pulse small. But the difference between a small pulse due to inelastic artery and one due to weakness is that in the former the pulse is hard and not weak or short or low as in the latter. Low resistance also makes a small pulse, but it is not weak. Weakness is the chief cause of all three forms of small pulse. Granted the power is constant, lack of hardness of the artery has more effect than lack of resistance, for there is nothing to prevent the artery from expanding.

§**1144** The temperament has not much influence unless the resistance be lowered.

12.7.2.3. The Resistance or Urge

§**1145** If the resistance be great, the power strong, and the artery inelastic, the pulse becomes swift. The swiftness makes up for lack of size of pulse. But if the power be not adequate and the pulse is therefore unable to become large, and therefore not swift, it necessarily becomes brisk, and this briskness makes up for the lack of volume and swiftness. Several beats of this kind would become equivalent to the effect of one adequately large beat, or of two swift beats.

§**1146** It is like a human being wishing to carry a very heavy weight. If he is able to do so, he will carry it in one journey, though with difficulty or he may divide it into two, thus making the journey more easily or, if he cannot manage even that, he will divide the load into many portions, and carry each one as leisurely or as quickly as he wishes. He need not rest himself between the journeys, though he may choose to linger. But if he were very weak, he would stop and rest awhile between the loads and as he becomes tired with the journeys would perform them more slowly.

12.7.2.4. Further Distinctions

§**1147** If the vital power be strong, and the artery responsive and the resistance moderate, the effect of the power would be to make the pulse more swift and of greater volume. But if they resistance were greater, there would be; briskness as well as larger volume and swiftness.

§**1148** The factors which go to make a large pulse also go to make a long pulse, if rise and fall are hindered in any ways For instance, a hard artery cannot widen, and tough flesh and skin, especially if the tissues be wasted, prevents the artery from rising to the finger.[27]

12.7.3. The Causes of Pulses Having Distinctive Names

§**1149** Emaciation may make a pulse appear broad. Emptiness of vessel also makes a pulse appear broad, because the two walls come into apposition. A very soft artery gives the same effect.[28]

§**1150** Hurried pulse: the causes of a hurried pulse are weakness; great resistance; heat.

§**1151** Sluggish pulse: the causes of a sluggish pulse are power relatively greater than resistance; great coldness due to resistance; great loss of vital power; approach of death.

§**1152** Feeble pulse: the causes of feeble pulse are loss of natural power because of lack of food; emaciation; excessive discharges; insomnia; too much exercise; solicitude; morbid change in the humors; movement of the humors, especially into a very sensitive member, or into a member which is in relation with the heart; any source of intemperament; pain (producing syncope); sadness, grief and other mental states or cares; any factor whereby the vitality is markedly depressed. (Note also: age, season, locality; temperament).[29]

§1153 Hard pulse: the causes of hard ("tense") pulse are: dryness of the arteries and great stretching of the arteries; intense cold. The pulse may become very hard at the crisis of an illness owing to the intensity of the conflict between the person and his disease, for all the members are implicated. (This pulse is usually also small, quick, and' sometimes frequent).[30]

§1154 Soft pulse: the causes of soft pulse are: "natural" agents with an emollient action such as aliments (more abundant diet; liquid food). Morbid states which tend to emollient effect: i.e., dropsy, sleepy-sickness, coma, disorders arising from or in a serous humor. Mental states, such as hilarity. Agents which rare neither "natural" nor morbid: like bathing (to excess).[31]

§1155 Irregular pulse: if the vital power be maintained, the cause will be heaviness [in substance] of the food, or of some humor. If the vital power be weak, it shows a contest between causative agent [of the illness] and the tissues. Other causes: (1) over fullness of the vessels. This would be remedied by venesection. (2) Viscidity of the blood. In this case the breath becomes choked in the vessels. This form of pulse is especially liable to occur when the breath is also imprisoned in the cardiac region—for example, by an over-full stomach, which produces this effect very rapidly, by anxiety or by pain.

§1156 If the stomach contain depraved humor, the irregularity increases until cardiac tremor comes on, and a thrilling pulse (tachycardia) results.

§1157 If the irregularity is orderly, it betokens lesser constitutional injuries; if disorderly, it shows that there are more serious constitutional defects to deal with.

§1158 Harsh pulse: this pulse shows a varying consistence of the artery which is produced by changes in the composition of the (circulating) humors, whereby decomposition products, "crudities," or products of maturation diffuse through the vessel wall and affect its mode of expansion. Inflammatory deposits fibro-muscular organs (like diaphragm, pleura: Rhazes) also render the pulse harsh.[32]

§1159 Dicrotic pulse: vital power is strong; the artery is hard; the resistance is considerable. The artery does not at once yield to the force. It suggests a person wishing to sever something at one blow, but failing to do so until helped out for instance by a sudden dire need to achieve it. (Significance: approaching crisis).

§1160 Mousetail: such a pulse is produced when the vital power is weak, as a person who ceases manual labor, or is resuming it after a rest. If it is constant, it shows that the loss of power is greater. However, as long as the pulsation is mousetail in type (and the similar forms) it shows that there is some vitality left. But it is apt to pass on to the terminal mousetail, then to continuous mousetail, and finally end in the grave "recurrent mousetail" ("swooning" pulse).[33]

§1161 Fading or falling pulse: the vital power is enfeebled or waning, and inadequate. It is also produced by a sudden change in the "nature" and in the mind.

§1162 The spasmodic or tense pulse: this is produced when there are non-natural movements in the vital power or when the artery is itself unhealthy.[34]

§1163 Thrilling pulse: here the vital power is strong; the artery is hard; the resistance is great. Without these conditions it cannot arise.[35]

§1164 Undulatory pulse: this usually means chiefly lack of vital power, expansion being hardly achieved, if at all, and then only little by little. If the artery is soft, this would itself suffice to produce the effect of waves, even though the power were not much reduced. A soft and moist artery does not respond to an impact, and does not allow every part to bet expanded whereas a dry and hard artery does, dryness being responsive to impact and tremor. An artery which is both hard and dry will transmit expansion at once; the soft and moist artery will only do so at the beginning of the pulsation, expansion and alteration of form of the vessel subsiding suddenly so that the other fingers do not perceive any movement.[36]

§1165 Vermicular and formicant pulse: these types are produced by great weakness, and so the pulse is sluggish, the intervals between the beats are short and the components are unequal. This is because the artery is unable to expand at once, but only little by little.[37]

§1166 Pulse of faulty rhythm: if this occurs during a time of repose, it is due to an increased resistance. If it occurs during exercise, there is an increased weakness (of vital power) or deficient degree of resistance. The pulse of exercise produced by swiftness of expansion is something different to this.[38]

§1167 The causes of full, empty, hot and cold, deep (high) and low pulses are evident.[39]

12.8. The Effect of Age and Sex on the Pulse

§1168 Male sex: the pulse is larger and much stronger, because the vital power and the resistance are both marked. The pulse is slower and more sluggish than in women because the degree of resistance is so great.

§1169 If the vital power is maintained, and the pulse is brisk, it must needs be swift. Swiftness comes before briskness. Hence the pulse of males is slow, and is necessarily also sluggish.

§1170 Late childhood (7-14): the pulse is softer because the temperament is moist at this period. It is weaker and more brisk because the innate heat is abundant. The vital power is not great, for growth has not yet become complete. Considering the small size of the body at this age, the pulse is large. This is because the artery is very soft and the resistance strong, and the vital power is not small—considering the small bulk of the body (at this age). Compared with the pulse of adult life the pulse at this age is not large but quick and more brisk (due to the resistance). This is because at this period of life there is a greater aggregation of "fumosities" (smoke or mist) consequent on eating so often and so liberally wherefore more frequent evacuation as becomes called for and "ventilation" of the innate heat is desirable.

§1171 Early adult life (21-35): The pulse is large, not very swift indeed inclined to be slower and less brisk; the tendency is to become sluggish. At the beginning of this period of life the volume of the pulse is greater; and at the middle of the period it is stronger. The innate heat, as we have stated, is about the same in adolescents and in young adults; there is, therefore, about the same resistance in each. The vital power is greater at this period, and the greater volume of pulse therefore compensates for the lack of swiftness and frequency. Vital power is the main reason for the pulse being large at this time of life. The resistance is next in importance, and the state of the arterial wall is the contributory factor.

§1172 Elderly persons: the pulse is here smaller because of the weakness of the vital power; then swiftness is lessened both because of this and because of the lessened resistance. Such a' pulse is therefore more sluggish.

§1173 Old age: in advanced years of life, the pulse becomes small, sluggish, slow. If it be also soft this is because of extraneous, and not natural, humors.[40]

12.9. The Pulse in the Various Temperaments

12.9.1. Hot Temperament

§1174 The resistance is great. If the vital power and artery correspond, the pulse will be large. But if one of them do not correspond, the pulse will vary in the manner already described.

§1175 If the heat is not due to an intemperament, but is natural, the vital power will be very strong, and the heat increases. But one must not suppose that the increase of innate heat, to however great an extent, will lessen the vital power. Odor, on the contrary, the power of the breath becomes greater, and the mental qualities show more boldness. If the heat arises from intemperament, the greater the degree of heat, the greater the weakening of vital power.

12.9.2. Cold Temperament

§1176 The pulse is reduced in breadth, and so becomes small, slow and infrequent (sluggish). If the artery is soft, the pulse increases in width, and also becomes slow and infrequent. But if the artery be hard, the breadth will lessen.

§1177 The weakness produced by a cold intemperament is

greater than that produced by a hot intemperament because the heat of the latter, for instance, is then more correspondent (i.e. in slowness or activity) than is the innate heat.

12.10.3. Moist Temperament

§1178 The pulse is here soft and wide.

12.10.4. Dry Temperament

§1179 The pulse becomes hard and wiry If the vital power be strong and the resistance great, the pulse will become dicrotic, or spasmodic, or thrilling.

12.10.5. Summary

§1180 These remarks will suffice in regard to the relation between the several temperaments and the simple types of pulse. The effect on composite pulses can be worked out from the principles already explained.

§1181 Its may happen that a person may have a dual temperament, one side being cold and the other hot. The pulse will then be different on the two sides, according to the heat and cold respectively. In the one case it will be like the pulse in hot temperament; in the other like that in cold temperament. From this we learn that the expansion and contraction of the pulse is not merely an effect of the ebb and flow of cardiac action, but there is also an expansion and contraction of the arterial wall itself.

12.10. The Effect of the Seasons on the Pulse

12.10.1. Spring

§1182 The pulse is equable in all respects except in strength, which is above the mean.

12.10.2. Summer

§1183 The pulse is quick and brisk, because of the resistance. It is small and weak because the vital power is dispersed by the dispersal of the breath (which in its turn is due to dominance of undue external atmospheric heat).

12.10.3. Winter

§**1184** They pulse is more sluggish, slow, weak and therefore small. This is because the vital power is lessened. In some people the heat is retained interiorly and aggregated together, thus making the vital power stronger. This is especially so if the temperament is hot, for then the external cold is overruled and prevented from; passing inwardly, as would otherwise occur.

12.10.4. Autumn

§**1185** The pulse is unequal and tends to a certain weakness. The inequality is due to the frequent changes of temperament which occur during this season owing to the fluctuations of temperature. The temperament is now hot, now cold accordingly. The weakness is due to two causes: (1) a contrary temperament always renders the injurious effect of a nocument greater than a similar but equable temperament would, although that be a morbid one; (2) autumn is a season antagonistic to life because at this period the innate heat is lessened and dryness dominates.

12.10.5. General Effects of Seasons on the Pulse

§**1186** At periods between the seasons the pulse corresponds to the adjoining season rhythm.

§**1187** The pulse at each season also has its own appropriate rhythm.[41]

12.11. The Effects of Locality on the Pulse

§**1188** Some regions are temperate and vernal; some are hot and aestival; some are cold and winterly; some are dry and autumnal. The character of the pulse will follow they statements made in regard to seasonal influences upon the pulse.

12.11.1. The Effects of Food and Drink

§**1189** Aliments (lit. substances entering the body from

without) alter the condition of the pulse according to their quality and quantity. (1) By quality one refers to the calefacient or infrigidant nature of the substance in question, which has a corresponding effect upon the pulse. (2) As regards quantity, if the amount of aliment is moderate, the pulse shows an increase of volume, swiftness and frequency, owing to the increase of vital power and innate heat resulting. This change in the pulse lasts a considerable time.

§1190 If the amount be unduly great, the pulse will become irregular and disorderly, because the burden of the food overrules the vital power; any overloading renders the pulse irregular. Archigenes thought that the; swiftness of the pulsed exceeded the frequency, as long as the excess of food existed. When the excess came to be less, the pulse would; show an orderly irregularity. If the amount be unduly small, the pulse becomes irregular both in volume and swiftness. In this case the duration of the change would be short because so small an amount of food would be rapidly digested.

§1191 If the vital power is weakened, whether the amount of food taken be small or large, the pulse corresponds in smallness and slowness until the digestion of the meal is completed. If the natural (vegetative, digestive, maturative) faculty be strong, the pulse will be equable.

§1192 The effect of wine on the pulse: wine has a notable effect on the pulse, in that if taken plentifully, being attenuated in nature, it gives rise to an irregular pulse, but not to so great an extent as other similarly nutrient aliments.) This is because its substance is too-rare, attenuated, and light. Being in actuality cold, wine, like other cold things, lessens the pulse-rate and makes it slow and infrequent in proportion to the rapidity with which it enters the body. Once it has become warmed by the initial effect it passes off as the heating effect of wine.

§1193 The heating effect which wine produces is not very different from that of the innate heat, for wine is rapidly distributed through the body, especially if taken warm, and it undergoes rapid dissipation or resolution. If taken cold, it exerts an injurious effect on the pulse of a kind not shared by other cold articles of food, for the latter become warm only gradually and do not reach the blood as quickly as does wine, and they are therefore warm when they do so. But wine is absorbed so quickly that it has to be warmed by the blood itself and this constitutes a noxa for such persons as are sensitive to cold. This injurious effect is not as great in degree if the wine is taken warm, because the natural faculty then counteracts it by breaking it up, distributing it through the body and finally dispersing it.

§1194 The cooling effect of wine. Wine has a cooling effect when it causes the natural power to fail, so that the pulse loses its strength before the wine has become broken up, distributed and dispersed.

§1195 Such is the manner in which the use of wine in quantity produces a heating or a cooling effect.

§1196 When we study the question of how the use of wine can make the pulse strong, other factors must be considered. Its own intrinsic character invigorates healthy persons, and enhances the vital power by securing a rapid accession to the "substance" of the breath.

§1197 Although the heating and cooling effects above explained are injurious to most persons, there are some whose temperament is suited by it. Cold things, for instance, are tonic for persons of hot intemperament. For, as Galen truly said, the juice of pomegranate is strengthening for persons of hot intemperament; wine is tonic for those of cold temperament.

§1198 Wine may therefore be considered to be hot in nature, in that it is a tonic for persons of hot temperament; cold in nature in that it is tonic for those of cold temperament. Still, this question is aside from our purpose. We are concerned with they fact that is speedily accedes to the breath, as an intrinsic property and that from that point of view it is always invigorating.

§1199 The pulse becomes stronger if either the invigorating effect is exerted or the warming effects. It becomes weaker if neither occurs. By warming the body the resistance [i.e. the blood pressure] is increased; by cooling the body the resistance is diminished. But the usual action is that the pulse becomes stronger. Moreover, resistance [blood-pressure] is never increased without rendering the pulse more swift.

§1200 Water has a similar invigorating effect to wine because it is the means by which the aliment is enabled to permeate all through the body. But as it induces colds rather than warmth, it does not increase the resistance as much as does wine.

12.11.2. The Effect of Sleep and the Act of Waking on the Pulse

§1201 The characters of the pulse during sheep vary according the stage of sleep and the state of digestion. At the beginning of sleep the pulse is small and weak because the innate heat is then in the process of retracting and withdrawing inwardly, instead of expanding and traveling to the surface.[42]

§1202 During the time of sleep, the innate heat is withdrawn inward by the vegetative drive in order to procure the digestion of the chyme and the maturation of effete substances. The heat is therefore, as it were, mastered and forced into service. The pulse is therefore more slow and sluggish in spite of the fact that the contraction and imprisonment of the heat in this region means a local increase of heat. For, in amount, this local heat is not so much as exists during the waking state, with its associated movements and exercise.

§1203 Thus, exercise is apt to create undue heat and "inflammation" up to an intemperamental degree, whereas there is only a moderate aggregation of heat when the innate heat is 'imprisoned, and so "inflammation" is less feasible. You know that this is so, because of the fact that exercise makes breathing labored (forced), and hurried, incomparably more than when the innate heat is constricted and imprisoned by some other agent similar to sleep. For instance, to be submerged in tepid water brings about such an imprisonment of innate heat, and produces rapid respiration, yet not nearly to the extent produced by toil and exercise. Careful consideration shows that nothing increases the heat as much as these do. But it is not the mere exercise which accounts for this as if resting would bring about a cessation of heat production. It is rather that the heat produced by exercise simply moves on the breath to the exterior parts, as long as generation of the breath takes place.

§**1204** During the stage of sleep, following the completion of digestion, the pulse becomes stronger. This is because vital power is added to by the digested aliment. The heat which had passed to the inward parts now returns towards the surface in order to regulate the nutrients passing thither, and also returns towards its source. This fact, and the fact that the temperament is made hotter by the products of nutrition, explains why the pulse becomes of increased volume, and the arterial wall is softer because of the addition of the appropriate nutrients. There is no increase in swiftness and briskness along with the increase of volume, because mere increase of volume does not alter blood pressure (lit. increase the resistance) either directly or indirectly; that is, by restoring the factors which directly raise the blood pressure (lit. increase the resistance).[43]

§**1205** If sleep continues after the completion of digestion, and the pulse again becomes weak because of the aggregation of innate heat and the choking of the vital power by the undue preponderance of those effete substances which now await evacuation by channels only possible during the waking state—namely exercise, and the insensible perspiration.

§**1206** If the body were fasting when sleep began, and there is nothing awaiting digestion, the temperament would tend towards coldness, and consequently the pulse would not only remain small, slow and sluggish but would become more so.

§**1207** The act of waking has certain effects on the pulse. When a sleeping person awakes, the pulse steadily gains volume and swiftness until it reaches the natural state for that person. But if the wakening is sudden, the change in the pulse will be sudden; it will become rapidly weak, because the act of waking overrules the vital power. The previous large volume will reappear later, and the pulse will become: quick, brisk and irregular (up to "thrilling"). The quasi-violent movement introduces great heat. The sudden stirring up of the vital power to meet the sudden change accounts for the irregularity and trembling of the pulse. However, the pulse does not remain long in this condition; it rapidly becomes regular again. Seemingly potent though the agent is, its duration is so short that all trace of its effect is soon lost.

12.11.3. The Pulse During Rigorous Athletic Exercise

§**1208** At the outset,[44] as long as the exertion is moderate, the pulse is large and strong. This is because the innate heat increases, and is strong. The pulse is also swift and brisk. This is because thee resistance becomes greatly increased by the exertion.[45]

§**1209** As exertion continues and increases, even if it be intense for only a short time, the pulse weakens, and, with the dispersal of the innate heat, becomes small. The pulse remains swift and brisk for two reasons: (1) the degree of resistance (i.e. blood pressure) is further increased; (2) the vital power progressively fails until it is insufficient. After this, the swiftness steadily and progressively lessen; and the briskness increases correspondingly to the lessening of vital power.[46] Still further prolongation of the exertion weakens the pulse until it becomes formicant and very brisk.[47]

§**1210** Finally if the exercise has been carried on to an extremely excessive extent, it leads to a state akin to death, acting like all resolvents—that is, it renders the pulse vermicular, very brisk, slow, weak and small.

12.11.4. The Effect of Bathing on the Pulse

12.11.4.1. Hot Bath

§**1211** If one bathes in hot water, the first effect is to make the pulse strong and raise the pressure. When the bath has brought about a dispersal of the vital power, the pulse becomes weak. Galen says it is small, slow in beat and sluggish. But while agreeing that it is weak and small, we say that the hot water acts first by increasing the interior heat of the body, like any extraneous heat, i. e. only temporarily After a while the water resumes its cooling effects—its natural quality. This cooling effect may persist. As long as its action as extraneous heat holds the field, the pulse becomes swift and brisk. But when its own natural character is resumed, the pulse will be slow and sluggish. If the incidental quality (of being hot) lead to so much loss of strength that syncope is imminent, the g pulse becomes slow and sluggish.

12.11.4.2. Cold Bath

§1212 If the cold-reaches to the interior parts, the pulse becomes weak, small, sluggish, slow. If it does not dot so, but has the effect of aggregating the innate heat in the interior, the volume of the pulse will increase as the power increases, and the swiftness fan briskness decrease.

12.11.4.3. Bathing in Natural Thermal Waters

§1213 If these have desiccant properties, the pulse becomes harder and its volume diminishes. If they impart warmth, the swiftness increases. If they dispel the vital power the pulse will come to be as described above.

12.11.5. The Pulse in Pregnancy

§1214 The resistance is specially great in pregnancy because the foetus shares in the mother's respiration. Both mother and embryo have their own resistance (blood-pressure), and there is as it were a double respiration. Nevertheless there is no doubt about the fact that the vital power is neither increased nor lessened, except to a degree consistent with a slight lassitude proceeding from the mere weight of the foetus. Hence the increase of resistance overrules the moderate amount of vital power, and the pulse is made of greater volume and becomes swift and brisk.[48]

12.11.6. The Pulse in Pain

§1215 Pain changes the character of the pulse according to (1) its intensity; (2) its duration; (3) its situation—whether the member affected is a vital one or not.

§1216 Pain at first stirs up the vital power, making it resist and counteract the pain; at the same time the cause of the pain increases the heat of the body. The pulse is, therefore, of large volume, swift and very brisk, the effort entailed in immobilizing the body [the reflex effect of the pain] accounting for the volume and swiftness. When the pain becomes less unbearable in one or other of the ways we have already explained, the pulse steadily declines in fullness until it has lost its size and swiftness; but these features are replaced by very marked briskness and smallness of beat, and hence the pulse becomes formicant and vermicular.

§**1217** If pain becomes more and more severe, it makes the pulse sluggish and finally extinct.

12.11.7. The Pulse in (Inflammatory) Swellings

12.11.7.1. General Remarks

§**1218** The formation of certain swellings is associated with fever, either because of their size, or because they affect some vital organ. The pulse varies with the changes induced in the body as a whole by the fever, as we shall explain in its proper place.

§**1219** Afebrile swellings alter the pulse of the member itself from their very nature. The pulse in the rest of the body may be altered secondarily—not because they are swellings, but because they produce pain (and restrict movement. Aeg.).[49]

§**1220** When an inflammatory mass causes a change of the pulse, it does so either according to: (1) the kind of swelling, (2) its phase, (3) its bulk, (4) the organ in which it occurs, (5) its associated effects.

12.11.7.2. The Relations to a Variety of Mass

§**1221** (1) If "hot," the pulse becomes harsh, and coarsely, and then finely thrilling; swifts brisk. (2) If, however, there is an antagonistic humectant agent at work, the pulse ceases to be harsh and becomes undulatory. It is also always tremulous—coarse or fine tremor—and swift and brisk. Not only are there agents which will alter a hard pulse, but there are also agents which make a harsh pulse more decided. (3) If the mass be soft, the pulse is undulatory. (4) If very cold, the pulse becomes slow and sluggish. (5) If hard, the harsh pulse becomes still more harsh.

§1222 When abscess formation comes on, the pulse ceases to be harsh and becomes undulatory. This is because suppuration goes with moisture and softness. The pulse also becomes irregular owing to the weight of the mass, and the rate of brisk ness lessens owing to the fact that heat-formation ceases with maturation of the pus.

12.11.7.3. The Relation Between Phase of Inflammatory Process and Character of Pulse

§1223 The larger the "hot" inflammatory mass becomes, the more harsh does the pulse become. The hardness and tension in the mass increases steadily and as the pain increases, tremor appears in the pulse. At the acme, all the features of the pulse become more marked, except those depending on force; the force of the pulse lessens and the briskness and swiftness increase. If the acme is prolonged, the swiftness lessens and the pulse becomes fornicant. After the swelling subsides, whether by natural processes or by surgical interference, the pulse becomes strong in proportion as the tension in the swelling lessens; and the pulse ceases to be thrilling because the pain ceases with the fall of tension in the tissues.

12.11.7.4. The Relation Between Bulk of Inflammatory Mass and the Pulse

§1224 A large mass denotes marked inflammation; the pulse becomes larger in all respects, and each beat is prolonged. When the mass is only small, the pulse is smaller and more sluggish.

12.11.7.5. The Effect of the Position on the Body

§1225 When the inflammatory process is situate in an organ or tissue rich in sensory nerves, the pulse becomes hard and approaches the "harsh" type. If the organ is rich in blood-vessels, there is an increase in size of the pulse, and in force and it is very irregular. If arteries predominate—as in the spleen and lung—the volume is not maintained unless the force is maintained as well. When it is situate in moist soft members (like the brain and lung) the pulse becomes undulating.

§**1226** Effect of secondary results; of inflammation and inflammatory mass in the lung has a choking effect, and hence the pulse becomes thrilling; in the liver, atrophy is produced and the pulse becomes like that found in wasting diseases; in the kidneys strangury is produced, and there is suppression of urine, which alters the pulse accordingly. In members which are rich in sensory nerves (stomach, diaphragm), the pulse becomes spasmodic and swooning.

12.11.7.6. The Effect of Various Emotional States on the Pulse[50]

12.11.7.6.1. Anger

§**1227** Anger stirs up-the vital power and causes the breath (*ruh*) to expand all at once. Hence the pulse is large, rises high, is swift and brisk. It is not necessarily irregular because the passion does not change—unless there is fear present as well, ill which case anger would prevail at one time, and fear at another. Irregularity may also occur if shame is associated for the intellect warns the person to be silent and not yield to If the same evil as did the person who has excited once to anger.[51]

12.11.7.6.2. Delight

§**1228** Here the movement is gradual and outward. The pulse does not become as speedy and brisk as in the case of anger, but its volume is adequate for the resistance, and therefore the pulse is slow and infrequent.

12.11.7.6.3. Joy

§**1229** Joy. The pulse is similar to the preceding, because usually large in volume, and soft; it becomes slow and infrequent.

12.11.7.6.4. Grief

§**1230** Here the heat is extinguished, or choked, nearly to obliteration, and the vital power is weakened. Hence the pulse is small, weak, sluggish and slow.

12.11.7.6.5. Fear

§1231 If of sudden origin, the pulse becomes quick, irregular, disorderly. If that state is prolonged, or more or less habitual, having begun insidiously, the pulse varies with the varying shades of anxiety.[52]

12.12. A Brief Summary of the Changes Produced by Agents Antagonistic to the Nature of the Pulse

§1232 When the pulse is changed by such agents, it is either: (1) because of an intemperament, and you know the effect of each of these upon the pulse; or (2) by confining the vital power, whereby the pulse becomes irregular. If the restriction be unduly great, the pulse becomes also disorderly and arrhythmic The degree of confinement varies with the amount of morbid material, whether there be an inflammatory mass or not; or (3) by the dispersal of the vital power, whereby the pulse becomes weak. Here belong such agents as: severe pain; affections of the mind which produce a profound loss of vital power; severe or protracted diarrhea.[53]

Lecture 13: The Signs and Symptoms (Diagnosis): Urine and Feces

13.1. Urine

13.1.1. General Remarks About Urine

§1233 The specimen of urine for examination should be collected complying with these conditions: (1) the urine must be passed in the morning.[1] It must not have been kept over from the night before. (2) The person must not have taken either food nor drink before passing it.[2] (3) The previous food must have been free from coloring agents like crocus and cassia fistula (these render the urine a greenish tint), and from salted fish (which renders the urine dark), and from intoxicating wines (which tend to render the color of the urine similar to themselves. (4) The patient should not have been given an agent which expels some humor (a cholagogue or phlegmagogue) by the urine. (5) In regard to physiological state, the patient should not have undertaken severe exercise or toil, or be in a preternatural mental state; for in each case the color of the urine may alter. I.e., fasting, wakefulness (the patient must have slept through the night), toil, anger, dread—for all these cause the urine to become more lemon yellow or redder in tint. Coitus also alters the urine, rendering it oily. Vomiting and defecation alter both color and texture of the urine. The same happens if the urine is kept standing a while. This is why some advise urine not to be left standing more than six hours before examination, for otherwise the significance is altered; the color changes; the sediment goes partly into solution; and the density increases. Personally I think that such changes begin within an hour. (6) The whole of the urine should be collected into one single vessel lest anything should be spilt out of it; one should allow it to settle before scrutinizing it. (7) The urine must be clean. For instance, alkanna will impart its color to the urine; this is a dye used by some people for tinting their skin and finger nails. (8) The vessel used for the specimen must be clean, and the previous sample must have been rinsed out of it. (9) The material of which the vessel is made should be clear, white glass or crystal. (10) The urine must not be exposed to the sun or wind or freezing cold until the sediment has separated out and the various characters have properly developed. The settling is not immediate even if the digestive processes are normal. (11) The sample must be inspected in a light place where the rays do not fall directly upon it, as otherwise the brilliant light would interfere with the colors and give rise to erroneous deductions. (12) The near one holds the sample to the eye, the denser does it appear. The further away it is, the clear does it seem. In this way one can distinguish urine from other fluids brought to the doctor in a falsified state.

§1234 In infants and children, the urine does not give any reliable indication because milk feeding hides the true color and consistency of the urine. The phlegmatic nature of the children also tends to hold the pigments within the body and excretes them in a small quantity. Since children are relatively weak and delicate, their urinary findings could be misleading.

§1235 The first and foremost object of observing the urine is to form an opinion about the state of the liver, the urinary passages and the blood-vessels.[3] The various disorders of these organs are revealed by it. But the most precise information to be obtained is that concerning the functional capacity of the liver.

13.1.2. The Examination of the Urine

§**1236** The points to be noted in the urine are quantity, odor, color, density or texture, transparency, clearness or turbidity, sediment, quantity, odor and foam or froth. Some try to include the feel and taste, too, but that would be both impracticable and undesirable. By color, it is meant the various shades of color perceived by the ordinary vision, i.e., whiteness, darkness and the intermediate shades. Density or texture refers to the coarseness or fineness of the urine. By transparency, clearness or turbidity we refer to ease or otherwise with which light traverses it (translucence). Turbid urine may be due to the suspension of particles of dark or some other color. There is a difference between texture and translucence for a urine may be coarse and yet as clear as egg-white or liquid fish-glue; and a rarefied urine may be turbid (as turbid water is more rarefied than white of egg). Transparency is the opposite of turbidity. Turbidity depends on the presence of certain variously colored particles—opaque or dark or tinted with other colors which are imperceptible to the sense of sight and yet are impervious. Sediment differs from turbidity in that the particles are readily visible to the eye, whereas particles cannot really be distinguished in the case of turbidity. Sediment appears immediately after the passage of the urine; turbidity does not clear up on standing. Turbidity differs from coloration in that the latter pervades the whole substance of the urine whereas turbidity is less intimately admixed.

13.1.2.1. The Significance of the Color of Urine

13.1.2.1.1. The Degrees of Yellowness

§**1237** The degrees of yellowness include: (1) straw-yellow; (2) lemon-yellow; (3) orange-yellow; (4) flame-yellow or saffron-yellow; that is a very deep yellow; (5) clear reddish-yellow. All except the first two denote a hot intemperament in degrees varying with the amount of exercise, pain, fasting and abstinence from water. The fourth variety denotes predominance of the bilious humor.[4]

13.1.2.1.2. The Degrees of Redness

§1238 The degrees of redness include: (1) rose-red or roseate; (2) very dark red; (3) purple red, which has a brilliance about it like a certain rose; (4) smoky red or dull red. All these denote dominance of the sanguineous humor, for dullness of color points that way. A flame-yellow shows the presence of more "heat" than dull red because it shows there is bilious humor in it, and this is hotter than sanguineous humor.

§1239 The urine tends to saffron-yellow and flame-yellow in acute maladies described as "burning"; but if the urine is at all inclined to be clear, it shows a certain degree of "digestion," namely that this process has actually begun, but its products have not yet appeared in the substance of the urine.

§1240 Deepening of color from lemon-yellowness towards a flame-yellow shade shows that the innate heat is steadily increasing. The color then ceases to be yellow, and attains a pure, clear red. If the urine now begins to clarify it shows that the (pathological) heat is beginning to subside.

§1241 In acute diseases of a hemorrhagic character, the urine may be tinged with blood without any evident rupture of blood vessels having occurred. This would indicate an excessive amount of plethora. A gradual loss of blood by the urine, associated with a bad odor, is a sign to be dreaded because it informs us that there is hemorrhage proceeding from congested parts. The prognosis is still worse if the urine is offensive in odor.

§1242 Admixture of the urine with blood may be a good for fevers, because it shows that the crisis is about to take place, and recovery will follow. The only exception is if the urine becomes suddenly transparent (its color becoming normal, i.e.) before the crisis is due. Such a phenomenon would be a forerunner of a relapse. Thin urine appearing before the crisis may be equally unfavorable unless the change has been gradual and progressive.

§1243 If the urine becomes of a deeper red until it is nearly black in jaundice, and its stain on linen can no longer be removed, it is a good sign; the better, the deeper the red. But if the urine becomes white or slightly reddish, and the jaundice is not subsiding, the advent of dropsy is to be feared. Fasting is among the conditions which render the urine high-colored and of marked acridity.

13.1.2.1.3. The Degrees of Greenness

§1244 The degrees of green color include: (1) a color approaching that of pistachios; (2) the color of verdigris; (3) rainbow green; (4) emerald green; (5) leek-green. The first denotes a cold intemperament, as do all things the shade of whose green is not (2) or (5). These (2, 5) denote extreme combustion, but (5) is not as unhealthy as (2). If it should be met with after physical labor it denotes "spasm." A green colored urine in adolescence points to the same condition.

§1245 Rainbow green usually denotes an extremely cold intemperament. In this respect, some say it shows: that poison was present in the fluid taken as drink, and that if there be a sediment present there is a hope of recovery; if no sediment, death is likely to take place. Verdigris green-color of urine forewarns of death (destruction of innate heat).

13.1.2.1.4. The Degrees of Blackness

§1246 The degrees of blackness include: (1) dark urine approaching blackness, through a saffron color. This occurs in' jaundice, for instance. It denotes (i) denseness and oxidation of the bilious humor; (ii) atrabilious humor derived from bilious humor; (iii) jaundice. (2) Deep-brown-black. This shows the presence of sanguineous atrabilious humor. (3) Greenish-black. This shows the dominance of pure atrabilious humor.

§1247 Speaking generally, dark or black urine denotes: (1) extreme oxidation; (2) great cold; (3) extinction of the innate heat (i.e. death); (4) crisis; (5) evacuation whereby the effete substances from the atrabilious humor are expelled.

§1248 The details about each of these are: (1) dark urine due to extreme oxidation is recognized by its causing scalding, and being previously yellow or red. The sediment is discrete (not coherent), not homogeneous, discontinuous, not very dark, but tending to a saffron, lemon-yellow, or dark brown. If the color of the sediment tends to be lemon-yellow, it strongly suggests jaundice. (2) When darkness of the urine is due to great cold, the urine would previously be tending to a green tint or a livid tint. The sediment is here slightly coherent, and looks dry, and is more purely black in color. If a dark urine is also very offensive, it shows that the temperament is hot. If it be odorless, or has only a slight odor, it shows that the temperament is cold. This is because no odor emanates from urine unless the innate heat overrules the cold. (3) When darkness of urine is due to extinction of the innate heat this is recognized by the dispersion of vitality. (4) When the darkness arises from a critical charge in a fever ("critical polyuria") one of the following conditions may be supposed: the termination of a quartan fever; the resolutions of a splenic disease; the termination of a fever associated with the atrabilious humor; the termination of a fever prevailing by night and by day; subsidence of pains in the back and womb; retained menses; retained blood in a case of piles—both the latter two occurring especially when nature is assisted by art. It occurs in women in whom the menses are retained, because the effete matters of the blood cannot be disposed of by nature. This is shown in the urine by its being watery previously. When the effete matters are anally discharged from the body, the urine is the same time becomes very abundant.

§**1249** Prognosis: if at the critical periods the urine does not become dark, it is an ominous sign, especially in acute disease the more so if at the same time: (1) the quantity of urine be small (for scanty urine is evidence that the humor has already become destroyed by oxidation); (2) the sediment be coarse-textured the coarser, the more depraved; the finer, the less. Dark urine is a good sign in acute diseases.

§**1250** If the urine is limpid as well as dark, and a deposit is left suspended in it at different layers, this denotes cephalalgia, waked fullness, deafness, mental confusion. If the urine is secreted only by drops, and a sediment forms slowly, and the odor is less pungent, and there is fever—all this would be strong evidence of the above. But when. there is wakefulness, deafness, delirium and headache such urine would show that epistaxis is pending.

§**1251** Dark or dull red urine, which is passed after drinking wine of that color or after taking certain medicines, need cause no alarm. The wine has simply passed unchanged through the body. Dark urine may be evidence of renal calculus. As Rufus says, "black urine is good in infirmities of the kidneys and inky if stone in the bladder, and also in maniacal cases, for they are diseases proceeding from gross humors. But it is a grave sign in acute diseases." On the other hand, he says that black urine is a bad sign in diseases of the kidneys and bladder if at the same time it is extremely scalding. Therefore one must take all such signs into consideration. When dark urine occurs in aged persons, it is not a good sign because in such persons, as you know, it can only denote great destruction of tissue. In puerperal women, the appearance of dark urine is premonitory in convulsions.

§**1252** In brief, the appearance of dark urine is serious at the onset of fevers, as well as at their close, if there is neither crisis nor any abatement of symptoms at the same time.

13.1.2.1.5. Whiteness

§**1253** The word "whiteness" is applied in two ways: mere translucence, as the laity calls anything which is translucent "white." Thus, clear glass, clear crystal, are white. Translucence implies absence of all color. Such urine is "thin" and translucent. Secondly, there is true whiteness, like that of milk or parchment. Such urine is not translucent.

§**1254** Whiteness in the first sense shows that the intemperament is altogether a cold one, and that digestion is good. If the urine be at the same time coarse, it shows that the serous humor is abundant. A urine which is white in the second sense is necessarily coarse.

§**1255** Variety of whiteness: the significance of mucilanginous is an excess of serous humor and crude humor. The significance of wax-like urine is liquefaction of adipose tissue; of greasy, soapy whiteness, liquefaction of serious humor or it may denote diabetes, active or latent. Musty whiteness tinted with blood and pus signifies ulcers discharging into the urinary passages. Musty whiteness not tinted with blood signifies great excess of crude non-matured matter; vesical calculus. Semen-like critical in form signifies a crisis in an inflammation arising in serous humor while not critical in form and no inflammation signifies apoplexy and palsy and continuous semen-like urine throughout a fever signifies the fever will soon become quartan. The significance of lead-white urine with no sediment is bad while milk-white urine in acute diseases is ominous. Previously colored in acute fevers signifies that bilious humor has descended to some member about to develop an inflammation (for example the abdomen or which is worse, the head. A sudden change from red to white urine in the course of a fever signifies the patient will become delirious. Whiteness persisting in a person apparently healthy signifies absence of digestion especially in the venous system and in diabetes. Whiteness like buttermilk in acute fevers signifies fatal issue or wasting.[5]

§1256 When the intemperament is hot because of the dominance of the bilious humor, the urine may appear white (contrary to expectation). When the intemperament is cold because of dominance of the serous humor, the urine may appear red [contrary to expectation]. If the bilious humor passes down the urinary passages without being admixed with the urine, the latter remains white. Therefore, it is necessary to study white urine with care. For, if its color were brilliant, and if the deposit is plentiful and coarse, and the urine itself is rather thick, it shows that the whiteness arises from a cold intemperament, with predominance of the serous humor. Again, if the urine be not clear and bright, and there is not much deposit, and if the whiteness tends to a brownish tint, it shows that there is bilious humor concealed therein. Whiteness in the course of an acute disease, the signs of recovery being present, with no fear of maniacal delirium, and the like, indicates that the bilious humor has passed out by some other channels such as the intestine, causing constipation.[6]

§1257 If urine is red in the course of “cold” maladies it means one of four things (1) that there is severe pain which disperses the bilious humor (i.e., colic without the signs off inflammation); (2) there is so much serous humor in the bile ducts as to give rise to obstruction there, and the bilious humor is in consequence diverted from the intestine into the urinary passages. (3) hieratic insufficiency, especially in regard to separating off water from the blood, as occurs in coldly dropsy. The urine comes to look like the washing of raw meat. (4) Some form of putrefactive process in the veins subsequent to obstruction in the ducts; here the serous humor in they vessels undergoes a change of color. The urine is rendered watery, and the sediment is of a kind already described faint in color, and not refulgent. The presence of bilious humor renders a color refulgent (i.e. dichroic).

§1258 Urine is often white at the onset of a disease, and becomes dark and offensive in odor later. So it is in jaundice.

§1259 Urine becomes white after a meal, and remains so until digestion is nearly completed. It then begins to assume color.

§1260 During the waking state, the urine is white—partly because of dispersal of the innate heat, but it is not refulgent. It tends to be dusky if there is an associated defective digestion.

§1261 Prognosis: a red color is better than a watery-white one, in the case of acute diseases. But a white color is better if intrinsic—not due to wateriness.

§1262 Redness due to blood is not as dangerous as redness due to bilious humor. Redness from bilious humor is not as serious if the bilious humor is quiescent; it is very ominous if it begins to move about.

§1263 Red urine is very bad in the case of renal disease because it is a sign that there is a "hot" inflammatory process there. If it occurs in diseases associated with intense headache, it portends delirium.

§1264 When a urine begins to turn red in an acute disease, and stays so, without forming a sediments, it is an ominous sign because it points to an inflammatory swelling in the kidneys. If such urine becomes turbid, and stays so, it points to an inflammatory mass in the liver, with lack of innate heat.[7]

§1265 So much for the simple colors of the urine.

13.1.3. The Compound Colors of Urine

13.1.3.1. Like Raw Meat Washings (Blood Stained)

§1266 Urine the color of raw meat washings means hepatic insufficiency due to plethora of blood or to any form of intemperament, resulting in deficient digestive power and dispersal of the vitality. Were the vital power adequate, it would show that there is plenty of blood, even to great excess; and in such a case, the secretory power would be hardly adequate for dealing with it.

13.1.3.2. Oleaginous Oily

§1267 Oleaginous oily indicates that the fat of the body is being destroyed. The appearance is like a lemon-yellow tinged with the greenness of the mistletoe growing on larches. It is called oleaginous because it is viscid and translucent, and also has the luster of fat, and shows a certain brilliance or refulgence in spite of a certain opacity. It is not a good sign in many states, not to say it is bad. For it shows there is neither maturation, nor a change for the better. In rare cases it indicates the critical evacuation of unctuous matter, but for it to mean this alleviation must follow. If such urine be also fetid and scanty in amount, it is a very ominous sign. It is also serious if it be admixed with material like meat washings, as might happen in the course of dropsy, phthisis, and intestinal obstruction.

§1268 If oleaginous urine replaces a black urine, it is a good sign. But if such a urine appear on the fourth day of an acute disease it forewarns of the patient's death on the seventh day.

§1269 In brief, there are three kinds of oleaginous urine: (1) all fat, throughout; (2) fat only in the lower part; (3) fat in the upper layers. The first is oleaginous only in "color"; it occurs in phthisis, hectic fever, and wasting diseases, especially at their outset. The second is oleaginous only in "substance." The third is oily in both respects, that is, in diseases of the kidney, at the acme and termination of phthisis.

13.1.3.3. Purple (Black)

§**1270** This is a very bad sign. It means oxidation of both bilious and atrabilious humor.

13.1.3.4 Ruddy Color Mixed with a Tinge of Blackness

§**1271** This occurs in composite fevers and in fevers arising from gross superfluities. If it clarifies, and the darkness settles down from the surface, it denotes an inflammatory mass in the lung.

13.1.4. The Signs Afforded by the Density, Quality, Clearness or Turbidity of the Urine

§**1272** Urine may be transparent or opaque, or intermediate in density.[8]

13.1.4.1. Transparent (Limpid) Urine

§**1273** Whatever be the state, a urine of limpid consistence denotes: (1) deficient digestion (lack of maturation); (2) venous congestion; (3) renal insufficiency (for the kidneys only separate out fine matter, or if they attract other matter, they fail to discharge it until it has been rarefied or rendered capable of excretion; (4) excessive fluid-intake; (5) a very cold or a dry intemperament.

§**1274** When it occurs in the course of an acute illness, it denotes deficient digestive power, and inability to complete digestion (absence of maturation). It may indicate that the weakness of the other drives is so marked that they cannot influence water at all, and hence it passes through the body unchanged.

§**1275** Prognosis: it is worse for urine to be very transparent at puberty than in adolescence, because during the former period of life urine is naturally more opaque than in adolescence. Being more moist in their temperament, their bodies attract moisture more readily, and, in addition, moisture is essential for their growth. Therefore, if acute fevers arise during the age of puberty, the urine is decidedly abnormal if it is transparent. Should it continue of that character, it would be a very ominous sign. Should it continue and favorable symptoms should not appear, and should the vitality not be maintained, it would be a sign that an abscess is forming below the liver.

§1276 If urine continue to be transparent for a long time without any variation in a person otherwise healthy, should he experience pain one will know that an inflammatory mass is forming in the situation of the pain. The pain is usually lumbar when the urine is of this character, and that is the usual site for an abscess.

§1277 If there is no localized pain in such a case, but a general pain and heaviness, this points to the widespread formation of small pustules.

§1278 If the urine is transparent at the crisis of an illness, contrary to rule, it forewarns of a relapse.

13.1.4.2.Opaque (Thick) Urine

§1279 If the urine is very opaque, it shows that maturation has failed to take place; or, more rarely, it denotes the maturation of "gross" humors, such as occur at the height (status) of humoral fevers, or after the opening of abscesses. In acute fears, the appearance of opaque urine is usually a bad sign though not as bad as a persistently transparent urine. The fact that urine is opaque shows that there is a certain degree of digestion proceeding, because digestion adds to the opacity of urine to a certain extent, and shows that there is some power of expulsion (of effete matter). But it is a bad sign in so far as it denotes the breakdown of, and abundance of, humors, and that the evacuation of the separated materials is hindered.

§1280 To ascertain which of the two is dominant, notice whether improvement or increased weakness follows.

§1281 Prognosis: When opaque urine is passed in the course of fevers, it is a less serious sign if it be poured out quickly and plentifully. When excreted slowly it denotes a redundance of the humors and an enfeebled vitality. A sign which is still less serious is that a urine of medium density should go with a simultaneous improvement in the general condition.[9]

§1282 When the urine is transparent in an acute illness, and then becomes thick, and there is no improvement in the condition of the patient, it denotes colliquation [of tissues].

§**1283** Persistent opacity of urine in a presumably healthy person forewarns of fever should headache and mental confusion arise. Opaque urine also occurs after excessive evacuations, after the opening of an abscess, growing to ulcers in the urinary passages. Transparent and opaque urine cannot both denote lack of digestion (maturation) unless there is an intermediate degree of density associated with the maturation. Dense substances are rendered thin or limpid by the process of digestion, and the urine changes from transparency to opacity.

13.1.4.3. Clearness and Turbidity

§**1284** Thick urine, as has been already stated, is sometimes clear and translucent, sometimes turbid and opaque; and yet there is a marked difference between thick and limpid translucent urine. When the former is shaken, it does not easily break up into little portions—it only forms large portions and the particles move slowly and if it makes a foam, its foam is composed of numerous bubbles which do not coalesce for a long time. Such a urine is the outcome of an adequate digestion of the serous humor, or of the vitelline bilious humor (if there be any tint suggestive of yellowness in it). The last-named variety is often found in the urine of epileptics.

§**1285** But a well-colored transparent urine owes its color not to digestion but to admixture with: bilious humor. For otherwise digestion would be supposed to affect only the "substance" until a mixture of colors had been brought about, whereas the process of digestion effects a change of "substance" first, and of color secondarily. Digestion concerns "substance," not "color." Hence if a transparent urine is yellow, and there is no abatement of the acute illness, that is a bad sign, for it shows the digestive faculties are dormant!

§**1286** The appearance of alternating redness and yellowness in a limpid urine points to inflammatory changes dependent on toil. If it be limpid and shows scale-like objects in it, and if the bladder is healthy, that is a sign of oxidation of the serous humor.

§**1287** In brief, a thick urine in acute febrile states may denote predominance of various humors, and at the same time point to colliquatiste processes (in the body). Should such processes persist during the whole phase of a disease, the urine would become more opaque (denser, thicker).

§**1288** Lastly, turbid urine denotes earthiness as well as the presence of Has and wateriness. For when these qualities are combined, turbidity is the result. When they are separated again, the urine becomes clear.

13.1.4.4. Three States to Note

§**1289** The following three states should be noted: (1) the urine is clear at the time of passing, and then becomes opaque. This shows that maturation is difficult; that the matter of the food has not yet succumbed to the vegetative powers ("nature"). It may denote colliquation in the tissues. (2) The urine is opaque when passed, but then becomes clear. The coarse matters settle and separate out. This shows that the vegetative powers ("nature") have already overcome the material of the food and matured it. The clearer it grows, the greater the amount of sediment, and the more rapidly the sediment falls, the more complete is the digestion. (3) A state between the above two. In this case the vegetative powers improve, as long as the vitality is maintained. It shows that maturation is not progressing to completion. But if the vitality is not maintained, it would mean that the maturative processes are not likely to reach completion. Should this condition persist a long time without the feared symptoms of loss of vitality appearing, then it is likely that headache will develop, for it shows that there is much gas formation.[10]

§**1290** It is a better sign for a clear urine to become turbid than for it to remain turbid for several hours after being passed. Urine may become turbid because of loss of vitality, apart from expulsion of "the nature."

§**1291** It urine is watery when voided, and remains so, it shows that digestion has entirely ceased.

13.1.4.5. Good Signs

§**1292** (1) Opaque urine easily voided, whose sediment falls easily when occurring in palsy, etc. (2) Urine opaque when voided belt then becoming transparent and plentiful. (3) Limpid plentiful urine following upon thick turbid urine or thick and scanty urine. (4) Opaque turbid urine passed at a slow rate, and then becoming suddenly abundant and easy to void. This means that recovery is about to take place, whether it be an acute fever or any other plethoric disorder, or plethora about to manifest as actual disease, but this kind of urine is rarely met with.

§**1293** If the urine is of natural color, and its opacity be great, it is evident that much effete matter is passing through, and that there is no hindrance to their outflow. But it is usually a bad sign because it shows that the humors are superabundant and the vitality deficient. Such a urine is scanty and difficult to void.

§**1294** Opaque urine is a good sign if it occurs at the crisis in splenic diseases and "minced" fevers, in which the emunctory powers cannot come into play, or equipoise be restored.

§**1295** Lastly, turbid urine denotes that the humors are overabundant and that the vegetative powers are inadequate for their digestion.

§**1296** Diagnostic points. Opaque urine, with a sandy sediment, denotes calculus. Opaque urine, with pus, a bad odor, and scaly particles separating out, denotes rupture of an abscess. A thick urine, with the clinical evidences of an inflammatory mass or of an ulcer in the bladder, kidney, liver or chest, shows that there is an abscess about to burst.

§**1297** If the urine prior to that were like the washings of raw meat, it would show that there is unhealthy blood flowing from the liver, and if the feces were also similar, it would show there is an inflammatory mass in the interior of the liver. If prior to this there was shortness of breath, with a dry cough, and a stabbing pain in the chest, then one knows that an abscess has ruptured which arose in the chest or around the aorta. If the pus is "mature," it is satisfactory.

§**1298** Discharge of urine resembling pus may benefit a person who takes no exercise and lives in an unhygenic manner. It clears the whole body, and removes the laxity resulting from the lack of exercise. It may be that there are obstructions in the liver and adnexa, and when the obstructions are removed, the urine which is voided is dense owing to the matter which passes out with it. Such "matter" is not "pus." It is only pus if it appears in the urine after the bursting of an abscess; the urine is then not only thick but dark. If at this time there be pain in the left side, then one knows that the abscess was in the spleen. If the pain is in the upper part of the abdomen, one knows the abscess was in the stomach. The usual site for the abscess is in the liver and in the urinary organs.

§1299 Turbid urine often denotes loss of vitality; coldness dominates in the temperament as much as if the whole body were exposed to external cold.

§1300 Turbid urine of the appearance of poor wine, or of chickpea water, may occur during pregnancy, and may be met with in persons with long standing internal "hot" inflammatory masses.

§1301 Urine which has the extremely turbid appearance of asses' urine or the urine of other cattle, arises from the very marked agitation which is going on in the humors, especially the serous humor, a certain amount of heat coming into play so as to set up that agitation. Hence this kind of urine is a forerunner of headache or [coryzal] catarrh in the head. If it persists, it forewarns of lethargia.

§1302 If the urine resembles the color of some member for some time, it forewarns that disease is about to arise there.

§1303 Some say that if the lower layers of the urine have a powdery or nebulous appearance, it means that the illness will be of long duration; and that if it persists throughout the whole illness, it presages death, or the formation of "crude" serous humor, which is distinguished from pus by its fetor.

§1304 If the urine separates into several layers, the more there are the stronger is the natural faculty and the more open are the pores.

§1305 Threads floating in the urine denote that it was passed immediately after completing coitus.

13.1.5. The Signs Derived from the Odor of the Urine

§1306 Some people assert that no sick person ever passes a urine which has a healthy odor. But we say that if the urine is quite odorless, it denotes: (1) a cold intemperament; (2) excessive "crudity"; (3) extinction of the innate heat in the case of acute diseases.

13.1.5.1. Fedid Odor

§1307 A fetid odor, with signs of maturation in the urine indicates ulcers in the urinary passages, or "scabies." These are identified from their own signs. If with the fetid odor, there are no signs of maturation, the cause of the odor may the merely putrefaction.

§1308 In acute fevers, without disease in the urinary organs, such a urine is a bad sign. If it is present in acute fevers, and there is a tendency to acridity, it denotes putrefaction in humors which are of a cold nature, when there is a predominance of the extraneous heat.

§1309 If such a urine appears in acute diseases, it forewarns of death by extinction of the innate heat and predominance of the extraneous cold.

13.1.5.2. Sweetish Odor

§1310 This denotes predominance of the sanguineous humor. If also very fetid, it denotes predominance of the bilious humor.

13.1.5.3. Putrid Odor

§1311 If the putrid odor tends to sourness, it shows predominance of the atrabilious humor. An extremely fetid odor of the urine which continues in spite of seeming health denotes: (1) that a fever arising from putrefaction is coming on; (2) expulsion of retained putrescent matters. The latter will show whether the case may be expected to recover. If a fetid urine appears in an acute illness, and then suddenly ceases to be fetid, without subsidence of the symptoms, it shows a destruction of vitality.[11]

13.1.6. The Indications Afforded by the Foam on Urine

§1312 Foam arises from the moisture and the gases forced into the urine as it is passed into the urinal. The vapor which leaves the body with the urine doubtless adds to the consistency of the urine, especially if gases predominate in it, as occurs in cases of obstructions. The urine then shows many bubbles.

§1313 One notices the following points in regard to the foam: (1) color: it is dark or reddish in jaundice; (2) size of bubbles: large ones indicate viscidity; (3) number of bubbles: if numerous, it denotes viscidity and much gas; (4) rate of bursting of the bubbles: if slow, it indicates viscidity and coarse glutinous humor.

§1314 Prognosis: therefore, if small bubbles persist in a specimen, in cases of kidney disease, it shows that the illness will be of long duration. In brief, viscous humors in the course of kidney diseases are of bad omen; they show that the humors are depraved and cold in temperament. The significance of small bubbles has already been stated.

13.1.7. The Indications Derived from the Diverse Kinds of Sediment

§1315 Definition: in the first place one must specify the meaning of the term "sediments." It is not "that which sinks to the bottom of the vessel." It is "that whole substance (denser in essence than wateriness)" which separates out from the wateriness regardless of whether it settles down or not, floats or not, sinks or not.

§1316 Therefore we may say that there are various characters pertaining to the sediment its "structure,"; its quantity and quality; the arrangement of its components; its position; duration; and mode of permixture.

13.1.8. Structure

13.1.8.1. Natural Sediments

§1317 A sediment is natural, laudable, evidence of normal digestion and maturation when it is white, sinks to the bottom of the vessel, and its particles are in continuity [i.e. not discrete], uniform, and all alike. In contour it is rounded. It is light, homogeneous, delicate, like the deposit which forms in rose water.

§1318 Its relation to the maturation of the various matters of the whole body is comparable to that to the maturation of pus. But whereas it is white, light, and of homogeneous nature and delicate in the former, in the case of pus it is coarse.

§1319 A sediment betokens good digestion even though devoid of color anal homogeneity.[12] But ancient physicians considered that homogeneity was a more important test than color. A homogeneous deposit even though not altogether white, or even if reddish in tint is a better sign than a deposit which is white but not homogeneous, and composed of coarse particles. The sediment may or may not assume the same color as the urine. If it does not, it is better that it should be white, next best red, then lemon-yellow or saffron-yellow, and the least good is that it should be like arsenicum in color or of a color like that of lentils.

§1320 However, I counsel you not to regard what others say. I say that—whiteness does not necessarily have a relation to the state of digestion; homogeneity is always related to the (efficiency of) maturation. A thorough mingling of gaseous constituents will produce a white effect.

§1321 If a sediment presents an unhealthy appearance, it is more favorable that it should be discrete than continuous.

§1322 Good sediments resemble pus and crude serous humor when they are tenuous. But pus is different in possessing fetid, while crude serous humor is different in rendering the deposit compact and not homogeneous. A good sediment differs from both because it is finely textured and light.

§1323 One would not expect to find such a deposit in a person who is healthy; it occurs in a sick person, because matters are kept back in his blood vessels, and they undergo putrefactive breakdown, if they cannot be subjected to maturation. In health, the blood need not necessarily contain a humor which ought to a be removed, but if there were such a humor present, it would be better if it were disposed of by way of the feces (the indigestible excess in the aliments) than if it emerge by way of they urine as a sediment whether such humor have undergone maturation or not.

§1324 In thin persons, the sediment of the urine is scanty and it sinks down differently according to the state of health, especially if the persons are accustomed to exercise or to practice laborious arts.

§1325 The sediment is abundant only in obese persons and in those is of bad habits.

§1326 Therefore one does not expect to find as much sediment in sick persons who are lean as in those who are stout. For disease in the former often resolves without any sediment forming at all. At most there maybe a tiny particle floating or swimming at in it. In other cases the sediment falls immediately after micturition unless there is good maturation in which case it very little deposit is to be expected.

13.1.8.2. Abnormal Sediments

§1327 Varieties include: (1) flaky or squamous; (2) fleshy; (3) fatty; (4) mucoid or slimy; (5) purulent (ichorous); (6) hair-like; (7) resembling pieces of yeast infused in water; (8) sandy or gritty; (9) cinerital; (10) hirudiniform.

13.1.8.2.1. Flaky or Squamous Sediment

§1328 Flaky or squamous is composed of large red or large white particles. They are usually supposed to come from the urinary organs. If white, they come from the bladder (ulceration, desquamation, erosions). If red or fleshy, they come from the kidney. If brown or dark colored or like the scales of fishes, they are a very bad sign, worse than all types we have named. They suggest the shedding of mucous linings. Particles[13] from the bladder or kidneys may not be of moment. In fact, if vesical, they are a sign of recovery. Some say that cantharides causes white flakes to appear, which are like the membrane within eggs. These dissolve when the specimen is shaken and impart a reddish tint to the urine. This would be evidence of healing and recovery.

§1329 Another form resembles the scrapings from intestines; the particles being less broad and of dense consistency. If reddish colored, it is called orobeal [or tare like or grumous] sediment; otherwise it is called furfuraceous. The former recalls the appearance of decorticated orobs [*ervum ervilia*], and are reddish; this indicates the presence of oxidized particles[13] which are derived from: (1) the liver; (2) the kidney; or (3) blood. When they come from the kidney, the particles are more continuous and fleshy, whereas in the other cases they are more friable. When the color is decidedly yellowish one knows that they are of renal origin; if dusky red, that they are of hepatic origin. However, sometimes particles of hepatic origin may resemble those of renal origin.

§1330 Another form, more strictly scaly, consists of small bodies like the husks or hulls of grain. Such a sediment denotes: (1) bladder trouble, or (2) grave colliquative disorder of the system as a whole. We diagnose (a) bladder trouble if: (i) there is itching at the root of the penis; (ii) the urine is fetid; especially if (iii) pus is passed first. Such a state is more probable if (b) there is other evidence of maturation in the urine; (c) if the veins over the bladder are healthy; and there is no macula there. We diagnose (d) liquefaction of humor if there is fever; weakness; difficulty of micturition; and the sediment is brownish in color.

§1331 Yet another form in which the deposit is like coarse particles of barley flour may mean one of four things: (i) oxidation of the sanguineous humor if there is a tendency to redness; (ii) colliquative changes in the membranes and their components—if it be white; (iii) local bladder disease—in a few cases. The difference between this and the others is readily made out from that which has already been said; (iv) oxidation of the blood, especially in the spleen. Here the color tends to be black.

§1332 Squamous deposits other than those of vesical or renal and urethral origin, occurring in acute diseases, have the gravest significance.

13.1.8.2.2. Fleshy Sediment

§1333 These, as you already know, are usually of renal origin. They are not so if the flesh is healthy and there is no breakdown in the body. If the evidences of complete digestion are present in the urine, it shows that the blood vessels are healthy. The urine can show evidence of maturation even if the kidneys are diseased, seeing that this process begins “above” the kidneys.

13.1.8.2.3. Fatty Sediment

§**1334** This, like the preceding, denotes colliquative processes in the body. It is more serious if it resembles "gold water" in appearance. There are two chief types—either it is abundant and discrete (this being derived from renal fat); or scanty and admixed (this being derived from the fat of a more distant place). There is no fever, in the former case.

§**1335** A white particle like a pomegranate seed may be seen in the urine. This will be derived from renal fat. It denotes that a sanious ulcer has formed, especially in the urethra, especially if the sediment sinks promptly.

13.1.8.2.4. Mutoid Sediment

§**1336** This denotes an unnatural humor which is too plentiful within the body and passes out either by it the urinary tract, or a critical hip gout, or joint pains. The distinction between them is made by the symptoms—whether they abate or not. A dense humor may become rarefied and tenuous, and a laudable sediment results. Therefore, in the course of acute disease, one must not depend on a laudable sediment appearing before the time when maturation of the disease is due, or before its signs have appeared. It may denote that there is a very cold intemperament of the kidneys, very mucoid and abundant sediment appearing at the end of an attack of gout or arthritis, is a good sign.

13.1.8.2.5. Ichorous Sediment

§**1337** This differs from a crude sediment in being fetid. It is preceded by the evidences of abscess. Its particles easily aggregate and separate again. It may be very thoroughly mingled with water; it may separate out quickly from the water. A crude sediment, however, is both turbid and thick. It does not readily aggregate, nor separate easily. The urine is not fetid. The signs of abscess do not precede.

13.1.8.2.6. Hair-like Sediment

§**1338** This is produced by the coagulation of any internal humor which has been exposed to the innate heat on its way from the kidney to the bladder. It is sometimes white, sometimes red. It clots in the kidney. The clots may be as long as the palm of the hand.

§**1339** A sediment having the appearance of yeast soaked in water is evidence of gastric and intestinal weakness and of depraved digestion (often due to milk and cheese having been taken).

13.1.8.2.7. Sandy or Gritty Sediment (Gravel)

§**1340** This is always a sign of calculus whether in process of formation or actually formed, or in process of solution. If red colored, it shows it comes from the kidneys; if white, it shows the origin is in the bladder. A gritty sediment, where there are large particles like those of ground grain, is a bad sign in fevers.

13.1.8.2.8. Cinerital Sediment

§**1341** This is a sign that serous humor or pus has altered in color through long stagnation and breaking up of its particles. It may be that it is due to having undergone oxidation.

13.1.8.2.9. Hirudiniform

§**1342** The sediment is of the appearance and color of leeches. If well mingled with the urine, this denotes hepatic insufficiency. If less closely intermingled with the urine it denotes a trauma in the urinary passages which breaks their continuity. If discrete, it shows that the lesion is in the bladder or in the penis. This subject is carefully dealt with in the third volume, under the heading of "haematuria."

§**1343** The appearance of bodies like red leeches in the urine, associated with evidences of disease in the spleen, denotes a destructive disease in that organ. (It would seem that strings of blood clot are here referred to, in which case nowadays we should think of a villous humor in the bladder. Tr.)

§**1344** Note, that in diseases of the bladder, there is generally not much bleeding because the blood vessels are few in number, are slender, and are deeply situated in its wall.

13.1.9. The Quantity of Sediment

§**1345** According as the sediment is abundant or scanty, the degree of the efficient cause is great or small. This has been explained under the previous heading. (It is more abundant in gross living persons than in those who are temperate. It is less abundant in active persons than in those leading a sedentary life. Therefore, it is liable to be more abundant in females than males, children than adults.)

13.1.10. The Quality of Sediment, Color, Odor

13.1.10.1. Black Color

§1346 This is a bad sign, but it is not so bad if the supernatural fluid is not black. (Haly Abbas says it is a fatal sign if it comes on after being intensely red).

13.1.10.2. Red Color

§1347 This shows dominance of sanguineous humor (sanguineous plethora); it occurs in fasting; and when digestion is imperfect. If it continues to be present for a long time it denotes inflammation of the liver.

13.1.10.3. Yellow Color

§1348 This denotes great heat, because it is produced by bilious humor. It may also show an insidious disease.

13.1.10.4. Green Color

§1349 This has the same significance as black sediment.

13.1.10.5. White Color

§1350 This is sometimes good, sometimes bad. That is, when it is mucoid, ichorous, or foamy, because this shows that the urine is not a completed secretion.

13.1.10.6. Odor

§1351 The indications from the odor have already been given in describing the other characteristics.

13.1.11. The Constitution, Coherence and Consistency of Particles

§1352 Softness and homogeneity of the sediment which is otherwise laudable is more healthy than when met with in a urine otherwise not laudable Discreteness of particles points to flatulence and impaired digestion.

13.1.12. Position

§1353 A laudable sediment may swim like a cloud or nubecula may float on the surface; or be suspended in the middle layers (which shows that maturation has proceeded further than in the first variety.) If it is rugose or fimbriate and tends to sink, it is better; if it sinks to the bottom it is a sign of still more advanced maturation.

§1354 When the sediment is not laudable, it is more satisfactory when it is light and rises to the upper layers; or, if in the course of an acute fever, it is black; when the humor is serous or atrabilious, it is more satisfactory when it is like a cloud than for it to sink to the bottom; the fact of its being like a cloud shows it is tenuous, unless by chance gas is making it rise.

§1355 If the sediment sinks below the surface, but not right to the bottom, it is more satisfactory. It is heat which makes it rise or float or it is gas which carries it upwards.

§1356 If a sediment made of coarse discrete particles should float, it shows it is light. A fine sediment, especially if heavy, will sink lower.

§1357 If the sediment remains suspended as a nubecula right through an illness from its beginning, it shows that crisis will come with suppuration.

§1358 A nubecula or suspended sediment may never appear in an illness if the person be slender, as we have stated.

§1359 A sediment which is between a cloud and an enaeorema—made of particles suspended or floating in the middle layers like a spider's web is an ominous sign. (Such particles may appear like the specks of oil which one sees in cooled broth; or like hairs.) But even a nubecula may be an anxiety, though it be the beginning of a change for the better. It sinks to the middle layers and ultimately to the bottom. In that case it is not a bad sign. But if a "bad" sediment appears after this, it is certainly ominous.

13.1.13. Time Occupied in Sedimentation

§1360 If the sediment settles rapidly, it is a good sign, showing that maturation is correct. If it settles slowly, it is not good, for it shows deficient or absent maturation, according to its amount.

13.1.14. The Form

§1361 The significance of this has been described in making mention of passing blood and fat with the urine.

13.1.15. The Signs Relative to the Daily Quantity of Urine

§1362 Generally speaking, oliguria means weakness of vitality. If the amount is less than the fluid consumed, it points to great loss by diarrhea or to a tendency to dropsy. Polyuria sometimes means colliquation, and the discharge of fluid effete matters from the body by the urine.

§1363 To assess these correctly, one must note the state of the vitality, as follows: if the urine be of bad color, it is a bad sign but the more plentiful it is, the more likely is recovery to take place. If the quantity excreted fails, the illness will increase, just as applies in regard to dark or coarse urine.

§1364 Variation of quantity is a bad sign if the urine is at one time abundant, at another scanty, at another suppressed. It shows that there is a hard conflict between the vitality and the disease. A plentiful urine in an acute illness, occurring without any abatement of symptoms, and, associated with copious sweats, shows hectic fever and may be followed by convulsions.[14]

§1365 A scanty urine, passed involuntarily, drop-by-drop in acute diseases, indicates cerebral disease, affecting nerves and muscles.

§1366 If a fever subside and there are other signs of recovery, one may predict epistaxis. Otherwise delirium will ensue and death is likely.

§1367 When a person is in apparent health, if the amount of the urine is diminished and it is tenuous in character, and if that condition persists, and if there is a sense of heaviness and pain in the loins, this shows that there is a hard inflammatory swelling in the kidney.

§**1368** When the urine is increased in a case of colic, this is a good sign, especially if it be white and easily voided.

13.1.16. A Description of Normal Healthy Urine

§**1369** The following are the characters of healthy urine. A medium consistency; a delicate tint, tending to straw-yellow; and, if there be any sediment, it is white, light, homogeneous, a rounded contour; the odor should be moderate, neither offensive, nor altogether absent.

§**1370** Some say that if a urine of this kind appear suddenly the end of the acme of an illness, health will be restored following day.

13.1.17. The Variations According to Age

§**1371** Infancy: the urine tends to the character of milk, considering the food and their moist temperament. Therefore, it is nearly colorless.

§**1372** Childhood: the urine is thicker and coarser than in adolescents, and more turbid. This has already been mentioned.

§**1373** Adolescence: the urine tends to igneity, and homogeneity.

§**1374** Later life: the urine tends to be white and tenuous, but it may be coarse ("thick") because of the effete matters which are now being evacuated to a greater extent by way of the urine.

§**1375** Decrepit age: the urine is whiter and still more tenuous. A similar coarseness to that of the preceding may occur, but this is rare. If the urine becomes very thick, it intimates liability to develop calculus.

13.1.18. The Variations According to Gender

§**1376** Women: the urine is always thicker, whiter and less pellucid than in males. The reason is fourfold: in women there is feebleness of digestion; abundance of effete matters; width of emunctory channels; and material discharged by way of the uterus, which draws similar material down the urinary passages also.

§1377 Men: when the urine is shaken, it becomes turbid and the turbidity ascends to the surface, though occasionally it remains throughout the whole bulk of the urine. When the urine in women is shaken, it does not become turbid because the particles are barely discrete, and there is usually a circular foam on top. Even if such urine becomes turbid, it does so only to a light extent.

§1378 If male and female urine be mingled, a filamentous network forms at once. (Filaments also appear in male urine if passed immediately after intercourse).

§1379 Pregnancy: the urine is clear and there is a surface cloud. The color may approach that of chickpea water, or be yellow with a bluish or iridescent tint in it. In either case there is a sort of "tinted cotton" in the midst of it. Occasionally there are granules present, which rise and fall. If the iridescence ("rainbow tint") be quite distinct, it is a sign that conception is beginning. When it gives place to redness, it shows that impregnation is completed, especially if the urine becomes turbid on being shaken.

§1380 Puerperium: the urine is often dark, as if there were a sootiness or shoemaker's black in it.

13.1.19. The Urine of Animals and its Difference from Human Urine

§1381 It is often desirable for a doctor to know something about the urine of animals, so that when he is tricked by a patient, he can quickly and truly discern it, difficult though it be to do so.

§1382 Asses: some say that the urine is like clarified butter as to turbidity and coarseness.

§1383 Beasts of burden: the urine is similar to the preceding, but clearer. The upper middle part of the urine is clear, while the lower middle part is turbid.

§1384 Sheep: the urine is nearly colorless, with a yellowish tendency approximating that of man. But it has either no "body" and the sediment is fatty, or it is like oil-less. The better the quality of the food eaten, the clearer is the urine.

§**1385** She-goats: the urine is like human and sheep urine, but a it has no "body," or sediment, and is clearer than sheep urine.

13.1.20. Fluids Resembling Urine and How to Distinguish Them

§**1386** Acetous syrup and all fluids compounded of water and honey, water and figs, resemble urine as well as fluids colored with saffron and the like—in all these, the nearer one holds them to the eye, the clearer do them seem, and the further they are held from the eye, the more opaque do they become. Urine is the opposite. The foam on hydromel is yellow.

§**1387** The sediment from fig water or from herbal decoctions lodges on the sides of the glass and not in the middle It has no definite contour, and does not move its position.

§**1388** So much suffices for the description of the states of the urine. All the individual varieties are discussed in the volume which deals with the special diseases.[15]

13.2. Feces

13.2.1. The Characteristics to Note

§**1389** The following are the characters to note: the quantity; the consistency; the color; the form or shape; and the time occupied in the passage of food through the bowel.

13.2.1.1. Quantity

§**1390** If greater than the amount of food taken, the reason lies in abundance of humors; if smaller in amount, the reason lies in deficient amount of humors, or in a retention of the food in the caecum or colon (in which case, it is the first step to obstruction). The reason may also be that the expulsive power is insufficient!

13.2.1.2. Consistency

§**1391** Moist excrement denotes defective digestion or

obstruction of some form; weakness of the mesentery, so that it does not absorb sufficient water from the food; fluxion from the head; some constituent of the diet which causes the dejection to be moist. If the fecal matter is both moist and viscid, this shows that there is colliquation in the tissues. Fetor is then present. It usually denotes an excess of depraved and viscous humors, and the fetor is then very great. It may denote the presence of viscous and "hot" constituents in the food, with defective digestive power.

§**1392** Frothy fecal matter indicates an admixture with flatulent vapors, or exposure to great (innate) heat.

§**1393** Dry stool results from: (1) severe toil; (2) dispersal of innate heat; (3) polyuria; (4) igneous heat; (5) dry aliments; (6) a long delay in the intestines—as will be explained in the appropriate chapter. When the fecal matter is both moist and hard, the dryness is due to: (i) undue delay in the intestines due to moisture which cannot escape; (ii) lack of bile, which serves to help in the excrement.

§**1394** If there has been no delay, and there is no evidence of moisture in the intestines, it shows that there is a continual dispersion of sanious and pungent effete matter from the liver into the intestine, until the latter has taken it all up.

13.2.1.3. Color

§**1395** The normal color is ruddy, owing to the presence of a slight fieriness. If this color is more marked, it shows that the bile is plentiful. If less marked it indicates defective maturation of the food. White stool points to obstruction in the biliary passages, and goes with jaundice, if there is also offensive sanious material present, it shows that an inflammatory mass has ruptured it. A healthy person who does not take exercise often passes a morbid sanious matter which acts as a purgative and produces a satisfactory evacuation. For by this means laxity of the tissues is avoided, which lack of exercise is liable to produce, as we have already explained when speaking of the urine.

13.2.1.3.1. Unduly Red Color

§**1396** Unduly red color of stool at the acme of a disease often denotes maturation; it often points to a depraved constitution.

13.2.1.3.2. Dark Colored or Black Stool

§1397 The significance of dark-colored or black stool are similar to those of dark or black urine. It means: (1) marked oxidation; (2) maturation of a disease due to atrabilious humor; (3) an aliment which colors it; (4) a medicament which procures the discharge of the atrabilious humor. The first is unfavorable; the second is merely a staining from admixture with black bile; this cannot be clearly discerned from color alone, but only by its acridity, bitterness and the; churning out of earthy matter from it. Moreover, among its peculiar properties is this, that it glitters (is self-luminous). The fact of black bile leaving the body, whether it be by the stool or by the vomit, is a bad sign.

§1398 Finally, the discharge of pure atrabilious humor per anum is usually a sign of impending death, while the exit of black chyme is beneficial because it shows that the tissues are active in oxidation, and their moisture is used up.[16]

13.2.1.3.3. Green Stool

§1399 This denotes extinction of the innate heat. The color is due to the verdigris-green type of bile.

13.2.1.3.4. Dark Colored or Livid Stool

§1400 This also denotes extinction of the innate heat; coldness; considerable mortification in the interior organs. It is a bad sign.

13.2.1.3.5. Parti-colored Stool

§1401 This is a bad sign. Reference to this is made in Book Four.

13.2.1.3.6. Fatty Stool

§1402 This is met with when the fat of the body is being dissolved out.

13.2.1.3.7. Glutinous Stool

§1403 In this case other tissues as well as the fatty tissue are being liquefied. It is a very grave sign.

13.2.1.3.8. Purulent Stool

§1404 The pus comes from the liver, or stomach, or bowel.

13.2.1.3.9. Intensely Yellow Stool

§1405 When occurring at the beginning of a disease it is due to bilious humor. If at the acme it is useful in that it purges the body (of undesirable substances).

13.2.1.3.10. Unusual Colors of Stool

§1406 Unusual colors in the stool, and the various colors which have a bad significance are spoken of in the special volume.

13.2.2. Form or Shape

§1407 If the feces are bulky like those of a cow it is because of flatulence, or gaseousness.

§1408 Time occupied in passage through the bowel. When the feces are passed out too rapidly it is a bad sign; it shows that there is an excess of bile in the gall-bladder, and also a weakness of the retentive power.

§1409 A delay in the passages of fecal matter through the body denotes a feeble digestion, coldness of the intestines, abundant moisture; taking too much sleep; flatulence.

13.2.3. The Characters of Normal Stool

§1410 The stool should be: (1) coherent; (2) homogeneous throughout, the water and solids being intimately admixed; (3) soft and honey like in consistency; (4) easily evacuated; (5) of a color tending to yellow (if the color should resemble that of the food it would mean indigestion); (6) of not very offensive odor, yet not odorless; (7) of a quality which is neither sharp nor biting; (8) it should emerge inaudibly, neither with gurgling, nor flatus, nor creaking, nor foamy; (9) passed at the time customary to the healthy person; (10) in bulk nearly equal to that of the food consumed.

§1411 Note that neither homogeneity nor softness is necessarily a laudable character in feces. These characters may be the result of violent maturation throughout the body, or of oxidation or colliquation. In such cases, these features would be unfavorable signs.

§1412 Note, too, that a consistency which tends to tenuity is not favorable unless there is no rumbling or discharge of flatus at stool; it should not then emerge bit by bit. But one must also be sure it is not being discharged in that form owing to the admixture of some irritant which prevents cohesion.

§1413 Many authors proceed from the discussion of urine and feces to other excretions, including sweat. I consider it more appropriate to deal with these under their appropriate headings in the volume on special diseases.[17]

Part Four
The Preservation of Health

Lecture 14: The Basis of Health and Disease and the Inevitability of Death

§1414 In the first part of this book it was stated that medicine comprises two parts, one theoretical, and one practical, though both are really speculative science. That which is specially named theory relates to the formation of opinions and the showing of the evidence upon which they are based, without reference to the mode of acting upon them. Thus this part deals with the temperaments, the humors, the drives, and with the forms, the symptoms, and the causes of disease. That which is specially named practical relates to the mode of acting upon this knowledge, and the prescription of a regimen.

§1415 For instance, it is that part of medicine which helps us understand how the health of the body is to be maintained in this or that state, and by what means we can heal the diseases with which the body is afflicted. Practical does not refer to the performance of surgical operations. It is the art which teaches us in what way to procure healing— the healing art.

§1416 Having expounded in the first and second parts of this work the various matters pertaining to this theoretical part of medicine, we now proceed to the study of the two subjects pertaining to the practical part—dealing with them in a general manner.

§1417 The two parts which belong to the practical side of medicine are: (1) the science of regulating the healthy body, so as to maintain it in health—the science of hygiene; and (2) the sciences of ruling the sick body so as to enable it to return to a state off health—the science of healing.

§1418 In this part then, we fully describe how health is to be maintained.

§1419 The human being takes its origin from two things: (1) the male semen, which plays the part of factor; and (2) the female menstrual discharge, which provides the matter.

§1420 Each of these is fluid and moist, but there is more wateriness and earthly substance in the female blood and female sperm, whereas air and fire are predominant in the male sperm. It is essential that at the outset of the congelation of the two components there should be moisture, even though earth and fire are found in the product. The earth provides the firmness and rigidity; the fire provides the maturative power. These give the coagulum ("*He created man from a clot*" Quran, 96:2) a certain hardness or firmness. But this hardness is not as great in degree as that possessed by a stone or glass. For these are either not soluble at all or only soluble to a degree imperceptible to our senses, however long one exposes them to solvents. Were the hardness comparable to this, the product of conception would never suffer injury however long or however persistently a solvent were applied. But that is not so. The act is contrary.

§1421 Our bodies are exposed to injury from two directions—externally and internally. The source of internal injury is the dissipation of the moisture from which we are created, and this dissipation proceeds in an orderly manner. The second source is the putrefactive breakdown and metamorphosis of the humor into a form such that the fermentative phenomena of life are no longer able to proceed.

§1422 The second source of injury differs from the first in that dryness is here introduced by virtue of depravity of humor;

and this dryness continues neutralizing the moisture of the body until the form ceases to have a capacity for life.

§**1423** Finally, the putrefactive breakdown disperses the vitality, because it first destroys the moisture and then disperses it, and simply dry ash is left behind.

§**1424** Therefore we see that these two sources of destruction [of the living product of conception] are different from those arising from other causes—such as, freezing cold, torrid heat, grave forms of loss of continuity, various maladies. But it is in regard to the first two named sources of destruction that we find the more important factors relative to the question of the preservation of health.

§**1425** Each of them takes its origin from extrinsic and intrinsic agents. The extrinsic agents are for example, the atmosphere, which is a solvent and putrefacient. The intrinsic agents are, for example, the innate heat, which is the agent within us through which moisture is dispersed: the extraneous heat generated within us from the aliments, and through other agents which cause putrefactive changes in the [native] moistures.

§**1426** All these agents mutually aid one another in rendering the body dry. And yet it is true that our perfection and soundness and the power to perform our various actions depend on a degree of dryness of the blood. But the degree of dryness becomes relatively greater and greater until we die. Therefore, this dryness is inevitable.

§**1427** If we were at the outset essentially composed of moisture, heat would have to overcome it or else the heat would be choked by it. Therefore the heat continues to exert its own effect, that is, it produces more and more desiccation. But whatever degree of dryness there might be at the outset (of life), it reaches equilibrium, and remains so until the limit of equilibrium in regard to dryness is reached. The heat remaining constant, the dryness is now relatively greater than before for the matter is less, and hence holds more. Therefore it is not difficult to understand that the dryness passes on beyond the stage of equilibrium, and goes on steadily increasing until the whole of the moisture of the body is consumed. Therefore (we may say) that the innate heat is the cause of its own extinction, for it is itself the reason for its own matter being consumed. We may compare it to the flame of a lamp; the light goes out when all the matter has been used up.

§1428 As the dryness increases, the innate heat diminishes. The loss continues unceasingly till death, and the moisture which is lost is not restored. The loss goes on more and more.

§1429 The dryness (of the body) is increased in two ways: by lessening of the power of receiving matter; by lessening of the native moisture resulting from dispersal of the (innate) heat. The heat becomes more feeble because dryness predominates in the substance of the members, and because the innate moisture becomes relatively less. The innate moisture is to the innate heat as the oil of a lamp is to the flame. For there are two forms of moisture in the flame: water, which holds its own, and oil, which is used up. So, in a corresponding manner, the innate heat holds its own in respect of the innate moisture, but is used up *pari passu* with increase of extraneous heat, due, for example, to defective digestion, which is comparable with the aqueous moisture of the flame. As the dryness increases, the innate heat lessens, and the result is natural death.

§1430 For the reason why the (human) body does not live any longer than it does lies in the fact that the initial innate moisture holds out against being dispersed both by the alien heat and by the heat in the body itself (both that which is innate and that derived from bodily movement). And this resistance is maintained as long as the one is weaker than the other, and as long as something is provided to replace that which has been thus dispersed, to wit, from the aliment. Furthermore, as we have already stated, the power or drive which operates upon the aliment in order to render it useful in this way only does so up to the end of life.

§1431 Therefore, we may say that the art of maintaining health is not the art of averting death or of averting extraneous injuries from the body or of securing the utmost longevity possible to the human being. It is concerned with two other things:

(1) the prevention of putrefactive breakdown; and (2) the safeguarding of innate moisture from too rapid dissipation and maintaining it at such a degree of strength that the original type of constitution peculiar to the person shall not change even up to the last moment of life.

§1432 This is secured by a suitable regimen, namely: (a) one which will ensure the replacement of the innate heat and moisture which are dispersed from the body as exactly as possible; and (b) a regimen which will prevent any agents which would lead to a rapid dessication from gaining the upper hand excluding agents which produce a normal desiccation; (c) one which safeguards the body from the development of putrefactive processes within it and from the influence of alien heat (whether extraneous or intrinsic) because all bodies have not the same degree of innate moisture and innate heat. There is a great diversity in regard to them.

§1433 Moreover, every person has his own term of life, during which the desiccation inevitable to his temperament (constitution) and the degree of innate heat, and of innate moisture can be withstood.

§1434 Nevertheless, factors may arise which assist desiccation, or are injurious in some other way. For which reason, many assert that the former are natural causes of death, whereas the latter are accidental. And under this view, the art of maintaining health consists in guiding the body to its natural span of life by paying attention to whatever things conduce thereto. There are two drives to be fostered by the doctor in striving for this object: (1) the nutritive drive whereby that is replaced which is constantly being lost to the body namely earthiness and aquosity; and (2) the sensitive drive (animal faculty), that is, the pulsatile faculty which is concerned with the replacement of that which is lost to the body by the breath namely air and fire. And since aliments are only potentially like the thing nourished, an alternative drive had to be created so that they could be changed actually into the likeness of the thing nourished. In this way the aliment becomes effective.

§1435 The instruments and channels necessary for this had to be created also—namely the means by which material is attracted, expelled, retained, and digested (sequence by sequence, turn by turn).

§1436 Therefore, we may say that the essential considerations in the art of preserving the health consist in maintaining equilibrium between all these various concomitant factors. But there are seven matters concerning which special care must be expended to ensure just proportion: (1) equilibrium of temperament; (2) selection of the articles of food and drink; (3) evacuation of effete matters; (4) safeguarding the composite; (5) maintaining the purity of the air respired; (6) guarding against extraneous contingencies; and (7) moderation in regard to the movements of the body and the motions of the mind, with which may be included sleep and wakefulness.

§1437 From all these considerations you will now perceive that there is no single fixed limit to which equilibrium or health is to be assigned. None of the temperaments enters into it. Health and equilibrium vary (in range) from time to time. That is to say, it is a state comprised—within two limits.

§1438 We therefore begin by discussing first the regimen appropriate to the period of infancy, in which the temperament is continuously at one extreme of equilibrium.

Lecture 15: Upbringing

15.1. Childbirth and Infancy

15.1.1 General Remarks

§**1439** Prenatal care of the mother during pregnancy and before confinement will be described in the volume on diseases of the various organs.

15.1.2. Treatment of the Cord

§**1440** Most physicians agree that immediately after birth the umbilical cord should be cut at a point four fingers breadth from the umbilicus and after this, tying a clean woolen thread so soft and lightly twined that it does not produce any injury. The end of the cord is dressed with a clean piece of cloth (gauze) soaked in olive oil. To assist healing, the cut surface should be dusted with a fine powder made of equal parts of turmeric, dragon's blood, sarcalla, cumin seed and lichen.

15.1.3. Care of the Skin

§**1441** The face and body of the newborn should be bathed in salt water to harden the skin and set the features. The best salt for this purpose is the one which contains a small quantity of seeds of Indian hemp, costus root, fumitary, fenugreek and origanum. Care should be taken to protect the nose and mouth while washing the face. The skin needs hardening because in the newborn baby, it is so soft, warm and delicate that everything which comes in contact with it is likely to be felt extremely cold, hard and rough. The saline bath could be safely repeated if the body is found to be still dry or covered with secretions. After the bath, the baby should be washed with lukewarm water. The nostrils should be cleansed with the tip of the little finger, provided the nail has been properly trimmed. A few drops of olive oil should be dropped in the eyes. The rectum should be dilated by introducing the little finger in the anus. Special care should be taken to protect the baby from chills. When the cord is separated—and it generally happens in three or four days—the navel is dusted with the ashes of oyster shell, burnt tendon of a calf's heel, or burnt zinc dissolved in alcohol.

15.1.4. Swaddling

§**1442** The nurse should handle the limbs gently and mold the various parts according to their shape, spreading out those which should be flat and thinning the ones which are to remain slender.

§**1443** The eyes should be carefully wiped with a soft silken cloth.

§**1444** If the baby tries to pass urine, it should be assisted with pressure over the bladder At the end of this procedure, the arms should be brought beside the knees and the head covered with a light turban or a properly fitting cap.

15.1.5. Sleeping Quarters

§**1445** The nursery should be warm and airy, but dark and shady rather than bright and glary. During sleep, the head should be kept slightly elevated and care taken to avoid twisting the body.

15.1.6. Bathing the Infant

§**1446** In summer, the water should be tepid and in winter lukewarm. Bath is best given after a spell of sound sleep and there is no harm if it is repeated two or three times a day. During summer, the temperature should be reduced gradually, but in winter it should be kept warm throughout. The bath may be continued safely as long as the baby remains warm and flushed. Care should be taken to avoid water entering the ears. While bathing, the baby should be held with both hands so that the chest rests over the left forearm and the right hand holds it from above in such a way that the baby's head and feet are hanging downward. When the bath is over, the baby is gently wiped with a soft cloth. It is first kept face downward and then turned over on the back. The various parts of the body are then manipulated into their proper shapes and the head tied up with a bandage. A few drops of olive oil dropped in the eyes would cleanse the eyes and lids.

15.2. Concerning Nursing and Weaning

§**1447** The following rules should be observed in infant feeding: The baby should be nourished as far as possible, from the mother's breast. Having received its nourishment in the womb from her menstrual blood, the mother's milk, which is really another form of the same, is naturally the most suitable for the further growth and development of the baby.[1]

§**1448** It is generally observed that the baby gets readily quiet after receiving the mother's breast. The baby should at first be breast-fed only two or three times a day. Large feeds should be avoided, especially during the first few days. In those early days, it is better that someone else should nurse the baby so as to give the mother time to regain her usual temperament.

§**1449** A little honey may be given to the baby before the initial feed. Before the morning feed, a small quantity of milk from the breast should be squeezed out and this should be done especially when the milk is abnormal. If the milk is inclined to be sour, breast feeding should be avoided, particularly when the mother is hungry or fasting. Gentle rocking and the customary lullabies help to induce sleep and strengthen the constitution. This should, however, be within the limits of tolerance of the baby as observed from his physical and musical responses. The former relates to the development of the body and the latter to that of the mind.[2]

15.2.1. The Inability to Nurse the Child

§1450 When for reasons of health or because of some abnormality in the milk, or for the sake of her own comfort the mother herself is unable to nurse the baby, a wet-nurse should be employed.

§1451 This nurse should of course be suitable in respect of her age, physique, morals, shape of breasts, quality of the milk, the time elapsed since her confinement, and the sex of her own child. If a nurse fulfills these requirements, she should be engaged and given good food such as wheat, millet, lamb, sheep or goats, fish which is neither hard nor putrefied; and lettuce; similarly almonds. Vegetables such as watercress, mustard, wild basil, and to some extent, even mint are best avoided, as they are not good for lactation.

15.2.2. The Character of a Good Wet-nurse

§1452 The age should best be between twenty-five and thirty-five years, when women are at the height of their youth and vigor. Her color and complexion should be healthy and the neck strong, chest broad and the body well-developed and muscular. There should be neither obesity nor leanness. The nurse should be cheerful and of good moral character and not liable to emotional outbursts of anger, grief or fear which tend to undermine character and affect the baby adversely in other ways. It is for the same reason that the Holy Prophet (peace be upon him and his descendants) prohibited the employment of mentally deranged women as wet-nurses. A nurse of bad character cannot be trusted to give conscientious care to the baby. Her breasts should be large and firm but not long and nor very big or hard. The milk should be moderate in quantity and consistency. It should be white rather than dark and never greenish, yellowish or reddish in color. The odor should be agreeable and not acrid or pungent. The taste should be sweet and not bitter, salty or sour. It should be homogeneous and plentiful and neither too watery nor too thick, cheesy or frothy.

15.2.3. Testing the Milk

§1453 A drop of the milk should be placed over the fingernail and allowed to run. If it flows freely, it should be regarded as being thin, but if it remains on the nail, even when the finger is turned, it should be taken as being thick. Milk can be tested also by adding a small quantity of myrrh to a small cup of milk. The relative proportion of cheese separated from whey would indicate the quality of milk. If the milk is of proper consistency, only a moderate amount of cheese would separate.

§1454 If the nurse is not of the requisite standard and breast feeding cannot be avoided, either the feeds should be modified or the nurse given proper treatment. Thus, if the milk is too thick or is of an unpleasant odor, it should be taken out (with a breast pump) and exposed to the air for a while before the feedings. If the milk is unduly "hot," the nurse should drink water before giving the feeds.

15.2.4. The Nurse's Diet

§1455 When the milk is too thick, she should be treated with some liquefying medicines such as decoctions of mint, hyssop, wild thyme and origanum. Also, salted fish and a little radish may be added to her diet. The nurse should be advised to have also emesis with lime juice cordial or warm water, and she should take moderate exercise before the meals.

§1456 When the nurse is of hot temperament, she should be given syrup of vinegar with or without some light beverage.

§1457 If her milk is too thin, she should take plenty of rest and avoid work and exercise. She should also eat things which tend to thicken the blood. If there are no contra indications, she should drink sweet wines and grape juice and have plenty of sleep.

§1458 When the milk is scanty, it may be due to abnormal heat in the breasts or in the temperament of the body as a whole. If the milk is scanty from abnormal heat in the temperament, it can be easily recognized from the signs already mentioned in the earlier chapters. Where it is due to excessive heat in the breasts, it could be ascertained from the feel of the breasts.

§1459 Abnormal heat should be treated with a diet consisting of things like barley water and spinach. If there are signs of coldness in the system, or when there is a tendency of stasis in the breasts or when there is evidence of inadequate absorption, the diet should include light warming things. Gentle cupping may also be given under the breasts. Carrots and carrot seeds are extremely beneficial for those with scanty milk. Where the scantiness of milk is due to malnutrition, the nurse should be fed on a broth made of barley, barley bran or some other suitable cereal. It is beneficial to have the roots and seeds of fennel, the seeds of dill or nigella added to the broth. According to some, the udders of sheep or goat may be taken raw with the contained milk. These are useful either because of the similarity of form or due to their specific lactogenic property.

15.2.5. List of Galactagogues

§1460 (1) One ounce of butter from cow's milk placed into a vessel of a beverage, taken as a drink. (2) Sesame ground up in a fine mill and mixed with a beverage; taken as a drink. (3) Local application of the oil cake of nard mixed with olive oil and milk. (4) Take one ounce of the interior parts of eggplant, dissolving it in a beverage by stirring and taken as a drink. (5) An especially good prescription consists of three ounces of powdered seeds of dill, one ounce each of the seeds of blue melilot[3] and leek and two ounces each of the seeds of alfalfa, lucerne, and fenugreek or mixed with fresh juice of fennel, honey and clarified butter. This is to be taken in small quantities at a time. (6) Massaging the breasts frequently with bland hands renders the secretion of milk plentiful.

15.2.6. Anti-galactagogues

§1461 When the secretion of milk is excessive and produces heaviness and fullness in the breasts, or when the milk is too thick, the food should be reduced in quantity and a less nourishing diet given. The breasts and the surrounding parts of the chest should be painted with a liniment containing cumin seeds and vinegar or a plaster made of pure clay mixed with either plain vinegar or vinegar in which lentils have been boiled should be applied. Saline waters may be given to drink after the meals. Mint may also be taken freely.

§1462 Resolvent measures should be adopted, such as a

bath on an empty stomach, venesection and plenty of exercise.[4] Massage of the breasts enhances the production of milk. When milk has an unpleasant odor, fragrant wines of good flavor and aroma should be given.

§1463 The nurse's own baby should neither be quite grown up, nor less than one or two months old. It would indeed be the best if her own baby, is also of the same age as her charge. The difference in the age of both the babies should not, in any case, be more than six weeks to two months. The nurse should be the one who has a male child. It is also important that the nurse should not have suffered from any abortions or miscarriages and should always have been having full term babies.

15.2.7. A Regime for the Nurse

§1464 The nurse should take moderate exercise and eat wholesome food which give good chyme like wheat, frumenty, lamb, kid of goats which are not putrescent or have hard flesh, lettuce, almonds, filbert-nuts, and mint. Potherbs which are deleterious include watercrest, mustard, or mountain balm for they cause the blood to undergo decomposition. She should abstain from sexual intercourse during the nursing period, as this activates the menstrual blood and makes the milk foul and reduces its quantity. It may also lead to fresh pregnancy which would be injurious both to the baby at the breast and the would be baby—the fetus in the womb. The baby suffers because the lighter blood gets diverted towards the fetus and the fetus suffers from inadequate nutrition as it has to be shared with the baby.

§1465 A small quantity of milk should be squeezed out before each feed and especially before the morning feed. This helps the flow of milk and saves the baby from unnecessary strain and exertion, and thus prevents troubles developing in the throat and trachea. A spoonful of honey, preferably with a few drops of wine (brandy) may be given before the feeds. Large feeds should be avoided as these produce distension of the abdomen and excessive flatulence and makes the urine white. The feeds should be small and frequent. If over-feeding produces any of the above mentioned symptoms, nursing should be stopped, the baby starved for a time and sleep encouraged to help the digestion.

§**1466** During the first few days, as mentioned earlier, no more than three daily feeds should be given the baby nursed, preferably by someone other than the mother. If the nurse becomes ill from some temperamental disease or disturbance or suffers from excessive diarrhea or severe constipation, nursing should be suspended and arrangements made with someone else to breast feed the baby. Feeding should also be interrupted when the nurse has to take some strong or potent medicine.

§**1467** After feeding, the cradle should be rocked gently rather than vigorously, to avoid splashing the milk in the stomach. A little crying before the feeds is generally beneficial to the baby. The normal period of nursing should be two years.

15.2.8. Weaning

§**1468** When the baby begins to ask for things other than milk, it should be allowed to take something suitable. When the incisor teeth begin to erupt, milk feeds should be gradually supplemented with things which are not too hard and difficult to masticate. It would be best to begin with bread which the nurse has softened by chewing. Later on, bread soaked in diluted honey or milk may be given followed by a little plain water as a drink. Sometimes, a little diluted wine may be given. Care should be taken that the stomach is not overloaded.

§**1469** If the baby suffers from heaviness and distension in the stomach or the urine begins to be white-colored, feeding should be suspended for a while. It is good for the baby to be fed after the oil rub and the bath.

§**1470** When breast feeding is stopped, light foods such as broths and easily digestible meat should be given, but special care is taken to introduce these gradually rather than abruptly. The baby may be comforted with sweet cones made of bread and sugar. If the baby keeps on crying for the breast, the nipple may be coated with a paste made of one drachm each of myrrh and the seeds of purslane.

§**1471** It may be summarized that preservation of health

amongst the children depends upon a regular supply of moist food, which is absolutely necessary for the nutrition of children, who have moist temperaments and a moderate amount of exercise for a sufficiently long time. This is particularly necessary in the transitional period between infancy and childhood.

15.3. Child Mobility

§**1472** When the child begins to stand up and toddle about, he should not be allowed to sit up and walk until he can do it himself, otherwise the legs and back might become deformed. When the child begins to crawl, he should be placed on a smooth carpet or skin to avoid injury from a rough ground. Sticks, knives and other sharp objects should be kept out of his way and care taken to prevent him from falling.

15.4. The Hygiene of Teeth

§**1473** When the canine teeth begin to erupt, children desire to chew things. These should not be so hard as to cause damage to the newly erupted teeth. The rubbing of rabbit's brain or chicken fat over the gums helps dentition. During dentition, the head and neck should be massaged with hot water containing olive oil. A few drops of oil may also be dropped into the ears.

§**1474** As soon as the child is able to bite, and this should be known from his attempts at biting his own fingers, a piece of licorice which is not very dry may be given to chew. Licorice benefits the gums because it prevents the formation of ulcers. The mouth should be cleansed regularly with a mixture of salt and honey.

§**1475** When the teeth have fully erupted, a piece of liquorice, which is not too dry or dried liquorice may be given to chew. Massage of the neck with olive oil or some other sweet oil is also beneficial during dentition. When the child begins to talk, the root of the tongue should receive regular massage.

15.5. Concerning the Diseases Which Afflict Infants and Their Treatment

§**1476** Diseases of infancy are best managed by attending to the mother. Thus, when the mother is suspected of plethora, she should have venesection or cupping. When there is a dominance of some humor other than the blood, appropriate measures should be adopted to eliminate it. Constipation, diarrhea, the ascent of vapors to the head, disturbances of the respiratory system, abnormalities of the temperament should all be corrected by regulating the food and drinks of the mother. If the mother develops diarrhea or has taken some purgative or suffers from vomiting or has taken an emetic, the baby should he nourished by someone else.

§**1477** The diseases which are common amongst the children will now be described.

15.5.1. The Disorders During Teething

§**1478** Gingivitis—inflammation of the gums, swelling of the temporal regions and trismus are common during dentition. In these cases, the inflamed part should be gently massaged with oil as mentioned in the section on dentition. Honey mixed with oil of chamomile or turpentine resin may be used. Decoctions of chamomile and dill may be poured freely over the head. For the burning pain in the gums apply oil and wax as an epitheme or use salted flesh which is a little high.

§**1479** Gums may be massaged with oil or oil mixed with wax. Salted and preserved meat used as a decoction would be a good mouthwash.[5]

15.5.2. Diarrhea

§**1480** Diarrhea is particularly common during teething. According to some, it is due to the indigestion caused by swallowing salty, purulent matter from the gums. This does not, however, appear to be a good reason. The real cause may well be that the system being occupied in erupting the teeth is unable to digest the food properly.[6] Indigestion may also be due to pain in the gums. A mild attack of diarrhea does not require any special treatment; but if it is profuse, foments made of rose seeds or celery, anise or cumin seeds may be applied to the abdomen or a plaster made of cumin seeds or rose seeds soaked in vinegar or millet boiled in vinegar may be used. If these things fail to relieve the trouble, a small quantity of *anfahah* from the stomach of a newborn kid [from which a paste is made to curdle milk] may be given in cold water. Since milk tends to curdle in the stomach, some suitable substitute like the yolk of a half boiled egg or soft bread or roasted and ground barley cooked in water should be given.

15.5.3. Constipation During Teething

§**1481** This may be treated with a suppository of solidified pure honey or honey to which a little mint or plain or burnt lily root has been added. A little honey may be given by mouth and a few grains of turpentine resin mixed with olive oil may be gently rubbed over the abdomen. Maidenweed and ox-bile may also be applied to the navel.

15.5.4. Convulsions During Teething

§**1482** These are particularly common during teething and are due to nervous instability and digestive disturbances generally associated with this period of life. They are more common in children with moist and robust constitutions. These are treated by rubbing the body with oil of iris, lily, alkanet, or mallow.[7]

§**1483** Sometimes children develop spasms. These are treated with water in which cucumber [or heliotrope] have been boiled or by oil of violets mixed with oil of cucumber.

§**1484** If the spasms are due to dryness, i.e., have followed febrile conditions, or severe diarrhea, or have appeared gradually, the joints should be rubbed with violet oil. The oil may be used pure or mixed with wax. In this condition, olive oil or violet oil should be applied freely over the head. Similarly, if the baby suffers from dry types of spasms, olive oil or violet oil should be beneficial.

15.5.5. Coughs and Colds

§**1485** In the case of coughs and colds, plenty of hot water should be poured over the head, and the tongue smeared freely with honey, and vomiting induced by pressing the back of the tongue with the finger. Expectoration of phlegm in this way would relieve the child. Gum acacia, gum tragacanth, powdered quince seeds, extract of licorice all mixed together with brown sugar are given daily in a small quantity with fresh milk.

15.5.6. Dyspnea

§**1486** Dyspnea may be treated with emesis or by rubbing olive oil over the roots of the ears or over the tongue or by simply pressing the tongue with the finger. Warm water should be given to drink and linseed mixed with honey used as a linctus.

15.5.7. Stomatitis

§**1487** Stomatitis is common in infants because the mucous membrane of the mouth and tongue is so extremely delicate that even sucking produces irritation. When the milk produces irritation, apthous stomatitis develops. The worst type of stomatitis is the one with black (gangrenous) ulcers (cancrum oris). This generally proves fatal.

§**1488** The white and red ulcers are not so serious. Stomatitis is treated with mild drugs listed under stomatitis in the volume on diseases of the individual organs. Sometimes, powdered violets alone or mixed with roses and a small quantity of saffron may be applied. Occasionally, carob beans are also effective. Night-shade juice, juice of lettuce, and purslane juice may also be needed. If the condition proves obstinate, bruised blue lily root may be used. If the gums are ulcerated myrrh, galls and frankincense bark thoroughly ground with honey may be applied. Occasionally, thick syrup made of sour mulberries or grapes may be used. It is often helpful to wash the mouth with honey water or wine before applying the various astringents mentioned above. If a more powerful remedy is needed, the mouth may be dusted with a powder made of six drachms each of turmeric, red blossoms and rind of pomegranate and fumitory, four drachms of galls and two drachms of alum all thoroughly powdered and mixed together.

15.5.8. Discharging Ears

§**1489** Discharging ears is a common complaint, because the body of the child and especially the brain are full of moisture. This condition is treated by dressing the ears with a wick (gauze) soaked in honey or wine (spirit) to which a small quantity of alum, saffron or niter has been added. Sour wine with a little saffron added to it is generally effective.

15.5.9. Earache

§**1490** Earache is frequently due to gas or excess of moisture. It may be treated with the ear drops of an oil in which berberine, origanum, rock-salt, lentil, myrrh, colocynth seeds or juniper has been boiled.

15.5.10. Inflammation of the Brain

§**1491** This is a hot inflammation of the brain which causes so much pain in the eyes and neck that the face becomes pale yellow. It may be treated with cooling and moistening measures such as the external application of cucumber or marrow peelings, juice of garden night shade, juice of fresh parsley which is almost a specific; rose oil mixed with a little vinegar or the yolk of an egg with rose oil. Whatever medicine is used, it should be changed frequently.

15.5.11. Hydrocephalus

§**1492** The treatment of hydrocephalus will be discussed under the diseases of the head.

15.5.12. Sore Eyes

§**1493** For sore eyes, berberine mixed with milk is applied over the lids. Later, the eyes are bathed with water in which chamomile and wild basil have been boiled.

15.5.13. Ulcers

§**1494** Sometimes, excessive crying produces white corneal opacities. These may be treated by applying the juice of garden night shade. Eyelids swollen from excessive crying may also be treated with the same remedy.

15.5.14. Fevers

§**1495** Fevers are best treated by attention to the mother's diet. She may be given such remedies as pomegranate juice mixed with honey and lemon juice or cucumber juice mixed with a little camphor and sugar. Sweating is induced by applying the juice of fresh green reeds over the head and feet. The rest of the body is kept covered with warm clothing.

15.5.15. Colic

§1496 Colic is often quite distressing and may force the child to cry and writhe in agony. The abdomen is fomented with warm water or oil mixed with wax.

15.5.16. Excessive Sneezing

§1497 Successive sneezing is sometimes due to inflammation near the brain. Its treatment is the same as of inflammation. Cooling measures should be adopted and cooling juices and oils applied to the head. Where sneezing is not due to inflammation, powdered seeds of the wild basil may be blown into the nose.[8]

15.5.17. Furunculosis

§1498 Boils which break up into ulcers and turn black are mostly fatal; but if they are white or red in color, they are generally not so serious. This is understandable because the black (gangrenous) ulcers often prove fatal even when they are in the mouth (cancrum oris). The appearance of multiple boils over the body may sometimes be beneficial. Boils should be treated by washing the body with an infusion of some mild astringent, such as of roses, myrtle, mastic leaves, or tamarisk. The oils obtained from these things may also be used as local applications. Simple boils should be left alone until they are ripe for surgical treatment. When boils break down into ulcers, white ointment should be applied. Washing with honey water containing a small quantity of niter is also beneficial. Ulcerative stomatitis can also be treated in the same way. If the boils are dirty and unhealthy looking, stronger medicines should be used, i.e., borax dissolved in water should be applied to prevent irritation. Vesicular eruptions over the face may be treated by bathing with a decoction of myrtle, rose, bog rush, and young mastic leaves. In such conditions, the mother's diet also needs regulation.

15.5.18. Umbilical Hernia

§1499 Umbilical hernia may be due to excessive crying or some other cause of rupture. Bishop's weed ground with the white of an egg should be freely applied to the navel and covered with a piece of gauze. The ashes of bitter lupin suspended in wine may also be applied. More potent medicines are: myrrh, bark and fruit of cypress, aloes and acacia fruit. Some other remedies have also been mentioned in the chapter on hernia which the reader may refer to for further information.

15.5.19. Inflammation of the Navel

§1500 Inflammation of the navel generally occurs soon after the cord is severed. It may be treated with celtic juice [a species of lotus]; turpentine resin melted in olive oil may be given in a small quantity by mouth and also applied locally.

15.5.20. Insomnia

§1501 Sometimes the child may become restless, sleepless and cry incessantly. In this case, sleep may be induced by applying a plaster of poppy or poppy seeds to the head. Lettuce oil or poppy oil may also be rubbed over the head and temples. If a stronger remedy is required, a prescription made of white poppy seeds, yellow poppy seeds, linseed, seeds of celery, parsley seeds, plantain seeds, cumin seeds, lettuce seeds, fennel seeds and seeds of anise all in equal parts, roasted and powdered with one part of roasted fleawort seeds and the whole mixed with an equal quantity of sugar, may be given in two drachm doses. If, however, a still more powerful remedy is desired, opium not more than one-third part of any single ingredient may be added to make the prescription more effective.

15.5.21. Hiccups

§1502 Hiccups may be relieved by giving a small quantity of coconut mixed with sugar.

15.5.22. Persistent Vomiting

§1503 Persistent vomiting is treated with four grains of cloves. A mild astringent plaster may be applied to the abdomen.

15.5.23. Indigestion

§1504 Indigestion is treated with a local application of wine of lily, myrtle and rose water. Conch and cloves with the juice of quince or four grains of conch with quince wine may be given.

15.5.24. Nightmares

§1505 Nightmares are often the result of an overloaded stomach. The resulting decomposition of food produces sensory disturbance in the stomach, which on reaching the brain excites the imaginative instinctive drive and produces fearful dreams. In such cases, the child should not be put to bed with a loaded stomach and honey should be given by mouth to assist digestion.

15.5.25. Inflammation of the Throat

§1506 Inflammation of the throat is a swelling of the region between the mouth and the larynx (pharynx). It may spread to the spine and muscles of the neck. The best treatment for this is a suppository in the rectum and a local application of mulberry syrup or some similar remedy.

15.5.26. Excessive Snoring

§1507 Linseed ground with honey or ground cumin mixed with honey are given as linctus.[9]

15.5.27. Infantile Convulsions

§1508 The treatment of convulsions has been described under diseases of the head. Four or five doses of the powder made of equal parts of castorium, origanum and cumin would be beneficial.

15.5.28. Prolapse Ani

§1509 The child should be seated in warm water in which equal quantities of pomegranate rind, fresh myrtle leaves, myrrh, chestnuts, dried roses, burnt hart's horn, alum, goat's hooves, pomegranate blossoms and galls have been boiled; when tepid, this water can also be used for an enema.

15.5.29. Enteritis

§1510 Sometimes, children may develop enteritis after exposure to cold. In such cases, the following prescription proves useful. Three drachms each of the nasturtium and cumin ground together, sieved and thoroughly mixed with cow-butter is given in small quantities with cold water.

15.5.30. Intestinal Worms

§1511 Children frequently suffer from tiny worms near the anus. Round worms are not common and the tape worms are generally rare. Round worms may be treated with a small quantity of absinthe water mixed with milk according to individual toleration. Sometimes embelia wormwood, ox-bile or colocynth pulp are applied to the abdomen as plasters. Thread worms are treated with a powder containing one part each of Roman ginger and turmeric mixed with two parts of sugar and given with cold water.

15.5.31. Intertrigo

§1512 A dusting powder made of ground myrtle leaves, lily root and dried roses or powdered galangale, and lentil or barley flour may be used.

15.6. Regimen for Older Children

§1513 From the age of four to seven, children should be carefully supervised and helped to develop healthy manners. Outbursts of unnecessary anger, fear and anxiety should be prevented. This is best ensured by considering the desires, wishes and aversions of the child. The natural tendencies of the child should be properly guided and encouraged. Things which arouse disgust should be discouraged. This kind of training is good both for the body and the mind. The mind is benefited by good habits and manners, which are permanently ingrained in the child's personality by early training. The benefit to the body is obvious from the way various temperaments produce different kinds of behavior.

§**1514** When some habit or trait is thoroughly established, it produces corresponding changes in the temperament. Thus, anger produces unusual degree of heat in the body, while sorrow produces undue cold and dryness. Similarly, mental torpor dulls the nervous and mental instinctive drives and makes the constitution phlegmatic. In short, a proper balance and moderation in the behavior underlie both mental and physical health.

§**1515** In the morning, the child should first have a bath and then be allowed to play for an hour or so before breakfast. After breakfast he may be left to play for a longer time and again have another bath before lunch. There should be no drinking of water during the meals, as this leads to the premature absorption of imperfectly digested food.

§**1516** At the age of six, the child should be sent to a teacher for necessary instruction. Care should, however, be taken not to burden the child all at once. By this time, bathing should be reduced and the amount of exercise and play before the meals increased. Children should not be allowed wine, especially when they are already inclined towards undue heat and moisture. The reason is that wine increases the bilious humor and excessive bile is particularly harmful at this age, as it cannot be removed by dieresis; moreover, there is no need in them for moistening of the joints. Normally, this humor is neither so much as to require special elimination, nor do the joints particularly need any moistening.

§**1517** Children should be allowed to drink as much of sweet and pure water as they like. The same regimen suitably modified should be continued up to the age of fourteen. During adolescence, the body fluids tend to decrease, thus, producing greater dryness and hardness in the tissues; hence, exercise should be gradually reduced at this time. Care should, however, be taken that the exercise is only moderate, neither too strenuous nor violent.

§**1518** After the age of fourteen, a regimen similar to that for healthy adults should be quite suitable. Hence, we should now consider the fundamentals of health preservation in the adults and describe exercise in the first instance.

Lecture 16: The Regimen for the Physically Mature

16.1. A Word About Exercise

§**1519** Since the regimen[1] for maintaining health consists essentially in the regulation of: (1) exercise; (2) food; and (3) sleep, we may begin our discourse with the subject of exercise. We may define exercise as voluntary movement entailing deep and hurried respiration.

§**1520** Once we direct the attention towards regulating exercise as to amount and time, we shall find there is no need for such medicines as are ordinarily required for remedying diseases dependent on [abnormal] matters, or diseases of temperament consequent upon such. This is true provided the rest of the regimen is appropriate and proper

§**1521** We know that this must be so when we reflect how in regard to nutriment, our health depends on the nutriment being appropriate for us and regulated in quantity and quality. For not one of the aliments which are capable of nourishing the body is converted into actual nutriment in its entirety. In every case digestion leaves something untouched, and nature takes care to have that evacuated. Nevertheless, the evacuation which nature accomplishes is not a complete one. Hence at the end of each digestion there is some superfluity left over. Should this be a frequent occurrence, repetition would lead to further aggregation until something measurable has accumulated. As a result, harmful effete substances would form and injure various parts of the body. When they undergo decomposition, putrefactive diseases arise [bacterial infections, Tr.]. Should they be strong in quality, they will give rise to an intemperament; and if they should increase in quantity, they would set up the symptoms of plethora which have already been described. Flowing to some member, they will result in an inflammatory mass, and their vapors will destroy the temperament of the substantial basis of the breath.

§1522 That is the reason why we must be careful to evacuate these substances. Their evacuation is usually not completely accomplished without the aid of toxic medicines, for these break up the nature of the effete substances. This can be achieved only by toxic agents, although the drinking of them is to a certain extent deleterious to our nature. As Hippocrates says: "Medicine purges and ages." More than this the discharge of superfluous humor entails the loss of a large part of the natural humidities and of the breath, which is the substance of life. And all this is at the expense of the strength of the principal and auxiliary members, and therefore they are weakened thereby. These and other things account for the difficulties incident to plethora, whether they remain behind in the body or are evacuated from it.

§1523 Now exercise is that agent which most surely prevents the accumulation of these matters, and prevents plethora. The other forms of regimen assist it. It is this exercise which renews and revives the innate heat, and imparts the necessary lightness to the body, for it causes the subtle heat to be increased and daily disperses whatever effete substances have accumulated; the movements of the body help to expel them conveying them to those parts of the body whence they can readily leave it. Hence the effete matters are not allowed to collect day after day and besides this, as we have just said, exercise causes the innate heat to flourish and keeps the joints and ligaments firm, so as to be always ready for service, and also free from injury. It renders the members able to receive the nutriment, in being free from accumulated effete matters. Hence it renders the attractive faculty active, resolves fibrosis in the tissues, rendering the members light and the humidities attenuated, and it dilates the pores of the skin.

§**1524** To forsake exercise would often incur the risk of "hectic," because the instinctive drives of the members are impaired, inasmuch as the deprivation of movement prevents the access to them of the innate breath. And this last is the real instrument of life for every one of the members.

§**1525** The value of exercise includes the following: (1) it hardens the organs and renders them fit for their functions; (2) it results in a better absorption of food, aids assimilation, and, by increasing the innate heat, improves nutrition; (3) it clears the pores of the skin; (4) it removes effete substances through the lungs; (5) it strengthens the physique. Vigorous exercise invigorates the muscular and nervous system.

16.1.1. The Varieties of Exercise

§**1526** There are two main forms of exercise: (a) that pertaining to the ordinary human undertakings; and (b) that which is undertaken for its own sake—namely, for the advantage accruing from its pursuit. [i.e., sports, athletics, gymnastics, etc.]

§**1527** There are differences between the two forms. One is strong and powerful, the other weak and light; one is speedy, the other slow. Athletics implies strenuous exertions combining swiftness with energy. Recreative exercise, undertaken for relaxation, implies leisurely movements. There are all grades between these extremes, and there is a mean between them [called moderate exercise]. List of the forms of exercise include:

16.1.2. Strenuous Exercises

§**1528** Strenuous forms include wrestling contests; boxing; quick marching; running, jumping over an object higher than one foot; throwing the javelin; fencing; equitation or horsemanship [hunting: Galen, Rhazes].[2] Also, clapping the two hands alternately before and behind, with a quick motion while standing on tip-toes [dancing[3] (Oribasius), swimming (*ibid.*)]. These are special forms of individual athletic exercises.

16.1.3. Mild Exercises

§1529 The following are recreative or milder modes of exercise: swaying or swinging to and fro, as when being carried in a litter; standing or reclining in small boats; fishing; sailing; being driven in horse-carriages or carried on camels or in palanquins or a horse-litter.

16.1.4. Vigorous Exercises

§1530 Among the more vigorous exercises are those performed by soldiers in camp, in military sports; field running: where a man runs on the field from end to end to and fro, lessening the distance each time until finally he comes to a stand in the middle; combat with one's shadow; exercise with the leather bag [which is filled with flour or sand, and hung to the level of the person's navel]; long jumping; high jumping; playing with a large ball [inflated skins or leather]; playing with a small, wooden ball on horseback [i.e., polo]; playing with a small wooden ball on horseback [i.e., polo] are also included along with stone-throwing; lifting heavy stones or weights, either while standing, or carrying them; scaling ropes; running galloping horses round in a circle; [leaping with a weight on the shoulders which exercises the spine: Galen].

§1531 There are various forms of wrestling. For instance, in one form, one of the wrestlers grasps the other and holds him by the tips of the hands. The other tries to get loose from his opponent. In another, one wrestler grips the right hand of his opponent and takes the left hand with his left, the two facing one another; then the one raises the other up into the air, and turns him round sometimes in the bent position, sometimes in the upright position. Again, the two wrestlers may press against one another breast to breast or one holds the other by the neck to pull him to the ground. Or, one may twist and press with his feet, twisting his legs round his opponent, or turn heel to heel. Various other movements of that kind are in vogue among wrestlers.

16.1.5. Brisk Exercises

§1532 Exercises involving swiftness include interchanging places with a partner as swiftly as possible, each jumping to and fro, either in time [to music] or irregularly. Another exercise is carried out with two stakes. The man jumps backwards repeatedly without moving his position, and plunges the two stakes on either side, one pace apart, causing the one on the right to go to the left, and the one on the left to go to the right. This is to be done as swiftly as possible.

§1533 Exercises involving vigor and swiftness should alternate with mild exercises, or with rest. The manner of the exercises should also be diversified, so that they are not always performed in the same way.

16.1.6. The Instructions for Exercise

§1534 There is an exercise which is appropriate for each individual. Gentle exercise (i.e., swinging: rocking in a swing) is beneficial for those who are debilitated by fevers or who are convalescing and can neither walk nor sit—for those weakened by a draught of hellebore and the like or for those whose diaphragm has been rendered enfeebled by disease. When it is done gently, it tends to induce sleep, and disperse flatulence, relieves various disorders of the head (i.e., stupor, forgetfulness) provokes the appetite, and favors movement of the bowels.

§1535 To ride in a litter [horse, camel, palanquin, etc.] is appropriate for those afflicted with semitertian fever, composite fevers, phlegmatic fevers, those who are dropsical, or have gouty pains or renal disorder. For this form of exercise renders effete matter in a condition favorable for excretion, and may be made gentle for the feeble, more vigorous for the more vigorous. Greater movement is produced in the humors by riding in a carriage, but when doing so one should face backwards, because this is better when the eyesight is weak, and it is an advantage to have the shadow in one's face.

§1536 Boating and sailing: to go out in a small boat, or in a larger sailing vessel is beneficial for lepra, dropsy, apoplexy, dilatation of the stomach and coldness of the stomach. For if the person is near the shore he is incited to vomit, and then when that subsides, the stomach is benefited. But to go on the high seas is more efficient for clearing up such disorders as we have named, because the mind is diverted by successive gladness and misery, and the organs of nutrition receive benefit in proportion to the exercise of the body itself.

16.2. The Exercises for Special Organs of the Body

§1537 Each member should be exercised in a manner appropriate for itself. (1) The hands and feet—the proper way to exercise these is obvious. (2) The organs of respiration, and the muscles of the chest. These may be exercised in various ways: (a) By singing and "vociferation." The voice is sometimes deep, sometimes loud, sometimes abrupt, sometimes used in all modes in one exercise. By this means the condition of the mouth, uvula, lips, tongue is improved. The muscles of the neck are improved in appearance. The color of the skin is improved. The chest is expanded. (b) Exercises in which the expiration is forced and the breath is held. These benefit the whole body, because they open up and purify the channels, including those of the breath.[4]

§1538 However, to use a loud voice for a long time is injurious because by continuing it vigorously too much air is taken in, which is itself harmful, and by continuing it too long, air must be expelled unduly, and this also is harmful. Therefore the rule is to begin gently, by reading aloud, speaking more and more loudly up to a certain point and then allowing the voice to sink by degrees. If the time occupied in this exercise is moderate, it is very helpful, but if the time is too long, there is risk of injury to health.[5]

§1539 Vision is exercised by inspecting minute objects, and sometimes by arranging that they are only poorly illuminated.

§1540 Audition is exercised by listening to faint sounds, or sometimes to loud ones.

§1541 Exercises appropriate to each individual member will be referred to when we speak of the maintenance of the health of each organ in the special volume.

16.2.1. *Important Instructions*

§1542 Whatever the exercise, one must ensure that its vigor or heating effect is not likely to affect some weak organ directly. Such an organ should only bear the brunt of the exercise secondarily. For instance, a person with varicose veins should not use an exercise in which the feet are much used. He should substitute an exercise which employs the upper parts of the body the neck, the head, and the hands. In this way the brunt of the effect of the exercise is borne first by the upper parts and by the feet last.

§1543 The exercise must be modified if the person is debilitated. If he is robust it should be made vigorous. You realize now that every organ has its own peculiar form of exercise. That the exercise for the eye is to gaze upon something delicate; that the exercise to strengthen and expand the chest is vocal, and consists of graduated singing exercises. Similarly with the teeth and the ear. Every member is considered in this way in the chapter specially devoted to it.

16.2.2. *The Time for Exercise*

§1544 The time to choose for beginning exercise is when the body is free from impurities in the internal organs and blood vessels so that there is no risk of unhealthy chyme being dispersed through the body by the exercise. Yesterday's food should have passed both gastric and hepatic digestion, and also intravascular digestion—the time for the next meal now approaching, as can be ascertained by examining the urine as to its substance and color.

§1545 If it is some time before the next meal is due, and there is a need for more nutriment, and the urine shows igneity (i.e., is high-colored), the natural yellowness having now passed off, it indicates that exercise at this time would be detrimental, namely by exhausting the strength.

§1546 For this reason, some people say that when vigorous exercise has to be undertaken, it is best that the stomach should not be quite empty: that there should still be a little food, and that this should be substantial in winter and light in summer.

§1547 Moreover, it is better to choose a time for exercise when one is not hungry, and when one is hot and moist rather than cold and dry. But the best time is when the state is between the two. Exercise in a man of hot and dry temperament may lead to illness, and he will benefit by avoiding it at such a time.

§1548 It is necessary, then, for a person who is about to take exercise that he should first get rid of the effete matters of the body by way of the intestines and bladder. Should friction be used in preparation for exercise, with the object of helping the bowels and opening the pores of the skin, it should be carried out with a rough towel and be followed by inunction with sweet (perfumed) oil made warm by being held in the hollow of the palm. This inunction is done according to rule until the limbs show a florid blush; the massaging should not be too forcible nor the penetration too great. It is done with the hands, which pass over many various positions in order to ensure that every part of the muscular system has been dealt with. When completed, the massage is stopped and exercise may begin.

§1549 In the spring, the best time for exercise is round midday and it should be done in a moderately warm room. In summer, the exercise should be done earlier. In winter, it should be delayed until evening, but there are other objections to doing so. Consequently, in winter, the place used should be made moderately warm, to enable the exercise to be carried out at a time when the aliment is digested and the effete matters have been expelled.

16.3. The Amount of Exercise

§1550 Three things must be taken into consideration: (1) the color—as long as the skin goes on becoming florid, the exercise may be continued. After it ceases to do so, the exercise must be discontinued; (2) movement—exercise may be continued as long as the movement is moderated; (3) the condition of the organs-exercise must not be continued after they show any puffiness. Should the insensible perspiration lessen and the visible sweating stop, the exercise must stop. Should the action of the skin have ceased, one applies a strongly-diaphoretic oil as an inunction, especially if the exercise were one which exerted the breathing.

§1551 At the conclusion of the first day's exercise, you will know the degree of exercise allowable and when you know the amount of nourishment the person can bear, do not make any change in either on the second day. Arrange that the measure of aliment, and the amount of exercise shall not exceed the limit ascertained on the first day.

16.4. Massage

§1552 Varieties: (1) hard massage: this stretches and contracts, and braces the body; (2) soft massage has a relaxing effect; (3) repeated massage diminishes the fat of the body; (4) moderately hard massage; (5) rough massage: this is done with rough towels. It draws the blood rapidly to the surface; and (6) gentle massage is done with the palm or with soft towels. It draws the blood together and retains it in one member.

§1553 The object of friction is to render thin persons heavier, and heavy persons thinner; to brace flabby persons, and to modify those who are not pliable enough (giving tone to the body).

16.4.1. The Preparatory Massage

§1554 Massage as a preparatory to athletics. The massage begins gently, and then becomes more vigorous as the time approaches for the exercise.

16.4.2. Restorative Massage

§1555 Massage as a sequel to athletics is called restorative friction. This produces repose. Its object is to disperse the effete matter formed in the muscles and not expelled by the exercise. It causes them to disperse and so removes fatigue [the feeling of lassitude]. Such friction is soft and gentle, and is best done with oil [or perfumed ointments: Aeg.]. It must not be hard, or heavy, or rough, because that would roughen the members. Young men would be hindered in growth. But for adults it is less harmful.

§1556 It is less detrimental to err on the side of hardness than on that of softness, because it is easier to correct undue dispersal [of effete matters] than to prepare the tissues (by soft friction) for the reception of effete substances. On the other hand, hard and rough friction to an excess in youths is a hindrance to their growth.

§1557 You will learn about this under the heading of the proper time for massage. For the present it will suffice to say that restorative friction should be begun vigorously at first, and with oil; that then it should be moderated, but not stopped, until all roughness has gone. It is best that many persons should do it together. The person, having been rubbed, now stretches out his massaged limbs to help to expel the effete matters from them, and a broad bandage or binder is applied over the regions to which the muscles concerned belong. He should hold his breath as long as he can, while relaxing his abdominal muscles if he should at the same time make his thoracic muscles tense, if he can. Finally, he makes his abdominal muscles tense again. In this way the intestines are given a certain amount of restorative massage. One may pause to take a breath between the exercises; or sometimes restorative massage may be given in the middle of the exercise. Thus, it may be omitted or resorted to according to whether the exercise is to be prolonged or not. A person who desires restorative massage does not need much preliminary massage, unless there is something about his condition with which he is not satisfied. If he does not desire restorative massage he will undergo more thorough preliminary massage. If fatigue should be experienced, inunction with oil will be employed, as we have stated. If he should experience a sense of dryness, the massage will be increased until the natural mean condition is attained.

§1558 Causing friction without massage (compression) is beneficial if sleep is due, because it cheers the body and prevents humid matters from flowing into the joints.

16.5. Bathing and Bath Houses

§1559 For the type of person whose regimen we are discussing, a bath which induces resolution is not required, because his body is inwardly pure. A person does not need the bath except in order to derive a gentle warmth from it, and a moderate amount of moisture. That is why such persons should not stay long in it.

§1560 If such persons employ a full length (copper) bath, they should stay in it only until the color of the skin becomes red, and the skin becomes puffy; they should leave it as soon as dispersal (of humors) begins. The surrounding air should be moistened by a sweet-water spray The actual washing should now be quick and the bath left quickly.

§1561 A person should not go into the bath immediately after exercise. He should rest properly first.

§1562 The forms of bath have already been referred to and are dealt with again in another place.

§1563 At this point we should state that all who propose to bathe should pass through the successive rooms of the bath-house according to rule, and not linger in the hot room long enough to cause harm; they should stay long enough in the rest-room to give time for the dispersal of the effete substances, otherwise there is a risk of weakness which will interfere with digestion and leave a susceptibility to the causes of septic fevers.

§1564 A person who wishes to become stout should take his bath after a meal, if he is not likely to develop obstructions in consequence.

§1565 If he is of hot temperament, he may guard against the formation of obstructions by drinking oxymel [a mixture of vinegar and honey].

§1566 If he is of cold temperament, he should take penny-royal and capsicum.

§1567 If it is desired to reduce fat, and to procure the resolution of the humors, the person should bathe while fasting, and stay a long time in the bath.

16.5.1. The Beneficial Effects of Baths

§1568 The benefits are (1) induction of sleep; (2) dilation of pores; (3) cleansing of skin; (4) dispersal of the undesirable waste matters; (5) maturation of abscesses; (6) drawing of nutriment towards the surface of the body; (7) assistance to the physiological dispersion and excretion of poisonous matters; (8) prevention of diarrhea; and (9) removal of fatigue effects.

16.5.2. The Injurious Effects of Baths

§1569 To ensure against impairment of health the bather should wait till after the gastric and hepatic digestions are both completed. Where there is any risk of the bilious humor undergoing fermentative decomposition, and one wishes to bathe fasting, the aliment should be attenuant. But a person of hot temperament, in whom the bilious humor is plentiful, should not enter the hot chamber at all. The best things for such persons to take are: bread soaked with the juice of fruits or rose-water. Cold drinks should not be taken either while in the bath or when leaving it, for the pores are now open, and coldness would speedily enter and pass towards the principal organs and damage their functional capacity. Articles which are, very heating (hot) should also be avoided, especially water because thereby there is a risk of the warmth penetrating rapidly to the principal organs and this predisposes to wasting and hectic. Further, such persons should take care not to leave the bath suddenly, or to uncover the head, thus exposing the body to cold. If it is winter, the body should be well covered with towels.

§1570 A person suffering from fever should avoid the bath at the febrile period. The same applies to a person suffering from any form of loss of continuity, or from inflammation.

§1571 From the above, therefore, it will be clear to you that baths have the following effects: warming, cooling, humectant, desiccants beneficial, harmful.

§1572 Injurious effects include the fact that the heart is weakened if the person stay too long in the bath. The bath produces syncope and nausea, sets stagnant humors in circulation, disposes them to undergo putrescence, and to pass down into the weaker members, with consequent inflammatory deposits in both internal and external members.

16.5.3. Bathing in Cold Water and Starting With It

§1573 The bath is only beneficial if all the proper rules are observed, and if the age of the person, his physique and build, are suitable, and the seasons is appropriate (i.e. the summer). The contra indications are: nausea, or a feeling of satiety associated with indigestion; vomiting; or diarrhea; or want of sleep; or nasal catarrh. The person must not be at the age of boyhood, nor at old age. [Therefore he must be in the prime of life.] The moment chosen for the bath should be one at which the body is light and the movements appropriate.

§1574 The object of bathing with cold water following upon one with hot water is to make the external parts stronger and to retain the natural heat. For this purpose the water used should not be very cold, but of a medium temperature.

§1575 Bathing with cold water after exercise. Here the preparatory massage should be more vigorous than usual. The customary inunction with oil is employed as well before the exercise, which must be less vigorous than usual. The exercise completed, the person plunges into the cold water tank, so as to harden all the members at once. He stays in the cold water in proportion to his lightness, and as long as he can without shivering ensuing. Then, having come out of the water, let him be rubbed as we have described (i.e. till the skin is red) and let him take more food than drink. The time which elapses before the natural color returns to the skin must be noted, because if the color returns rapidly, the duration of the cold bath was reasonable, whereas if there is delay, it shows that the stay in the water was too prolonged. In this way the person will know the proper duration of the bath for the future.

§1576 Should the person wish to reenter the water after the massage, and after regaining his color and normal heat, he must on this occasion enter the water gradually, and on a hot summer's day before the hottest part of the day, and when no wind is blowing. He must not do so when in a state of lassitude after coitus, or after a meal which has not had time to digest, or after emesis, or after evacuation of the bowels or after gastro-enteritis, or insomnia, or if the body or stomach be enfeebled.

§1577 Cold bathing should not be done after exercise except in the case of the very robust. Even then the rules which we have given should be followed. To use cold baths in the ways we have named drives the natural heat suddenly into the interior parts, and then invigorates the strength so that the person should leave the bath twice as strong as when he entered.

16.6. Concerning Food

§1578 In seeking to maintain health care must be taken that the essential basis of the meal is not in medicinal nutrients like potherbs, fruits, and such-like. For things which are tenuous in character over oxidize the blood, while those which are dense render the blood phlegmatic and the body heavy.

16.6.1. Menu

§1579 The meal should include: (1) meat especially kid of goats; veal, and year-old lamb; (2) wheat, which is cleaned of extraneous matter and gathered during a healthy harvest without ever having been exposed to injurious influences; (3) sweets of appropriate temperament; (4) fragrant wine of good quality.

§1580 Any other kinds of food can only be regarded as a sort of medicament or preservative.

§1581 The more nutritious fruits are: figs, grapes (ripe and sweet), dates from countries and regions in which they are indigenous. But if superfluity arises after partaking of these fruits, speedy evacuation should be procured.

16.6.2. The Appetite

§1582 A person should not eat unless hungry. Nor should he delay his meal until the appetite has passed off. This rule does not apply in the case of the fictitious appetite met with in drunkards or the subjects of nausea. If fasting be continued the stomach will fill up with putrescent humors.

16.6.3. Hot Meals

§1583 In winter the food should be hot; in summer cold or only slightly warm. A food should not be served either hot or cold if it is likely to be spoiled thereby.

16.6.4. The Quantity of Food

§1584 Nothing is worse than to eat to repletion during a time of plenty after having been in a state of starvation during a time of famine, and vice versa. But the transition period is the worse. For we often see many people who lack food at a time of famine, and eat to repletion when a fertile year comes with fatal result. Great repletion is very dangerous in any case, whether in regard to food or to drink. For how often do not people overeat, and perish from the consequent choking of the channels of the body?

16.6.5. The Order of the Meals

§1585 An error in eating or drinking any of the medicinal nutrients is to be corrected according to the digestion and maturation thereof. The person must be protected from the intemperament which is likely to arise. To effect this, one takes the contrary substance until the digestion is completed. Thus, if the aliment was cold (i.e., cucumber, gourd), temper it with its opposite (i.e., onions, leek). If the aliment was hot, temper it with the opposite (i.e., cucumber, purslane). If the aliment is binding, take some food which will open and evacuate, and then fast for a suitable period. A person in this state—and this is true for all who wish to maintain their health—should not partake of food until there is a definite appetite, and unless the stomach and upper small intestine have emptied themselves of the previous meal, because there is nothing more harmful to the body than to super impose digestive matter upon incompletely digested food. There is also nothing worse than nauseative indigestion especially when this is the result of bad foods. If these are gross, the following symptoms and illnesses arise: pains in the joints, in the kidneys; dyspnea, podagra, indurative enlargement of the spleen and liver, illnesses in which the serous or atrabilious humors are concerned. If the foods were attenuated, then acute fevers, malignant fevers, and grave acute inflammatory disturbances would develop.

16.6.6. Aids to Digestion

§1586 However, it is sometimes really necessary to give a food or a substance like food, on the top of another food, by way of medicine. For example, if one has taken sharp and salty nutrients, one may further take humectant aliments which have no flavor, before the former have digested completely The chyme by which the body is nourished is then rectified. This is a suitable measure for cases of this kind, and the use of exercise is not indicated. The contrary holds good in the case of those who partake of gross foodstuffs and afterwards admix with them something which is speedily digested and acrid in taste.

16.6.7. Food and Exercise

§1587 A small amount of movement or activity after a meal allows the food to descend to the fundus of the stomach, especially if after this there is a desire to sleep. Mental excitement, emotion or vigorous exercise hinder digestion.

16.6.8. Seasons and Food

§1588 In winter, feebly nutrient foods like pot-herbs are not to be eaten. The aliments should be stronger and more solid in texture such as cereals, legumes, and the like. In summer, the contrary is true.

16.6.9. The Size of Meals

§1589 In regard to the quantity of food taken at a meal, no meal should be bulky enough to completely satisfy the appetite, One should rise from the table while some appetite or desire for food is still present for such remnants of hunger will disappear in the course of an hour. Custom is to be regarded in this regard, for a meal is injurious when it brings heaviness to the stomach, and wine is injurious when it exceeds moderation, and swims in the stomach.

§1590 If one ate to excess one day, one should fast the next, and a longer sleep should be taken in some place which is neither hot nor cold. If sleep refuses to come, one should take gentle walking exercise and allow neither rest nor recumbent position. A little pure wine should be taken. Rufus say: "Walking after a meal is gratifying to me, for it gives a good preparation for the evening meal."

16.6.10. Food and Sleep

§1591 A short sleep after a meal is useful; one should lie first on the right side, then on the left, and finally turn back again to the right side. If the body be covered with a number of wraps and the neck be raised, this will aid digestion. The limbs should slope downward and not upwards.

§1592 The standard size of the meal depends on usage and vigor. A normally robust person should take as much as will not produce a sense of heaviness, or a sense of tightness of the hypochondria. There should be no subsequent rumbling in the stomach or splashing of the food on bodily movement. Nausea should not be experienced, nor a canine appetite, nor loss of appetite, nor great disinclination for exertion, nor sleeplessness. The taste of the food should not repeat in the eructations. If the taste of food lingers in the mouth a very long time after the meal it shows that the latter was too heavy.

16.6.11. The Quantity of Food

§1593 Indications that the meal was moderate: the pulse does not become full; the breathing does not become shallow. The latter only occurs if the stomach is compressing the diaphragm, thus making breathing shallow and short. The pressure to be met by the heart increases after a large meal, and as the force of the heart does not diminish, the pulse becomes large and full.

6.6.12. Food and Temperament

§1594 The following should be observed: a person who experiences a sense of heat and flushing after a meal should not take a whole meal at one sitting, but partake of the food in small portions at short intervals to avoid the effects of repletion such as shivering followed by a sense of heat like that in a sthenic fever. This is due to the heating effect of the food; a person who cannot digest the amount of food appropriate for him should increase the number of articles of diet, but diminish the quantity; a person of atrabilious constitution needs a diet which is very humectant but not very heating; a person of choleric constitution needs a diet which is humectant and infrigidant; a person who generates hot inflammable blood needs feebly nutritious articles of food, which are cold. One who generates phlegmatic blood needs feebly nutritious articles of diet which are hot and attenuant.

16.6.13. The Order of the Dishes

§**1595** The order in which the components of a meal are to be taken—a person who is desirous of maintaining his health needs to be watchful of this matter. Thus, one should not take a tenuous food, which is rapidly digested, after taking a very nutritious dish which is slowly digested. An exception to this rule has been named above. The reason is that the first article of food will be digested first and therefore float over the other, unable to enter the blood. Consequently it ferments and decomposes, and in addition sets up decomposition of the food next taken. The reverse order, therefore, is the one to adopt, so that the labile food will pass on with the other into the intestine, and then undergo complete digestion.

§**1596** Fish and similar articles of food should not be taken after laborious work or exercise, because they undergo decomposition and then decompose the humors.

§**1597** Some persons may be allowed to eat an article of food in which there is a styptic property as a preparatory to the actual meal.

16.6.14. The Prescription of the Diet

§**1598** Some persons have an idiosyncrasy of the stomach in which the foods leave it very rapidly and do not stay in it long enough to undergo gastric digestion. This explains the necessity for taking the idiosyncrasy of the stomach and its temperament into consideration [along with other factors when drawing up a diet].

§1599 There are some persons in whom tenuous food, instead of being digested quickly as it should, undergoes decomposition in the stomach, whereas less rapidly digestible foods are digested more readily. The stomach of such a person is designated igneous. But other persons are exactly the opposite. Therefore the rules to be given must be adapted to the peculiarity of each patient.

§1600 The countries in which people live have also their own natural properties, which are distinct from the ordinary rule. This must also be borne in mind, and a test must be made to ascertain what the rule should be. Thus, a food which is often used, though injurious to a certain degree, may be more appropriate for a given individual than a food which he does not often take, though its character is good.

§1601 Then again, there is a food which is to be regarded as appropriate to everyone's physique and temperament. To change from such a diet would prove injurious and detrimental to him. Good and laudable foods may be injurious to some. They should therefore avoid them. But persons who are able to digest a bad foods should not be deceived, because (for all they know) they will some day give rise to bad humors and the consequent obstinate ailments.

§1602 Good food may often be allowed liberally in the case of persons in whom the humors are unhealthy, so long as diarrhea from intestinal weakness does not supervene in consequence. But if the person be of spare habit, and liable to have the motions loose, the diet should consist of moist aliments, because they are digested quickly, even though it is a fact that such persons can tolerate various heavy foods, and are less liable to be affected adversely by intrinsic noxae, and are more susceptible to the antagonistic influence of extraneous noxae.

16.6.15. The Excess of Meat

§1603 An active person accustomed to take much meat needs frequent bleeding. A person inclined to be frigid in temperament should drink substances which cleanse the stomach, intestines and the (mesenteric) veins including confections of spices and myrobalan electuary.

§1604 It is a bad practice to combine nutrients of diverse character in one meal and so prolong it. For by the time the last portion has entered the stomach, the first portion is already digested, and therefore the various contents of the stomach are not all at then same stage of digestion.

§1605 Palatability—one should remember too that aliment is best which has the most agreeable flavor for the walls of the stomach and the retentive faculty jointly apply themselves better to a food of good substance and the efficiency of the retentive power is assisted when the principal members all mutually concur the temperament of one being not more divergent from that of another than natural. That is the requisite condition. The conditions are not fulfilled, for instance, if the temperaments are not normal, or alike in the respective members. Thus, the temperament of the liver may differ to an unnatural extent from that of the stomach. Among noxious influences arising from the taste of aliments is that if very gross aliments are tasty, a person may be tempted to eat too freely of them.

16.6.16. The Number of Meals

§1606 In taking successive satiating meals, it is best for a person to take only one on one day and two on the next (morning and evening). But one must not be too strict in this rule, for if a person is accustomed to have two meals a day, and then takes only one, he will be weakened and his digestive faculty will suffer. A person of weak digestion should take two meals a day lessening the amount partaken. On occasion he may eat once a day. A person who is accustomed to take one good meal a day will, on resuming the habit of two meals a day, suffer from weakness, lack of energy, slackness. If he should take no food at bedtime, he will feel weak; and if he should take a late meal he will not be able to digest it, and will have acid eructations, nausea, bitter taste in the mouth, loose bowels and become moody, or irritable. This is because he has put into the stomach something to which it is not accustomed, and so he is liable to show some of the symptoms which befall a person whose aliment is not fully digested and these you are now acquainted with.

§1607 Among the symptoms arising when a person does not take a late meal are: subjective sensations at the cardiac orifice of the stomach, gnawing pains, a sensation of a void in the stomach so that all the interior organs and intestines feel as if they were suspended and, therefore, all clumped together. He passes scalding urine, and the feces produce a burning sensation as they are passed. There may be a feeling of cold in the extremities owing to the bilious humor being poured out into the stomach and irritating it and making it congested. This is more likely in persons of bilious temperament, and in those who have bilious humor in the stomach but not to an undue extent in the rest of the body; these suffer from loss of sleep, and keep turning over from one side to the other [in bed].

§1608 Persons then in whom the bilious humor is apt to accumulate in the stomach should take their meals divided, thereby taking the food quickly; the meal is taken before bathing. In other persons, exercise should be taken first, then the bath, and then the meal. The meal should not precede the bath in these cases. If circumstances demand that the meal betaken before the exercise, the food should consist of bread only, and to an amount no greater than can be easily digested. As it is necessary that the exercise should not be gentle if taken before food, so it is necessary that the exercise should be mild and gentle if it is taken after the meal.

§1609 When the appetite is depraved so that it prefers sharp tasting things to sweet or unctuous things, nothing is better than to procure emesis with such as oxymel with radish after fish.

§1610 A person who is stout should not eat at once after a bath, but should wait and take a little nap. He is best advised to take only one meal a day.

16.7. The Rules to be Observed After Meals

16.7.1. Exercise

§1611 One should not go to sleep immediately after a meal with the food still swimming in the stomach, and one should, as much as possible, abstain from much exercise after a meal, lest the food pass into the blood before it is sufficiently digested, or glide out of the stomach without being digested at all, or undergoes decomposition, since the exercise disturbs the gastric temperament.

16.7.2. Water and Meals

§**1612** Nor should much water be drunk after a meal, for it causes the food to leave the coats of the stomach and float about. One should wait, and not drink fluids until the food has left the stomach which is evidenced by the sensation of lightness in the upper part of the abdomen. However, if there were urgent thirst one may take a modicum of cold water through a straw, and the colder it is the less one will require. Such an amount would soothe the stomach and keep the food together. To sum up if a person must drink, it is better only to take so small an amount at the end of the meal (not during the meal), as will spread over and moisten the food, and therefore not be injurious.

16.7.3. Hunger

§**1613** To go to sleep while thirsty is beneficial to cold and moist temperaments, but is injurious to those in whom the temperament is too warm, because of the bilious humor being too plentiful. The same is true as regards going to sleep while fasting.

§**1614** Bilious humor comes to predominate in persons who fast and therefore flows into the stomach. Therefore when they eat any food it decomposes, and the same symptoms occur in them, whether asleep or awake, as when food corrupts. And, further more, there is loss of desire for food.

§**1615** When there is loss of appetite for food something needs to be given to counteract this and relax the bowels. For this purpose something mild, like prune, should be given, or something which does not suggest nausea, like a laxative fruit juice (manna). Meals may be resumed after the appetite has returned. Those whose tissues are moist in virtue of natural humidity are liable to speedy aperierat action, and are in consequence not able to fast as long as those whose tissues are dry in virtue of only a small (degree of natural) humidity: unless the latter should by rich in humidities other than those inherent to the substance of the tissues, for these are proper, good and receptive, and in consequence the natural faculty is able to change them completely into (true) nutriment.

16.7.4. Beverages

§**1616** To take wine after a meal is very unsatisfactory, for it is rapidly digested and enters the blood quickly and carries food on into the blood before it is properly digested. Obstructions and decompositions in this imperfectly digested aliment ultimately arise.

16.7.5. Sweets

§**1617** Sweet things readily produce obstructions in the channels of the body because the attractive faculty-draws them into the blood before they have been properly digested. Obstructions culminate in various diseases of which dropsy is one.

16.7.6. Contamination of Food

§**1618** Heaviness of the air or water, especially that of summertime, favors the decomposition of food. In this case, then, it is not harmful to take a tempered wine after a meal, or hot water in which xylaloes and mastic have been toiled.

16.7.7. Excessive Heat in the Stomach

§**1619** If a person whose alimentary tract is hot and strong eats heavy food, it will give rise to flatulence in the stomach and fermentative ailments.

§**1620** When a person takes a tenuous article of food upon an empty stomach, the latter contracts on it, and if he then takes something heavy, the stomach abandons the tenuous food and ceases digesting it, and it undergoes putrescence in consequence. This would be avoided by allowing an interval of time to elapse between the two kinds of food. Undcr these circumstances it is best to take the heavy food slowly, because then the hold which the stomach has on the tenuous food is not broken.

16.7.8. Dyspepsia

§1621 When a state of over repletion exists in regard to some meal, whether as a result of exercise (which causes undue hunger), or because a draught has been taken as well, then there will be a need for rapid emesis. If this should fail, or one cannot vomit, the person should sip hot water until the repletion is displaced and sleep supervenes. The person should therefore lie down to sleep. Let him sleep as long as he will. But should this not suffice, or should he be unable to go to sleep, reflect whether the natural course of events is likely to save you from procuring emesis. If so, good. If not, assist the natural power by any gentle laxative, such as myrobalan electuary, confection of roses, or origanum prepared with sugar or honey; or by the use of such things as cumin, spiced candies, asphodel and cabbage ptisan. It is not as bad to be replated with wine as with solid food.

§1622 Among the (aperient) remedies which are suitable after food are: aloes to the bulk of three chick-peas; or half a drachm of aloes, half a drachm of mastic, and a sixth of a drachm of niter.

§1623 Mild remedies are: turpentine resin to the amount of two or three chickpeas; niter in an equal quantity, or less, if necessary. Another much praised remedy is to use an epitheme with wine.

§1624 If none of these remedies succeed, let the patient sleep for a long time, and abstain from food for a whole day. Then, if he feels better, let him bathe, and place a hot blanket over the abdomen, and see that the aliments are tenuous.

16.7.9. Fullness of the Stomach

§1625 If the food is still not properly digested, in spite of all these measures, and heaviness, distension, and lack of energy are experienced, you may know that the veins are already overcharged with effete matters. Bulky and unneeded nutriment, even were it digested in the stomach, would hardly undergo the proper changes in the veins, and so would remain "crude" within them, and stretch them, even to bursting point. This is the explanation of the lack of energy, the heaviness, the desire to stretch oneself and the yawnings. The treatment in such a case consists in securing the release of the superfluities from the blood vessels.

§1626 If these are not the symptoms, but there is only a transient weariness, followed later by another form of weariness, this should be treated in the manner to be described.

16.7.10. Age and Diet

§1627 If a person should be very advanced in years, and his body does not derive as much benefit from the food as it did when he was young, and if his aliments become simply effete matters, then he should not eat as much as he used to do.

§1628 If a person is accustomed to a heavy diet and then lightens it by the use of attenuant foods, the new food material is unable to keep the channels of the body as full as bearer on resuming the heavy-foods, obstructions are brought about.

16.7.11. Ill Effects of Food

§1629 The injurious effects of heating or calefacient foods can be corrected by the use of syrup containing acetic acid, especially when made with seeds, for then the syrup is more efficient. If honey is used however, the simple syrup will suffice. The injurious effect of "cold" foods is corrected by the use of hydromel, and its syrup, and caraway.

§1630 Heavy and light foods—to correct aliments which are heavy, a person having a hot temperament should use acetous syrup made of strong seeds; a person with a cold temperament should use a little capsicum or peppermint.

§1631 Tenuous foods are better for the health, but less valuable for the vegetative faculties and strength. Heavy foods have the opposite value. Hence, for a person in need of a tonic, aliments which make strong chyme are necessary and-such as antagonize the hunger-feeling. But they should not be taken in greater quantity than can be digested. Heavy foods are better borne by those who take plenty of exercise or are accustomed to heavy work. Probably the deep sleep which this favors helps the digestion. But on the other hand they lose much by sweating. And as their livers seize whatever of the aliment has not yet digested fully, this paves the way for fatal illnesses towards the end of life, or at the beginning of life, the more so because they trust in their digestive powers too much. This power is really due to the deep sleep which is customary, and that is lost by old age.

16.7.12. Fruits

§**1632** Fresh fruit is only good for those who carry out hard work, or take much exercise, or for persons with plenty of bilious humor, or during the height of summer. Fruit should be taken before a meal, namely, for instance, apricots, mulberries, melons, peaches, and prunes. But it is better to regulate oneself by using other articles of food than these, for they render the blood too watery, and so it is apt to ferment.

§**1633** Hence the juices of fruits, unless taken at a seasonable time, pave the way for putrefactive processes. So, too, any food which comes to burden the blood with "crude" humor has this effect, though it is true that sometimes such a food may be beneficial. That is why people who make use of such aliments, even though they are primarily infrigidant, are likely to develop febrile diseases.

§**1634** You will also realize that it is when watery humor is not dispersed, but lingers in the blood-vessels, that it usually becomes toxic. However, when exercise is taken before such aquosities have become aggregated, and exercise is taken immediately after eating the fruit, these aquosities will disperse and the noxious effect of the fruits is thereby lessened.

§**1635** Note too that the presence of a crude serous humor or of wateriness in the blood prevents the nutrient part of the food from adhering to the tissues, some of the nutritive value of the food being lost as a consequence.

§**1636** A person who partakes of fruit must (therefore) take walking exercise afterwards, and then eat something which will cause the (aquosities) to flow out.

16.7.13. VEGETABLES

§**1637** Aliments which give rise to (1) wateriness; (2) crude, raw, immature humor and (3) gross humor and bilious humor, give rise to febrile diseases. This is because: (1) the watery parts permit putrescence to occur in the blood; (2) viscous gross substances close the orifices (of the juice-canals); and (3) the increase of bilious humor adds to the heat of the body, and renders the blood sharp.

§**1638** Bitter pot-herbs are sometimes very advantageous in winter time, just as tasteless herbs are beneficial in summer time.

§**1639** Correctives of unwholesome foods—if a person is bound to partake of unwholesome aliments, he should do so seldom and sparingly, and should counteract their action by combining with them something of a contrary effect. Thus, if a certain sweet food is injurious, he may counteract it by a sour aliment like vinegar, and pomegranate, and an acetous syrup prepared with sour wine and quince and the like, and also by procuring evacuation. Should it be a sour aliment that is injurious to him, he may follow it up with honey, or old wine, taking this before the maturation and digestion of the former are complete. If it be an oily aliment that is injurious, this can be corrected by (a) pungent articles, like chestnut, myrtle-seeds carob bean of Syria, the fruit of the lote tree, medlar; (b) bitters, such as conserved elecampane; (c) salt and sharp substances, such as capers, onions, garlic [that is, articles usually belonging to the second course of a meal], and other contraries.

§**1640** If the body is in a state of repletion by unhealthy humors, this state may be counteracted by a liberal allowance of commendable attenuant aliments. If the body is one which is easily purged, moist and easily digested food should be made use of.

§**1641** Galen says that a humid article of food is nutrient when it is separated from all other qualities, and is as it were tasteless-being neither sweet nor sour, bitter nor acrid, pungent nor salty.

§1642 A heavy food which is divided up into small portions will be better borne than one which is taken solid.

§1643 If dry aliments be taken plentifully, the strength will fail and the color will fade, and the nature become dry.

§1644 Fatty food produces lack of energy and vim, and creates a false appetite. Cold food produces lack of vim and is infrigidative (or attenuant). Sour food has the same effect as old age; it dries the body and makes it lean. Sharp and salty food is injurious to the stomach. Salty food is bad for the eyesight.

§1645 If an appropriate aliment is oily, and is followed by an uncommendable aliment, the latter will decompose it.

§1646 Viscous aliment experiences delay in passing through the intestine.

§1647 Citrul [a species of cucumber] passes down the intestine more rapidly if the rind is taken, as well, than if first peeled. Bread also passes down more quickly if the crust be taken as well than if it be deprived thereof by crumbling it through a sieve.

§1648 If a fatigued person, who is accustomed to a mild regimen should take heavy foods as for instance, a dish of rice with soured milk after a long fast, it will come about that his blood becomes sharp in quality and as if ebullient. Hence reducing his regimen would be indicated (e.g., blood-letting), though only to a moderate extent. A similar remedy is applicable when a person is angry. (Quick-tempered, the bilious humor easily becomes dominant or astir).

§1649 Note, too, that sweet aliment accelerates the nature before the food is matured and digested, and the blood is tainted in consequence.

16.8. Dietetic Aphorisms

§1650 Certain rules must be noted in regard to combining various articles of food. Indian observers and others have long taught that (1) milk must not be taken with sour foods; (2) fish must not be taken with milk for in that case chronic ailments such as leprosy[6] may develop; (3) pulse must not be taken with cheese or radishes or with the meat of flying birds; (4) a polenta[7] of barley-meal should not follow on a dish of rice made with soured milk;[8] (5) eatables should not have oil added, or oil which has stood in a brass vessel; (6) meat should not be taken when it has been roasted over live coals (with certain herbs).

§1651 To have several courses to a meal is injurious for two reasons: (1) the rate of digestion is diverse, for the part that digests more speedily is admixed with a part which is not yet digested; (2) a person may eat too much of one dish. Already in ancient times, too, persons who had been exercising themselves avoided this error, being satisfied to partake of meat alone in the morning, and bread alone at supper-time.

§1652 During the summer it is best to take the main meal at an hour when the temperature is cooler.

§1653 During a period of fasting the stomach sometimes fills with unhealthy humors.

§1654 Note further that when meat is roasted, and taken with onions and eggs [a special recipe kabab],[9] it is very nutritious; but it is slow in passing through the intestines, and lingers in the caecum. White soup [a Syrian dish containing rice, honey, onions] is nourishing, and when onion is added it dispels flatulencies; if onions are omitted, borborygmi arises.

§1655 Some people consider that grapes are good to take after roasted meats; but the contrary is really the case; they are very bad indeed. So too, is a dish containing dates, figs, and the like. But (dry) pomegranate seeds are good.

§1656 Fowl—the flesh of partridge is dry and constipating; but that of chicken is moist and relaxing to the bowels. Roast fowls are better if they have been prepared (stuffed) in the belly of a kid or lamb because that preserves their moisture. Chicken-broth tempers the humors strongly; more so than fowl-broth, though the latter is more nutritious.

§1657 Kid of goat is better when cold than when warm because the steam quiesces it. The flesh of lamb is better when hot because its unsatisfactory odor is thereby dispersed.

§1658 Meat boiled in water and vinegar [a Persian dish] should be served hot, and then needs no saffron in it. But if served cold saffron must be introduced.

§1659 Honey confections may be made with dates or wheat flour (sweetmeats); but they are unhealthy because they cause obstructions and evoke thirst.

§1660 Bread is an unsatisfactory food when it does not digest, more so than meat when it does not digest.

16.9. Concerning Water and Beverages

16.9.1. Water

§1661 Water is more suitable for attempered constitutions when it is moderately cold, than when it has been cooled by the addition of snow, especially if the snow were not pure. Even with good snow, there remains the objection that that which passes out from it is harmful to the nerves and the organs of respiration and all the internal organs. Moreover a person cannot tolerate it unless he is very full-blooded, and it will do harm sooner or later, even after the lapse of years.

§1662 Certain empirics assert that one must not mingle well-water with river-water, except by taking the one after the other has passed out of the stomach.

§1663 We have already spoken about the properties and choice of waters and how to correct them when bad. Addition with vinegar rectifies unhealthy waters.

§1664 One should remember that it is very harmful to drink water while fasting, or after exercise, or after the bath, especially when either of these was carried out on an empty stomach. It is also harmful to gratify the false thirst of the night, like that from which drunkards or topers suffer, or when the vegetative power strives to accomplish digestion in the face of a preceding satiety with water. If the thirst be very urgent, the water should be such as has been exposed to cool air, and rinse out the mouth with cold water. If this is not effective, some water may be taken out of a vessel with a narrow mouth. This is sometimes agreeable to a toper, who would not be hurt by drinking while fasting. If a person cannot avoid drinking while fasting, let him take water; especially if he has been taking exercise. In this case, let him first drink wine diluted with hot water.

§1665 False thirst is relieved by going to sleep without quenching it with fluid. For during sleep the natural power disperses the matter which is the cause of the thirst, and it does this more effectively if the thirst was not yielded to by a draught. To attempt to allay false thirst by a draught is to interrupt the digestive power, and the false thirst will return later because the humor giving rise to it is still there. When there is false thirst, water should not be taken rapidly and greedily, but through a straw.

§**1666** It is bad to drink much cold water. If it is very imperative to do so, defer it till after a sufficient meal. Tepid water evokes nausea. Water warmer than that, if drunk frequently, weakens the [tone of the stomach. But when taken infrequently, it washes out the stomach and opens the bowels.

16.9.2. Beverages

§**1667** White light wine is best for those who are in a heated state, for it does not cause headache. But sometimes it is humectant. It may relieve a headache when that is due to heat in the stomach.

§**1668** Instead of a light white wine, one may use a wine which has been clarified by infusing honey or bread in it, especially if this is done two hours before the wine is required.

§**1669** Heavy wine, if it is sweet, is best for a person who wants to put on weight and become strong. But he must beware of developing obstructions. Old red wine is best for a person of cold phlegmatic constitution. It is bad to drink wine after any of the various dishes, for the reason we have already explained. It should not be taken until after digestion, the food having passed into the small intestine. To drink wine upon food forming bad chyme, either during the meal or before it has digested, is bad because it causes the bad chyme to be absorbed and pass into the remote parts of the body. The same is true if wine is taken after fruit, especially melons.

§**1670** It is better to begin with a small amount than a large one. To take two or even three glassfuls upon a meal is not hurtful to anyone accustomed thereto, or to a healthy person who has been bled.

§1671 Wine is beneficial for persons with a predominance of bilious humor, because it gets rid of the excess of this by provoking the urine. It is good for persons of humid temperament because it brings humidities to maturity. The better its aroma (bouquet) and taste, the more beneficial.

§1672 Wine is also very efficient in causing the products of digestion to become disseminated through the body. It cuts phlegm and disperses it. It separates of the bilious humor and draws it on into the urine. It renders the atrabilious humors more mobile and able to leave the system. It counteracts the harmful influence of this atrabilious humor by contrariety, and it breaks up all entanglements without the necessity of extraneous heat. The varieties of wine have been already enumerated in the proper place.

§1673 Wine does not readily inebriate a person of vigorous brain, for the brain is then not susceptible to ascending harmful gaseous products nor does it take up heat from the wine to any degree beyond what is expedient. Therefore it renders his mental power clearer than before; other talents are not affected in such an advantageous manner. The effect is different on persons who are not of this calibre.

§1674 A person who is weak in the chest, to the extent that wintertime is trying to the breathing, cannot [wisely] take much wine.

§1675 A person who wishes to take much wine should avoid taking much food beforehand, and the components of the meal should include diuretics. If he should become replete with food or wine, he should procure emesis and take hydromel (honey and water); then procure emesis again; then wash out the mouth with vinegar and honey, and apply cold water on the face.

§1676 If wine has an injurious effect on the body and is heating to the liver, the diet should include some dish containing for instance the juice of (sour) unripe grapes, and the like, and the articles of food which are generally served with the wine after the end of a meal (dessert) should include such as pomegranate, and tart things like citron.

§1677 If the wine is liable to go to the head, one should take less and take it dilute and clarified. After the meal, he should take such as quince with his wine.

§**1678** If the harmful effect of wine consists in being heating to the stomach, the dessert should include toasted myrtle seeds and one should suck a few camphor lozenges and other astringent and acrid things.[10]

§**1679** As you know, old wine is like a medicine. It is only feebly nutritious. New wine clogs the liver and produces a hepatic dysentery by giving rise to much gas. The best wine to take is that which is clear, white, tending to a red tinge, of good bouquet, and neither tart nor sweet in taste, neither old nor new.

§**1680** A good drink which is widely known is made as follows: take three parts of marjoram, and one of water. Mix well. Boil to a fourth.

§**1681** If a gnawing feeling come on after taking wine, take pomegranate, cold water and syrup of absinthe next morning. Enter the bath after partaking of a small meal.

§**1682** Wine which is thoroughly diluted softens the stomach, makes it humid and allays thirst. Diluted wine intoxicates quickly because the watery constituent takes it quickly into the blood.

§**1683** The wise person will avoid drinking wine when fasting or before the limbs have been refreshed in warm water, or after vigorous exercise; for both these entail a strain on the brain and nerves, and render a person liable to develop cramps and amentia; they produce either actual illness or at least undue heat.

§**1684** Frequent intoxication breaks down the constitution of the liver and brain, weakens the nerves and tends to produce diseases of the nervous system, apoplexy, and sudden death.

§**1685** When wine is taken to excess it is changed, in the case of some persons, into a bad kind of bilious humor or, in the case of others, into pure vinegar. In both cases, the changes in the stomach are very injurious.

§**1686** Some persons claim that it is an advantage to become intoxicated once or twice a month, for, they say, it allays the animal passions, inclines to repose, provokes the urine and sweat, and gets rid of effete matters.

§**1687** The most detrimental of the effects of wine is that upon the brain. That is why those who are not strong in that way should take but the very least amount of wine, and diluted.

§1688 If called to a person who has drunk wine to excess, emesis should be procured as speedily as possible. Failing that he may drink a considerable quantity of water, with or without honey. When emesis has been procured, he should bathe in a full length bath. Then he should be thoroughly rubbed with oil, and left to go to sleep.

§1689 To give wine to youths is like adding fire to a fire already prepared with matchwood. Young adults should take it in moderation. But elderly persons may take as much as they can tolerate.

§1690 Wine is borne better in a cold country than in a hot one.

§1691 If a person wishes deliberately to take his fill of wine, he must take no food, or anything sweet. The [Persian] white broth [made of meat, onions, butter, cheese, etc.] may be allowed; also grated bread steeped in broth made with fat meat cut into pieces. He should have an inunction. He should avoid physical labor or exercise. Then after the meal, when he wishes to drink, he should accompany it with almonds, salted lentils and a condiment prepared with salted capers.

§1692 It is an advantage to include in the menu cabbage boiled with meat; olives boiled in water, and the like. For this conduces to drinking more wine. Anything which lightens the fumes of the wine is also helpful for instance the seeds of Syrian beet; cumin, dry rue, pennyroyal, Nabathean salt, cardamoms; and more particularly, any aliments which are viscous and glutinous, for they aggregate the fumes (i.e., oily, sweet and viscous articles of food) and prevent inebriety in spite of drinking so much wine, by restraining the rapidity with which the wine enters the blood.

§1693 Inebriation is rapid: (1) when there is weakness of the brain; (2) when there is an abundance of humors; (3) when the wine is strong; (4) when the food is scanty; (53 when the regimen is itself depraved; and (6) when the wine is taken continuously (for a long time).

§1694 When the cause of the ready inebriation is weakness of the brain, the remedy is to use the epithemes named in the chapter on catarrh, give sedatives, and avoid fluids.

§1695 The following syrup averts inebriety: one part of juice of white cabbage; one part of juice of unripe pomegranate, a half-part of vinegar. Simmer. Take one ounce before taking the wine. The following is another remedy: pills containing salt, rue, black cumin. Eat pill by pill. The following is another: take seeds of Syrian beet, cumin, peeled bitter almond, pennyroyal, absinthe, Nabathean salt, cardamom, dry rue.

§1696 A person who is not afraid of a hot mixture may take two drachms by weight in a draught with cold water, fasting.

§1697 For agents which restore from inebriety, let the person take water and vinegar several times one after the other, or whey water and junket. Let him sniff at camphor and sandalwood. Put cold repercussives over his head, such as rose oil and wine vinegar.

§1698 The treatment of inebriety is discussed in Volume III.

16.10. Concerning Sleep and Wakefulness

§1699 If it is desirable to get a person unconscious quickly, without his being harmed, add sweet smelling moss to the wine, or lignum aloes.

§1700 If it is desirable to procure a deeply unconscious state, so as to enable the pain to be borne which is involved in painful applications to a member, place darnel water into the wine; or administer fumitory, opium, hyoscyamus (half-drachm dose of each); nutmeg, crude aloeswood (4 grains of each). Add this to the wine, and take as much as is necessary for the purpose. Or, boil black hyoscyamus in water, with mandragore bark, until it becomes red. Add this to the wine.

§1701 The causes of natural sleep and of lethargy; their opposite states (the waking state, and insomnia); their effects; the remedial measures applicable when they are baneful; the significance of each; and all other points about them, have been dealt with in brief in the appropriate place. The special treatment will be discussed later.

§1702 Physiological effects of sleep—at present we may say that sleep in moderation: (1) assists the vegetative drives in their functions; (2) brings the sensitive drives into repose and in so doing (3) renews and restores them and thereby (4) arrests the dissipation of the breath (the vital power). Hence, the digestion of the food in the several stages we have named is accomplished. Sleep also remedies the weakness due to the dispersal of the breath (vital power) in various ways; namely, by bodily fatigue, by coitus, by anger or violent emotional disturbance, and the rest.

§1703 Furthermore, a moderated amount of sleep brings about an equilibrium in regard to quantity and quality of the humors, and therefore it has a humectant and warming action, which is specially advantageous for the aged, who need their moisture preserving and renewing. That is why Galen said: "Every night I partake of a little packet of herbs and lettuce combined with aromatics; the former because they induce sleep, the latter because they rectify the coldness of the lettuce." And he said: "I am now careful to obtain sleep because I am an old man, and the humidity which sleep brings is beneficial to me."

§1704 This then is the way to obtain sleep. And if a bath be taken after the digestion of the meal has been completed, and plenty of hot water is poured over the head, this will be an additional help. A still more efficient method will be mentioned under medicaments.

§1705 Conditions to observe regarding sleep—healthy persons should pay attention to the subject of sleep: it must be moderate, properly timed, and excess must be avoided. And on the other hand they must avoid the injury resulting to mental and all other faculties from remaining awake too long.

§1706 However a person is often driven to keep awake, and refrain from sleep owing to a dread of syncope and loss of strength. The best sleep is that which is deep; and that which occurs after the food has passed on from the upper part of the intestine, and after the flatulencies and eructations which may have followed have subsided; for to sleep on this is detrimental in many ways, though the person himself may not know it; it keeps him turning from side to side in his sleep; it hinders digestion; and it does injury. For this reason, if the passage of the food out of the stomach is delayed, he should take a walk for a little while, and then retire to sleep.

§1707 It is also bad to go to sleep on an empty stomach, as this is weakening. It is bad to go to sleep after repletion, before the food has left the stomach, because sleep cannot be deep under such circumstances, and the sleeper will keep turning from one side to the other all the time. For when the natural drives are busy with the work of digestion at a time when it is accustomed to be asleep, the fact of being prevented from waking up is disturbing to the natural drives; so they become dulled and the process of digestion is disorganized

§1708 It is also bad to go to sleep during the day, for in this case illnesses depending on humidity and catarrhal states are brought about; the color of health passes off, the spleen becomes heavy, the nerves lose their tone; lack of vim and a poor appetite are noticed, and inflammatory conditions and fevers often appear.

§1709 Among the reasons for the injurious effects are: liability to sudden interruption of sleep whereby the natural drives become dulled.

§1710 Among the good qualities of sleeping by night are that it should be continuous and deep. If a person is accustomed to sleep during the day, he should not suddenly discard this custom but do so gradually.

§1711 Posture in sleep—the best way to sleep is to begin on the right side, and then turn round to the left. If one begins by lying face downward, it greatly helps the food to digest, because by this posture the innate heat is conserved and magnified.

§1712 It is a bad practice to sleep on the back. It courts the development of grave maladies like apoplexy, paralysis, and nightmare, because the effete matters then tend to accumulate in the tissues of the back, where they are held and prevented from entering the natural channels which are in front, such as the nostrils and palate. Persons who are accustomed to sleep on their backs often become debilitated, for their muscles and members become weakened; also because one side cannot alternate with the other, seeing that such persons quickly return to the supine position, the back being more powerful than the sides. The consequence is that such persons sleep with their mouth open, for the muscles which keep the jaws closed are too weak to maintain them in that position. (A special chapter is given on this subject in the special part).

16.11. Matters Which Are Best Described Later

§1713 We leave over until later the discussion of coitus and its constitution, and the measures to be taken to correct errors in this function, though strictly they belong to this place. It is discussed in the special part.

§1714 At this point also, one would discuss the agents for procuring evacuation of the bowel, and how to deal with any antagonistic influences towards them. We reserve this subject to the section dealing with treatment and the chapter on purgatives. However, we may say here that a person who wishes to maintain his health should procure evacuations by the bowel, the urine, the sweat, and the sputum.

§1715 We shall also explain how one may assist and regulate the menstrual flow of women, in order that you may become familiar with this.

16.12. Strengthening, Fattening and Enlarging Weak Organs

§1716 Members (limbs) which are weakly and undersized may be strengthened and caused to grow and develop during the period of growth, up to the final limit for growth, by the use of a suitable degree of massage and of a suitable form of exercise, steadily persisted in. Also by the use of pitch plaster. An exercise consisting of holding the breath [according to proper rules] is also effective, especially for the respiratory organs (thorax, lungs).

§1717 For instance, let us suppose the legs to be underdeveloped; the person takes a short running exercise; then a certain amount of massage is given; then a plaster of pitch is applied. Next day the running exercise is prolonged a little, but the amount of massage remains the same as on the first day. On the third day, the massage given is to the same extent as before, but the exercise is still further lengthened, taking care to stop short of distension of the vessels, for this would show matters are lodging in them which might be antecedent to some inflammatory process or repletion specifically met with in them: varices, and elephantiasis being an instance of such. Therefore, should there be any suspicion of anything of that nature, shorten the exercise to the original degree, reduce the massage; enjoin rest in the recumbent position; raise the affected member. Thus, if the persons have a wasted (lit. dried up) leg, raise it by the foot, and apply massage from its distal towards its proximal end.

§1718 To carry this method out for parts related to the organs of respiration the thorax, for example we proceed to apply a bandage to the lower parts, making it moderately tight, and of uniform breadth. Then we instruct the patient to exercise his arms, and to breathe as deeply as possible, uttering a loud sound the while (this may be assumed to a singing exercise, a sustained note being produced for as long as possible at each breath), light massage being applied as well. (This subject will be fully discussed in the Special Part on Beauty Culture, God willing).

16.13. The Types of Fatigue Affecting Exercise Management

§1719 There are three kinds of lassitude, and we may add a fourth. There are two modes. The three varieties are: the ulcerose (painful), the tensive (cramp-like), and the inflammative (congestive). The fourth variety which we add is the chapped, dry, and thin.

16.13.1. Painful Fatigue

§1720 Painful fatigue or ulcerose lassitude is a form in which the subject experiences the sensation of ulcers upon the body or in the depths of the skin. The deeper the sensation the greater is the lassitude. The sensation may be evoked by contact with the skin; or it may be evoked by movement. Sometimes it gives rise to the sensation of pricking with needles, with a dread of movement, and the subject lies extended because of the weakness of his shoulders and arm-pits. If the degree of lassitude is still greater, there is a goose-skin. When it is still greater, tremors and fever appear.

16.13.2 Cramp-like Fatigue

§1721 The cause of this kind of lassitude consists in an abundance of tenuous and pungent effete matters, a liquefaction of the flesh and fat in consequence of the over-vigorous exercise, and, lastly, the presence of depraved humors in the vessels, which results in changes in the blood, whereby it loses its healthy character; these abnormal products pass into the skin and affect it. This form of lassitude is the lesser evil which such substances produce. If they should become mobile, gooseskin will result. If they move about still more actively, tremors result. Sometimes the pungent humors detach themselves from the others, leaving the crude humors in the vessels. Sometimes the crude humors are situated in the flesh.

§1722 With cramp-like fatigue there is the sensation of the body being broken, of heat, of tension or being in a stretched condition, and has a dread of moving himself or straightening his back from the bent position. This is specially the case when the condition follows physical labor. This condition arises from the retention of waste matters in the muscles which are otherwise in themselves normal; it is not due to acridity or gaseous matters in them. The fibers are separated from one another, and there is a state of lightness or heaviness. This is often the result of want of sleep. When not associated with want of sleep, the case is different and more serious. Here the muscle fibers are stretched lengthways.

16.13.3. Congestive Fatigue

§1723 With congestive or inflammative fatigue, the body is hotter than usual. The part is as if distended, being swollen, and of corresponding color. Distress is felt when the part is touched, or when the patient tries to move, for this brings out the tension or stretching which is like the sensation in an inflamed or bruised tissue: Aeg.]. The deep-seated pain is called ostealgia. The cause is abundance of waste matters in the muscles.

16.13.4. Dry Fatigue

§1724 This is a state wherein one feels a sensation of being dried up in an unusual degree. It follows (a) undue exercise, the chyme being normal; (b) twisting the body back sharply; (c) sometimes it is owing to dryness of atmosphere; (d) deficient nutrition; (e) fasting too much. [There is great disinclination for any movement: Aeg.].

16.13.5. Complex Fatigue

§**1725** The two modes of lassitude. (a) That following exercise; this is less serious. It is rectified by suitable measures. (b) Spontaneous; this is a forerunner of illness. Special measures must be used for its cure.

§**1726** These two forms or modes may be combined, the matters which give rise to each being present together, both those which arise spontaneously, and those which result from exercise.

§**1727** The regimen for the simple form is known to you. That for the compound form entails the following rules: in the first place pay most attention to avoid the danger of the condition by dealing with the underlying cause. There may be three sources of danger: severity, the nobility (of the organ), and the substance involved. If two, or three are concurrent, the condition is more serious unless the one of them which outstays the other is more potent and therefore overrules them. For instance, inflammative lassitude is more severe, and the ulcerose form is nobler; but if the substance underlying the ulcerose is far from equilibrium and from the natural course, it forms a restraining influence over the two modes of the inflammative lassitude, by virtue of this nobility and strength, and takes precedence over it. But if the relation be not so very remote, the inflammative lassitude would take the precedence.

16.14. Stretching and Yawning

§**1728** Stretching comes on when effete substances have accumulated in the muscles. For this reason the desire to stretch oneself is often experienced after sleep.

§**1729** If these humors become superabundant they give rise to goose-flesh and trembling and shivering. If they increase to a still greater degree, fever develops.

§**1730** Yawning is really a form of stretching, when this

takes place in the muscles of the jaws, lips and chest. Should it arise without any apparent reason in a person seemingly healthy, and not at an appropriate time, and to an unusual degree, it is bad. In such a case, it is best when it comes on at the end of digestion, because then it is due to the effete substances being expelled.

§1731 Stretching and yawning may be due to external cold, to thickening of texture of the skin, whereby exit of certain humors becomes restricted; to being awakened from sleep before it has finished; to postponing the evacuations.

16.15. The Treatment of Fatigue After Exercise

§1732 Moderately diluted wine is good for this condition, provided there is no contra-indication.

16.15.1. Painful Fatigue

§1733 We may say that the chief object to be attained in treating lassitude is to prevent it from being followed by many diseases, including fevers. Ulcerose lassitude is dealt with by reducing the amount of exercise if that be the cause. If at the same time there is an over abundance of humors, they need to be expelled. If there be a transient sensation of nausea and satiety these effects are counteracted by fasting, evacuation through the bowels, and dispersal of the humors in the subcutaneous tissues by the use of plenty of light massage, carried out with oil devoid of astringency. Exercise is then resumed. On the first day the nourishment should consist of the usual quality of foods, in lessened amount. On the second day the diet should consist of humectants. If the vessels be patent, and there be crude serous humor in the mesentery, friction may help to mature it, especially if one could bring the virtue of calefacient medicines (digestives) to bear on it. Very good (calefacients) are: willow oil, oil. anethi; oil of chamomile; and the like. A decoction of beet roots in oil, prepared in a double-vessel; ointment of mallow roots; oil of the roots of cucumber asininus and of bryony; oil of sweet-scented moss; and any oil in which the latter (moss) has been incorporated. [Galen recommends discutients and restorative exercise.]

16.15.2. Cramp like Fatigue

§1734 In regard to cramp like or tensive lassitude, the object in view in treating this is to relax the indurated tissues by means of a little gentle massage with oil heated in the sun; tepid baths in which the patient stays a considerable time; or, better, to take the bath once or twice a day, followed each time by an inunction; complete rest. If it becomes necessary to procure an abstersion of the vessels, or if the oil of the inunction has become dried up, repeat the inunction and administer moist foods in only small amount. It is more important that the amount should be small in this case than in that of ulcerose lassitude. Exercise is sufficient to disperse this kind of lassitude, and cleanse out [the substances which cause it].

§1735 If tensive lassitude have arisen simply by the presence of gross superfluites, these must be evacuated. If it has arisen from flatulencies, it is dispersed by the use of such as cumin, caraway, and anise.

16.15.3. Congestive Fatigue

§1736 In regard to congestive fatigue or inflammatory lassitude. There are three aims in treatment of this condition: to relax the tense parts, to cool the heated parts, and to remove the superfluities. These are achieved by the use of plenty of tepid oil, by vigorous light massage, by a prolonged stay in a bath of tepid water (on the warm side), and by sufficient repose [and by repeated inunction: Aeg.].

16.15.4. Dry Fatigue

§1737 With dry fatigue or arefactive lassitude, the first day: the normal regimen for maintaining health is to be continued, save that the bath water should be hotter, because very hot water has a contracting effect upon the skin. This action is not as detrimental as that of cold water, for in this case there is a risk of the cold penetrating into the body, already dry. The cause of the wasting (wrinkling, shriveling of the skin) may also lie in the fact that the skin is usually relaxed.

§1738 The second day of the restorative treatment consists in the use of gentle restorative exercise of a light character. The bath should be carried out in the same way as on the first day and the patient should then plunge into cold water, to make the skin shrivel, and to reduce perspiration to a minimum. In this way the skin keeps moist. For water will come in contact with the body as soon as there is sufficient heat in it to counteract the dryness of the skin. And these two factors mutually assist one another in combating the injurious effect of the cold. The injurious effect is greater if the person comes quickly out of the water into which he has plunged.

16.16. General Principles

§1739 Those affected with lassitude need wholesome food, which must contain little moisture, and should be taken at the end of the first morning hour. Friction may be given on a later occasion, towards evening. The supper must then be taken later still.

§1740 The removal of superfluities from the body must also be procured, using massage with sweet, or willow oil [cf. the modern oil. betula oil, or oil of wintergreen]. The abdominal muscles are not touched unless lassitude is present in them. In that case, give light inunction and increase the amount of such food as is not too heating.

§1741 One should take care that exercise should stop short of producing any sign of lassitude. Then proceed to reversion exercise in order to draw matters towards the skin by the moderate amount of movement. Having reached the skin, massage during the time of resting between the exercises will finally disperse these substances.

§1742 As regards bathing, person's condition is the guide. If the bath should induce tremor, the last degree of lassitude has been reached. How much more is this true if fever comes on after the bath. In such a case the bathing must be stopped, and recourse must be had to evacuation [of various kinds] and the rectification of the temperament. As long as the water is moderately hot, and the bathing produces none of these adverse symptoms, one knows that it is beneficial to bathe.

§1743 If there were non-matured humors in the vessels, the first measure to take would be to apply whatever was suitable for the lassitude, and the next would be to endeavor to make the crude humors mature and become attenuated, and then to expel them. If they were plentiful, order rest; forbid exercise, because rest is the great digestive. Avoid bleeding because by this means both pure and crude matters are expelled.

§1744 It is injurious to procure purgation before maturation. There is no harm in inducing dieresis. But avoid drugs which are very heating, for otherwise the crude humor would be caused to diffuse throughout the body, and facilitate its action.

§1745 Diet: include pepper, capers, ginger, vinegar of capers, vinegar of garlic, vinegar of spurge, and dried dates, and the well-known confections (i.e. of quince, apples, prunes, etc.), according to measure. The appearance of a sediment in the urine informs us that maturation has occurred. One may now order wine to complete the maturation and to procure dieresis. The wine must be delicate and clear, and must not excite vomiting.

16.17. The Management of the Side Effects of Exercise

16.17.1. Physical Conditions Which Follow Exercise

§1746 We may first speak about the states, and then pass on to the subject of the regimen applicable for lassitude of autogenous origin.

16.17.2. Flabbiness

§1747 Rarefaction of the skin: very often this is the result of insufficient massage, and of bathing. The treatment consists in dry massage, tending slightly to rough, using an astringent oil for the purpose.

16.17.3. Hardness

§1748 Thickening of the skin (induration, constriction, tightness, tenseness, shriveling, sclerosis, corrugation may be the result of: (a) cold; (b) an astringent bath; (c) over-abundance of effete matters, (d) thickening and aggregation of coarse particles of effete matters; (e) change in the effete matters [or immatured humors] in the direction of viscidity in consequence of which they cannot pass through the pores of the skin, and so block them; (f) exercise, for this draws the humors out from the deeper (or remote) tissues, if no other cause for this has previously been in operation; we (g) residence in a dusty place; and (h) too rough and vigorous massage.

§1749 When it is due to cold and astringency, the color of the skin is pale [because it is stretched hard and tight], and the bodily warmth returns only slowly; sweating is delayed. The skin becomes red again on resuming exercise. Such cases should be treated thus: the stay in the cold room of the bath must be very short, and the water must not be very cold; then go into very hot water; turn the patient from side to side, then on to the belly, then on to the back. The slab on which he lies the while must be of medium heat. Do this until perspiration sets in. Then anoint with thin [sweet: Aeg.] oils of a hot and resolvent character [oil of dill, of black poplar: Aeg.].

§1750 Cases due to exercise are distinguished by the absence of the above-named sign. The skin is discolored by sweat and sordities. Such cases are treated by getting rid of such superfluities as may be present, and then carrying out a bath and inunction regimen of resolvent character.

§1751 Cases due to exposure to fine dust, or due to the use of too much rough massage, are much more in need of the bath than of inunction with oils. Soft massage is to be employed both before and after the bath.

16.17.4. Excessive Moisture

§1752 Rarefaction of the skin may be associated with weakness (asthenia). This may be the result of (a) excessive exercise, especially if subsequent massage were insufficient; (b) overindulgence in coitus; (c) too frequently repeated baths. The treatment of such cases therefore consists in the use of restorative exercises, and of dry massage, for which an astringent oil is used in order to obtain a hardening effect. The diet should include humectants in small amount, which are moderately calefacient or moderately infrigidant or slightly inclined to be hot.

16.17.5. Excessive Dryness

§1753 The same sort of treatment is used for asthenia, wakefulness, sadness, dryness in the nerves (or the state which follows on anger). In such cases, if the patient finds the digestive process of the food is depraved, the reversion exercises are not good; indeed no exercises are to be recommended.

§1754 When the cause of the weakness is an over indulgence in baths, in eating and drinking, and inactivity, the patient suffers from undue humidity in the tissues (especially the tongue), and the activity of the limbs is impaired. Should this depend on some antecedent cause, the special treatment for that will become necessary.

§1755 In the case of any other causes which we have named—wine, undue inactivity, undue moistening effect of the bath—the best thing to do is to anoint the body, use vigorous exercise, employ rough dry friction without oil, or a massage with the aid of a small amount of a calefacient oil.

§1756 When a person experiences undue dryness of the skin of the hands, this belongs to the category of arefactive lassitude. The treatment is the same as for that condition.

16.18. The Treatment of Spontaneous Fatigue

§1757 The ulcerose state is recognized when the humor upon which it depends is within or without the vessels. The humor is shown to be within the vessels by: (1) the urine being fetid; (2) the nature of the previous diet, for some articles of diet give rise to an undue proportion of superfluous matters in the blood; some articles of diet give rise to too few superfluous matters; or these matters are expelled too speedily, or medicinal treatment may become necessary for them; and (3) the character of the fluids taken if wine, whether clear or thick.

§1758 From all such data one comes to the conclusion that the site is within the vessels; if it is not found, the condition is extravascular.

§1759 In cases where the lassitude from superfluities is of extrinsic origin, and the vessels are unobstructed, it is sufficient to carry out reversion (restorative) exercises, and follow the regimen, to an increased degree, which we have indicated for cases of ulcerose lassitude due to exercise. But if the case belongs to the other group, one should not order exercise, but inactivity, sleep, fasting. Then, towards each evening, the abdomen should be anointed with oil, followed by a bath in moderately hot water, if his condition is such that he will stand the bath.

§1760 The diet should be of the character already stated: one which makes good chyme, fluid or semi-fluid [lit. able to be sucked, e.g. through a tube or spout], not viscid, and not particularly nutritious. Examples of such foods are: barley, frumenty, game (provided it is delicate), *syrupus acetous* with honey, mead, light white wine. A wine which is matured and diuretic need not be forbidden, but to begin with one would prefer to administer a wine which is slightly sour or rather yellow. Afterwards one changes to a white and light wine.

§1761 If this regimen proves ineffective it will show that the excess of humor present needs evacuation. Should it be the sanguineous humor, do a venesection [or scarify the ankles: Aeg.]. Otherwise, procure purgation, making your choice between them according to the proportion of sanguineous humor which you judge to exist. But take care not to do either if the vitality is low.

§1762 To ascertain the kind of humor concerned, one considers the character of the urine and sweat; and the tendency towards sleep or wakefulness. It is a bad sign if sleep is banished in spite of a good regimen.

§1763 If one has ascertained that there is a deficiency of good blood in the body, and that the immature acrid humors are in excess, one must not bleed the patient or purge [or let him bathe (Aeg.)], but procure complete rest. Order attenuant foods and fluids; avoid any fluid nourishment which is calefacient, but choose such as has a sharp or biting or incisive quality: e.g. *syrupus acetous*, with honey [acid wines, capers with vinegar and honey: Aeg.]. If it be necessary to increase the power of the attenuants, put a little pepper into the food, and into the barley-water [especially as there is generally hypogastric flatulence: Aeg.]. Cumin and pepper may be needed to counteract the immaturity of the humors (i.e. acrid matters which have not been properly digested) administering them either before or after a meal, or at bedtime, according as seems best to you. The dose is a small tablespoonful. Pennyroyal is not so good, for it is overheating.

§1764 Now if one is absolutely certain that the immature humors are not it the vessels but in the tissues (lit. roots of the members) one orders massage; laxative oils, especially in the mornings; heating drinks—whose heat passes to the skin; a long rest; then a moderately hot bath. Prescribe pennyroyal fearlessly, whilst being sure to give it before meals and exercise.

§1765 If it be necessary to aid the gastric digestion before a meal, do not give a strongly penetrative remedy like pennyroyal, but choose cumin and pepper in small dose. Quince may also be used. One could administer more of the latter, if one decides that the extraneous heat of the body would not be much greater in degree by giving it. Beneficial remedies: inunction with oil of chamomile, of aniseed, of sweet marjoram, etc.-whether given alone or combined in wax. Their action is increased by resin, alone or with twice its volume of its oil.

§1766 When one has ascertained that the immature humors are in the vessels, and at the same time outside them, one would become more anxious. Do not lessen your efforts in consequence. If there be as much within as without, first aim at procuring the maturation of the humor; pepper may be used for this purpose. To that, if one wishes, one may add parsley, and an equal weight of anise. In this way a greater degree of dieresis will be procured. Or, if one so desire, one may admix with it a little pennyroyal, and at the same time lessen the amount of cumin and pepper. These are lessened step by step until at last there remains simply nothing but pure pennyroyal. As soon as the (foreign matter) in the vessels has become digested, and has passed on out of them, one has to deal with that which is exterior to them. Pennyroyal will be useful for this purpose, whereas it was impeditive at first. Where the two conditions occur concurrently one must take special care not to attract the impure matter forcibly towards the surface of the body, or to the interior organs either. Therefore, one should not risk producing emesis too soon, or purging before the humors are rendered tenuous, and have been cut and matured. Exercise is also not ordered.

§1767 When the lassitude has passed away, and the color of the skin is more healthy, and the urine normal (mature), plenty of massage is given and exercise in small amount. One considers whether there is any chance of a relapse, for in that case one would pause in these measures. If it appears that a relapse will not occur, the customary life with regard to bathing, inunction, massage, exercise, is gradually resumed. Finally the strength of the ointments used is brought back to the customary.

§1768 If a relapse is threatening, with a sensation like that of ulcerose lassitude, the regimen must be taken up again. If the relapse threatens without that sensation of ulcerose lassitude, the treatment is by reversion-exercise.

If the signs are ambiguous, and the sensation of lassitude is not marked, order rest.

§1769 The cause of pensive lassitude is repletion without depravity of the humor. If the temperament is unhealthy, order venesection and an attenuant regimen. In the type of person of which we speak, the treatment is by attenuants and a certain amount of incisives; after that one helps the cure by using appropriate agents.

§1770 Treat inflammative lassitude by venesection. The choice of vein depends on the part most affected with lassitude or the part in which the condition began; if it be the head, use the cephalic vein; if the chest or back, use thee basilic vein; if the other members are chiefly affected, or there is no distinction of priority, bleed from the median vein of the arm. It may be necessary to bleed on the second or even the third day On the first day, one bleeds as soon as the lassitude appears, otherwise the condition may become established. The proper time to bleed on the second or third day is sunset.

§1771 On the first day, the diet should consist of barley water alone, or juice of frumenty as long as there is no fever. If there is fever, give barley water alone. On the second day give a cooling or attempered oil like almond oil. On the third day give a salad made with lettuce or cucumber (or, members of the gourd family), or garden mallow [or, beet, Aeg. or sorrel in cold broth: Aeg.], and give rock fish in white broth (i.e. a special dish or recipe) and forbid drinking [cold: Aeg.] water as much as possible during this day.

§1772 If by the third day, the patient feels nausea, or, if he has an appetite but the stomach cannot digest the food, let him have mead, or a light white wine, or an attempered white wine. After the evacuations, take care not to give a great deal of food all at once, for undigested food will be drawn into the blood. This is due to three factors: (i) when there is not much food, the stomach greedily holds it, and its retentive power—is antagonistic to the attractive power of the liver. When food is plentiful, the stomach is not greedy of it, and then its expulsive power helps the attractive power of the liver. The same holds good with each receptacle in turn in regard to that which comes next into play; (ii) when there is much in the stomach, it does not get digested as well; (iii) the presence of plenty of food means that there will be much nutriment for the blood, and the vessels [greedily absorb the chyle before it is digested: (Aeg.) and they themselves are incapable of digesting it.

16.19. Concerning the Bodies of Those With Abnormal Temperaments

§1773 The temperament (constitution) of the body may be defective either from some deleterious influence, or from the natural course of events beginning from birth. In the former case the temperament was appropriate for a certain length of time, until persistent faulty regimen has produced a change which itself remains persistent. In the latter case the defective constitution has been present from the outset (of conception).

§1774 In the first group of cases, the error is in quantity or in quality, and the nature of the case is revealed by a study of the form of the body. The remedy is to have recourse to the corresponding contrary.

§1775 The second group of cases shows a depravity of the state of the body in that there is a change either in the original constitution or in the course of advancing years of life.

§1776 We therefore begin the subject by going into the regimen of the elderly.

Lecture 17: Concerning the Elderly

17.1. General Remarks About the Elderly

§1777 In brief, the regimen appropriate for old people consists in giving those forms of aliment, drink, and baths which render the body warm and moist (i.e., moistening, calefacient food; warm or hot soft water baths). There should be plenty of sleep, and the time spent on the couch should be liberal—more than is legitimate for adults. The flow of urine should be continually assisted by diluents; the mucus should be helped out of the stomach by way of the bowels and urine. The nature is too soft, and this needs correcting.

§1778 Massage: massage with oil, moderated both in quantity and quality so as to fall short of occasioning lassitude, is beneficial.

§1779 Exercise: Walking or horse-riding is taken after the massage. The choice depends on which is too fatiguing. If both forms of exercise are fatiguing, repeat the massage once or twice (instead).

§1780 Sleep: the air of the room: some pleasantly redolent aromatic should be used to perfume the air which is breathed, using one which is moderately hot.

§1781 After sleep, the body should be anointed with oil in order to stimulate the sensitive faculties. After this the horse-riding or walking exercise may be taken.

17.2. The Diet for the Elderly

§1782 Food should be given in small amounts at a time. There may be two, or three, meals a day, divided up according to the digestive power, and according to the general condition-whether robust or weakly. In the latter case, at the second or third hour they may partake of well-baked bread, and honey. At the seventh hour after the bath, they may partake of some one or other of the foods we shall name later, which are laxative in action. At bed-time, some laudable nutriment may be allowed.

§1783 When they are robust, old persons may have a rather more liberal supper as long as they avoid any gross aliment which is likely to give rise to atrabilious or serous humor, and avoid all hot, sharp, or desiccative foods, such as dishes made with vinegar, salt or hot aromatics, seasoning, pickles, etc. These may, however, be allowed as medicaments.

§1784 Should some article of food in the first group have been taken which should have been avoided such as salted foods, eggplant, dried salted animal-game-meat, fish with tough flesh, smoked fish, then this must be counteracted with water-melon, and cucumber.

§1785 Should one of the other group have been wrongly taken dishes made with vinegar, salt and strong aromatics (like fish jelly, dishes with pickles, savories) the remedy is to use the contraries, and select only attenuant articles if one knows that there are superfluities in the body.

§1786 When the bowels have been opened, give humectant foods, followed by slightly attenuant foods, as we shall explain. Olive oil may be given before the meal.

17.3. Beverages for the Elderly

§1787 For persons who like and can digest milk, it is beneficial. One knows that it is well-borne if it does not cause fullness over the liver and epigastrium, or itching, or pain. Milk is good for old persons because it is nutritious and humectant. Goats' and asses' milk are best. Asses' milk is recommended because among its properties is this that it is not cheesy, and it passes quickly through the intestines, especially if salt and honey have been added to it. However, one must be sure that the pasturage is free of pungent herbs, or sharp or bitter herbage and marshmallows, or very salty herbs.

§1788 The wine which is best for elderly persons is old, red, with warming effect, and diuretic. New and white sweet wine should be avoided, unless a bath is taken after a meal at which such wine is taken, and unless there is thirst. In that case it is allowable to take white wine which is light without much body in it, thus taking the place of plain water.

§1789 Elderly persons must shun sweet wines which are likely to prove oppilative [but wines prepared with honey may be allowed even in cases where gout is threatened: Aeg.].

17.4. Alleviating Constipation in the Elderly

§1790 Potherbs and fruits specially suitable for old persons: beets, celery [which is good for persons with a gouty tendency or tendency to calculus: Aeg.]; also a little leek, which may be dished up with tasty aromatics to help: digestion; also olive oil [and pickles, olives, damascenes seasoned with salt: Aeg.]. This is specially chosen to take before the meal, in order to obtain a laxative effect. It is also an advantage to partake of such at bedtime, for they dispose one to sleep.

§1791 Ginger, which is really a medicine, is a good condiment for old persons. And there are various other medicines which may be taken as heating confections made with liquid extracts, taking them in sufficient amount to be warming without causing indigestion or being desiccative. It is essential that the nutrients should be humectant, without any likelihood of exerting a drying effect, and that they should be calefacient and help digestion.

§1792 Among the foods which may be enjoyed are such as are laxative, and congenial to the elderly body namely, game birds boiled with water and salt and flavored nicely with condiments, and served with oil; polypody root, which has been placed in chicken-broth or beet-broth, or in cabbage broth.

§1793 Articles of food which have a laxative action, appropriate for elderly persons—for summer: figs and prunes; for winter: dried figs cooked in water and in honey. They must be taken before food, to have the laxative effect. [Ripe figs are preferable, unless they cause unpleasant symptoms in the right hypochondrium: Aeg.]

§1794 If the individual has the peculiarity of being one day loose, and the next bound, solvent foodstuffs may be omitted. If the bowels are loose one day, and bound for two days, it will be sufficient to take such articles of food as cabbage water, and a (Persian) ptisan of barley containing bastard saffron, or turpentine gum, to the amount of one, two or three hazel-nuts. All these have the property of relaxing the bowels, and cleanse the interior organs without harm. Another good medicine is one compounded of the kernel of bastard saffron and twice its amount of dried figs. The dose is the size of a nut; take in a draught.

§1795 Purgation in elderly persons—another good remedy is an oil enema, for it empties the bowel as well as lubricates the bowel-walls, especially if sweet oil is used for the purpose. The rectum may simply be lubricated with oil. Strong clysters must be avoided because they dry the intestine. A moist unctuous clyster is very beneficial in cases where the bowels have been constipated for several days.

§1796 There are also other remedies for procuring gentle motions, and we shall specify these in the formulary.

§1797 The evacuations in the elderly must be procured with as little depression as possible, for it is greatly to their advantage to have the bowels opened gently.

§1798 If phlegm is engendered in the stomach, remove it by appropriate remedies, and then at once resume the diluent diet. If serous and mucoid waste matters accumulate, remove them by dieresis, and give oil before the meals.)

§1799 Obstructions are very liable to result from the use of white wine. These may be cleared by the use of pennyroyal, capsicum, and by sprinkling pepper on the wine. Onions and garlic may be taken for the same purpose, if the person is accustomed to take them. Theriaca is also good, especially if the obstruction is recent.

§1800 These remedies are to be followed by a bath, by oil, and such aliments as meat-broth with frumenty and barley. Mead is beneficial both when there are actual obstructions or they are merely threatened, and is useful for averting joint-troubles. If there is a sensation of a block in a given member, or if there is a premonition of such, one should combine some diuretic remedy with it, like celery seed.

§1801 In cases where the (ureter or) urethra is blocked by a calculus something stronger is advisable, like parsley. For obstruction in the lung, use hyssop, maidenhair, cassia wood, and the like.

17.5. Massage for the Elderly

§1802 Massage must be moderate in amount and quality; feeble or tender parts must not be touched. Between the times of massage, the parts may be rubbed with rough towels (binders), or with the bare hands [i.e. without oil], in order to ensure that the members concerned shall not become enfeebled.

17.6. Exercise for the Elderly

§1803 The factors to consider in regard to exercise in old age are: (1) the different bodily states [of different people]; (2) the sequelae likely to arise from their ailments; (3) their previous habits in regard to exercise.

§1804 For if, towards the end of life, the body is still equable, it will be right to allow attempered exercises. If one part of the body should not be in a first-rate condition, then that part should not be exercised until the others have been exercised. For instance, if an ailment begin in the patient's head (like vertigo, or epilepsy), or if there is catarrh [nose, throat, etc.]) or there is a liability to suffer from the ascent of vapors to the head and brain then the exercise should not entail bending the head down; the exercise should be of walking, running, horse-riding, and other exercises involving the lower parts of the body. On the other hand, if the ailment were in the feet, the exercise should employ the upper limbs: for instance, rowing, throwing weights, lifting weights. If the ailment be in the trunk (spleen, liver, stomach, intestines) the extremities should be exercised, supposing there is no contra-indication. If the ailment is in the chest, the lower limbs should be exercised. If the ailment is in the kidneys and bladder, only the upper limbs may be exercised. In these cases the exercises are not to be graduated strictly, as if the members were to be strengthened. In this respect the exercising differs from that for other periods of life. In early old age the same principles apply as for ordinary old age. In other periods of life the weaker members are progressively strengthened by the adoption of exercises for the purpose.

§1805 The exercise of members is sometimes allowable in the infirm, sometimes not. Thus it is not permissible if the members are hot or dry, or if there are matters (in the body) which might be drawn down into the limbs by the exercises, and fail to undergo resolution in them.

Lecture 18: Concerning the Regimen of Those Whose Temperament Is Abnormal

18.1. The Management of Excessively Hot Temperaments

§**1806** We may say that in the case of a hot intemperament (i.e. bilious habit or disposition), either there is an equilibrium of the two passive qualities, or there is either dryness or moisture.

§**1807** When the two passive qualities are balanced, the degree of heat will come to a limit; it will never be predominant, for that would lead to dryness. If dryness is associated with the heat, the intemperament may be maintained over a long period of time whereas if the heat is associated with moistness, the intemperament will be of short duration because the moisture becomes predominant and obliterates the heat. However the heat sometimes comes to predominate and obliterate the moisture, producing desiccation. Consequently, the condition of a person whose temperament shows a preponderance of moisture will become improved towards the attainment of adult life, and then become equable, whereas later in life the extraneous moisture begins to increase and the bodily heat to diminish.

§1808 Therefore we may summarize the principles upon which the management of persons with hot intemperament is to be conducted in these two intentions: (1) to restore equilibrium; and (2) to conserve the existing state of health.

§1809 To secure the first a patient needs training during the early years of life, the passions being subdued in a willing obedience to orderly discipline during all that time. Unless the discipline is orderly there will be a liability to illness. This intention is also gained the more easily if care be taken that the aliment is appropriate for their particular intemperament because in this way the health recovered is also conserved.

§1810 Individuals with a hot intemperament who are attempered in respect of the two passive qualities, are nearly normal in health at the commencement of life so that this kind of intemperament makes the teeth erupt early and the hair grow quickly; such children will be ready of speech, clear in utterance, and quick walkers. As they grow older, the hotness becomes dominant, dryness increases, and the temperament biting [sharp-tempered]. Bilious humor is formed to excess in many of such individuals [as they grow older].

§1811 Accordingly, the regimen during the early years is the same as that of attempered constitutions, and as the temperament changes the regimen must be correspondingly changed, seeking to provoke the urine, and help the choleric humor out of the body either by the bowel, or by emesis [and by the urine]. For if nature (i.e. the action of the bowels) alone does not suffice to get rid of the excess of humor, emesis by mild remedies may help to do so using such as plenty of warm water, either alone or with wine. The action of the bowels is secured by the use of such things as conserve of violet, confection of tamarinds, manna, and Persian manna. Exercise should be lightened. The only food that should be allowed is such as yields good chyme.

§1812 If baths are necessary, they may be taken daily or every third day. But in that case nothing heating should be allowed (in the food). If the bath be taken after a meal, and it does not cause distension or heaviness over the liver or epigastrium, there need be no anxiety. But if such symptoms should arise, an aperient should be given. For instance, infusion of absinthe; a mixture containing aloes, anise, bitter almond, and oxymel. The bathing after food should also be stopped [and the diet should be light, with deobstruents and viscid articles of food (Galen)]. These aperients are to be given at the end of the first stage of digestion, and before the second stage is completed.

§1813 But there should be a certain interval of time between the aperient and the next meal—namely the interval between the morning exercise and the time for the bath. Inunction with oils is required, and a light white wine should be given. Cold water has a useful influence.

§1814 All these suggestions apply specially to those whose temperament has been hot and dry from birth.[1]

§1815 Those who have a hot and moist temperament show a tendency to (abnormal) decompositions in the various matters, which also tend to descend into the limbs. Such persons should take exercise of a kind which will favor dispersal (of humors), but is mild enough not to prove over-heating. A degree of activity likely to cause ebullition in the humors must be avoided.

§1816 A person who is not accustomed to much exercise should eschew it. Exercise should be taken after the bowels have been evacuated. Baths should be taken before the meal. Care should be taken to get rid of all superfluities (quickly). When spring approaches, moderation should be observed in bloodletting and purgation.

18.2. The Management of Cold Temperaments

§1817 There are three kinds of cold intemperament: (1) When there is a balance between the two passive (qualities the intention is to produce more innate heat by means of (a) hot aliments which are moderately moist and dry; (b) calefacient inunctions; (c) large electuaries; (d) evacuation of the corresponding humors; (e) baths likely to induce sweating; and (f) exercises contributory to sweating. (2) At some periods such persons may be attempered in regard to humidity, and yet it sometimes happens that the coldness gives rise to humidities. (3) In those individuals in which there is dryness as well as the cold intemperament, the regimen should be prescribed as for old age.[2]

18.3. The Management of Increased Susceptibility to Disease

§1818 When persons are prone to illness, it is because of (1) repletion, or (2) the presence of immatured humors. In the former, the quantity requires modification; in the latter the quality of the humors needs modification.

§1819 (1) The quantity of humors is modified by modifying the amount of food taken; by increasing exercise; by massage before the bath (if the person is accustomed to exercise and massage; otherwise these must be mild); by dividing the meals so that the food is not all taken at one time, and to satiety. If the skin acts very readily) and the inducing of sweating is customary, this may be procured. If the fact of the meal being taken slowly does not result in the pouring out of bilious humor into the stomach, the meal may be taken after the bath. But if it should do so, the meal should be taken before the bath. In the former case, the proper time for the meal is after the fourth hour.

§1820 But if bilious humor pours into the stomach, the meal is taken before the bath, and further, if there are symptoms of congestion in the liver, those among the above-named aperients which are appropriate to the temperament are administered. Should there also be symptoms pointing to (congestion in) the head, walking about is of assistance. If the food undergoes putrefaction in the stomach, and then passes, no matter; but if it does not pass, one must administer cumin, or figs mixed with bastard saffron seeds. An electuary of this is cited [in the Formulary, Volume V].

18.4. The Treatment of Leanness

§1821 The chief cause of emaciation, as we have said, is a dry intemperament, dry mesentery, and dry atmosphere. When the mesentery is dry, it will not absorb nutriment, and this renders the degree of dryness and wasting still greater.[3]

§1822 Before taking the bath, the skin is rubbed with linen cloths to a degree between rough and gentle, until the skin becomes red. The rubbing may then be more vigorous. After that, a pitch plaster is applied[4] [for three or four days: Aeg]. The object of the massage before the application of the pitch plaster is to prevent the puffing of the tissues from subsiding again. Exercise is to be moderate. The bath follows at once. The skin is dried with towels. Then massage is given, using [emollient (H. A.)] oils. Lastly, a meal of suitable type is given [fat meat, pulse, almonds, bread: Haly Abbas].

§1823 If the age, season, and custom allow of it, cold [tepid: Aeg.] water may be douched over the person.[5]

§1824 The above regimen is almost identical with that which we have spoken of for increasing the bulk of an undersized member. The completion of the subject will be found in Volume IV, when discussing beauty culture.

18.5. The Treatment of Obesity

§1825 The regimen which will reduce obesity: (1)procure a rapid descent of the food from the stomach and intestines, in order to prevent completion of absorption by the mesentery. [One may take saltish things of laxative nature: Rhazes]. (2) Take food which is bulky but feebly nutritious. (3) Take the bath before food, often. [Do not take food immediately after the bath, and a short sleep; follow up the bath with massage; make a long stay in the bath: Haly Abbas]. (4) Hard exercise. (5) Resolvent oils. [Rub in oil containing root of wild cucumber, marshmallows, gentian, all-heal root, birthwort root, poley, and theriaca; volatile ointments; oil of dill: Aeg.] (6) Electuaries: the lesser myrobalan electuary; electuary of lacca; theriaca. (7) Take vinegar, and salt while fasting. (The subject is further discussed under the heading of beauty culture.)[6]

Lecture 19: Changes in the Atmosphere

19.1. Seasonal Regimen and Changes of Air

19.1.1. Spring

§**1826** At the onset of spring one has recourse to bleeding. Cathartics are taken according to requirements and custom. Emesis should be induced. [Spring fills the system with humors (Rhazes)]. Diet: avoid very heating and moistening meats and drinks; use attenuant articles of food. Exercise: in moderation, but in greater amount than is proper in summertime.

§**1827** Too much food should not be taken at a time; the meal should be divided over a period. As to drinks, take diuretic syrups. Avoid hot, bitter, salty, or sharp things.

19.1.2. Summer

§**1828** Summer dissolves the humors and weakens the vitality (Rhazes). Eat sparingly of foods. Moderate the drinks. Moderate the exercise. Take sufficient rest. Use diuretics plentifully. If emesis is possible, it is advisable. One should keep in the shade, under cover. The food should be infrigidant. [Avoid wine and venery (Rhazes).]

19.1.3. Autumn

§1829 Autumn is the season when the weather is changeable and unsettled. Autumn engenders bad humors, bilious sanguineous (Rhazes).] A more liberal regimen is here needed if health is to be preserved. Avoid desiccant agents; sexual intercourse; drinking much cold water; cold shower baths; sleeping in a cold place (cold enough to excite gooseflesh); retiring to sleep on a full stomach. It is advisable to protect oneself from the midday heat and the early morning cold breezes. Fruits are to be avoided, or at least taken only in small quantity [they supply bad chyme, and engender flatulencies (even figs and grapes do this) unless taken before food]. In bathing, only tepid water may be used. [Exercise should be moderate.]

§1830 During the time of the autumnal equinoxes, evacuations should be procured in order to ensure that the excrementitious particles shall not be held back in the system all winter. Although for some persons it is better to see that the humors are kept on the move, it is usually best they should keep in repose.

§1831 As the age advances, emesis must no longer be procured in autumn lest fever should be encouraged to develop. Wine must be well-diluted, and restricted as much as possible.

§1832 You may be assured that if the autumn is a wet one, there will be little likelihood of the usual autumnal disorders coming on.

19.1.4. Winter

§1833 There should be plenty of physical work. Eat liberally, if the prevailing wind is northerly. If southerly, increase the exercise but diminish the amount of food.

§1834 Diet—the bread should be made heavier in winter than in summer. The same applies to meat, roasted meat, and the like. Potherbs: take cabbage, beet, celery; avoid orache, red barley, purslane, endive.

§1835 When the body is healthy, illnesses are unlikely to come on during the winter. Should they do so, however, the appropriate treatment should be used, including purgation if that is necessary.

§1836 Illness will only arise under strong provocation, the agents being usually of a hot quality. The reason is that the innate heat, which is the determining factor, is very strong during the winter, because the cold prevents its dissipation, and collects it among the interior organs. Furthermore all the vegetative faculties are more efficient at this season.

§1837 Hippocrates favored purgation to blood-letting. He was against procuring emesis during winter, though approving of it during summer, on the ground that the humors of the body are now on the move whereas in winter they tend to stagnate. One may use this fact as a pattern.

§1838 When the atmosphere becomes pestilential in character, the body should be given a desiccant regimen, and the dwelling-house should be constructed so as to be able to be kept cool and dry. When contagious diseases are abroad, the air should be warm, and charged with agents which prevent decomposition of the air. Things which emit pleasing odors are good, especially if they are contrary in temperament to that of the atmosphere. Besides this, during times of pestilence, one should not allow draughts, but ventilation should be secured slowly, by means of small fans and ventilators.

§1839 Very often air is contaminated from the soil. In this case it is well to sit on couches (instead of on the ground) and to seek out dwellings on ground which is as elevated as possible, so that the winds traverse them.

§1840 Very often, too, the air itself is the seat of the beginning of the decomposition changes either because it is contaminated by adjoining impure air, or by some "celestial" agent of a quality at present unknown to man. In that case it is best to retire to underground dwellings, or to houses enclosed in walls on all sides, or to caves.

§1841 Fumigants may be used to purify the air: sedge (or, galangale), frankincense, myrtle, rose, sandalwood.

§1842 During the time when pestilences are about, one may use vinegar in both food and drinks, for this preserves one from the danger.

§1843 Other details will be discussed in the special part of this work, in order to complete the subject.

19.2. The Symptoms Premonitory of Diseases[1]

§1844 Those prone to attacks of palpitation of the heart should have immediate treatment if a sudden death is to be avoided,

§1845 Those suffering from nightmares and vertigo should be treated with the elimination of humors to prevent convulsions and coma.

§1846 Twitchings of the body require elimination of the phlegm to prevent rigidity and coma.

§1847 Elimination should also be carried out when plethora is associated with drowsiness and weakness and there is a fear of rigidity and coma developing.

§1848 If sensory loss develops, phlegm should be eliminated immediately to prevent paralysis.

§1849 Twitchings of the face should be treated with elimination to prevent facial paralysis.

§1850 Excessive congestion of the face with watering and running of the eyes, photophobia and headache should be treated with venesection and purgation to prevent delirium.

§1851 Anxiety and depression for no apparent reason should be treated by eliminating the burnt humor (black bile), lest melancholia should follow.

§1852 A red puffy face with pigmentation is a sign of leprosy.

§1853 Heaviness and lassitude in the body with associated plethora need venesection to prevent rupture of the vessels and thus, apoplexy and sudden death.

§1854 A swelling of the face and eyelids which spreads to the hands and feet points to a disturbance of the liver or kidneys and should be treated to prevent the development of ascites.

§1855 Stools of an offensive odor indicate putrefaction in the blood which should be treated to prevent fever. A foul smelling urine is not so bad in this regard.

§1856 Fatigue and aching of the body are generally prodromata of fever.

§1857 Loss of appetite or excessive craving for food is a prodromal sign of disease.

§1858 In short, when any of the functions are abnormal in some way appetite, defecation, urine, sexual desire, sleep, action of skin, itching, keen mental faculties, violent temper, unusual tastes, nocturnal pollutions—whether the abnormality is an increase or a decrease of function, or of quality or of character, one may be forewarned that some disease is on the point of supervening.

§1859 Unusual events have the same significance. For instance, bleeding of piles, menstrual flow, vomiting persisting, nose-bleeding, craving for something, whether bad, or apparently good because in a way natural.

§1860 For this reason one should not abstain from desired foods or things unless they are entirely bad and even then, the abstention should take place gradually.

§1861 Some special symptoms denote particular conditions. Thus, persistent severe headache, and dilation of the pupil warn of cataract.

§1862 The following are also forerunners of the same disease: imagining that there are bodies like insects, etc., in front of the face when one is sitting still and motionless; great impairment of vision.[2]

19.3. General Remarks Concerning the Regimen of Travelers

§1863 A person who is about to make a long journey must accustom himself to do without many things which are available in his own home, and must be prepared for hardships and pains. He must therefore take precautions against many illnesses {including fevers: Rhazes] to which he is exposed, if God will. He must be specially careful about diet and to avoid lassitude (a consequence of fatigue).[3]

§1864 Preliminary measures: (1) Bodily state. One should not set out upon a journey when in a state of sanguineous or other plethora. A purge should be taken first. [If the journey is likely to be arduous, a bleeding should be done also: the body is rubbed with oil (Haly Abbas).] If there is a sense of nausea, due to indigestion, one should fast, and then sleep till the nausea has passed off, before proceeding on one's journey. (2) [Hygiene of body: it should be anointed with oil (*ibid.*). (3) Dress: a binder should be worn. This is at least five cubits in length, and six or seven fingers breadth. This is applied round the loins, and the hollow of the ribs. The head must be covered. Take also a staff, as a help both in descending and ascending hills. (Haly Abbas); (4) Care of the eyes (from snow and dust): expose them to the vapors produced by pouring wine on a heated stone or to those of chamomile, dill, or marjoram [Rhazes]. (5) Care of the feet. Wrap them in cloths smeared with calefacient oils. (*ibid.*)

§1865 Sleeping and fasting—if it is necessary to travel on without sleeping, the habit of doing with little sleep should be acquired by preliminary practice. Similarly, if there is a likelihood of long fasts and of long abstinence from fluids, a habituation to this should be made first. One should also accustom oneself to the kinds of foods one is likely to be able to obtain during the journey foods of high degree of nutritive value, and taken in concentrated form.[4]

§1866 Exertion. The exertion which a journey entails should be met by making the first day's work very little more arduous than that customary; and so grade the exertion day after day.

§1867 Diet. The food must be concentrated and of good substance, and allotted into rations which are not too bulky, so that digestion will be well completed, without leading to the accumulation of effete matters in the blood. Should hunger be very pressing, let the traveler take a snack of a quality appropriate for his temperament, and unlikely to induce thirst. This rule applies whether the journey be by night or by day.[5]

§1868 Potherbs and fruits are to be eschewed, as also any articles likely to engender crude humors, unless such articles are required for medicinal purposes.

§1869 The traveler should not resume riding immediately after a good meal, because the food would then undergo decomposition, and thirst would arise. Then, after quenching the thirst, rumblings and distension of the stomach would supervene, and there would be nausea with satiative indigestion. Therefore, instead of so doing, one should wait until the time for alighting at the hospice, unless there is some special reason for doing otherwise, as presently to be stated.

§**1870** A person may have to fast so long that the appetite is lost. To aid one in submitting to this, the following are useful: cold foods prepared from roast livers and the like, pills prepared with viscid or glutinous substances, strong fluid fats, almonds, and almond oil. Certain fats like that of beef will stave of the feeling of hunger for a long time. There is a story of a man having swallowed a pound (12 ozs.) of oil of violets in which fat had been dissolved until the oil was of the consistence of a plaster; he is said to have been free of desire for food for ten days.

§**1871** Precautions against thirst—one may adopt a similar plan (to the preceding) when one knows one will have to suffer long from thirst. It is therefore advisable to inform oneself of those medicinal drinks which will abolish thirst, and are named in Volume III, in the chapter on thirst. Especially good medicine of this kind is furnished by dissolving three drachms of purslane seed in vinegar.

§**1872** Avoid any foods which are likely to evoke thirst. Namely, such as fish, capers, salted foods, sweets.

§**1873** Converse as little as possible. Make the rate of walking gentle.

§**1874** If there is a shortage of water, it is a good plan to add vinegar to it, for this allays thirst.[6]

§**1875** Fatigue: Lassitude. This must be treated according to the chapter on that subject.[7]

§**1876** At the end of a journey, take a comfortable apartment; do not go near the fire. Rest; do not go to sleep for an hour. After that, a bath may be taken. Massage is then given till the skin is all ruddy. Then the traveler may go to sleep on a soft couch. (Rhazes).

19.4. The Prevention and Management of Exposure to Heat

§**1877** The things to guard against are: asthenia, loss of bodily vigor, muscular weakness; insatiable thirst; sunstroke.

§**1878** Therefore the head and body must be protected from the sun. Those who are journeying must protect the chest, using an application composed of such things as mucilage of fleawort; purslane juice. It is advisable to partake of such things as we have named in small amount and wait awhile to give them time to pass out of the stomach, and so ensure that there will not be any splashing about of its contents.

§1879 One should use oil of rose and violets on the journey, anointing the back with them from time to time.

§1880 The injurious effect of traveling in the heat may be alleviated by having a swim in cold water, but it is best not to plunge in suddenly. One should wait a while and enter the water gradually.

§1881 If there is a risk of bad winds, the nostrils and mouth should be covered, and one should go about in that way. Before being exposed to such a danger, one may eat onions with buttermilk and without butter; or, better still, onions infused for a night in the milk; and one may eat onions by themselves as well, and take the buttermilk after them. Before steeping the onions into the buttermilk, deep incisions should be made into them.

§1882 Another remedy is to make use of some fragrant substance like rose oil, and the oil of gourd-seeds. The latter may be sucked because it mitigates the ill-effects one fears.

§1883 If sunstroke has already occurred, let cold water be thrown over the limbs, and lave the face with it. Pour cooling oil like rose oil over the head, and also willow oil, and cold juices like that of house leek. Then lave. Sexual intercourse must be avoided. The rations should consist of cold pot-herbs. Salted fish is also appropriate, the person resting the while. Diluted wine is advantageous. If there is no fever, milk is the best food of all. But if there is fever (not of a putrid type, but of a one-day type), sour buttermilk should be given. If there is thirst after sunstroke, rinse the mouth with cold water. Water should not be swallowed to repletion, because of the risk of sudden death [from shock] thereby. The rinsing of the mouth should be done with moderation. If, however, there is an excessive craving for fluids, allow the patient to sip a little at intervals. Such thirst being due to the previous exertions, let him rest, and then drink. But it would be better to take rose oil with the first portion of water, and take the ordinary water after that.

§1884 In brief, when exposed to heat stay in a cool place; lave the feet and hands with cool water. If thirsty drink cold water by sips. The food should be such as is readily digestible.

19.5. The Instructions for Those Traveling in Cold Weather

§1885 I consider that it is a very fearsome thing to travel in intense cold even if one takes great care and protects oneself by every possible precaution. So how much the more is it fearsome if the person has made no preparations at all?

§1886 How many travelers have taken every possible precaution and have yet died from the exposure to cold, and the cold winds, worse because there is no rain-dying in convulsions, or tetanus, or were frozen to death; or died with apoplexy, or died in the manner of persons who have been poisoned with opium or mandrake?

§1887 And even if the condition to which they are reduced is not fatal, they often experience the pangs of hunger, as what is called bulimia the treatment for which has already been described in the proper place, along with that for other disorders of the same class. The best thing to do is to plug the nostrils and other apertures, and protect the mouth so that the cold air does not enter at once (into the lungs). The exposed parts must be protected in the way we shall describe [see §2042].

§1888 When the traveler in bitterly cold places has reached his halting-place, he should not approach a very hot fire at once, but gradually by degrees, beginning with a slight warmth, and slowly going nearer to the fire, though it would be better not to do that at all. However, even though the need of warmth is very great indeed, the approach must be still made gradual.

§1889 The traveler may push on quickly if he so wish, if the exposure to cold is not affecting him adversely, or depriving him of energy.

§1890 Frostbite—a person who has become frostbitten must be attended to without delay; he must be warmed and the vitality restored by calefacient oils, especially those which possess the properties of theriaca) such as oil of lilies.

§**1891** When the traveler has reached an inn, and is an hungry, let him partake of something warm; he will get wonderfully warm, with fever-like heat.

§**1892** Provisions to take—certain kinds of provisions enable the traveler to endure the exposure to cold more easily. Thus, any prepared foods containing plenty of garlic, nuts, mustard: asafetida are good. Lactic cheese made up with barley (meal a special recipe) may be added in order to impart a pleasing taste to the garlic and nuts. [Pickled onions may be chewed (Rhazes).] Butter is also a good thing to take especially if wine be drunk afterwards. Wine should be taken instead of water. One should take rest until the wine has come to rest within the body, and gives the sense of warmth. He may then mount and continue his journey. No one should go out into the bitter cold on an empty stomach; he should have taken plenty of nutriment.

§**1893** Asafetida is among the things which have a warming effect, when one is frozen with cold; especially if wine is given at the same time. The initial dose is one drachm (12=1 oz) of asafetida to 1 lb. weight of wine.

§**1894** The body may be protected from injury by the external cold by the use of epithemes, made with oil (pitch or tar). [The loins, spine, and chest may be bound with a long swathe to protect them (Aeg.).] Garlic (as an epitheme) is among the things useful for those exposed to a cold atmosphere. For care of the eyes and feet see [index].

§**1895** The limbs should first be rubbed until they grow warm. Then use a warm liniment compounded with pleasantly smelling oils like that of lilies, and oil of myrobalan (benzoin). syrup of lily flowers combined with aromatics. If this is not to hand, take oil, especially oil into which pepper, or pyrethrum, or euphorbium, or asafetida, or castorium have been placed. Epithemes may be applied to the limbs to protect them from the cold, using galbanum, garlic, aided by *pix liquida*, for instance.

§**1896** The foot-wear must not be so tight as to compress the feet, for freedom of movement is the best means of protection from cold, whereas restriction of movement interferes with (the circulation) and makes the limbs cold. It is also a good plan to cover the feet with parchment, and wear fur over that.

§1897 If the hands or feet are not aware of the surrounding cold, so that one does not take the proper precautions against it, it is a sign that the sensation is already being lost, and the frost is already exerting its harmful action upon it. In such a case there must be no hesitation in action. For you know that once the freezing cold penetrates into a member, not only is the innate heat extinguished, but the very substance on which that heat depends is destroyed. The tissues are then at the mercy of putrefaction. So there is an urgent need for all those measures which have been discussed in the chapter on ulcers, especially the grave eroding ulcers. If the degree of action is still short of the stage of putrefaction, the best thing is to place the limbs in snow water, or into water in which figs have been boiled, or cabbage, or myrtle (i.e., odoriferous things)) or into dill water, or chamomile water. All these are beneficial.

§1898 A good local application is made with pennyroyal. Wormwood of Pontus, betony, and turnip are also good medicaments for the purpose.

§1899 One must avoid exposure to direct heat. It is also necessary to walk about quickly, moving the feet and limbs, doing exercises with these, and also applying friction, and inunction. Warm water may be poured over the part from a height, along with the other aforesaid measures.

§1900 It is important to realize that to allow the limbs to be still and motionless in the cold air, without exercising them in any way, is the surest way to subject them completely to the intense cold. Some people, however, actually make use of cold water for the purpose of overcoming frostbite, taking away the ill-effects of the cold just as is done with frozen fruits. For the plunging into cold water has the effect of drawing out the ice, and of washing it away, and melting the tissues and restoring them to a normal temperature, whereas exposure to heat would simply lead to decomposition. However it is done is no particular concern of the doctor.

§1901 If the extremity begins to become dark in color an incision should be made into it, let the blood out of it the limb is then placed into warm water to prevent the blood from congealing and so failing to run out of the tissues. The flow is allowed to continue till it stops of its own accord. After that an epitheme is applied, using Armenian bole and vinegar blended together, for this antagonizes the injury done. *Pix liquida* is also a good adjuvant to this both at the commencement and at the conclusion.

§1902 When the darkness goes on to blackness or greenness, showing that the mortification is increasing, no time must be lost in stepping the process, for otherwise the healthy parts adjoining will become implicated and undergo putrefactive changes which will surely spread on into the interior organs. The measures to adopt under these circumstances are described in the appropriate chapter.

19.7. The Care of the Complexion

§1903 The face should be treated by applying epithemes to it, which are prepared with viscid substances, such as mucilage of fleabane, mucilage of purslane, gum tragacanth in water, gum arabic in water, white of egg, and such things as rusks of the finest wheaten flour dissolved in water, Qaritan lozenges. When the face is exposed to biting winds, or cold or the action of intense sun, the measures to be adopted are those given in the section on beauty culture.

19.8. Protecting the Traveler from the Ill Effects of Bad Water

§1904 The traveler is more exposed to illness from the diversity of the drinking water than he is from the diversity of foods. Hence it is necessary to be particular about correcting the bad qualities of the drinking water, and expend every effort in purifying it. (1) Procure the rapid passage of water through the body by inducing sweating. (2) Boil the water, for as we have already pointed out, boiling sometimes clarifies the water and separates off the impurities which are admixed with the intrinsic substance of the water. (3) The best measure is to distill the water. This may be done by making a wick out of twisted wool, one end of which is placed in the full vessel and the other into an empty vessel. Water will then escape from the one to the other drop by drop. This is a good way of clarifying water when it is necessary to do so frequently. When the water is bitter and altogether unwholesome, one should boil it, and add pure sand to it while it is boiling. It is then distilled over drop by drop by using the wool as mentioned above. It amounts to the same thing if the water be shaken with clean sand, especially when this material has been burnt in the sun. When the sand has settled, the water will be harmless. (4) Drink wine with the water, for that removes such injurious matter as is of feeble penetrative power. (5) If water is scarce and not attempered, it should be taken with vinegar, especially in summer time, because that prevents one from drinking too much.

§1905 Salty water: take vinegar with it, and *syrupus acetous* into which has been placed pulse and various species of myrtle and medlar.

§1906 Bitter aluminous water—take aperients afterwards. It is also beneficial to take wine after it.

§1907 Sour water—take sweet things and oily things, mixed with julep afterwards. Chick-pea water, taken previously to the water, will make it harmless before one could wish. The same is true if one eats chick-peas first.

§1908 Stagnant and marshy water—theses are putrescent. Do not take warm foods before drinking it. Afterwards take astringents made with cold fruits and potherbs, such as quince, apple, and sorrel.

§1909 Thick and turbid waters—garlic should be taken after such waters. Among the reagents which will clear these waters is rock alum.

§1910 Other things which remove the harmful properties of various waters: onions, because these act on them like a theriaca; especially onions and vinegar; garlic; and, among cold things, lettuce.

§1911 Another good rule in regard to the diversity of waters which travelers are likely to encounter is this: to carry some of the water from his home, to mix with it the earth from the inn in which he has stayed last; then carry some of the water to the inn to which he goes next, and mix that with the water he has brought; and go on in this manner until he reaches his destination. Similarly he may take some of the clay (sand) from his own home, and use that to mix with each successive specimen of water, shaking them with it, until it has cleared them.

§1912 One should be sure to pass all the drinking water through a cloth, in order to make sure there are no leeches or other creatures in it, or any minute particles of evil nature suspended in it.

§1913 It is a good rule also to take a sour, thickened fruit juice with pulp when traveling to mix with the various waters one is likely to have to drink.

19.9. Travel by Sea

§1914 Those who travel by sea often suffer from scotoma and vertigo, and the motion brings on nausea and vomiting, especially during the first few days of the voyage, after which it subsides. It is not wise to allow nausea and vomiting to continue longer than is required for getting rid of superfluities.

§1915 Measures to prevent sea-sickness—it is justifiable to endeavor to prevent sea-sickness. Thus, take fruit such as of quinces, apples, and pomegranates. Parsley seed made into a drink will prevent nausea as long as one lies quite still; and if one cannot lie still, it soothes the sense of nausea. Absinthe has the same effect.

§1916 Among the things which prevent seasickness are: nourishing the mouth of the stomach with tonic acetous substances, and such things as prevent vapors from rising into the head. Namely, lentils in vinegar (or dried and boiled with a little pennyroyal, or boiled till soft and then triturated and dried and kept in an earthen vessel: Aeg.); juice of sour grapes; a little pennyroyal, thyme; bread broken up in weak and fragrant wine, or in cold water. Thyme is sometimes added to that.

§1917 The nostrils should also be smeared over on the inside with white lead (cosmetic) ointment.

§1918 Persistent sea-sickness—avoid all food. Take a little vinegar and honey with water in which thyme has been infused, or pennyroyal water with some fine polenta; or take some weak fragrant wine, with fine polenta. Take antibilious remedies. (Rhazes).

§1919 Simple precautionary measures: (1) Counteract the disagreeable smell of the ship by sniffing at quinces, thyme or pennyroyal. (Aeg.) (2) Do not look at the sea. (*ibid.*) (3) Beware of the drinking water (*ibid.*) (4) Note the diet already mentioned. (5) Have remedies against vermin. Mercury, oil, long birthwort or wearing wool smeared with oil or mercury ensures against lice. (Haly Abbas).[8]

PART FIVE
GENERAL THERAPEUTICS

Lecture 20: The Treatment of Disease

20.1. General Remarks

§**1920** The subject of treatment comprises three headlines: that of the regimen and diet (dietetics), that of the use of medicines (pharmaceutics), and that of manual or operative interference (surgery).

§**1921** By the word "regimen" we understand the systematic management of the several factors which we have enumerated as being essential to health, and among them diet has an important place. The prescription of a regimen is based upon data pertaining to the qualities of the nutrients to be selected, as well as those belonging to the qualities which determine the choice of medicines.

20.2. Dietetics

§**1922** In regard to diet, the first question to decide is as to the quantity of each article of food which should be allowed. Sometimes a given article of food is to be forbidden; sometimes lessened; sometimes no change need be made; sometimes the amount taken is to be increased. The physician only forbids a food, or all food, if he intends that the digestive faculties throughout the body shall be left entirely free to complete the maturation of the humors. He prescribes a lessened amount of a food if he wishes the digestive powers to be conserved. The very fact of taking nutriment is a tax on the digestive faculties; therefore the withdrawal of a certain amount of food means a corresponding alleviation for them.

§1923 The physician must also be watchful in regard to two dangers: (1) that the natural powers should become too enfeebled; and (2) that an illness should become too grave.

20.2.1. How to Reduce the Diet

§1924 A diet may be reduced in two ways: lessen it either in amount or in quality. In fact, by combining these two ways, one has a third method at one's disposal. To explain more exactly, an aliment may be bulky but poorly nutritious with such things as pot-herbs or fruits. A person may eat plentifully of these without receiving much nourishment.

§1925 On the other hand, an aliment may be small in bulk, but highly nutritious. For example, eggs or the testicles of fowls. It is, for instance, necessary to lessen the nutritive value of food and increase its bulk in cases where the appetite is altogether excessive and "crude" humors enter the blood. So we lull the appetite by filling up the stomach, and yet see to it that only a small amount of nutritive matter enters the blood, thereby enabling the digestive products already in the blood to become "matured" or be properly disposed of. And there may be other reasons. On the other hand, it may be desirable to increase the nutritive quality without adding to the bulk of the food; namely, when we wish to increase the bodily strength or vitality and when the digestive power of the stomach is inadequate.

20.2.2. The Function of Foods

§1926 Diminution in the amount of food, or stopping food altogether is usually the line of treatment in acute illnesses. But sometimes we decrease the amount of food in chronic maladies, also, though not to the same extent as in acute ones. The reason is that in the case of chronic maladies it is more necessary to see that the bodily strength is maintained, for we know that a long time will elapse before there can be a crisis or restoration to health. So unless the strength be maintained, the patient will not hold out until the time for crisis comes, and he cannot digest anything which takes a long time to digest. But in the case of acute illnesses, the crisis is near at hand, so we may confidently expect the vitality to hold out until that time. If we have any doubt about this, we should see to it that the diet was not lowered too much.

§1927 It is not so necessary to diminish the amount of food in the earlier stages of an illness when the symptoms are not very marked. In this way one conserves the natural powers. But as the illness progresses and the symptoms become more severe, so the amount of food is to be lessened according to the principles already stated. In this way the digestive powers are helped at the critical hour of struggle.

§1928 The regimen must also be made definitely attenuant during the height of the disease. The more acute the malady, and the nearer the crisis, the more attenuant must the regimen be made, unless there should happen to be contra-indications such as we shall name in the special part.

§1929 Aliment possesses two functions besides mere nutrition: (a) rate of penetration, or absorption—rapid penetrative power, as for instance, wine; slow penetrative power, as for instance, roast meats and fried meats; (b) compactness of the substance of the digestive products in the blood, and consequent retention (i.e., this is the feature of the digestive products from veal); or attenuation of substance, with consequent speedy dispersal as is the feature of the digestive products of wine and figs.

§1930 We need to make use of an aliment of rapid penetrative power when we wish to remedy a loss of vital power so as to revive it when there is not sufficient time or digestive power to justify waiting till the aliments are digested in their ordinary course, slow as that may be. We have also to take care not to take easily digested food after food which is only slowly digested, lest the result of the mixture be undesirable in the way already explained. We should also take care to avoid foods of solid texture, since we know for a fact that these give rise to obstructions in the ducts of anal tissue channels as well as in the intestines.

§1931 Therefore, when we wish to restore the strength of the patient and make him fit to undertake strenuous exercise, we will select highly nutritious foods which digest slowly. We select a feebly nutritious food for a person whose pores are choked with dense matter.

20.3. The Treatment With Medicines

§1932 There are three rules to follow in selecting medicines: (1) according to quality—whether hot, cold, moist, dry; (2) the amount to be given (the dosage). There are two subdivisions of this: (i) measurement in terms of weight; (ii) measurement in terms of quality—degree of hot, cold, etc. quality; and (3) the rules relating to the time of administration.

20.3.1. The Quality of Medicine

§1933 In regard to (1) above, the selection according to quality, the decision depends, strictly speaking, on one's knowledge of the type of illness to be treated. Once one knows the quality of the illness, the appropriate medicine is that whose quality is exactly opposite just as in health, it is the like which is to be maintained.

20.3.2. The Quantity of Medicine

§1934 In regard to (2) above (the selection according to quantity), there are two factors to consider in order to arrive at an arbitrary measure: (i) the nature of the organ; (ii) the degree of illness. Beyond this are factors determining the suitability and fitness of the treatment, namely, species, age, custom, season, geographical position, occupation, strength, physique.

20.3.3. The Nature of the Affected Organ

§1935 To understand the nature of the organ or member, one must know these four things about it: (1) its temperament; (2) its structure; (3) its position and relationship to other organs; and (4) its strength.

20.3.3.1. The Temperament of the Organ

§1936 If the normal and original temperament of the affected organ is known, it will be easy for the physician to determine the degree of abnormality and its proper dosage for a cure. Thus, if the affected organ is primarily of a cold type and the disease is a hot one, it will denote a gross abnormality of the organ necessitating strong cooling doses. When, however, the original temperament is hot and the disease is also of the same nature, only mild cooling doses will suffice.

20.3.3.2. The Structure of the Organ

§1937 There are four structures of an organ, as already referred to. In addition, it is necessary to be aware that (1) certain organs have been constructed with openings of easy ingress, with ample spaces (receptacles) at the entry and exit of the channels[1] so that the waste products can be expelled readily by appropriate tenuous and attempered or weak medicines. There are others which are not so formed and in these cases stronger medicines become necessary. (2) Some organs are loosely constructed while others are dense in texture. For the former, tenuous medicine will suffice whereas for the latter a powerful remedy is necessary. The strong medicine is the more necessary in cases where there is neither cavity nor receptacle—either internally or externally.

20.3.3.3. The Position and Relationships to Other Organs

§1938 This includes consideration of the site and relationship of the effected organ with the neighboring organs.

§1939 A knowledge of the mutual anatomical relations of the organs is helpful in selecting the route to administer the medicines and the mode of elimination of morbid matters, that is, if a morbid matter is in the upper part of the liver, it is to be eliminated through the kidneys, but if it is located in the lower part, it is better to eliminate it through the bowels. This is because the former is related to the kidneys, while the latter is related to the intestine.

§1940 The site and position of the affected organ are helpful in three ways:

20.3.3.3.1. The Accessibility or Remoteness of the Organ

§1941 If the organ is easily accessible, the medicine can reach it directly. Thus, the stomach can be easily effected even with mild drugs while remote organs like the lungs require more powerful medicines, because in their case the milder drugs would lose their potency long before reaching the affected organ. In case the organ is remote and the drug has to reach there earlier, it should be somewhat more potent than usual, i.e., the plaster for treating sciatica should be a little stronger.

20.3.3.3.2. The Specific Relation of the Affected Organ

§1942 One must know what substances to admix with medicines in order to bring them rapidly to the affected organ. For instance, one must admix diuretics with a medicine for the urinary tract; and saffron with medicines intended for the heart.

20.3.3.3.3. The Site of Disease

§1943 One must know by what route the medicine is to be brought to the affected part. Thus, if we have ascertained that there are ulcers in the lower bowel, we inject remedies by the rectum; whereas if we know that the ulcers are in the small intestine, we give the remedies as fluids by the mouth.

Sometimes it is advantageous to consider both situation and relations to other organs at the same time. This applies in the case where the whole of the morbid matter has been discharged into the member, or when it is in process of being so discharged. For as soon as we know that it is in process of descent to the particular spot, we may draw it out of the body altogether by making use of the following four principles:

20.3.3.3.3.1. The Rule of Diversity of Parts

§1944 If the morbid matter is on the right side, it should be withdrawn from the left; when it is above, it should be diverted downward.

20.3.3.3.3.2. The Rule of the Physiological Relationship

§1945 Menstrual bleeding can be arrested by cupping the breasts because blood tends to travel towards its related organ.

20.3.3.3.3.3. The Rule of Directness

§1946 In diseases of the liver, venesection is carried out from the right basilic vein, but in diseases of the spleen, it is from the vein on the left side.

20.3.3.3.3.4. The Rule of Distance

§1947 The organ to which the morbid matter is to be diverted must not be too near the one diseased.

§1948 If by chance the whole of the morbid matter has already been withdrawn, both sides of the body may be used together. For we may, if we desire, draw the material into the member itself, or first draw it into an adjoining physiologically related one, and then from that. For instance, we open both saphenous veins when treating maladies of the uterus and we open the one median vein under the tongue when treating double quinsy.

§1949 When you wish to draw morbid matter to another organ to that from which you are drawing it first allay the pain there. And take care that in so transferring the matter you are not crossing a vital organ.

20.3.3.4. The Strength of the Organ (Functional Capacity)

§1950 This is a guide to treatment in three ways:

20.3.3.3.4.1. The Vital Nature of the Organ

§1951 The value of assessing the strength of an organ lies in three directions: (1) it enables us to direct the treatment in the order of nobility of organs. Thus, one must not use potent drugs which might act on the principal vital organs to so great an extent as to risk producing a harmful effect all over the body. When it is necessary to withdraw matter from the brain or liver, one would not attempt to do so at the same period of the disease and one must not apply infrigidants too assiduously.

Again, when we wish to apply external applications over the liver and at the same time introduce resolvent medicines, we must take care to combine astringent drugs of aromatic character with them so as not to risk interfering with the functional capacity of the organ. The same rule applies when giving fluid remedies. In applying these rules, the order of importance of the organ is: heart, brain, liver.

20.3.3.4.2. The Normal Function of the Organ

§**1952** The treatment is directed to an organ of physiologically related function provided the organ selected is not a vital one like the stomach and lung. For instance, one does not give very cold water in cases of fever when the stomach is weak. You are aware, too, that to administer undiluted remedies, which are relaxing to vital organs or to organs closely related to them, is simply to imperil life.

20.3.3.4.3. The Sensibility of the Affected Organ

§**1953** One takes the sensibility of an organ into consideration—whether it is keen or dull. That is, one must beware of giving drugs possessing injurious (mordant, pungent or toxic) qualities to very sensitive organs or organs of special sense—for instance, plants belonging to the Euphorbia group.

20.3.4. The Degree of Illness

20.3.4.1. According to the Severity of the Disease

§**1954** There are three kinds of medicines in the administration of which we must be very cautious. Those which are extremely resolvent; those which are cooling; and those which are contrary in property. Examples: lead, copper salts, and the like.

§**1955** This, then, is how one chooses medicines according to the nature or character of the organ to be treated.

§**1956** Choice of medicine according to the severity of the illness—for example, when the degree of morbid heat of the body is unduly great, it must be counteracted by means of a medicine of strongly infrigidant character. But when the abnormality consists in a marked degree of coldness, this is met by exhibiting a strongly calefacient medicine. If the degree of abnormality is not marked, remedies of weaker quality will suffice.

20.3.4.2. According to the Stage of the Disease

§1957 Choice of medicine according to stage of the disease—when we know the stage at which a disease is, we adjust the treatment accordingly. Thus, if an inflammatory focus is in the initial stage, we shall apply a remedy which will act upon it alone. If the disease is near the terminal stage, we may apply a remedy which will resolve it at that phase. If the disease is between these two stages, we should combine both forms of remedy which will resolve it (at that phase). If the disease is between these two stages, we should combine both forms of remedy. If the disease be acute, we should at first aim at attenuation by means of an attempered regimen; but at the later stage we should seek to procure attenuation. In the case of a chronic disease, we should not aim at attenuant treatment in the early stages and we should use a modified attenuation at the later stage, though it is true that an attenuant regimen disperses many chronic maladies besides fevers. Again, if a malady is due to active fermentation of the humors, we procure evacuation including venesection at the early stages without waiting for the matter to undergo maturation. But if the fermentation is only moderate in degree, we wait until maturation is complete before undertaking the evacuant measures.

20.3.5. Other Factors

§1958 You can easily recognize which factors are favorable to the end in view (and how to adapt them accordingly). Thus, air is the most important of all such and one needs to take care that it shall assist the action of the medicinal treatment and not contribute to an aggravation of the illness.

20.3.5.1. The Management of Drugs

§1959 In the case of maladies where any delay in treatment might entail a loss of vitality, or where one wishes to do more than merely alleviate, we shall begin with a strong medicinal agent. But if there is no fear of such an eventuality, we may proceed in orderly fashion using a milder remedy first and the stronger one if that proves insufficient.

§1960 Further, you must not forsake the direct rule of treatment if you find that there is only a tardy response to it; and, on the other hand, you must not commit the fault of delay when there is no contraindication. In addition, you must not confine yourself to one single medicinal remedy throughout the treatment, but you must interchange the medicines all the time because when the tissues are accustomed to one they cease to respond and moreover, the same tissue or member or the body as a whole may react to one given medicine at one time or phase and not at another.

20.3.5.2. Leaving It to Nature

§1961 When you do not know the nature of a malady, leave it to nature; do not strive to hasten matters. For either nature will bring about the cure or it will itself reveal clearly what the malady really is.

20.4. The Treatment of Pain

20.4.1. General Remarks

§1962 When the malady is accompanied by pain, whether the pain is the cause or the effect, as in the case of blows or falls, the first thing to do is to allay the pain. If it is necessary to induce a stuporose state, do not go beyond the use of such as white poppy. Its anodyne action is well-known.

§1963 When the member is hypersensitive, nourish it with such things as render the blood viscid, as for instance, cooked grain. If this is not sufficient, and there is no reason to be afraid of infrigidation, such things as lettuce may be used.

20.4.2. The Psychological Factors

§1964 Remember, too, that among the advantageous contributory factors in treatment is the help afforded by anything which exalts the sensitive and vital drives: for instance, joyfulness. In consequence, one sets out to please one's patient, and even tranquilize him by anything which can reasonably gratify him. Sometimes one may advantageously arouse his sense of shame, making him blush, and so leading the sick person to avoid what is harmful for him.

§1965 A measure which is akin to the preceding is that of removing from one country to another, from one climate to another, or a change made from one external form to another. To do this, one particularizes the various forms and movements which will act upon the given member, or alter its temperament. Thus one may advise a youth with disorders of vision to avoid very close writing and looking at very bring objects; a person with squint should look into a narrow mirror so held that the effort of turning towards it will help remedy the malposition of face, forehead or eye.

20.4.3. Omit Strong Measures

§1966 Another rule to be observed is to omit strong measures of treatment at the strong seasons, as far as possible. For instance, one refrains from violent purging, from provoking emesis, or from opening a part, or applying cautery, during summer or winter.

§1967 Gentle treatment is to be applied when two maladies are conjoined into one, such that contrary measures have to be carried out at the same time. For instance, if the malady is infrigidant, and its cause is warming or conversely the malady is to be treated with calefacients and the cause is to be treated with infrigidants; i.e., fever requires infrigidation, and the obstructions in the channels which give rise to the fever need the application of heat. Again, the indications in colic are warmth, incisives, and attenuants; but the pain to which it gives rise needs cold, and analgesics.

20.4.4. A Liberal Regimen

§1968 Remember, further, that not every case of plethora is to be treated by its contrary, namely, evacuation by purging or by venesection, nor is every intemperament to be treated by inducing a contrary temperamental state. As a matter of fact, a liberal and good regime will often suffice by itself to remedy plethora or intemperament.

Lecture 21: The Treatment of Disorders of Temperament

§1969 When an intemperament occurs without abnormal, unhealthy matter, the treatment is to alter it; but if there is abnormal matter, this has to be evacuated. Usually a single evacuation will suffice to amend the previously existing intemperal state; but sometimes it is not sufficient for the purpose, and the intemperament will then require rectification after evacuation has been procured.

§1970 We may therefore state that the treatment of intemperament comprises several modes of procedure.

§1971 An intemperament is either chronic (longstanding), in which case the treatment is strictly by contrary, and a complete cure is achievable thereby; or it appears at the terminal phase of an illness, in which case the treatment is by anticipation. Thus, treatment by contraries is instanced by the giving of theriaca for the putrefactive processes associated with quartan fever, and of ice cold water to abolish the fever of tertian fever. Treatment by anticipation is instanced by the use of evacuation, namely, by hellebore in the case of quartan, and by scammony in the case of tertian. The hellebore applies to atrabilious humor; the scammony to bilious humor. Our object is thereby to prevent or forestall the morbid changes.

§1972 If in any given illness you are in doubt as to whether heat or cold is responsible, and you therefore desire to put the matter to the test, you must be careful not to overdo this, and not to be misled by secondary super-imposed symptoms. You must note that the appropriate moment is the same for infrigidation as for calefaction. But one is more apprehensive regarding infrigidation, for heat is the friend of "nature." One is as apprehensive of moistening as of dessication, but the period during which the former is permissible is longer. Moreover, the state of moistening and desiccation is, in each case, maintained simply by fostering the factors which give rise to them, and they are modified simply by re-inforcing the contraries of those factors.

§1973 Heat is reinforced by the agents already expounded. Putrefication of the passages is carried out next, by procuring the expulsion of wastes, the removal of plethora, and by opening up obstructions. Finally the heat is to be conserved by preserving a moderate degree of moisture.

§1974 Cold is reinforced by assisting any factors which bring it about, by repressing the bodily heat, and by dispersing the heat unduly to which dryness contributes by its essence and heat secondarily.

§1975 In treating undue heat by removing obstructions, one must guard against producing too much infrigidatory, for in that case there is a risk of rendering the obstruction still greater by conversion of the matter into a stone. One must also take care not to render a hot intemperament more marked. Hence the treatment by abstergents should be entered upon gradually. It is advantageous to use an abstergent which is sufficiently cooling (i.e., barley water and endive), but if this be not adequate, one makes use of an agent which is neither "hot" nor "cold"; and if this is inadequate, one employs an agent which is warm and tenuous. One need not be anxious in making use of such a remedy, for it lends further assistance by provoking diaphoresis, which renders the body cooler, thereby causing more good than the heating effect can harm. Anyway, it is easy to remove the heating effect once the pores have been opened.

§1976 It may happen that the innate heat is so much reduced by such measures that the digestion of the morbid humors is interfered with. Yet there are some who boldly pursue this wrongful method and ignore the fact that undue reduction of the innate heat means loss of vitality, which is especially to be expected in persons much weakened by illness. This result occurs even though the matter is rectified in some other way, and other maladies follow on, either in the form of simple intemperaments, or by arising out of "cold" matters which are opposite in quality to the temperament. When a cold intemperament is established, it is as difficult to render it warm as it is easy to do when it is only beginning. To render a cold intemperament warm at the outset is easier than to render a hot one cold at the outset. But to render a hot one cold at the end of the process, though difficult, is nevertheless easier than to render a cold one hot at the end of the process. The reason is that excess of cold itself implies complete, or nearly complete, destruction of the innate heat.

§1977 Infrigidation is sometimes associated with desiccation, sometimes with moistness, and sometimes occurs independently of either. But dryness is more persistent if associated with infrigidation and moisture is more conducive to the supervention of coldness. All the factors producing calefaction aid desiccation if they are preponderant. All the factors producing infrigidation aid humectation if they are preponderant. Nothing is so likely to have this effect as inactivity, and constant use of the bath, even the full-length bath. We have already made this known to you. Diluted wine is also strongly humectant.

§1978 You must note also that if it is an old man who needs infrigidation and moistening, it is not enough to reduce the temperament to equability. One must continue till the temperament is cold and moist beyond the normal, because such a temperament is acquired secondarily, though quasi-natural to the old person.

§1979 Note, too, that when changing the quality of a temperament, it is often necessary to reinforce it by admixing with the remedy something of contrary quality. Thus, we give vinegar with medicines which are hot towards a given member, because then their virtues can penetrate into the member. We give saffron with cardiac infrigidants, because saffron carries such remedies to the heart.

§1980 Oftentimes it happens that a medicine which produces a very marked change of temperament does not have a lasting effect; this is because it is so tenuous that its action does not pass on to completion. In this case we must admix with it something which will render it less tenuous and more stable, even though one risks the production of a contrary effect. Thus, we mix wax with balsam, and so on. The one remedy is thereby preserved long enough to ensure its proper action being accomplished.

Lecture 22: The Use of Eliminants: Purgation, Emesis, Cupping, Venesection, Leeches

22.1. The Indications to Determine the Manner and Moment of an Eliminant

§**1981** There are ten indications which show when it is right to procure "evacuation" [i.e., blood-letting, wet-cupping, purgation, enemas, diaphoresis, use of leeches, etc.]: (1) plethora, (2) vitality, (3) temperament, (4) appropriate symptoms (thus, we need not evacuate the bowel in a case of diarrhea), (5) habit of body or physique, (6) the age of the patient, (7) the time of the year and the state of the atmosphere, (8) the geographical situation, (9) the patient's mode of life regarding "evacuation," and (10) his occupation.

§**1982** Evacuation should not be carried out when there are contra indications in these respects.

22.1.1. Plethora

§**1983** If the state is the opposite of plethora (vacuousness), evacuation is obviously contraindicated.

22.1.2. The Strength of the Patient (Vitality)

§1984 Weakness in any of the three primary faculties is a contra-indication. Nevertheless, we may decide to act in spite of such a weakness if more harm is likely to accrue from neglecting evacuation. This applies to the sensory and motor drives since we are more anxious to avoid injuring them if they are weak. In fact, the same applies with all the drives.

22.1.3. The Temperament

§1985 Contra indications are: hot and dry temperament; or cold and moist temperament, in which there is little or no heat. One may act vigorously, however, if the temperament is hot and moist.

22.1.4. The Symptoms

§1986 Certain unfavorable symptoms are contra indications such as endemic diarrhea and cramps (spasmodic diseases).

22.1.5. The Physical Development

§1987 Excessive leanness or spareness of build is a contra-indication because the breath is so readily dispersed. For the same reason, when a person is weak and lean, and has much bilious humor in the blood, he must be treated blandly, and evacuation avoided. The aliment should be such as will engender good blood, making it incline to coolness and moistness of quality. In this manner the temperament of the humor will be corrected, after which the patient will perhaps be strong enough to tolerate evacuant measures.

§1988 Similarly, one must not venture to "evacuate" a patient who is accustomed to eating sparingly; or, at least, one should postpone such a measure as long as possible.

§1989 Obesity is a contraindication, because one runs the risk of making the frigidity dominant, and of allowing the flesh to compress the vessels up to occlusion, thus blocking the flow of innate heat, or of forcing out the effete matters from the vessels and driving them inwardly.

22.1.6. The Age of the Patient

§**1990** Avoid evacuant measures when the fullness of growth has not yet been reached, or when the patient is nearing the end of decrepitude.

22.1.7. The Season

§**1991** Avoid evacuant measures if the time of the year is extremely hot or extremely cold.

22.1.8. The Geographical Position

§**1992** A southerly country which is very hot is contra-indicative, for persons with diarrhea are usually hot temperament ("hot-tempered.") The association of two adverse conditions [the extraneous heat and the evacuation] is badly borne, because the bodily faculties are enfeebled by the dispersal of vitality, and because the extraneous heat draws the matter outwardly, and the medicine draws it inwardly. Being thus drawn in two opposite directions, it tends to remain where it is.

§**1993** Avoid evacuant measures in very cold, northerly countries.

22.1.9. Habits

§**1994** Avoid evacuation when the habit is to have evacuations infrequently.

22.1.10. Occupation

§**1995** Avoid evacuant treatment when the occupation is one which in itself is evacuant in effect, e.g., bath-attendants, porters; all toilsome or arduous physical labor.

22.2. The Aims and Objectives of Elimination

§**1996** In procuring evacuation there are five points to consider: (1) Removal of that which is to be evacuated, followed by rest to the parts unless there is atony (lassitude) in the receptacular spaces or overheating of the blood whether in the form of ephemeral fever or of other accompanying maladies. Thus there may be excoriation of the mucosa, which brings about diarrhea; or ulcers in the bladder. Such things may be advantageous, and yet not appreciated as such by the patient because of the pain and suffering they cause him until the symptom has been removed. (2) To choose which organ is to be "evacuated": thus nausea is removed by emesis; burning pain in the abdomen is eased by purgation. (3) To use as member of egress that which corresponds to the organ to be evacuated. Thus for maladies of the liver the right basilic and not the right cephalic must be used. To make an error in such a matter might be harmful. The member chosen for the site of evacuation must be less important ("noble") than that which is to be evacuated lest the morbid matter pass down into the more important organ. The channel of exit should also be the natural one; thus for the blood-vessels of the liver the urinary tract; for the ducts of the liver the intestinal tract. Sometimes the organ to be evacuated is itself the one to take as the site for evacuation, and yet it is the seat of chronic or acute disease. In this case it would be risky to induce the humors to traverse it, and they should be diverted to another organ instead. Sometimes there is a risk of superimposing another malady on the first, by inducing a superabundance of the humors in the second part. For instance, if the morbid matter is drawn downward from the eye to the throat, choking [edema of glottis] might result, and therefore one must proceed with such a measure carefully and with gentleness. Nature herself [i.e., the vegetative soul], often acts on the same principle, and protects a weak member by effecting the evacuation through a part other than that which would be the normal one for that member. Very often the part at which the evacuation actually occurs is quite distant, and opposite in position, and it comes to be a matter of doubt as to which member is being drained in this way. Thus the head may be drained by the anus, or the leg or the foot, and one could not say whether the evacuation is of the brain as a whole or only from one ventricle. (4) To decide on the proper moment to evacuate—in chromic maladies, as Galen rightly says, one does not wait for maturation. You know what is meant by the term "maturation." Therefore one should give attenuant drinks such as water of hyssop, of thyme, and herb seeds, before commencing to carry out the evacuant treatment, and after the maturation stage has been reached. But in acute maladies, it is best to wait until the maturation stage has been reached, especially as long as the humors are stagnant. Once they appear to be on the move, one must hasten to drain them away, because the damage accruing from their movement is greater than that which one risks by evacuating immatured humors—especially if the humors are tenuous, and especially if within vessels and not in the tissues in which they arise. When the morbid humor is confined to one particular member, it will certainly not move out of it until maturation has occurred in it, and its character has become modified as has already been explained for you in the proper place. Again, if we feel doubtful as to whether the vitality (of the patient) will hold out until the time for maturation has arrived, we shall proceed to procure evacuation noting carefully whether the material to be evacuated is labile or viscid. In the latter case we must first render the material tenuous. And we shall know that it is viscid by the fact of the premonitory dyspeptic nausea having passed by, or by the existence of tensive pain under the hypochondrium, or by the development of an inflammatory swelling inwardly. We must also carefully make sure that the passages are patent. Having taken these precautions you will be able to drain the morbid matter by the bowel before it has become purulent. (5) The amount to be evacuated—this is judged from: (a) the quantity of material already evacuated, (b) the strength of the patient, and (c) the symptoms which remain afterwards. If symptoms should still remain, we must either reduce the amount of evacuation according to the amount already estimated, or we consider whether the symptom is itself to be treated, as would apply for instance in the case of plethoric spasmodic disorders.

§1997 There are two ways of evacuating morbid material and eradicating it from the place where it has lodged: (1) by attraction from a distant place; and (2) by attraction to a neighboring place. And the most appropriate time for carrying out the treatment is when there is no sort of plethora of the humors in the body, and they are not moving downward into the member to which there is attraction.

§1998 Let us suppose, for instance, that there is a considerable flow of blood from above the mouth in a man, or from piles in a woman. To remedy this we may proceed to do one of two things. Either we draw downward towards a neighboring part of diverse character: that is, we cause the blood to flow down into the nostrils and emerge from them, in the one case; and provoke the menstrual flow from the uterus in the other. Or we draw to a distant part of diverse character: that is, in the former example we bleed from veins in the lower parts of the body, in the case of the male, and bleed from veins in the upper parts of the body, in the case of the female.

§1999 When the attraction has to be made from a distant part, one need not undertake to do so from both sides of the body, but just from that which is corresponding. Thus if the material is at the upper end on the right side, one would not draw it away to the lowest part on the left side, but to the lowest part of the right side (and indeed this would be the most necessary), or to the upper part of the left side, supposing there were as much distance between the two as there is between the humerus and the other, and not a matter of just the two sides of the head itself. For one would draw morbid material from the right side of the head down to the lower parts of the body, and not to the opposite side of the head.

§2000 Suppose one wishes to draw morbid material to a distant part. One first allays the pain in the part, for this will itself lessen the amount of material by attraction, since pain exerts an attracting effect. But, if it does not move to the part as soon as desired, avoid violent measures; for while it is true that violence would procure the desired movement, yet the material would become attenuated and not amenable to the attracting influence, and would simply pass right into the painful part.

§2001 It may prove sufficient to draw the material away without actually evacuating, because the very attraction arrests its progress to the desired member. But even so, our object in securing attraction may still have been attained, supposing that one would be satisfied to have accomplished the attraction downward without the additional evacuation. This is done when one bandages up the opposite member, or applies cupping glasses, or rubefacient medicines in short, any measure which allays pain.

22.3. The Time for Elimination

§**2002** Morbid materials are more readily evacuated when they are in the vessels than when in the tissues and joints, for sometimes it is difficult to remove them thence, and evacuate them. And in evacuating them from such situations one inevitably evacuates other things with them.

§**2003** A person from whom diseased matter has been evacuated must not partake of much food or unhealthy articles of food and anything which has an indigestible nature. If by chance one is for some reason obliged to do so, one should do so gingerly and cautiously, in small portions, so that that which enters the body may be digested and prove harmless accordingly.

§**2004** The drawing of blood is a special method of evacuating morbid humors which are all increased equally or proportionately. It is not the removal of one humor which is simply increased in amount or has its own particular quality destroyed.

§**2005** To carry out evacuant treatment to an undue degree is to bring about febrile conditions.

§**2006** If the bowels, previously usually loose, are bound, this condition will give rise to some other malady, and it will be proper to treat it by repeating the evacuation. For instance, supposing the discharge of sanious matter from the ears or mucous passages of the nose should cease, leading to vertigo, then, if the flow be restored, the vertigo will be removed.

§**2007** It is less injurious to leave a little of the morbid matter behind than to strive to evacuate everything to the most minute fragment, thereby risking a dispersal of the vitality. Nature herself often removes the last remnants.

§**2008** When the humor is of the kind which necessarily

exists, you need not be afraid of how much blood you take as long as the sick person is able to sustain it. For sometimes one is bound to evacuate (bleed) up to syncope.

§2009 When the person is robust, and the humoral matter plentiful and depraved, evacuation must be done gradually. Further, if the morbid material is extremely viscid or widely diffused, or admixed with much blood, it cannot be emptied at one sitting. This is true in the case of sciatica, longstanding arthritis, cancer, old-standing skin diseases and obstinate furuncles.

§2010 Remember also that purgation draws morbid matters from the upper parts of the body and discharges them below. Purging is, therefore, an attractive force in two different directions to the near and to the remote region of the body. It is most useful when the morbid material is stagnant. Therefore, when the morbid matter is either above or below, one may draw it to the opposite direction, away from the position in which it has lodged. Attraction is procured by emesis; eradication by the converse.

§2011 Furthermore, one varies the kind of blood letting according to the positions from which the blood is taken up as has been explained.

§2012 A person accustomed to a good diet, and having a healthy digestion, is less in need of evacuant measures than are most men.

§2013 Persons residing in hot countries need little in the way of evacuant treatment.

22.4. The General Rules for Emesis, Purgation and Their Mode of Action

22.4.1. Before Emesis or Purgation

§2014 Whenever purgation or emesis is to be procured, the food sufficient for one day should be divided up into portions to be partaken of in installments. The aliments and drinks are diversified accordingly. For under the circumstances the stomach acquires the desire to expel what is in it, either upwards or downward. The stomach is greedy for foods that are not diversified, and if no other food be taken in addition it holds its contents very stubbornly, especially if the amount be only small

This must be borne in mind by those who are naturally "loose." Emesis and purgation and the like do not apply for those who follow a good regimen. This is because a person who controls himself properly will not need anything but mild attention, and may be excused even from exercises, bathing, and massage. If such a person be in a plethoric state, the humors concerned will be healthy, i.e., sanguineous. Consequently, such a person requires letting if indications for cleansing should arise.

22.4.2. The Strong Purge

§**2015** If both blood letting and purgation (by hellebore and similar violent medicines) are needed, begin with the blood letting, because this precept of Hippocrates in his *Book on Epidemics* is sound. If, on the other hand, the plethora is of phlegmatic humors admixed with sanguineous humor, so that they are viscid and "cold," one would begin with purgation, because blood-letting would make the humors still more coarse, and more viscid.

22.4.3. Further Elimination Required

§**2016** In short, if the humors are in balanced proportion, blood-letting is preferable. Then, if a plethoric condition still persists, purgation is undertaken.

§**2017** If the humors are not in balanced proportion, first purge the superabundant humor until balance is restored, and then proceed with the blood letting. If the patient should have taken medicine before the blood letting (which was an error on his part), he should defer the subsequent blood letting for a few days. If purgation is needed within a short time after the blood-letting, the appropriate medicine may be given then. Sometimes, however, the person who has (improperly) taken the draught of medicine, instead of first undergoing a blood-letting will develop fever and restlessness before it can be done. If the restlessness is not allayed by the usual remedies (sedatives), the blood letting should be done.

§**2018** Evacuant treatment is not necessary in every case of excessive plethora. It may be indicated by the severity of the malady, or by the quality of the plethora, rather than its degree.

(Indeed, a good regimen will often make such measures unnecessary: marginal reading).

§2019 It may happen that there is a need for evacuation, but something intervenes which forms an adequate substitute, such as fasting, sleeping, correcting the unhealthy state of the temperament which has been produced by the plethora.

§2020 Then there is a form of evacuation which itself serves to protect one for instance from an attack of gout, or from an epileptic seizure which one knows will occur on a certain date, especially in spring. In this case one must apply the evacuant measure before the time is due, choosing the appropriate method; that is, choosing between blood-letting and purgation, according to the kind of things to be evacuated in the given malady. It may be also wise to apply desiccants externally, and to use absorbents for the purgation as one does in the case of those afflicted with dropsy.

22.4.4. Remarks About Purging and Its Rules

§2021 Sometimes the medicine to be chosen as purgative must have a quality corresponding to that of the humor to be evacuated. Thus, scammony is needed for evacuating bilious humor. A drug which is of a different quality should be mixed with it as an adjuvant for the purgation without preventing proper evacuation. For instance, myrobalan. Should the temperament afterwards become unhealthy, one must just correct it.

§2022 Emesis should be procured in cases where there is an internal inflammatory mass, because such cases are difficult to purge. But if purgation becomes essential, use such agents as pellitory, seed of safflower, apozema of polypody, cassia fistula, and the like.

§2023 Hippocrates also says that the best way of cleansing a person of spare habit, and of a nature—such that vomiting easily takes place, is to procure emesis; and this should be done in summer, spring, or autumn, but not in winter. But if he is of medium habit, it is better to purge. If evacuation by emesis is necessary, it is better to wait until summer, avoiding it altogether if it is not really necessary.

§2024 Prior to procuring purgation or emesis, the humor to be evacuated must be attenuated, and the channels of exit must be widened, and their outlet opened, in order to save the body from trouble. The last-named is achieved by an aperient regimen. That is, the patient accustoms himself to obey the calls of nature, and to maintain the motions loose. The actual medicines for purgation and emesis are reserved till later. Moreover, it is difficult, wearisome, and dangerous to procure purgation when the belly is wasted.[1]

§2025 An emetic may be given at the same time a purge: (1) when the stomach is strong; (2) when taken during a state of prolonged fasting; (3) when gastro-enteritis is present; (4) if the bowels tend to be loose; (5) when the patient is not accustomed to emesis; and (6) if the medicine is itself actually heavy (weighty) and passes down the intestines quickly as a result.

§2026 A purge will act as emetic: (1) if the stomach is enfeebled; (2) if there is much dryness of the stool; (3) when the medicine is very unpleasant; and (4) when it produces nauseative dyspepsia.

§2027 Should a purgative not act, or should it not remove the mature humor by its action, it will cause the humor to be distributed throughout the body. The result will be that other humors will become changed into the same kind of humor, and the body will be flooded with it.

§2028 There is one of the humors which readily responds to emesis, namely, the bilious; and there is one which is resistant to emesis, namely, the atrabilious. The serous humor occupies a middle position in this regard.

§2029 In the case of fever, it is better to purge than to procure emesis. When the humor is passing downward, as in a case of lienteric diarrhea, emesis is not advantageous.

§2030 Among purgative medicines, that is most harmful which is compounded from drugs which show marked variation in their rate of purgation; for the result is simply confusion.

§2031 The drug acting more speedily comes into play before the next, and sometimes the one will expel the other before it has come into operation at all.

§2032 Should a person take some drink which has a purgative action or is emetic, at a time when the bowels are emptied, he is sure to develop vertigo, or colic, and distress. That which finally is expelled will leave the body with the greatest difficulty.

§2033 Lastly as long as a given drug gets rids of the superfluities, it will cause no restlessness. If it should cause restlessness, one would know that something more than superfluity is being discharged. Moreover, we shall know when the superfluous humors have actually been gotten rid of by the fact that the humor lost by emesis or by purgation is now changed into another kind of humor. The cleansing process of the body will have passed on to a harmful degree if the lining of the intestines is beginning to be lost, and the stool is black with a fetid odor. Also, if a prolonged sleep allows the purging or emesis, it will show that the evacuation is complete, and salutary. Also, if there is great thirst after purging or emesis, it shows the purgation is maximal and satisfactory.

§2034 Purgative medicines expel humors in cooperation with the attractive faculty concerned with the given humor; maybe attracting the coarse and rejecting the subtle humor. This happens in the case of expulsion of atrabilious humor.

§2035 He who asserts the purgative itself gives rise to that which it attracts, or that it attracts first that which is tenuous, is in the wrong. It is true that Galen says so, yet he says accurately that a purgative medicine which is not poisonous, will, if it does not purge or undergo digestion, give rise to the same kind of humor as it ordinarily attracts. However, an assertion of that kind is hardly relevant. It would seem that Galen, in making this assertion, considers that there is an agreement in substance between the attracting drug and the attracted humor, and that that is why they mutually come together. But it is not true to say so, for if like attracted like, then a larger bulk of iron would attract a smaller, a larger bulk of gold would draw a smaller bulk of gold to itself. To discuss this is not in the province of the doctor.

§2036 You should note that it is the humors in the blood vessels which become attracted by the purgative or emetic. This attraction goes on until they reach the stomach and intestines, which finally expel them by virtue of their own nature (i..e., the natural expulsive faculty). It is only rarely that humors which are drawn out by a purgative should ascend into the stomach; if they did, they would be expelled by vomiting. If they should fail to ascend into the stomach, it would be because of one of two reasons either: (1) the purgative medicine has passed on speedily into the intestines; or (2) having taken the purgative drink, the "nature" proceeds to drive it from the mesenteric vessels to the lower parts of the abdomen and not to the upper parts because to do so is nearer and simpler, and because there is nothing beyond which will mechanically impede their progress [i.e., the distal parts of the digestive tube will not compress or block the proximal parts]. This indeed will be evident, considering that the "nature" will act by the shortest route of exit.

§2037 If the medicine possess an attractive power which will hold the humor, then the expulsive power may still overrule, assuming that the drug only attracts towards the route indicated. An emetic is different in this respect. When it reaches the stomach, it lingers there, draws the humor towards itself out from the intestines, and, by its own power, overcomes the resistance offered by the natural power of peristalsis downward.

§2038 The humors which medicines draw out are usually in the vessels or neighboring structures because it is in the veins that the seat of attraction lies. But medicines also draw humors out which are not in vessels, i.e., the lungs; in this case they are drawn to adjoining organs like the stomach and intestines but not via the vessels.

§2039 Remember, too, that it is possible to draw humors from the body by the use of desiccant medicines using the attraction, for instance, by way of the nostrils. This applies, for instance in the case of dropsy.

§2040 In the preceding chapter we have shown that the way to prepare the body for the purgative to be administered is to cause the pores to dilate and the "nature" to relax. This applies especially in the case of "cold" illnesses.

§2041 In brief, the rule: "soften the nature before purging" ensures safety in all cases except that of gastro-enteritis. In that case, nothing is to be done because the disease is itself the cause of the superfluity present.

§2042 Something of an emetic character must be admixed with the laxative agent to prevent the latter from leaving the stomach before it has done its allotted work. Or, rather, the two ingredients should be so balanced in power that their respective functions shall both come into play in the right order—the purgative action in the one direction, the emetic in the other.

§2043 People who lisp are liable to gastrointestinal catarrh and such people do not stand strong purges, as a consequence. All the same, many do run the risk of gastroenteritis because of the materials which flow down (rheums) from the head.

§2044 It is dangerous to administer a purge when the fecal matter is dried up within the bowels; in such cases it is best to get rid of it by means of an enema or by an emollient broth.

22.4.5. Bathing and Purgation

§2045 The use of the bath for several successive days before purgation is a good preparative measure, as it is attenuant. There must be no contraindication, however. A small interval of time should elapse between the bath and the draught of medicine, and one should not take a bath afterwards because the effect of that would be to draw morbid material to the skin. The bath is only of use for binding the bowels, especially during winter; for at that season one need not be afraid of going straight into the first room; the heat will not interfere with drawing out the humors, and in fact assists in virtue of its emollient effect.

§2046 Lastly, one should not take the purgative medicine, while in the hot room of the bath lest the medicine should give rise to sweating and a sense of oppression. This is one of the precautions which must be noted.

§2047 Other adjuvants, or preliminary measures, are massage and the inunction of oils.

§2048 Avoid the use of violent purges for persons who are not accustomed to take medicine, or to drink it.

§2049 Do not administer a medicine to persons who are in a state of "dyspepsia with nausea," or whose humors are viscous, or who have distension of the hypochondrium or inflammation or obstruction [of channels] in the inward parts. In all such cases, the condition must first be rectified by ordering emollient aliments, the bath, rest (in bed), and by avoiding anything likely to arouse disturbance of, or inflammation in the humors.

§2050 Persons who are accustomed to drink stagnant water and have enlarged spleens, will need strong aperients.

22.4.6. Sleep and Purgation

§2051 If the purgative used be strong, it is advisable to take it overnight, for by sleeping after the dose, it will act more efficiently. If the purgative be a mild one, it is better not to sleep after the dose, because the vegetative faculty would digest it. Whether the medicine be strong or weak, one should not go to sleep when it is about to act.

§2052 On the other hand, a person should not immediately begin to walk about after taking an aperient. He ought, at any rate, to rest [long enough] after it to enable the "nature" to embrace it and insinuate itself into it. For unless this insinuation takes place, the "nature" will not be influenced.

22.4.7. Nauseating Aperients

§2053 When a medicine has a nauseating odor, one should make use of aromatic agents in order to prevent nausea occurring. Examples of these are: mint, rue, celery, quince, Khorasan earth (Lemnian earth: marginal reading), sprinkling rose water and a little vinegar on them. If a person greatly dislikes the odor of a medicine, let him compress his nostrils. If he dreads the medicine in any case, let him first chew a little tarragon (Artemisia dracunculus), or pellitory (pyrethrum) to dull both taste and smell. If he is afraid of being sick after it, the limbs may be bandaged up, and an astringent taken after swallowing the medicine. In the case of pills, some doctors give them a coating of honey, or boiled honey, or boiled sugar. Another useful artifice is to coat the pills with wax softened in a little oil. Another expedient is to fill the mouth with water or the like, and then swallow the pills with it. Various expedients may be adopted to meet various temperaments or personal proclivities, thus enabling the patients to swallow the drug without being aware of it being a medicine.

§2054 Decoctions should be taken tepid. Pills should be taken with tepid water. If the temperament is cold, the abdomen and feet should be kept warm.

§2055 When the patient's mind has become soothed in this way, he should take graduated exercise, for bodily movement favors the action of the medicine. After an interval of time, he may take warm water, but not enough to dilute the medicine, or get rid of it or weaken its strength, unless the time has come to arrest the aperient action. The use of hot water lessens the harmful character of the medicine.

§2056 If the patient has a hot temperament, a weak conformation of humors, and a weak stomach, the medicine should be preceded by some bland tenuous drink, such as barley water or pomegranate juice. Or, speaking generally, the stomach should contain light, tenuous aliment. Otherwise it is better to take the medicine fasting.

§2057 If the purgative is given in summer time, fever may develop. Therefore when the person has taken the medicine he should not eat or drink until the medicine has exerted its effect. And if the action is delayed, he should go to sleep unless he wishes to stop its action altogether.

§2058 If a person cannot tolerate food owing to the stomach being in a choleric state, bile readily pouring into it, or if he has had a long extended fast, it is well to take a little bread which has been soaked in a little wine after he has taken the (purgative) medicine and before the bowels have acted. This measure will help the action of the medicine. The anus should be laved with hot water and not with cold.

§2059 Some people assert that if pills are to be administered with decoctions, one should select those of like character. Thus, if one orders pills to expel choleric humor, the decoction to go with them must be such as fumitory. Pills chosen for expelling the atrabilious humor require a decoction, for instance of dodder or polypody, or the like. Pills for getting rid of serous humor need a decoction of such as century.

§2060 When the body to be evacuated is dry in nature with firm flesh, a strong medicine like hellebore and its allies, will be needed, taking great care to associate it with unctuous aliments to exert a humectant.

§2061 Finally, powerful medicines like hellebore are to be avoided because they produce convulsions if the bowels are empty at the time, and also produce irregular, disorderly movements in the moisture if the bowels are over-loaded, besides drawing into the intestine things which are difficult to expel. Sour milk will remove the harmful influence in the case of purgative herbs having poisonous milky juices, like mezereon and spurge (euphorbia group).

§2062 A medicine often leaves its odor behind in the stomach making it appear to be still there. The remedy for this is to partake of a barley ptisan or barley-meal cake, for this will have the effect of cleansing the stomach, and is more efficient than any medicinal powder. Moreover, the ptisan is the best beverage to take if the medicine fails to act, or if one wishes to make the action of the bowels mild and gentle. But if one were afraid about this, it would be better to administer mead, or syrup of honey, or a solution of niter in water, giving either a collyrium or an enema.

22.4.8. The Causes of the Failure of a Purgative to Act

§2063 The following are causes of failure of action of a purgative: (1) Constriction of the passages due to (i) the kind-of temperament, (ii) some lesion of the neighboring parts. Thus, in the case of persons afflicted with paralysis or apoplexy, the passages of ingress and egress for the medicines are constricted and purgation is rendered difficult in such persons. (2) It is dangerous and unprincipled to give two purges on the same day. (3) Affinity—every purgative medicine which has a specific affinity for a given humor will produce agitation and confusion if it does not reach the humor, and the purgation will be difficult. The same thing happens if a contrary be prescribed with it. The immediate action of a purgative medicine is to draw out the humor for which it has affinity. It then draws out whatever humor comes next in amount and in degree of attenuation and so on in turn with others, with the exception of blood itself for nature retains and stores up the blood to the very last. (4) Remoteness of humor—it is difficult for a medicine to draw out a humor from a distant part of the body. (5) One should see to it that there is not much salt in the food if one wishes to take a purgative medicine. If there is a risk of nausea or faintness after taking the purge, it is well to take radish-water as an emetic for two or three days before, and to eat radishes.

§2064 A draught of medicine may induce nausea, oppression, faintness, fluttering of the heart, griping, especially if it fail to purge or induce sweating. But it is often necessary to induce emesis also, and an astringent is then unnecessary. Barley water may be taken after the purging because it removes the evil effect of the medicine and cleanses out whatever remnants may have been left behind in the bowel.

§2065 Persons of cold temperament, in whom the serous humor predominates over the others, should follow the purgation by nasturtium which has been rinsed with hot water and oil.

§2066 Persons of hot temperament may take fleawort with cold water, oil of violets, conserve of roses, or julep.

§2067 Persons of equable temperament may take linseed after the purging.

22.4.9. The Undesirable Consequences of Purgation

§2068 Undesirable consequences of purgation include: (1) Armenian bole and pomegranate juice remove the risk of excoriation of the intestines by the purge. After the medicine has acted, the things we have named should be taken, though they may not be retained. (2) If fever follows the medicine (mixture), barley water is the best thing to take. Syrups: a sour syrup should not be given for two or three days after the purging, because it is excoriative, and one must wait until the intestines have regained their original strength. But the bath may be entered on the second day after the purging, for if there should happen to be any residual humor, the bath will get rid of it. If you find that the idea of a bath is pleasing and that it is agreeable, you will know that the last remains of humor have been gotten rid of and nothing more need be done; but if the patient does not like the bath, and finds it sets up disorderly movements (or restless feeling) of the bowels, it shows there is still something to expel. (3) Remember that if the intestines are weak, purgatives excite an unduly violent and unduly prolonged action, so that a great deal of medicine is needed to arrest it. The same is true for old persons, in whom purgation is liable to be injurious. Fever and agitation of the bowels will follow purgation, if wine be taken after the medicine. (4) Pain in the region: of the liver may follow both purgation and blood-letting. This is relieved by a draught of hot water.

22.4.10. The Time for Taking Purgatives

§2069 Purgatives should not be taken at the time of rising of the greater Dog-Star; and the season during which snow still stays on the mountains; or the season of extreme cold. Medicine should be taken during spring and autumn. Spring is the season during which the snows melt from the mountain tops. Then comes the summer which is a period during which attenuant agents should not be taken. Autumn is the contrary to spring, and is an appropriate time for the use of attenuant agents. If a person has to take an aperient in winter, he should at any rate make sure the wind is in a southerly direction. Some say that the opposite rule should hold for summer, but there is a difference of opinion about this.

§2070 Care should be taken not to acquire a habit of taking medicines as emollients for the bowels, for it will prove disadvantageous in the end. Strong purgatives depress those of dry temperament. Exercise should be avoided after a mild medicine, lest its potency be impaired. Of weak purgatives, the best are violets with sugar.

§2071 When the purgative which a sick person requires does not act, he should not move about more, but less. Purgation may excite movement of the sanguineous humor or make it agitated, and give rise to fever. Venesection or blood letting may be well under these circumstances.

22.4.11. On Excessive Purgation and the Proper Time for Using Astringents

§2072 Thirst is one of the indications that catharsis is to be ended. Therefore, if diarrhea from drugs persists without any thirst, one need not be afraid the action is excessive.

§2073 Thirst may develop, not from undue purgation, or excessive purgation, but: (1) because the stomach itself is hot or dry or both, for these conditions soon lead to thirst; (2) because of the character of the medicine—it may be pungently hot; or (3) because the material itself is hot as, for instance, bile. In the case of material of this kind, it is not long before thirst comes on. The contraries of these causes delay the appearance of thirst. If, therefore, you find that the thirst is excessive and the bowels are acting freely, you may apply astringents, especially if factors which cause thirst to develop quickly are not present. But if these factors are present, one should not delay, but use astringents as soon as thirst is evident.

§2074 Sometimes the time to apply astringents is shown by the fact of that which was intended having been discharged. Thus, if the bile has been discharged and mucus begins to emerge, this shows that the medicine has already acted too much. How much more certain is it that the action has been too prolonged if ordinary bile in the stool has given place to the appearance of atrabilious humor or to that of blood—which is still more dangerous?

§2075 If the medicine has given rise to colic, one should proceed to carry out what is said in the chapter on colic.

22.4.12. The Remedy for Excessive Purgation

§2076 The exhaustion which arises from excessive purgation is accounted for by: (1) weakness of the vessels; (2) undue patency of their orifices; (3) the laxative cleansing out the orifices; (4) some unhealthy state; (4) some unhealthy state of temperament arising from the purgation; or (5) other such causes.

§2077 Therefore when the purgation has been too free, bandage up the upper limbs and the lower ones, beginning at the axillae and groin respectively. Give a drink containing a little theriaca. If possible, let the patient be made to sweat in a bath or in steam, the head being free, the rest of the body under blankets. After copious sweating has been produced, give a massage and let the patient take astringent drinks. Fragrant aromatic liniments should be prepared using myrtle water, sandalwood, camphor and fruit juices.

§2078 The exposed members should also be rubbed, and heat should be applied in the form of dry cupping over the lower ribs, and between the shoulder-blades. If deemed necessary, one may apply plasters prepared with roasted bruised barley and astringent waters over the stomach and intestines. Oils may be used in like manner for instance, quince oil or oil of mastic.

§2079 The patient should be protected from cold air because that helps out the contents of the bowels and induces purging; and he should be protected from over-warm or hot air because that is enfeebling. He should also be invigorated by the use of fragrant perfumes, by sipping astringents and by giving plain biscuits or rusks soaked in wine of mild bouquet. But all these should be given hot, and before giving them, give bread with pomegranate juice, and various kinds of dishes prepared with roasted barley meal and the ground cortices of white poppy.

§2080 A tried formula of this kind is as follows: three drachms by weight of nasturtium seeds are toasted and boiled in buttermilk until they have clotted. This drink is extremely beneficial. Astringent aliment such as is made with the juice of sour grapes and the like, and made cold with snow is to be advised. In addition, any measure which helps to restrain the movement of the bowels for instance, the induction of emesis with warm water, keeping the limbs warm with hot water, and not allowing the extremities to get cold. Faintness may be averted with wine, and if this fails to have that effect, narcotics may be given as a last resource, and other powerful medicines which are noted in the chapter on arresting diarrhea.

§2081 For all that, it is far wiser for the doctor to anticipate all such events by having ready lozenges and pungent powders against any need for them, and also to have at hand the appliances for giving an enema.

22.4.13. The Procedure When a Purge

Fails to Act

§2082 When a laxative fails to act, and induces colicky pains and abdominal distress so that the patient feels ill, uneasy, and suffers from impaired vision, dizziness and migrainous headache, with yawning and stretching, one must have recourse to enemas, suppositories or a drink of two drachms or three *qirat*s of mastic in tepid water.

§2083 The medicine also sometimes behaves in this way because the patient has taken astringent drinks, or has eaten such things as quince, apples. Such things cause tightness of the cardiac sphincter, allay nausea, and forcibly drive the medicine downward instead of upwards, and they also reinforce the natural faculty.

§2084 If the enema is ineffective, and such bad symptoms appear as rigidity, eyeballs moving outward, or retching, then blood letting will become necessary.

§2085 Even if unwanted symptoms do not appear in spite of the purgative failing to act, it would still be well to do a blood-letting in two or three days, lest the morbid humors should pass into one of the vital organs.

22.4.14. The States (hal) of Purgative Medicines

§2086 Some purgative medicines are very malignant in character. For instance: black hellebore, the yellowish kind of turpeth (which is not good, like the white variety); agaric—the blackish kind instead of the white and pure kind; mezereon.

§2087 Inasmuch as these are harmful, if they are taken and evoke bad symptoms, it is best to get rid of the medicine out of the body as soon as possible, by means of emesis or diaphoresis, and give antidotes such as rotted yellow turpeth. The evil character of many of these drugs and the mental disturbance they give rise to, may be removed by taking excessively cold water or by sitting in it.

§2088 Beneficial for this also are medicines which antagonize the acuity of the purge by glutinosity, unctuousness, and soothing character.

§2089 Some medicines are compatible with certain temperaments, but not with others. Thus, scammony will act only feebly if at all, when the patient is living in a cold climate, unless a large dose be administered; so this is usually done in the land of the Turks. In some countries, too, one must introduce into the body only the properties of the medicine, and not the actual substance.

§2090 Medicines of pleasing odor must be mixed with purgatives in order not to risk loss of strength in the members. Cordials are good adjuvants, for they reinforce the vital breath in every member in addition to their action by virtue of their tenuous nature and ease of penetration.

§2091 Two medicines are sometimes combined, one of which expels its corresponding humor rapidly and the other slowly. In this case the one will complete its action after confining the other in its corresponding humor, and then impairing its power. When, in due time, the second comes into play, it does so in a feeble manner, so that ineffective straining movements occur. Something must therefore be admixed to help and hasten its action. Ginger will serve in the case of turpath, because it does not dull its action. You must learn how to mix them properly in order to produce this effect.

§2092 Besides this, you must take into consideration all those principles which we have set forth in speaking of the properties of purgatives (laxatives), under the heading of the general principles regarding the use of simples.

§2093 Purgatives act by virtue of five kinds of property: (1) a specific resolvent property (i.e., turpeth); (2) power of expression (i.e., myrobalan); (3) lenitive property (i.e., manna); (4) lubricant quality (i.e., mucilage of fleawort; prunes; [liquid paraffin!]; (5) a certain poisonous character, in the case of the violent purges which itself produces the purgation by direct aggressive action upon the natural drive. Consequently such properties should be met by associating medicinal agents endowed with the virtues of bezoar stone [specifically antidotal for poisons]. Bitterness, sharpness, pungency, astringency, and sourness help the action of a medicine in which that particular kind of property is present. Thus, bitterness and sharpness help the resolvent property; pungency and astringency help the expression; sourness helps the incisive property (i.e., of mucus) and paves the way for lubrication.

§2094 To ensure a lubricant action, one must not combine the drug with one having expressive power in such a way that both properties are simultaneous and equal; they must be arranged so that the one property does not come into action until after the other. Thus of two medicines, the lenitive one should be able to exert its own function before the one with the function of expression; the latter will then act after the lenitive effect has been produced. The same principle applies to the other cases.

22.4.15. Topics Dealt With Elsewhere

§2095 Purgative and lenitive epithemes and potions, and so forth, are deferred to the Formulary (Volume V). Under "Simples" we give the rules for modifying the respective simples according to the age of the patient, how to assist their action, and how to administer them in fluid form.

§2096 Pills must not be given if they have become so dry as to be as hard as stones; and they must not be given in a soft state lest they should be absorbed and held within the body. The proper time to give them is when they are just beginning to get dry, and yet yield to the pressure of the fingers.

22.5. On Emesis

22.5.1. General Remarks

§2097 Contra indications of emesis include people who are difficult subjects for the procuring of emesis: (1) due to nature, contracted chest, bad method of breathing, long, thin neck, [prominent chest, Rhazes], lean habit for in such persons the bile should be adequate, liability to haemoptysis, liability to throat inflammations [i.e., pharyngotonsillitis], persons with poor digestion, ("weak stomach"), very obese subjects,; those with weakness of vision, epileptics: in such cases it is better to use purges instead; (2) due to custom—such persons are not accustomed to be sick, and if vomiting be induced by powerful emetics, the effect will not last, and the vessels in the respiratory organs will be liable too burst, and "phthisis" will develop.

§2098 Another contraindication includes pregnancy,

because the menstrual superfluities in such a person will not be gotten rid of and the great exertion entailed in the emesis may lead to restlessness. One must allay the vomiting should it occur during this period. In other cases, vomiting may be encouraged.

22.5.2. Objectives

§2099 The immediate intention is to empty the stomach alone and not the intestines. The remote intention is to relieve the head and finally the whole body of humors which are drawn down and gotten rid of from the upper parts. And you know that the emesis has been beneficial when it is followed by relief, good appetite, good breathing, and normal pulse; and by noting the condition of the other functions of the body.

§2100 The following chronic maladies are benefited: dropsy, epilepsy, [jaundice: Aetius], melancholy, leprosy, [arthritic diseases: Aetius], gout, sciatica.

22.5.3. The Procedure

§2101 When one is unaware as to how a given person will respond to an emetic, one should first give a mild one and not venture on a strong one like hellebore and the like until after the effect of the former has been observed. Should the first one not agree, and it be still necessary to administer an emetic, one should adopt preparatory measures in order to get him accustomed to it. Thus, one orders some emollient articles of food made unctuous and sweet; and then to desist from exercise and then take oil with wine; then give good food, especially if vomiting is difficult to induce for if it fails it is better than the food still in the stomach should be good than bad. The patient should not masticate the food much which he is taking before intending to procure emesis.

22.5.4. The Rules Regarding the Food to Be Taken After Emesis

§2102 If the vomiting continues even after the contents of the stomach have been emptied, the next meal should be postponed until the patient is very hungry. The thirst should be allayed with a drink of undiluted syrup of apple or the like but not with julep or a sour syrup because these would themselves have an emetic effect.

§2103 An appropriate dish is the special one prepared with fowl; viz., first boiled awhile and then roasted before the fire. Three glasses of wine should be taken after it.

§2104 The meal should be postponed to midday and be preceded by a drink of hot rose water if the vomitus be unusually sour and the pulse is suggestive of fever.

§2105 Should the vomitus be very dark bile, a sponge soaked in hot vinegar should be applied over the stomach and the next meal should consist of something different from the foods taken to procure vomiting because to use the same kind of food would simply fill up the stomach and excite it to discharge the food.

§2106 If the vomiting has been copious, the best thing to give is small birds such as chickens or pigeons which are just beginning to walk. But the patient must take care not to eat up the leg-bones for these are heavy in the stomach and will remain in it a long time.

22.5.5. Articles of Food Which Facilitate or Induce Emesis

§2107 Almonds dipped in honey and the like; barley water taken with its wax and honey, fresh pennyroyal, confection of bruised beans, decoction of radishes, decoction of narcissus bulb, herb rocket, cucumber root boiled in honey, green marjoram, leeks, meat fat swallowed in lumps (Aeg.), oil of privet (Aetius), old pickles [onions, ptisan of pulse made with honey, rocket, moistened pumpkin seeds and cucumber seeds pounded with honey, sweet cakes, sweet wine, tepid drinks, (Aegineta)]; tepid chamomile tea, water with butter, and the like; a special dish prepared with unleavened bread, oil, melon, cucumber in its seeds or the roots well-ground up and infused in sweetened water; soup made with radish.

§2108 A person may elect to use intoxicating wine to procure emesis, but it will not do so unless a large quantity be drunk. It also may act as an emetic provided it be combined with honey, and be taken after a bath. It will also prove purgative as well.

§2109 A strong emetic like hellebore should be taken fasting, unless there is some special contraindication, and it should be taken after the second hour, and after the bowels have been emptied.

22.5.6. The Methods of Assisting the Act of Vomiting

§2110 The use of a feather will incite the movement. If so, good; if not, the patient should walk about a little; and if that fails, he should go into the bath. As midday approaches, let him do running exercises. The feather with which vomiting is induced should be anointed with, for instance, henna oil. [The throat may be tickled simply with the finger, which should be smeared with iris ointment. Aeg.] Should distress in the stomach, and spasms arise, let the patient take a draught of hot water or of olive oil, for that will either bring on vomiting or empty the bowels.

§2111 Another way of helping it on is to apply warmth to the stomach and extremities, because this will induce nausea.

§2112 At the time of vomiting, it is a help to bandage the eyes with a double turn of bandage and a light binder may be applied round the abdomen.

§2113 If the effect of the medicine comes on precipitately, the patient should keep still, inhale pleasant odors, have his limbs rubbed and compressed; a little vinegar should be given as a drink, and he should chew apple and quince with a little mastic.

§2114 Moving about makes vomiting worse; repose lessens it.

§2115 Nausea is the first premonitory symptom. Then profuse salivation.

22.5.7. Ill-effects Produced by Vomiting

§2116 The worst effect which may happen is intense spasm of the stomach and a burning in the stomach This occurs if a violent emetic like hellebore be taken. It first produces salivation, after which a copious discharge of watery fluid appears, and finally a viscid or slimy fluid. The colicky pain persists, and the other symptoms pass on to nausea and distress, which increases. The bowels may begin to act after the movements of the stomach have quietened down and the patient has lain down to rest.

22.5.8. Ill-effects Produced if the Emetic Fails to Act

§2117 If vomiting does not occur, distress increases, distension occurs, and the eyes start out, and get very red, and profuse sweating comes one and the voice fails, death will ensue unless something is done.

§2118 The best thing to do in this case is to give an enema, which you must have ready beforehand, and a dose of honey prepared with hot water. In his drink, the patient should have some oil of antidotal character, such as oil of lilies; and this should be persevered with until emesis occurs; he will not choke with it.

§2119 Difficulty of vomiting may arise because the humors are too tenuous. In such a case, they must be thickened. Barley meal is taken which has been made into a cake with cooked pomegranate seeds.

22.5.9. Ill-effects Often Resulting From Vomiting in Any Case

§2120 Sordes form in the mouth and round the teeth. Deafness may come on. While emesis benefits the body, it is injurious for the eyes.

§2121 The sign that the cause of the nauseative satiety is passing down away from the stomach is that it is being expelled by the bowel after the vomiting is over.

§2122 If purgation is followed by vomiting, it shows there is something still to be expelled.

§2123 Blood-letting must not be done consecutively upon emesis. One should allow three days to elapse, especially if there is any heaviness in the pylorus or if there is a humor lodged there.

22.5.10. The Proper Time for Procuring Emesis

§**2124** The summertime is the most appropriate season for inducing emetic treatment, and if a person had to undergo a course of emesis, whose physique is not appropriate for this kind of treatment, the summer is the best time in which to undertake lt.

§**2125** The best time of day in summer is midday because the air is then hottest.

22.5.11. The Treatment for Arresting Vomiting

§**2126** The procedure to follow in order to arrest vomiting is to rinse the mouth and the face with water, to which vinegar or sour wine has been added, for this relieves the aching of the head. A little mastic may be taken in apple juice or cider. He should abstain from food and water. He should take a long rest. The abdomen should be anointed [or a mustard plaster applied over the epigastrium. Aeg.] He may enter the bath, perform the prescribed bath rapidly, and leave it quickly.

§**2127** If it is necessary to give any food, let it be of good flavor, substantial, and readily digestible.[2]

22.5.12. The Advantages of Therapeutic Emesis

§**2128** Hippocrates advised vomiting to be induced monthly and for two consecutive days. The difficulty of the first day is obviated on the second day and that which has entered the stomach is fully emptied. Hippocrates claimed that health was conserved thereby. To exceed this would be harmful.

§**2129** Emesis carried out in this way gets rid of mucus and bile, and cleanses the stomach. For in the case of the stomach there is no cleansing secretion like that for the small intestine where the bile cleanses the mucous membrane as it passes down the bowel.

§**2130** Emesis clears heaviness of the head; clears the vision; removes nauseative dyspepsia. It benefits persons in whom it is apt to pass into the stomach and decompose the food. If vomiting precedes the meal, the latter will always enter the stomach without being contaminated, and so the sense of loathing is removed which proceeds from oiliness of food, as also the depraved appetite—namely, the longing for sharp, sour, or pungent things.

§2131 Emesis is also beneficial for flabbiness of the body and for ulcers of the kidneys and bladder. It has a powerful effect in (anaesthetic) leprosy; in persons with unhealthy color of skin; in gastric epilepsy, jaundice, asthma, tremor, hemiplegia. It is also an effective treatment in cases of impetiginous skin diseases in which there are ulcers covered with scabs.

§2132 It should be procured once or twice a month after a heavy meal. It is well not to follow fixed time intervals.

§2133 Emesis is a great help for persons whose temperament is primarily bilious and who are lean of habit.

22.5.13. The Evils of Too Much Emesis

§2134 To procure emesis to an undue degree is injurious for the stomach, weakens it and renders it susceptible to noxious matters. It is prejudicial to the thorax, to the vision, and to the teeth. It is harmful in cases of long-standing pains in the head, except when these are due to gastric disorder; and in cases of "epilepsy of the head " when the cause of this is not in the lower limbs.

§2135 The superfluity which explains the excessive emesis is injurious for the liver, the lung, and the eye, and it may lead to rupture of blood-vessels.

§2136 The custom of some people of eating to excess—even beyond that which the stomach will tolerate—and then procuring emesis [to enable more to be taken] is one of the things which ends in chronic disorders. Such persons must be advised to cease the habit of repletion, and must take measured amounts of food and drink.

22.5.14. How to Remedy the States Incident on Emesis

§2137 We have already given methods for arresting vomiting.

§2138 Tightness and pain under the hypochondrium are relieved by applying upon the stomach-region cloths wrung out of hot water, by the use of lenitive oils, and by dry cupping (using fire).

§2139 Persistent spasm of the stomach is relieved by taking greasy, easily digestible broths; the area should be anointed with oil of violets admixed with oil of mallows [variety not stated] and a little wax.

§2140 Hiccup: If this is persistent, give a sternutatory, and sips of hot water.

§2141 Hematemesis: This is referred to in the next chapter.

§2142 Lethargy, spasmodic diseases (including lockjaw), a "cold" maladies, loss of voice—in such cases bandage up the extremities tightly, apply a cloth over the epigastrium wrung out of oil in which rue and cucumber have been boiled, and administer honey in hot water as a drink.

§2143 Drowsiness or swooning (trance) are treated in a similar way, and the oil is also instilled into the ear.

22.5.15. Concerning Excessive Vomiting

§2144 Let the sufferer sleep as long as he can. The extremities should be bandaged in the same way as one does for arresting diarrhea. Over the stomach apply invigorating astringent plasters.

§2145 If the vomiting is so violent that humors are continually being discharged and even blood comes, milk should be given mixed with wine to the amount of four glassfuls, because this antagonizes the evil quality of the medicine, and arrests hemorrhage, and soothes the "nature." If you wish to clear the blood from the breast or stomach so that there is no risk of it clotting, administer syrupus acetosus in small doses, mixing it with honey or sugar and making it icy cold by means of snow.

§2146 If you are afraid a person has taken too much medicine of any kind, purgative or otherwise, procure emesis.

§2147 Emetic medicines are to be selected according to their degrees of potency, and according to the mode of administration applicable to each. These points, and especially the use of hellebore, are dealt with in the Formulary (Volume V) and under simplex.[3]

22.6. On Enemas

§2148 The enema is an excellent agent for getting rid of the superfluities in the intestinal tract, as well as for allaying pains over the kidneys and bladder, and for relieving inflammatory conditions in these organs; for relieving colic; and for drawing superfluities from the vital organs of the upper parts of the body. Such acute superfluities impair the function of the liver, and are apt to produce fever.

§2149 Among the advantages of enemas is the fact that by their means the remnants or residues of the evacuants, which are left behind, are cleared away.[4]

§2150 Form of enema; for the method of giving an enema see the chapter on colic in Volume IV.

§2151 Best posture for giving an enema is to first lie the patient supine; then turn him over on to the painful side.

§2152 Best time for administration is when the air is cold because heaviness, pain, restlessness and nausea do not then supervene; or, if present, they will decrease.

§2153 The use of the bath in regard to the administration of enemas. The purpose of the bath is to arouse movement in the humors so that they may disperse. The property of the enema is to draw out gases and the imprisoned humors. For this reason it is best that the bath should not precede the enema. In the case of intestinal ulceration, if a bath were necessary to relieve the fever or any other symptom, the risk which there is of the enema being retained would be met by applying a poultice of hot millet or frumenty over the epigastrium and umbilicus, or over the anus and thigh.[5]

22.7. On Liniments

§2154 Liniments are among those useful remedies which reach the diseased condition itself. They belong to two groups: (1) fluid, and (2) viscid. The former are more often required than the latter. If the viscid variety is used to modify the consistency of the fluid variety, a plaster results. The fluid portion will then penetrate to the affected part, the viscid portion remaining behind. It is the penetrant part which is beneficial. Example: making a plaster with coriander and crushed barley for application upon scrophulous lesions.

§2155 Plasters are akin to liniments, but are solid, whereas the latter are fluid. Cloths may be impregnated with liniments, and then applied over the important organs (liver, heart) if there is no contraindication. Cloths impregnated with crude xylaloes are useful, for they impart an agreeable odor which helps the efficacy of the liniment.

22.8. On Douching and Spraying

§2156 Douching over the head, usually is a method of treatment applicable when there is something to be dispersed from the head or other members. It is also applicable for the purpose of altering the temperamental state of a person when that is necessary.

§2157 In applying the douche in cases where superfluities have not passed into organs or members, one first prepares it with hot water, and afterwards with cold water, in order to produce an astringent effect. If the state of affairs is otherwise, the cold application is used first.[6]

22.9 On Blood Letting (Venesection)

§2158 Blood letting is a method of general evacuation. It removes the excessive quantity of humors present in the blood vessels.

22.9.1. General Indications

§2159 General indications include the following. Blood letting is only applicable: (1) when the blood is so superabundant that a disease is about to develop; and (2) when disease is already present. The object in both cases is to remove the superabundant blood, to remove unhealthy blood, or both.

§2160 Cases coming under the first category are such as the following: incipient sciatica, podagra, or any arthritic disease due to an abnormal blood-state; danger of hemoptysis from rupture of a vessel in a rarefied lung, for superabundance of blood then makes the vessel liable to give way; persons on the verge of epilepsy, apoplectic seizure, melancholia with super-abundant blood, pharyngotonsillitis, internal inflammatory masses, hot ophthalmia, persons with piles which generally bleed but now do not; women who fail to menstruate, but do not show the two colors indicative of a need of venesection, because they are so dusky or pale or greenish. Persons who suffer weakness from the hot temperament of the interior organs (in these cases it is best to do the blood letting in the spring).

§2161 Cases of severe blows and falls need bleeding for fear of an inflammatory mass developing because there is a risk of causing the latter to burst before it has matured provided there is no urgency and not too much blood in that part.

§2162 Remember, too, that blood letting is safer when the maladies to be feared have not yet befallen the patient. It must be avoided in the initial stages of a disease because it renders the humors tenuous and makes them become dispersed throughout the body and come to be admixed with healthy blood.

§2163 Sometimes it happens that the venesection does not remove what was desired and it would have to be repeated, which would be enfeebling. Once the maturation stage has been passed, the disease having passed its initial stage as well as acme, blood letting is to be done unless there is some contra-indication.

§2164 Phlebotomy is necessary in the case of a person who sweats profusely from repletion.

22.9.2. Contra Indications

22.9.2.1. Age

§2165 Blood-letting should not be done before 14, or after 70. Young adults should be gradually introduced to it by beginning with small blood abstractions.

22.9.2.2. Physique

§2166 Those who are very emaciated; those who are corpulent; those who have flabby muscles; those whose color is white or yellow; those who have often been ill. An exception may be made in the case of adolescents and old persons, if they have firm muscles, full veins, have a red color.

22.9.3. Physiological States

§2167 The following physiological states are contra indications: (1) A state of repletion with food; the stomach full of food; the bowels still loaded with feces; a state of nauseative satiety; a state of sensitiveness of the pylorus, or weakness of the sphincter. Explanation: if the stomach is full, the effect of the venesection will be to draw imperfectly digested matters into the veins to replace the loss from the vein. If the bowels are full, the veins of the intestines will suck in putrid matters from the feces. In the former case, one waits till the food has had time to pass on; in the second case, the bowel is emptied by emollient enemas. In the case of nauseative satiety, one must wait till it passes off. (2) Avoid blood letting when the patient is in a state of fasting, the pylorus is relaxed and the bile runs into the stomach, producing gastric pain, persistent nausea, vomiting, and a bitter taste in the mouth. By these signs you know of the condition. (3) Tenderness of the pylorus is another contraindication. One knows that this tenderness is present, because pain is felt during the passage of acrid substances through it. (4) Pregnancy. Avoid letting blood from a pregnant woman unless there is grave necessity, such as the need for arresting hemoptysis, and even then not unless the strength is sufficient. (5) Miscellaneous. A resolvent bath should not have been taken shortly before. Coitus should not precede. A cold temperament is a contra-indication. Caution is requisite in the case of persons living in cold countries.

22.9.4. Pathological Conditions

22.9.4.1. Humoral

§2168 It is not necessary to let blood every time you find the signs of plethora which we have given, or rather where there are signs of repletion with immatured humors. In such a case venesection would be very disadvantageous, because blood letting would incur the risk of their not maturing, with consequent risk to the life of the patient.

§2169 It is a good practice to let the blood of a patient with excess of atrabilious humor, and to follow it up with a purge. But you must carefully watch the color to judge of the patient's condition, and also the tension, because it is from the state of tension in the whole body that one can best judge of when to employ venesection. So if a person's blood is good and scanty, and his body contains many bad humors, venesection would extract the good blood and leave the bad humors behind. If the amount of bad blood were scanty and something passed down into a member which markedly interferes with the downward passage of the bad blood into it, and it became necessary to do a blood letting, one should only take a little, and give the patient good food, repeating the blood letting after a few days. It will then be possible to abstract the bad blood and leave the good behind.

§2170 If the blood contain unhealthy bilious humors, the proper thing to do first is to purge with a tenuous laxative, or use an emetic, or give sedatives and order rest and inactivity.

§2171 If the humors are gross, the ancients advised the patient to take a bath, and pursue his ordinary occupation. Both before and after venesection, and before any other form of depletion is undertaken, he was to take drinks of an attenuant sour syrup, in which hyssop and thyme had been boiled. If done unnecessarily phlebotomy simply sets the bilious humor in motion, shown by dryness of the tongue, etc.

22.9.4.2. When the Disease is on the Move

§2172 Neither venesection nor purgation is to be done when the disease is on the move, because that is the time when rest is to be ordered, and sleep is to be aimed at; it is the time when the malady will bestir itself.

22.9.4.3. Febrile States

§2173 Note that blood letting may be quite unnecessary in fevers. If there is not much matter, the nature will overcome it unaided. One ascertains whether this is likely by studying the aspect of the patient, his age, his strength, and the like. When the fever is high or when there is inflammation, blood letting is avoided. It is also avoided if there is a severe rigor, if there is spasm or if there are convulsions. In all such cases, bleeding would deplete the treasury of blood with resultant weakness.

Moreover, another febrile state would be if a febrile person with a headache suddenly develops a diarrhea, Phlebotomy, though likely to benefit up until then has become superfluous.

22.9.4.4. Critical Period of an Illness

§2174 When the crisis has been reached and it is of long duration, one must in no wise remove much blood. If possible, procure rest. If that is not possible, a small blood letting may be done, reserving the treasury of the blood for a subsequent venesection if such prove to be necessary, and also conserving the patient's strength for undergoing the critical stage. If a long time has elapsed since the blood letting was done and if there be a complaint during the winter season, of a feeling as if one is broken in pieces, one would just do a blood-letting without touching the main bulk of the blood for the present.

22.9.4.5. Enfeebled Strength

§2175 If the strength is enfeebled by having much recourse to blood letting, it will result in the formation of many humors.

22.9.5. The Proper Time of Day for Venesection

§2176 There are two occasions when venesection may be done. There is the time of election, and there is the time of necessity.

§2177 The time of election is before midday, after digestion is completed and when the bowels are empty. In the other case, the need for the relief of venesection is too urgent to wait for the other favorable conditions.

22.9.6 The Vessels Used for Blood Letting

§2178 Both arteries and veins may be used for blood letting. But arteries are avoided because of the risk of not being able to stop the blood, and if a small hole be made, an aneurism may result. When there does not appear to be this risk, the use of an artery gives better results in some diseases unless they are situated in the vicinity of the artery to be tapped, for that would make the blood thin and hot. The artery to be selected must be near the diseased part in the case of chronic conditions, in the opposite region in acute cases (Aeg.].

22.9.6.1. The Veins of the Upper Extremity

§2179 Six of the veins of the upper extremity are made use of: the cephalic, the median, the basilic, the funis brachii, the vein between the middle and ring finger and that between the thumb and index finger. The cephalic is much the best to use. The parts drained by these various vessels are as follows: The cephalic vein drains from the neck, and parts above that, but very little from the parts below, and none from the liver and hypochondrium, or from the lower limbs. The basilic vein draws blood from the abdomen and parts below. The median vein draws blood from regions intermediate between those drained by the cephalic and basilic. The funis brachii drains the same parts as does the cephalic. The vein between the right middle and ring finger is used for conditions of the liver. The left one is used for disorders of the spleen. The blood from these veins readily clots, so the patient should put his hand into hot water to keep the blood flowing longer, and to help it to emerge better if inclined to come out too scantily. The incision in these two veins should be longitudinal.

22.9.6.2. The Veins Between the Thumb and Index Finger

§2180 The vein between the thumb and index finger, on the right side is used for similar purposes as the basilic. It is useful in cases of chronic hepatic pain, and very efficient in disorders of the diaphragm (as Galen perceived). An artery may be used which goes to the inner part of the palm, and is nearly as effective.

22.9.6.3. The Veins of the Head

§2181 The veins of the head include: (1) The frontal veins between the two eyebrows. Phlebotomy in this situation benefits heaviness of the head, especially occipital heaviness; heaviness of the eyes; long-standing headache. To make these veins swell, apply fomentations, and also a bandage round the neck, placing a finger oyer the windpipe to prevent suffocation. (2) The supraoccipital veins: bleeding here is beneficial for megrim, and ulcers of the scalp. (3) The temporal veins, which are tortuous. (4) The two veins at the lachrymal angle of the eyes. These can only be rendered visible by compression of the neck in partial suffocation. Use of these two veins is indicated with headache, migraines, chronic ophthalmia, pannus, trachoma, blepharitis. Precautions include not to cut deeply lest a fistula be set up, by striking the bone. Moreover in such an event very little blood will emerge. (5) Three small postauricular veins, found at the point which the tip of the ear touches when pressed back against the hair. One of the three is more conspicuous than the others, and this is opened in cases of glaucoma, ulcers of the ears, neck and back of the head. (6) The veins behind the ears below the nuchal protuberance are beneficial for chronic eye diseases due to thin blood, and for chronic headache. (7) The vein at the tip of the nose may be made obvious by pressing the finger upon the tip of the nose so as to make if groove into two. Very little blood will come from it. It is used for freckles, for dimness of vision, pimples in the nostrils, itching of the nostrils; for piles. Its ill effects include a permanent serpiginous redness of the tip of the nose which may result. It can spread out over and disfigure the face, so that the remedy is worse than the disease. (8) Labial veins of which there are four. Use of phlebotomy here for ulcers of the gum; aphthae; (septic) gingivitis, flabby gums, ulcers, fissures and fistula in the gums. (9) The sublingual vein is used in cases of angina, and tonsillar abscess. Supra and sub-lingual veins are used in cases of heaviness of the tongue due to congestion. The incision must be lengthwise as other wise it is difficult to staunch the blood. (10) A vein at the lowest part of the lip. This is opened in order to relieve fetor of the mouth. It is situate between the chin and lower lip. (11) Veins of the gums: these are opened when wishing to act on the mouth of the stomach. (12) The jugular veins. The instrument to use here is one with a sharp point. Technique: draw the head to the opposite side until the vein is stretched like a cord. Consider in which direction the vein is likely to slip, and then make the opening accordingly. The incision must be transverse. This is used at the onset of lepra; in severe angina; in dyspnea, in "hot" asthma, in hoarseness in abscess of the lung; in dyspnea due to superabundance of "hot" blood, in diseases of the spleen and side.

22.9.6.4. The Arteries of the Head

§2182 The following arteries of the head may be open: (a) The temporal arteries. These are sometimes phlebotomized, sometimes incised, sometimes drawn out, sometimes cauterized. The object is to influence watery matters in glaucoma. (b) The two postauricular arteries. This is for treating some forms of ophthalmia, incipient glaucoma, pannus, dimness of vision, and long-standing headache. There is always the risk that coagulation will be very slow.

22.9.6.5. The Veins of the Trunk

§2183 There are two veins of the trunk to be found coursing over the abdomen. One runs over the hepatic region, and the other over the splenic. The former is opened in cases of dropsy, the latter in diseases of the spleen.

22.9.6.6. Bleeding from Vessels in the Lower Limbs

§2184 (1) The sciatic vein is opened in the region of the malleolus. The bandage is applied above, anywhere between the prominence of the hip and the instep. It will have to be applied tightly. The limb should be bathed in hot water first. The incision must be longitudinal. Contingencies include: a deep artery, or one difficult to find. In this case use one of the branches, such as that which runs between the little and second toe. They are used in cases of sciatica, podagra, varices, and elephantiasis. As for repetition, it is difficult to do a second phlebotomy. (2) The saphenous vein is opened over the internal malleolus, above the instep. It is more conspicuous than is the preceding. The incision must be transverse. It is used for emptying the blood from the organs below the liver and for causing the blood to descend from upper parts to lower ones. It is a powerful aid for the menstrual flow. It opens up the pores of piles. While one would expect either vessel to be equally efficacious, experience actually shows that the use of the sciatic vessel is more beneficial for sciatic pain. (3)The popliteal vein is opened behind the bend of the knee. It is as effective as opening the saphenous vein. For exciting the menstrual flow, however, it is even more efficient, as well as for pain from piles, and pain in the anus. (4) The use of the vein over the heel is similar to that of the saphenous of which it is a branch. (5) The vein over the inner toe may be used in cases of sciatica and uterine disease.

§2185 In brief, the veins of the lower extremity are used in cases where matters descend from the head, and for disorders connected with the atrabilious humor.

§2186 Phlebotomy from the feet is more weakening than that from the arms.

22.9.7. The Procedure in Blood Letting

22.9.7.1. Preoperative Treatment

§2187 The stomach requires to be previously fortified, as there is a risk of death otherwise. If the stomach is weak and sensitive, give pieces of bread soaked in a rob made with a vinegar of good odor. If the person is also of cold temperament the bread should be dipped in sugar water with aromatics, or a syrup of spearmint perfumed with musk. If bile is regurgitating into the stomach, induce vomiting with plenty of hot water containing oxymel. Then give the soaked bread, and do not delay with the operation. It is disadvantageous to take a bath prior to the blood-letting because it makes the skin thick and soft, and the operation is difficult unless the blood is thick.

22.9.7.2. Make the Veins Stand Out

§2188 A band is tied round the limb for this purpose. The artery may swell also, in which case the tourniquet should be loosened, and the swollen vessel rubbed. If the swelling reappears on tying the band, abandon that vessel and turn to the vessel running over the elbow. On the other hand, a bandage may obliterate the arterial pulse and lead to a risk of opening this in mistake for the vein. If the vein remains difficult to see, relax and tighten the band alternately. Rub the vein down and up, up and down, using two fingers for this, because then the stationary finger feels the blood run in which the other finger forces down. With very thin veins this will need repeating several times. The band must be adapted according to the coarseness of the skin, the amount of fat and size of the muscles. If the band conceals the visible part of the vein, a mark should be made along the line of the vessel, to enable it to be found afterwards.

22.9.7.3. The Incision

§2189 Take hold of the scalpel between the thumb and middle finger, so as to leave the index finger free to feel the place to incise. Grasp the knife by the middle and not by its end, so as to have proper control of the blade The point should be so sharp that it will enter the vein by a gentle coaxing. To have to keep on poking the knife about to find the vein will only do injury. The blade should have been dipped in oil, and the area of skin should have had oil gently rubbed into it.

§2190 The incision into the vein should be longitudinal, to render clotting less likely. The opening should be well above the level of the joint. If made at the level, the blood would not come out freely, and the risk of injuring the nerves and arteries is great.

22.9.8. Possible Mishaps

22.9.8.1. Injuries to the Opened Vein

§2191 Since venesection has to be repeated on some future occasion, the vessel must not be unduly injured: Repeated blood-letting is likely to injure it, hence a second operation should be done at another spot, thus averting risk of inflaming of the part.

22.9.8.2. Injuries to Other Structures

§2192 When using the median vein, the nerve is in danger. There may be two nerves in the way. Hence one should cut downward and lengthways. The nerve may lie over the vein, tense like a string, and injury to this, thinking it is the vein will lead to permanent numbness of the fingers. The more distended the vein the more prominent is this aberrant nerve.

22.9.8.3. Injury to a Nerve

§**2193** Should the mishap take place, the measures to adopt are those for wounds of nerves given in the Volume IV. Take care not to let any infrigidant agent touch the wound (like nightshade and sandalum), but rub warm oil all round. The large basilic vein has arteries, nerves and muscle beneath it. There are sometimes two arteries with it, and in thinking one avoids the one, one hits the other. The nerve may also be mistaken for the vein. Hence in this case it is best to go as low down the arm as possible, as then the artery is out of the danger zone.

22.9.8.4. Injury to an Artery

§**2194** The sign that one has entered the artery by mistake is that thin red blood comes out and cannot be staunched. Pressure will stop it. One must quickly put rabbit hair into the wound, with a little powdered frankincense, dragon's blood, aloes and myrrh, and a little zinc sulphate. Apply a cold compress and bandage tightly. If this arrests the bleeding, keep it so for three days, and even then be very cautious about loosening the bandage. Apply a styptic plaster instead. When the artery is hit deep down, the flesh may close over it and stop the bleeding. But usually death from hemorrhage will result. Some have died of the great pain produced by a ligature sufficiently tight to arrest the bleeding, or from the mortification of the limb produced by the tight bandage. Note that the veins may bleed alarmingly freely.

22.9.8.5. Inability to Find the Vein

§**2195** Do not keep on making attempts to puncture the vein, especially if the hand is being used; repeat a trial at some other level, or use some other vein, or wait a day or two. Remember that a tight bandage may have the effect of emptying the vein instead of swelling it. In the case of fat persons, however the veins are so slack that it requires a tight bandage to make them show.

22.9.8.6. Poor Flow of Blood

§**2196** If fat gets into the orifice, do not cut into it, but push it gently aside.

22.9.9. Other Points

§2197 Some maintain that the operation is less painful if the parts are made numb with a tight bandage for about an hour previously.

22.9.10. Amount of Blood to Be Removed

§2198 There is a proper time for arresting the flow in various cases. Some persons, even though febrile, can bear losing five or six pounds of blood, whereas others cannot stand losing even one pound, though apparently in health.

§2199 One must consider three points: (1) An impetuous exit of blood or a sluggish flow. (2) The color of the blood: it is permissible to go on drawing blood as long as it is black and thick. But if it turns pale and is thin, its flow must be quickly arrested lest dangerous results ensue. It may be pale and watery at first, so that one might think one should stop the operation even though one knows there are signs of plethora. For the color of the blood does not always correspond to what would be expected in cases of plethora. The color of the blood is also misleading when there is an inflammatory mass from which the blood is coming. (3) The state of the pulse. If the flow of blood fails, and the color alters, and the pulse becomes weak, stop the bleeding. Also, if yawning and stretching, hiccup, or nausea come on. Watch the pulse if the color changes quickly and the flow is free, so as to be on guard against syncope.

§2200 A limited venesection is a great conserver of the strength and yet it entails the flow of tenuous and sometimes clear blood, with retention of the thick and opaque blood. Liberal venesection is very liable to cause syncope, but is more cleansing; it clots more slowly, but is more efficient in those cases in which it is done prophylactically, and in obese persons. It is better to do a liberal venesection in winter, as the blood does not clot; it is better to do a limited one in summer, if it is needed then at all.

§2201 When the blood letting is done to stop hemorrhage by drawing blood away from the site of bleeding (e.g., epistaxis, uterine hemorrhage, hemoptysis) draw only a small amount, and employ several sittings rather than one single one, unless the case is very desperate.

22.9.11. Syncope

§2202 Syncope rarely occurs during the flow of blood, unless a great amount is lost. One only bleeds up to syncope in cases of synochal fevers, in incipient apoplexy, in extensive angina or inflammatory swellings, or in cases of severe pain. Even in such cases one would make sure the strength of the patient is adequate.

§2203 The persons liable to faint as a result of blood letting are those of hot temperament, and with lean and flabby bodies. Those with equable temperament, and with firm flesh, are not likely to faint unless a large amount of blood is withdrawn. Watch the pulse.

§2204 The first blood letting may be accompanied by syncope if it is carried out quickly on a person not accustomed to it therefore emesis should first be procured to guard against that, and it may be repeated at the time of the blood letting.

22.9.12. After Treatment

22.9.12.1. Washing the Part

§2205 When washing the part, the skin must be deflected by means of one's finger, so that the site of puncture is no longer over the aperture in the vein. Then wash, dry carefully, and apply a compress. Then allow the skin to return to its natural position.

22.9.12.2. Diet

§2206 The loss of blood is replaced by grilled meat with its gravy. Allow only small quantities, for the stomach will not be able to digest much. Light food should be given first, and the full dietary only resumed} gradually.

22.9.12.3. Other Points

§2207 The patient should lie supine. A resolvent bath must not be taken. Exercise must be avoided. Suppuration of the wound. The wound may become inflamed. Apply a plaster of ceruse, and dress with cold, wet infrigidants. The other arm would have to be used if venesection has to be repeated subsequently.

22.9.13. Repetition of Venesection

22.9.13.1. Indications

§2208 The operation may be repeated often if the humors are much in excess, for the operation sets them in motion (causes them to boil). But if the blood be rich in atrabilious humor, the blood letting should be infrequent. Though soothing at the time, it results in undesirable disorders, including apoplexy, especially in old persons.

22.9.13.2. Proper Time Interval Before Repeating the Blood Letting

§2209 This depends on the degree of weakness. If there be no weakness, it may be repeated within an hour, in which case the blood is prevented from clotting by applying bread soaked in oil with a little salt over the wound, and keeping it in place with a bandage. If much blood has to be taken wait a day. Two or three days is the limit for reopening the wound.

22.9.13.3. Technical Details Regarding the Reopening

§2210 Technical details regarding the reopening. Another vein may have to be used, especially if the hand was used previously. The same place must not be used if a palsy was accidentally produced previously. Some force may be needed to get into the vein next time. If the second blood letting was to be done within an hour, or during the same day, the first incision should have been transverse; but if a day or more elapse, a longitudinal cut is best. The movements of the fingers will keep such an opening patent. The scalpel should be narrow.

22.9.13.4. Treatment Between the Operations

§2211 Sleep hastens clotting and prevents the superfluities from getting into the blood, because they pass into the interior parts of the body during sleep. Sleeping on the side from which the blood-letting was done tends to damage the tissues. The strength of the patient must be maintained proportionately to the amount of blood evacuated. The bowels must be kept clear.

22.9.14. Precautions Regarding Blood Letting in Fevers

22.9.14.1. Indications

§**2212** When the fever is septic, and the inflammation is not great, the ten rules already given are to be followed. Note the urine. If the urine turns thick and reddish, and if the pulse is large, and the face swells, and the fever does not quickly improve, blood letting may be done, and it should be on a fasting stomach. But if the urine becomes thin and "fiery," and if the face wastes from the outset of the illness, avoid blood letting. Blood letting may be done during an apyrexial period. When the fever does not arise from putrefaction, bleeding without depleting the treasury of blood will resolve it. But bleeding may kindle up a fever.

22.9.14.2. When to Operate

§**2213** If the indications are present, take no notice of those who assert it should not be done after the fourth day of the illness. It may be done any day, even after forty days, avoiding only the moment of a fever paroxysm. Otherwise follow the ten rules already referred to.

22.9.14.3. Quantity to Remove

§**2214** Do not remove much blood at first in hemorrhagic fevers, and take plenty at the stage of maturation, for this itself will often put a stop to the fever. Stop the flow if you find the blood is pale and watery. Phlebotomy often disperses fevers, and resolves putrefaction. When the febrile person is enfeebled, one should divide up the venesection. Note that as venesection draws contrarily, it has a constipating effect.

22.10. Cupping

22.10.1. General Remarks

§**2215** The operation of cupping cleanses the particular part of the skin more effectively than does venesection. It withdraws the rarefied rather than the more viscid blood. It is not much use for persons with bulky coarse bodies, with thick blood, for it does not withdraw any blood from them even that component which it is desirable to withdraw. It only removes such matters as are extremely tenuous—and even these only with difficulty. It also produces weakness in the member to which the glasses have been applied.

22.10.2. The Proper Time for Using Cupping Glasses

§2216 The proper timed for using cupping glasses. Some authorities advise against applying cupping-glasses at the beginning of the lunar months because the humors are then not yet on the move or in a state of agitation; also against applying them at the end of the (lunar) month, because at that period (of the cycle) the humors are less plentiful. The proper time (according to them) is the middle of the month (when the humors are in a state of agitation) and during time when the moonlight is increasing (when the humors are on the increase also). During that period the brain is increasing in size within the skull, and the river water is rising in tidal rivers.

§2217 The time of day proper for using cupping glasses. The second and third hours are best. One must take care not to apply cupping glasses after the bath, except in the case of the blood being thick. If so, the bath is taken first; then wait an hour; then apply the cupping glasses.

22.10.3. Points of Application

§2218 (1) Forehead: most people have a horror of applying cupping glasses here, as they believe that the senses and intellects will suffer thereby.

§2219 When the cupping is done with it, whether with or without scarification, it is more efficient. But cupping with scarification is more efficient, especially in cases of flatulence of various kinds. Cupping without scarification is more applicable for cold swellings and whenever the cups are to be moved about over various place.[7]

22.10.4. Some of the Purposes For Cupping

§2220 (1) To move materials away from one part to another. Thus menstrual flow will be arrested if the cupping is done over the breasts. (2) To draw an inflammatory process from deep parts towards the surface and so render it accessible to some medicine. (3) To divert an inflammatory process to a neighboring and less important organ. (4) To render a member warm and draw blood into it and disperse vapors from it. (5) To restore a member to its proper position (i.e., inguinal hernia). (6) To allay pain. Applied over the umbilicus, cupping relieves violent colic and flatulent distension of the abdomen and the uterine pain due to movement of the menstrual fluid, especially in young women.

§2221 There are three points to note in regard to wet cupping: (1) the evacuation from the member itself, (2) the safeguarding of the basis of the life-breath so that the latter shall not leave the body with the humor which is being evacuated, and (3) the evacuation must not be made from a vital organ.

§2222 In wet cupping, the scarification must be deep to ensure drawing the humors from the deep parts. Such cupping must not be done over the breasts themselves for fear menstrual flow and epistaxis should be set up.

§2223 If the region to be cupped is covered with ointment, one should not delay the scarification. The first point of application should be made light and the cup removed quickly. As the part is accustomed to the cups, they may be left longer.

§2224 The site of the cup may afterwards develop inflammation, and thus render it difficult of removal. To avoid this, a cloth or sponge soaked in tepid or nearly hot water should be used as a fomentation around it.

§2225 Cupping of the upper parts of the body ensures that morbid materials will not pass down into the lower parts of the body.

§2226 One should not begin to apply cupping to infants until they are in their third year. Cupping should be quite unnecessary in the first year of life. It is altogether contraindicated after the sixtieth year.

22.10.5. After Treatment in Regard to Food

§2227 In ordinary persons a meal may be taken an hour after the cupping has been completed. Persons of bilious type should be given the following foods after being cupped: pomegranate juice with the seeds, endive juice with sugar, and lettuce and vinegar.[8]

22.11. About Leeches

22.11.1. General Remarks

§2228 The Indians have specified which leeches are venomous. One should beware of using those with large heads of antimonial and black color, or green color; those with down on them, like eels (snake fish), and those upon which have fine streaks of bright color, or are chameleon-like in color. All these are poisonous, and would give rise to inflammations, hemorrhage, fever, syncope, paresis of the limbs, and intractable ulcers.

§2229 One should not employ leeches taken from unhealthy water or those whose excrement is black and muddy, and whose movement immediately darkens water, and renders it offensive in smell. Take leeches from water whose surface is covered over with duck weed and in which frogs live. Pay no attention to those who make out that leeches are bad to use if they come from water in which frogs live.

§2230 The color should be greenish (like duck weed), and there should be two longitudinal lines having the color of lemon-yellow and ruddy; they should be rounded and liver-colored. One may accept leeches that look like little locusts, or like mouse tails, with very small heads. But do not accept those with red bellies and green backs, especially if they were collected from running waters.

§2231 The blood which leeches remove from the body comes from deeper down than that obtained by wet cupping.

22.11.2. Procedure of Application

§2232 Leeches should be kept a day before applying them, and they should be squeezed to make them eject the contents of their stomachs. If feasible, they should be given a little lamb's blood by way of nourishment. The slime and debris from their bodies should be cleansed off, with, say, a sponge.

22.11.3. Site of Application

§2233 The place where the leeches are to be applied must be well waved with niter-water and rubbed till red. Dry carefully. Dip the leeches in fresh tepid water, cleanse and apply with one's freshly-washed hand or with a soft towel or in a test-tube called a "leech-glass," especially if the place in question is the palate or gums. The point of application may be smeared with clay or moistened with sugar-water or milk or scratched with a needle until blood appears, in order to coax them to take hold.[9]

22.11.4. Removal

§2234 When the leeches are full, and you wish to let them come off, sprinkle a little salt over them, or pepper, or ashes or niter, or burnt bristles, or flax, or burnt sponge or burnt wool. They will then fall off.

§2235 Do not detach leeches forcibly or else there may be violent hemorrhage.

22.11.5. After Treatment

§2236 After the leeches have fallen off, the place should be sucked by cupping it, in order to extract some of the blood at the spot and thereby get rid of the toxic substances left in the wound. If one wishes to keep the blood flowing anyway, one applies warm, dry cloths to the part, or a warm poultice, or a sponge soaked in warm water. After the bleeding has stopped, apply a soft, dry compress.

§2237 If the blood will not stop flowing, dust the spot with finely powdered burnt galls, quicklime, ashes, ground-up earthenware and similar styptics.

§2238 The use of leeches is beneficial in subcutaneous maladies like serpiginous ulcers, morphea, impetiginous ulcers, and the like.[10]

22.12. The Retention of Substances Due to be Discharged

§2239 Substances which are due to be discharged may be retained within the body for the following reasons: (1) The material may be withdrawn from the part, but not from the body itself. (2) The material may be retained, although an evacuation or discharge is actually taking place at the same time. (3) The retention of these substances itself aids evacuation. The substances here meant are infrigidants, styptics, glutinous medicines, caustics. (4) Stricture.

22.12.1. Materials Are Retained

§2240 Materials are retained because attracted to a certain place, and no (outward) evacuation occurs. E. g., the application of cupping to the breasts, this relieves uterine hemorrhage. The action is more decided if the pain in the (diseased) part is first relieved.

22.12.2. The Retention of Substances

§2241 The retention of substances although an evacuation is taking place. For instance, venesection from the basilic vein may serve to arrest emesis in a case of purgation; or purgation in a case of emesis. Or again, cessation of both discharges if the sweat is (strongly) provoked at the same time.

22.12.3. The Retention of Material

§2242 The retention of material helps evacuation in the case where one cleanses the stomach and intestines from glutinous unhealthy humors by giving lubricant laxatives, using quassia; or where one procures as thorough cleansing of the cardiac orifice of the stomach by emesis, or cutting up of the material which remains behind in the stomach. Styptic medicines aggregate abnormal matter, and contract up the lumen of the passages. Infrigidant medicines clot the material, and cause the orifices to tighten up and become narrow. Glutinous medicines choke up the orifices of the channels of the body, and if they are desiccant as well, and sharp or hot, this action will be still more decided.

§2243 Caustics produce a scab which stays on the orifices of the passages, and becomes hard and closes them. But the obstruction may be harmful. The scab may get loose or break, and the underlying aperture would thereby become enlarged.

§2244 Some caustics have a styptic action (i.e., copper sulphate) and some have not such an action (quicklime). The styptic caustics are required when one wants a firm scab; the others are used when one wishes the scab to come off before long.

22.12.4. The Retention of Material by Stricture

§2245 Retention of material by stricture. There are two varieties. In one the foramen is closed and contracted so that the adjacent parts are fused together. This happens for instance when the artery is opened in mistake for the basilic vein in doing venesection. The other is where the outlet of a wound is blocked, and the channel itself is blocked, as when we insert rabbit hairs into a wound.

22.12.5. Brief Summary of Cupping

§2246 We may say, in brief, that if blood is flowing out because the orifices of the veins are open, we must use styptics to tighten them up; but if it is flowing because of rupture of the vessel, glutinous styptics must be used, such as Lemnian earth. If it is due to ulceration (erosion), one must incite the development of granulations by adding something which will cleanse away the corrosive substance.

Lecture 23: The Treatment of Obstructions and Swellings

23.1. General Remarks

§2247 Obstructions are due to the humors being thick, or viscid, or over-abundant.

§2248 If the humors are simply overabundant, their injurious effect is removed by evacuating them either by venesection or by purgation. If the humors are thick, they must be rendered thin. If they are viscid, and tenuous, incisives are required.

§2249 You have now learned the difference between a thick or coarse and a glutinous quality. It is the difference between melted glue and clay. Thick or coarse humor requires attenuation by a resolvent to make its expulsion easy; viscid or glutinous humor requires an incisive which is able: (1) to cut its way between the fluid and that to which it adheres [the wall of the passage], thus parting one from the other; and (2) to break the fluid into small fragments, because glutinous matter obstructs both by adhesion to its surroundings and by the cohesion of its particles.

§2250 In resolving thick humor there are two opposite conditions to guard against. On the one hand, if the resolution is not sufficient it will render the material watery and at the same time increase its volume so much that it cannot be resolved at all, thereby making the obstruction greater still. On the other hand, the resolution may be carried too far, in which case the attenuated portion will dissipate altogether, leaving the sediment behind as a calcareous mass.

§2251 Therefore, when vigorous resolution is necessary, one helps the action by the use of lenificant tenuous matter free of coarse particles, and moderately "hot," for this will assist in removing the whole of its obstructive action.

§2252 Obstructions in the veins are worse than others. Obstructions in the arteries are still worse. Obstructions in the vital organs are the worst of all.

§2253 Therefore it is better to combine astringency and attenuation in an aperient, because the former will counteract the damage which attenuant substance does to the member.

23.2. The Treatment of Inflammatory Swellings

§2254 As has been explained, some inflammatory swellings are "hot," some are cold and soft, and some are cold and hard. Their causes are either immediate or remote. Plethora is a remote cause; blows, falls and bites are immediate causes. Some of these causes may befall a body which is in a state of plethora, or one in which the humors are in balanced proportion.

§2255 Inflammatory swellings due to remote cases or to immediate causes associated with plethora occur either in organs which are adjuncts to vital organs; namely, emunctory organs or not. If they are not present in such organs, one must not at first apply any of the resolvent agents, but simply relieve the special emunctory organ concerned, if there is one. If the particular vital organ has not its own emunctory the whole body requires attention with a view to influencing the affected part by recoil [i.e., using a "repercussive"], drawing the material to a different organ, and also introducing an astringent influence. Owing to a difference in the member, an attraction may occur for something placed in the opposite side, whether by using some appropriate exercise, or by applying something heavy over the part. Thus, inflammatory matter may often be drawn away from the hand by keeping something heavy over the place for an hour.

§2256 For acute inflammatory swellings, astringent repercussives must be purely cold in temperament. But if the swelling is "cold," the remedies must be combined with something possessing a heating property in addition to being astringent, such as *adhkhar* (a kind of green grass) and *azfar al-tayyib* [a pungent plant beneficial in cases of warts and malignant sores].

§2257 During the stage of maturation of the inflammation, the retentive quality of the treatment must be kept down, and it must be combined with something resolvent. When the height has been reached, the two classes of remedy may be given in equal proportions. Then, during the stage of declination, the remedy should be simply resolvent and relaxing. Cold relaxing remedies have a more desiccant effect than hot ones.

23.3. Inflammatory Swellings Produced by Immediate Causes

§2258 Inflammatory swellings produced by immediate causes in a person who is not plethoric require an initial treatment with relaxant and resolvent remedies, otherwise the treatment is as before.

§2259 The inflamed organ may be the emunctory of a vital organs as is the case if the glands of the neck are inflamed, for these are related to the brain; or the glands of the axilla, which are related to the heart; the glands of the groin, which are related to the liver. In all such cases one must certainly not employ repercussives—not because it is a wrong treatment for inflammation in these situations, for it is not wrong but because in this case we do not wish to touch the inflammation itself. Our aim is to direct our energies to enlarging the swelling and convey morbid material to it from the vital organ itself. We can do no good as long as there is disease in the vital organ, and our efforts must be directed towards relieving that. Were we to employ repercussives, we should risk returning the morbid material back to the vital organ, and finally make its state so bad that we cannot possibly mend it. That is why we aim at drawing the unhealthy material down to an ignoble member, so relieving the vital organ of which it is emunctory, and we encourage the inflammatory process in the ignoble member, even to the extreme of applying cupping or calefacient plasters which will draw the inflammation thither.

§2260 When the inflammatory mass has in this way become fluid, it may burst of its own accord, especially if it be in an emunctory organ; the promotion of maturation will help to bring about this result. Sometimes both maturation and incision must be done together. Maturation is favored by the use of an agent which both obstructs and agglutinates, for in this way the heat of the part is maintained. In carrying out such measures one should watch to see when the innate heat is feeble or the tissues are breaking down. At that moment, the agglutinative and oppilative remedy must be removed and an aperitive medicine given, making a deep incision. After that, resolvent and desiccative medicines are to be applied which we shall specify in the special part.

§2261 When the inflammation is deep-seated it must be drawn towards the skin, even if to do so we must employ dry cupping.

23.3.1. Hard Inflammatory Masses

§2262 When these are at the end of the first stage, the treatment is to soften with remedies which are "hot" and not very "dry," because one must not make it so dense as to undergo calcification. The aim is to dispose the mass to resolution, increasing the resolvents up to a point, and if one is then afraid that the dispersal of the resolved portion will lead to calcification in the residue, the softening; process is resumed. These alternations are repeated time and again until the whole is dispersed by the alternate softening and solution.

23.3.2. Gaseous Swellings

§2263 Gaseous swellings are treated by agents which have a calefacient effect and rarefy the gaseous substance, and open up the pores. This treatment depends on the view that the swellings are due to coarseness of the gaseous particles and to closure of the pores. In addition one must take measures to prevent the appearance of the material from which the gaseous matter arises.

23.3.3. Inflammatory Swellings with Ulceration

§2264 Examples are like vesicular or herpetic ulcers. These require infrigidants. If they are like phlegmon, they do not need humectants, but desiccant treatment, because the secondary state the ulceration of the inflammatory mass which one feared has actually happened, and the proper treatment of ulceration is by desiccants, not humectants.

23.3.4. Internal Inflammatory Masses

§2265 The morbid material in such swellings must be removed by venesection and purgation. The following must be forbidden: use of baths, wine, bodily exercise or movement, avoidable mental emotions such as anger and the like. In the early stages repercussives must be given and a minimum bulk of food, especially if the organ affected be the stomach or liver. As the time of resolution arrives, one must not omit introducing astringents of agreeable odor in the manner in which we have set forth for you in preceding pages. This principle is more important for the liver and stomach than for the lungs.

§2266 Emollient medicines or mild aperients are to be given to those cases in which maturation is taking place, because they are beneficial to inflammatory processes. An example would be nightshade, cassia fistula. Nightshade has the power to disperse acute inflammations in the internal organs. One should give only light food, and not even then either at the beginning of an attack or during it, unless the patient is very feeble. The signs of a collection of pus in the internal organs, associated with loss of strength, indicate that the patient is on the road to death unless nutriment is given to sustain his vitality. But the giving of food is very risky. Therefore, it will be well if the disease should resolve of itself, and if the abscess bursts, i.e., into the alimentary tract, such things as honey water and sugar-water may be given to lave the parts, following them with remedies which favor maturation and are desiccant. Finally, one administers desiccants alone.

§2267 This subject is fully dealt with in the special part under the appropriate headings.

§2268 Internal inflammatory swellings in the abdomen may give rise to errors in diagnosis. If the condition is not inflammation but rupture, there is a danger of perforation. Such swellings are not usually in the omentum, but in the intestine itself [e.g., appendix], and it is dangerous to give aperients.

Lecture 24: On Making Incisions

24.1. General Remarks

§2269 When one decides to make an incision or opening (into the diseased part) one should take into consideration the various small and larger folds of the skin. In the case of the forehead, however, one would act otherwise, because an incision along the folds there would divide the muscles and cause drooping of the eyelids. Similar care must be taken in the cases where the muscular fibers take a different course to the surface folds. The surgeon must therefore know the anatomy of the nerves, the veins, and the arteries, so as not to sever any by mistake. He also needs various drugs for stopping the blood, plasters to allay the pain, and the appropriate instruments handy—namely Galen's remedy, rabbit-hair, spider's web, white of egg, and the cautery. With such agents one is able to arrest the flow of blood whether due to an accidental injury (by the surgeon), or the result of emollient medicines which provoke hemorrhage.

§2270 Having opened the abscess and extracted its contents, one should avoid applying oil or water or a plaster containing oil, or basilican. One should use a plaster made with vitriol, if something has to be applied. A sponge soaked in astringent wine may be applied to the part.

24.2. Gangrene Excision

§2271 When decomposition occurs in an organ, whether involving humoral matter or not, owing to some depravity of the temperament, and when wet-cupping or the usually effective epithemes particularized in the special books fail to benefit, then one must remove the corrupt flesh. If this can be done without the use of the cautery iron so much the better, because that is injurious to the nerves supplying the muscles and goes more deeply into the flesh. Excision becomes necessary and one must burn the place with boiling oil to antagonize the virulence of the disease and prevent hemorrhage. The flesh will fill up again but the skin will shrink and resemble flesh in its hardness.

§2272 When you are about to excise the gangrenous part, cut along the bones where the flesh is adherent, and still healthy, and the pain is greatest, this being the indication of the healthy margin. Any part that is flabby belongs to the gangrenous part and must be excised with it.

§2273 Should the part you propose excising entirely surround the bone, involving the foramina where gangrene is taking, place, excision and the use of a saw is required. If you decide to do this, go in between the place for excision and the site of perforation and flesh, to avoid causing pain. If bone is projecting into the part to be excised, and is irreducible, and there is a risk of the tissues next to it undergoing gangrene as well, we should raise up and tear off the flesh from it, stretching it by bandages to an adjoining part or using any device for the purpose which seems best for the occasion. The object is to separate the diseased part and its fasciae from the healthy tissue as far as possible, after which it can be wholly excised.

§2274 If the part affected is large, and with nerves, arteries and veins in the vicinity (for instance, the thighbone), and if the gangrenous change is very great, the doctor should leave the case severely alone.

24.3. The Treatment of Loss of Continuity

24.3.1. *Fracture*

§2275 This includes ulcers, blows, bruises, dislocations, i.e., fracture. Loss of continuity in large members [i.e., fracture of a long bone] is treated by securing apposition and applying bandages in a suitable manner as described in the special instructions given in the appropriate section. The part must be kept at rest. The diet should include conglutinant foods which will supply chondrogenous nutriment to the seat of injury and bring about the closure of the edges of the fracture and make the bone continuous again. Food of this kind can be prepared from the feet of animals. When a person has reached the prime of life there is no other way of procuring reunion of the bone. But further details on restoring continuity are given in the special part.

24.3.2. *Wounds*

§2276 There are three principles to follow when treating loss of continuity in fleshy tissues: (1) stabilize the part which is insufficiently firm, arrest the bleeding, and if there be a discharge strive to reduce its amount; (2) make the immobilized part consolidated by administering appropriate medicines and suitable articles of food; (3) prevent sepsis [lit. putrefaction] as much as possible.

§2277 If all three cannot be achieved, concentrate on the two which can. You know from what has already been said how the arrest of bleeding is achieved. Consolidation of the part is secured by apposing the edges of the wound, and by applying desiccant remedies which tend to reduce the amount of discharge, and by taking agglutinative foods.

24.3.3. *Ulcers*

§2278 In treating ulcers, the aim is to procure dessication, so that the exposed surface shall dry up. Septic changes are treated with caustic medicaments such as yellow or green vitriol (an impure copper sulphate), unslaked lime, arsenic. If these do not succeed, a cautery may be needed, and an application prepared with verdigris, wax, and oil; the verdigris is cleansing; the oil and wax counteract the undue causticity; and so we have a medicine suitably modified or attempered.

§2279 All ulcers are either simple or compound. They are simple when they are of small size and there is so little loss of substance that the margins can be reunited, the union being secured by seeing that no oil or dust gets in between the margins during the process of healing. The fact that the opposite sides will meet ensures that there will be no loss of substance. When the ulcer is so large that the two sides cannot be brought together, and there remains a mark, depression, or gap which is full of sanious matter, there being already an actual loss of substance, the treatment must be desiccant.

§2280 If there is loss of substance, then healing will necessarily be by cicatrization. This is induced in the first place by means of astringents, and in the second by applying acrid [or escharotic] substances, for instance yellow and green vitriol [cf. "red lotion"], because these assist desiccation and the formation of a scab without producing further corrosion, and consequent enlargement of the area of the ulcer.

§2281 If the loss of substance be of flesh, as happens with deep wounds, we cannot hurry the cicatrization. The thing to do is to encourage the formation of fleshy granulations and this will not occur unless the "dryness" be hardly more than of the first degree. One keeps a lookout for any conditions which will expedite recovery. Thus: (1) the state of the temperament of the organ concerned as compared with that of the ulcer itself, because if the organ in question is very "moist" in temperament and the ulcer not very moist, a small amount of desiccation, namely, to the first degree, will be sufficient, for the malady is very nearly the same in character as the member affected. But if the member in which the ulcer is situated is dry in temperament, and the ulcer very moist, desiccation to the second, and even the third degree will be needed before the temperament of the lesion can be restored to the normal. Cases which are between the two extremes will need equalization of the respective states. One must also consider (2) the temperament of the body as a whole. If the body is of very dry temperament, and the diseased member is more humid than normal, we aim to reduce the humidity to one more nearly approaching equipoise. One applies desiccant remedies. The converse applies if the temperament of the body were more humid and the affected limb were drier. If both the body as a whole, and the affected part are increased in the same direction, more decidedly dessicant treatment is indicated if the excess be on the side of humidity and less desiccant treatment if the excess be in the direction of dryness. One must also consider (3) the potency of the desiccants. All desiccants promote the formation of granulation tissue (lit. flesh), but a powerfully desiccant action is not required. All that is needed is to hold back any material which is of a character likely to contribute to the formation of granulations in its passage down into the affected part. Therefore one searches for a desiccant agent which is useful for promoting cicatrization rather than the formation of “flesh,” but one also prefers one which is abstergent and cleanses away the sanious matter to one which promotes desiccation. The ideal desiccant promotes cicatrization, consolidation of the part and restoration of continuity. All remedies which are desiccant, without any caustic action, can be included among those which promote the formation of granulations.

§2282 Ulcers in situations which are not fleshy, and round ulcers, cannot be made to heal quickly. Internal ulcers require the admixture of purifying agents like honey, or special remedies for the affected part (i.e., diuretics for ulcers in the urinary passages) with the desiccant and styptic preparations needed in any case.

§2283 To promote cicatrization one may use a remedy which is viscous as well as astringent or styptic, such as Lemnian earth.

24.3.3.1. Conditions Which Frequent the Healing of an Ulcer

§2284 These include: (1) Unhealthy temperament of the

affected part. One must endeavor to rectify this. (2) Unhealthy temperament of the blood supplied to the part is to be remedied by diet, choosing that which will produce good chyme. (3) Undue abundance of blood entering the part, rendering it too humid, is counteracted by purgation, by a diluent diet, and exercise as tar as is permissible. (4) The only remedy for disease of the underlying bone whereby sanious matter is constantly flowing over the ulcer is to deal with the bone-disease: massage can help to get rid of the diseased bone, otherwise it must be excised. (5) Adductive plasters are often required for the treatment of ulcers to enable the fragments of bones and foreign objects lodged in the flesh to be withdrawn for otherwise they prevent healing. More nutritive food may be indicated, in order to provide strength to the tissues, and, yet, the nutriment may need to be curtailed in order to lessen the discharge of sanious matter from the ulcer. Therefore, there is a certain difficulty in adjusting these contrary objects, for sanious discharge is debilitating, and the remedy for this is to supply more nutritious food; yet, to make the diet more liberal entails increasing the amount of sanious discharge. The doctor has therefore to make his decision according to circumstances.

24.3.3.2. Bathing

§2285 When an ulcer is forming, the patient must not enter a bath, or use hot water, because this will attract matters to the ulcer which will lead to the formation of an inflammatory swelling. But when the ulcer reaches a stationary stage and discharges sanious matter, it may be permissible.

§2286 If an ulcer recurs soon after being healed, it needs consolidation and is on the way to becoming a fistula. One must therefore watch the discharge very carefully, and also the color of the edges of the ulcer. If the discharge increases apart from an increase in the amount of food, it denotes maturation.

24.4. Dislocations

§2287 We speak now of the treatment when tissues are torn, as by dislocation. That is, we speak of cases in which there is a loss of continuity deep down under the skin. In such cases, it is evident, the medicinal agents must be more potent than when the lesion is exposed to view. These deep tissues are rich in blood, and therefore the congestion needs relieving, but this must not be at the risk of undue desiccant action, for in that case the tenuous parts would be dispersed, and the thick residue would become a stone.

§2288 When we have procured as much dispersal as is necessary, we apply a consolidative of desiccant character to enable material to escape, instead of lodging in the cavity and finally giving rise to a stone; in such a case it might either decompose or be removed in some other way, allowing the continuity to be restored.

§2289 If the lesion is still deeper, the place is scarified to enable the medicament to get in better.

24.5. Contusions

§2290 If a contusion is associated with loss of continuity, venesection may suffice. But if the dislocation is associated with a severe crush, the latter must be alleviated first with appropriate medicaments. If the contusion be extensive, desiccants are used. If it be circumscribed, as in a stab, it need not be troubled with unless the wound is a poisoned one or there is great pain or the nerves are involved or if there is a risk of suppuration supervening or if aneurysm develops.

24.6. Sprains

§2291 A soft bandage is enough if the condition is not painful. Appropriate medicaments are applied over the dressing.

§2292 In cases of falls and blows, venesection is to be done in some part of the body, and the diet must be light; meat and the like must be avoided. Treat with decoctions and potions.

24.7. Cauterization as a Therapeutic Measure

§2293 Cauterization is a very useful method of treatment, for: (1) it prevents the spread of a destructive lesion, (2) has an invigorating effect on a member whose cold temperament we wish to rectify, (3) breaks up putrefactive matters imprisoned in a tissue, and (4) it restrains the flow of blood. A cautery is best made of gold.

§2294 The place to be cauterized may be exposed to view, in which case the cautery can be applied without more ado; or it may be deeply situated, for instance, in the nose, the buccal cavity, the anus. In this last case a special appliance becomes necessary in the form of a hollow cannula, enclosed in some material. Around this, one places cloths wetted with extremely cold rose-water or certain juices, and the instrument is introduced so that these coverings make a little pit to receive the cautery, whilst protecting the tissues around from injury, as well as the walls of the meatus down which the cautery will pass. The diameter of the cautery itself should be less than that of the cannula, so that when dexterously introduced, it will reach the exact spot to be treated without touching the sides of the cannula.

§2295 The person applying the cautery must take care not to expose nerves, or fasciae, or ligaments to the brunt of the burning. For arresting hemorrhage, great heat is required, with vigorous cauterization, so that a firm thick eschar is produced which will not readily come off. It is this crust forming under the eschar which stops the blood flow. Therefore, if it became loose, the condition would be worse than ever.

§2296 If the cautery is being applied to remove dead flesh or tissue, pain will show you when you have reached the healthy tissue.

§2297 If the cautery is being applied to the bone under the dead flesh, one must prolong the time of cauterizing the area till the dead matter is all completely destroyed.

§2298 If the cautery is to be applied to the skull, the application must be gentle, so as not to risk roasting the brain, or shriveling up the membranes of the brain. In the case of other bones, there is no need to be so anxious.

Lecture 25: The Relief of Pain

25.1. General Remarks

§2299 You have already learned that the causes of pain may be comprehended under two headings: (1) sudden change of temperament; and (2) loss of continuity. You have also learned that the first of the headings comprises hot, cold, moist or dry intemperaments and the second occurs apart from deposition of matter or as the effect of the presence of chymous, gaseous or inflammatory exudate.

§2300 The relief of pain, therefore, depends on making use of the contraries of these causes. What the contrary of each is, you have also already learned, and you have learned the way in which an intemperament, inflammation, and gaseous deposits are treated.

§2301 When the pain is too intense, it may cause death, this resulting in the first place from coldness of the body, and secondly from tremor of the heart, with a small pulse, which finally fails, thus bringing death.

§2302 In brief, pain is relieved either by altering the temperament or by dispersing the material which produces it, or by producing insensibility. The last named destroys the power of sensation in the part concerned. Insensibility of a part is only produced (1) by making it very "cold," or (2) by exposing it to the toxic properties which interfere with its functions. Agents which act by producing relaxation, and have a gently soothing effect are such things as dill, linseed, melilot, chamomile, celery seed, bitter almond, and anything which is hot in the first degree, especially if combined with a drug of glutinous character such the gum of prunes, starch, lead carbonate, saffron, gum-resin of cristus, marshmallow, cardamom, cabbage, turnip, and their decoctions, pharmaceutical adipes, fresh hyssup, and the oils specified in the Formulary, laxatives, and all forms of evacuant.

§2303 Laxatives are to be given after other methods of evacuation have been tried, if evacuant treatment is needed, until you have prevented any further material from passing down into the affected part. For it is just that that brings an inflammation to a head, or makes it burst open.

§2304 The most powerful of the stupefacients is opium. Less powerful are: seeds and root-bark of mandrake; poppy; hemlock; white and black hyoscyamus; deadly nightshade; lettuce-seed; snow and ice-cold water.

§2305 One must not overlook an extrinsic cause of pain by mistake. Thus, external heat, external cold, a faulty posture in bed, falls during epilepsy or during intoxication, etc. Search for intrinsic causes must be otherwise made, by looking for the signs of plethora, which you now know, or for the causes likely to produce plethora.

§2306 A source of pain which was at first external may come to be internal and persist. Thus, drinking of icy water will cause severe pain in the stomach and liver-region. In such a case evacuant treatment and the like may not be particularly indicated. The use of a bath and a good sleep after it may be enough. Or a person may eat something heating, and a severe headache may result from it. For this it is enough to drink cooled water.

25.2. The Selection of Remedies

§2307 Sometimes the method used for alleviating pain acts so slowly that there is a risk of its becoming unbearable before the remedy has come into effect. Thus colic may be cured by purging the small intestine of the material giving rise to it, but this requires time. On the other hand one may give relief speedily, but only at the risk of worse harm in the end. Thus, it is possible to apply remedies which will in a case of colic at once make the painful part insensible. The doctor is therefore in a dilemma in such a case, and requires good judgment so as to decide which is more harmful, to preserve the strength or to allow the pain to persist. He has to decide which is worse, the pain, or the danger liable to arise from inducing insensibility of the part. He has to decide which is the more important to avoid, or which is the lesser of the two evils. For, should he allow the pain to continue, there is the risk of it increasing so much as to prove fatal; and if he makes the part insensible, this danger is averted and yet some other part is affected adversely. However, one may be able to remedy that, and then if the pain returns in consequence, one may repeat the process.

§2308 In addition to all this, one must select the stupefacient remedy according to its own temperament, and the ease with which it exerts its effect. One might administer it in the form of a compound in theriaca (made with it), unless there is particular need to secure a powerful action.

25.3. Internal Medication for Pain

§2309 Some members, like the teeth, cannot be treated even by the local application of narcotics, because this is not a final cure. In this case better relief is obtained by internal remedies. So, in painful diseases of the eyes, less harm would result this way than from local application of the remedy.

§2310 In the case of other organs, the harm done them by taking a draught is easily rectified. The harmful outcome would be increased, for instance, in a case of colic, because the cold The narcotic is "cold" increases the amount of " matter," and solidifies it and encloses it.

§2311 Stupefacients often relieve pain because they produce sleep, one of the factors whereby pain is relieved, especially if the patient is fasting, and there is a material cause of the pain.

§2312 Stupefacients are safer when they are compounded with other drugs as diluents (i.e., theriaca) as for instance philonium, aromatic electuary or lozenges. But their efficacy is not as great. The fresh lozenges are more efficient than older ones, and very old ones have no action at all. Those which are between the two extremes are intermediate in efficacy.

25.4. The Pains of Flatulence

§2313 The pains of flatulence are very severe and are yet easy to relieve at certain times. Sometimes it is sufficient simply to pour hot water over the part, though one must take care the pain is not due to an inflammation (which simulates the pain of flatulence) before doing so. It would be a serious mistake, especially at the beginning of (suppurative) inflammation to administer a hot water douche (shower). Sometimes such treatment makes the condition worse, should it not disperse the gases, or cause them to expand.

25.5. Poulticing

§2314 Another sort of remedy for flatulence is a poultice. A poultice may act better if it is combined with a desiccant such asmillet. Poultices are not applicable to some members; for instance, the eye. In that case cloths are used

§2315 Some poultices are made with hot oil. The most efficient poultices are those made with flour of orobs boiled in vinegar and dried before use. Weaker ones are made with bran, treated in the same way. Steamed salt is burning (scorching); steamed millet is weaker, and better. A safe and easy way of steaming a part is from boiling water in a vessel, but it requires careful control to avoid any of the mishaps we have referred to above.

25.6. Dry (Hot) Cupping

§2316 Dry (hot) cupping comes under this heading as a powerful means of allaying the pains of flatulence. By repeating it over and over again the pain will be entirely abolished. But this is at the cost of those unwanted effects we have already described.

25.7. Other Means of Allaying Pain

§2317 (1) Walking about gently for a considerable time. The movement softens or relaxes the tissues; (2) fats of thin consistency, and the oils already named; (3) agreeable music especially if it inclines one to sleep; (4) being occupied with something very engrossing removes the severity of pain.

25.8. The Priority of Choice of Methods of Treatment

§2318 When several maladies occur together we should deal first with that which fulfills one of the following three conditions: (1) When one must be cured before the other can be relieved. For instance, if inflammation and ulceration occur simultaneously, the former must be attended to first until the intemperament on which it depends is remedied. The ulcer will never be healed until that is put right. The ulcer is then treated. (2) When the maladies are related as cause and effect Example: obstruction and fever. The former must be treated first. If the obstruction will only yield to a "shot" remedy, are shall not be able to cure the fever. We; may treat phthisis (inflammation of the lung) with desiccants, but we shall not cure the fever, because its cause is beyond our reach. The cause would be amenable to desiccant treatment, but this would keep up the fever. (3) When it is absolutely essential to deal with one of the maladies. Thus suppose relapsing fever and palsy should occur concurrently. There is no question about treating the former, and venesection is the proper treatment. But this will not cure the palsy.

§2319 The disorder and the symptom to which the malady owes its name may occur together. In such a case one would begin by dealing with the malady itself. But if the symptom became urgent, we should turn our attention to it and leave the disease itself alone for the time. Thus, in a case of colic, we should turn our attention first to relieve the violent pain, even though the condition causing it is thereby adversely affected. Again, we should postpone a venesection (otherwise indicated) if the stomach be in a feeble state or if there be diarrhea, or nausea.

§2320 Sometimes we should do a venesection (for instance) without hesitation even though that would not remove the whole trouble. For instance, in a case of spasmodic disease, we should not empty out all the morbid humor, but should leave some behind rather than risk losing some of the healthy humor, in the hope that this itself will cure the spasmodic movements.

*****

§2321 This brief account of the General Principles of Medicine should suffice for the present. I would now close this account and take up the subject of Simple Drugs. God willing, that volume would also be completed in due course.

The Seal of the Work and an Act of Thankfulness

May this our compendious discourse upon the general principles pertaining to the science of medicine be found sufficient.

Our next task will be to compile the work
on Simples, with the permission of
God. May He be our
aid, and Him do we
thank for all His
innumerable
mercies.

Notes to the Introduction by Laleh Bakhtiar

1 Seyyed Hossein Nasr, *Three Muslim Sages*, pp. 23-24.

2 The Islamic medical tradition is the part of reference of this great textbook of Avicenna (Ibn Sina) which served to heal millions of people as this was the only medical textbook for 700 years in Europe alone. Translated into Latin, it served as the basis for Shakespere's psychology, among others. St. Thomas Aquinas has said: Anything Avicenna says is correct.

3 Nader Ardalan and Laleh Bakhtiar, *The Sense of Unity*, p. 11.

4 *Ibid.*, p. 11.

5 *Ibid.*, p. 13.

6 *Ibid.*, p. 13.

7 *Ibid.*, p. 19.

8. R. A. Nicholson, *Rumi, Mystic and Poet*, p. 31.

9. Nader Ardalan and Laleh Bakhtiar, *op. cit.*, p. 19.

10 *Ibid.*, p. 19 which quotes S. H. Nasr, *Three Muslim Sages*, p. 112.

11 Seyyed Hossein Nasr, *Islamic Science: An Illustrated Science*, p. 161.

12 According to the Ayurvedic system, there are three bio-energies called *dosha* (*arkan*). They are *vatha* [nervous spirit]: driving force. It relates mainly to the nervous system and the body's energy; *pitta* [animal spirit, fire] relates to digestion, metabolism, enzymes, acid and bile; *kapha* [natural spirit] relates to mucous membranes, phlegm, moisture, fat and lymphatics.

Seyyed Hossein Nasr points out: "It is worth drawing attention to the similarity between the words *ruh* and *rih* (the wind or air) in Arabic and to the Galenic doctrine that through the air breathed by the organism the life-force enters the body. It is also of significance to note that in Arabic as in many other languages the words for breath (nafas) and soul (nafs) are related. Therein lies a profound cosmological principle which is also related to the invocation of the Name of God (dhikr) as the central technique of Sufism for spiritual realization." *Islamic Science: An Illustrated Study*, p.

13 Seyyed Hossein Nasr, *Science and Civilization in Islam*, pp. 223-224.

14 Called *prana* or energy of life in the Ayurvedic system, it is comprised of energy which changes according to our circumstances, our diet, our lifestyles and the world around us. Some are positive and some are negative. We have to live in a way to attain energy balance. Energy controls the functions of every cell, thought, emotion, and action.

Notes to the Introduction by O. Cameron Gruner

1 This was actually Gruner's conclusion, but because it explains the content of *The Canon* so well and because today we have grown so distant from

Avicenna's concepts, we have placed it before Gruner's original introduction, which follows and expounds the differences between Avicenna and "modern medicine."

2 Altounyan, *Lancet*, I928, ii, 684.

3 St. Thomas Aquinas, *Summa Theologica*, p. 177.

4 See Introduction by O. Cameron Gruner, Doctrine of "the Constitution"

5 See notes to Lecture 8, Details Regarding the Emotions.

6 See §1307-1309.

7 See §57.

8 Notes to Lecture 3, Application of the Doctrine; notes to Lecture 8, Details Concerning Some of the Drives; List of Terms Applicable to Mental Faculties.

9 Notes to Lecture 8, List of Terms Applicable to Mental Faculties.

10 St. Thomas Aquinas, *Summa Theologica*, p. 203.

11 See Chapter 7: The Breath.

12 For other cycles see Lecture 10.

13 See Introduction by O. Cameron Gruner, Doctrine of "the Constitution."

14 Notes to Lecture 2, Change in Vibration-rate.

15 Vallery-Radot, *Precis de Pathologie Medicale*.

16 *Uruj* (ascent), *nasul* (descent), *jalal* (majesty), *jamal* (beauty), *qada* (fate), *qadr* (destiny).

17 Cf. Bechold 112, Sckade 137, Pearson and Wyllie 160 and many other authorities.

18 See §1313.

19 See §1266.

20 See §1307-1309.

21 See §74.

22 Many other points are noted in Part Two.

23 See §2064.

24 M. O. Stanton, *An Encyclopedia of Face and Form Reading*.

25 Sir A. Garrod, *The Huxley Lecture on Diathesis*.

26 See Notes to Lecture 9, Classification of Types of Disease.

27 St. Thomas Aquinas, *Summa Contra Gentiles*, ii, 75, p. 204.

28 *Ibid.*, 205.

29 See Part Two.

30 F. Hartmann, *The Life of Paracelsus and the Substance of His Teachings*.

31 See Part Three.

32 J. Bauer, Int. Med., ii, 127.

33 The essay entitled "Progress," was Gruner's Appendix.

34 See Introduction by O. Cameron Gruner on knowledge.

35 See Part Four.

36 This is the beginning of Gruner's original Introduction.

37 *Les Grands philosophes*, p. 156.

38 Ameer Ali, *The Spirit of Islam*, p. 392.

39 For instance, at Cairo, established in 684 A.H. by the daughter of the Mameluke Sultan Malik Taher.

40 Ameer Ali, *The Spirit of Islam*, p. 392.

41 *Lehrbuch der Geschichte der Medizin*, i. 662.

42 *Arabian Medicine and Its Influence on the Middle Ages*, p. 57.

43 Ameer Ali, *ibid.*, p. 517.

44 Old saying quoted by Ameer Ali, *ibid*, p. 125.

45 *Many Days in Morocco*, pp. 32, 61.

46 Somerset Maugham, *On a Chinese Screen.*

47 Sir Henry Howarth, *History of the Mongols.*

48 Forke, *The World-conception of the Chinese.*

49 Others include Brucell, Wilhelm, Ging, *Das Buch der Wardlungen aus dem chinesische.*

50 See Avicenna's Introductory Words, §4.

51 See Avicenna's Introductory Words, §1.

52 See §27.

53 See §45.

54 See §45.

55 *Ibid.*

56 See §28.

57 J. P. Bruce, *Chu Hsi: Philosophy of Human Nature*, p. 168.

58 *Chuang Tzu*, Giles translation, p. 170.

59 *Ayurveda*, 1924, i, I.; and see also Weber, *History of Indian Literature.*

60 Forke, *Chinesische Mystik*, pp. 242, 243.

61 *Lancet*, 1927.

62 Cf. Forke, *ibid.*

63 Hume quoted by Maher, *Psychology*, p. 238.

64 Kempis, *Imitatio Christi*, ii, II.

65 St. Thomas, *Summa Contra Gentiles*, i, 53.

66 *Gulshan-i raz*, couplet 299, p. 30.

67 *Essays in Zen Buddhism*, p. 185.

68 *Ibid.*, p. 200.

69 *Ibid.* p. 306.

70 *Rose Garden*, 1st ed., p. 120.

71 J. P. Bruce, *Chu Hsi: Philosophy of Human Nature*, i., 182.

72 The real authorship of the Libellus on the power of the hearts is disputed. Arnold of Villanova translated it into Latin (ca. 1235-1312).

73 Huineng, Susuki, *Essays in Zen Buddhism*, p. 203.

74 *Ibid.*, p. 223.

75 Kempis, *Imitatio Christi*, i., 5.

76 St. Thomas Aquinas, *Summa Theologica*, Dominican translation.

77 *Ibid.*, liv; lv. 2; lviii. 3,4; vol. 3, p. 51-87; Pegues, *Catechism of the Summa Theologica of St. Thomas Aquinas*, p. 18.

78 F. Hartmann, *The Life of Paracelsus*, p. 217.

79 Ed. Hughes, *Lancet*.

80 Sauvage, *Catholic Encyclopedia*, xii., 313.

81 Mercier, *Manuel of Modern Scholastic Philosophy*; Logique, 1904; de Wulf, *Catholic Encyclopedia*, xii., p. 26.

82 Maher, *Psychology*, p. 520.

83 Cf. Maher, *Psychology*, pp. 35, 36; and especially Wundt, *Catholic Encyclopedia*, xii., p. 35.

84 Maher, *Psychology*, p. 9.

85 In. Met. I., lect. 2.

86 *Summa Theologica*, II-III, q. 45, art. i.e.

87 *Ibid.*, ad. 2.

88 *Ibid.*, q. 9, a. 2, ad 3.

89 St. Thomas Aquinas, *Summa Contra Gentiles*.

90 *Ibid.*, ii. 3, I. p. 5.

91 Catechism of the Council of Trent, 1545-1563.

92 *Summa Theologica*, especially Part I, Questions i., 32; art. I; p. 570.

93 By Lillie may be quoted from the *Times*, Oct. 24, 1927, p. 19.

94 See Notes to Lecture 2, footnote 7.

95 St. Thomas Aqunas, *Summa Theologica*, p. 25.

96 *Ibid.*, Inayat Khan, p. 53; Cardinal Mercier, *Manual of Modern Scholastic Philosophy*, pp. 302, 306.

97 Lecture to Notes to Lecture 2, footnote 7.

98 The relation between character and physique was scientifically studied by the Chinese 450 BC (cf. Wieger).

99 Cf. Wieger who is generally opposed by academic medicine; as is voiced by F. v. Muller, 1921, quoted by Kolle, Mitt. Geb. Med., 1926, 40, 371.

100 J. P. Bruce, *Chu Hsi: Philosophy of Human Nature*, i., p. 162.

101 Cf. Paracelsus, *de viribus membrorum* in F. Hartmann, p. 219. "Moreover, each individual is a member of the great organism of the world. . . "not a separate being isolated from nature" (*ibid.*, p. 50). Individual: human world: one leucocyte: one human being.

102 *Mathnawi*, p. 169.

103 438th Arabian night.

104 See notes to Lecture 2, endnote 1.

105 See notes to Lecture 2, endnote 7.

106 See notes to Lecture 2, endnote 7.

107 *Ibid.*

108 Chinese Thought, p. 34.

109 Forke, *Chinesische Mystik*, pp. 239, 269.

110 *Description of China*, p. 104.
111 Wieger, p. 309 on Su-Wen.
112 See 4, §103.
113 See §106.
114 See §98, 99.
115 See notes to Lecture 9, Errors of Development.
116 See §1300.
117 Ind. Med. Services.
118 *Ayurveda*, 1924, 2, i., 1.
119 Sontheimer, *Zusammengesetzte Heilmittel der Araber*, p. 91.
120 F. Hartmann, *Chinesische Heilmethoden*, Munch. Med. Woch., 1927; June 3rd, 935.
121 See Lecture 12, endnote 3.
122 See Lecture 12, endnote 4.
123 The following paragraphs are interesting among many others: §1276; §127; §152.
124 *Arabian Medicine*, p. 34.
125 *Die Augenheilkunde des Ibn Sina*.
126 *Arabian Medicine and Its Influence on the Middle Ages*, p. 139.
127 E. G. Browne, *ibid*., p. 26, 27.
128 *Manuel of Modern Scholastic Philosophy*.
129 Maher, *Psychology*, endnote, p. 31.
130 J. B. Bruce, *Chu Hsi and His Masters*, p. 137.

Notes to Part One

Lecture 1: The Scope of Medicine and Its Topics

1 "Whoever has mastered the first book of *The Canon*, to him nothing will be hidden of the general and fundamental principles of medicine" E. G. Browne, translator, *Chahar maqala*.

2 Joannitius (Hunayn ibn Ishaq al-Ibadi) defines medicine as "the science which informs us about the states of the human body in health or when it deviates from health, how to retain health, how to regain it." E. G. Browne, translator, *Chahar maqala*, p. 147. Medicine is concerned with that which is integral in the nature of the human being. The seven notes of the healthy human being—four being material, essential and three formal. The four "accidental" notes, that which is apart from the nature of the human being, and the abnormal to which belong the diseases, their causes and signs. [This note from Gruner is not clear. Adapter.]

The underlying motives include medicine as an exterior life or career; and medicine as an interior life.

(1) Medicine as an exterior life or career—

(a) The pursuit of a science. Medicine may be taken up as a science in itself, for the sake of science—namely, "that science which treats of the prevention or cure of disease. . ." This work entails the study of cognate sciences.

Love of knowledge may be the chief motive; that is, it is an intellectual pursuit; through other motives may be associated.

Many branches of medical science are separated off as distinct pursuits—external, internal, state, psychological, pathological, legal, medicine, etc. As a career, it may be orthodox, that is obedient to the laws about practice, etc.; in which case it is also obedient solely to the microbic theory of disease—or unorthodox in various degrees, through following different "systems," many of which are unauthorized, and lead to some form of illegal practice.

If medicine be regarded as concerned with the nature and constitution of the human being (as a matter of the first importance in learning how to maintain health and alleviate the distresses of ill-health), it is defined virtually in the same way as Avicenna, and conforms also to modern scholastic philosophy. In this case, the practitioner would center his attention on the individual, the patient himself, rather than on some disease or infection, or over and above the disease or infection; the constitution being primary in causation.

(b) The pursuit of a practical art—the scientific aspect is here made subsidiary to practical utility and success. (i) In the primary motive, this form of pursuit is, of course, the pursuit of a livelihood, and a medicine is a form of commercial life. Its success would then be measured by the bank balance. Admittedly this is seldom of the degree called wealth. After a long life of hard work, such a one might grieve at his lack of success did he not simultaneously have motive; (ii) for these words then apply: "the only compensation which medicine offers to wealth is the spiritual pleasure of sacrifice, that solemn sweetness which floods our being when we see the fruit of our pain. The dependence of the soul on the Creator brings our obligation to Him in dealing with those under our care. This is what makes the weary dispensary clinic blossom with a fullness of solace surpassing all expectations" (P. J. Flagg, *The Patient's Point of View*). (iii) Pursuit primarily for humanitarian motives—the alleviation of suffering, especially of physical pain; and of various disabilities. (The actual cure of disease is often supposed to be within human scope, though an impartial judgment must surely modify such an idea). Preventive medicine is based on the same motives.

(2) Medicine as an interior life. Motives in the strict sense:

(a) Worldly motives—the pursuit as a means of satisfying a certain egoism or ambition on the part of the doctor himself or of his relations; pursuit as a trade or business.

(b) As a form of devotion to fellow-men. Philanthropy: (i) the relief of pain, disability, suffering, etc.; (ii) socio-political motives—the efforts of legislation and research: sanitary medicine; state medicine; industrial medicine; organization of team work both for research and the panel. The devotion is more to the human being in the abstract, the individual not receiving personal contact, as he does under (1).

(c) As a form of devotion to God: (i) the study of medicine may be made the means of studying God both in nature and in the human being, and indeed in all life, to perceive the purpose of God therein; (ii) the pursuit of practice: (a) as a penance or means of mortification "in the cell of your heart." So Avicenna, the Sufi, seeing through the Quran how daily life is a disciplinary (L. Massignon, *La Passion d'al-Hallaj, martyr mystique de l'Islam*, ii, p. 515).

(b) A means of reaching personal perfection: "every soul is on the way to sanctification, after all, and God leads each according to the means He selects as best" (Ad Tanquery, *Precis de Theologie Ascetique et Mystique*, p. 976). This is the practitioner's "unitive way." To achieve one single act in the whole life would be to achieve the desire.

(c) A means of realization of the love of God—"the fear of the Lord is the beginning of wisdom" (medicine as a "religious life" being capable of inclusion under this title)—culminating, not through personal will, but through divine will, in a consciousness of the presence of God throughout every organ and tissue, so that the state (*hal*) of recollection may finally become actual.

(d) A means of expiation—it is possible that expiation may be accomplished through the instrumentality of the physician, and without his being aware of the fact. He may be the instrument whereby the patient is released from illnesses arising from causes indicated in [Lecture 10, endnote 45]. On the other hand, he may fulfill a deeper intention, especially when both skill and devotion are great, for in him the devotion of God to the human being may become capable of expression, he may become the vehicle of God's intention. As the master virtuoso is just one voice of God heard from among the sea of musicians, and is only able actually to utter one or two of the voices of thousands of composers in his recital, so also is the utterance of that expiation rare and restricted. One wave alone comes into prominence and then breaks, but it is with thorough purpose, not at random. Even so, God, in that wave, may wish to express Himself in that manner if only once and through one individual in one generation.

This, the highest aim of the pursuit of medicine as an art receives a dual reward: the subtle intangible, but far-reaching influence upon the patients, benefiting them unknowingly; the influence upon the physician by the spirit of divine love whereby is imparted the gift of insight into the realms of absolute realities—into that which underlies deeply the appearances of this kaleidoscopic world; the gift of ability to counsel the patient along the road of their own life, whereby those for whom this counsel is intended shall proceed towards the common goal of the human being. Neither physician nor patient may be conscious of this gift. Yet the former may recognize in the illnesses or persistent ill-health some decree, some divine purpose related to that particular soul, which it may be for the physician to intervene or not, whether he perceives the holy ground on which that patient momentarily stands or not. No treatment will cure until the expiation is accomplished.

To the despondent and over-tired and weary practitioner, these motives reveal the same life and vision of paradise as belonged to the author of *The Canon*; once viewed, its warmth and happiness may still accompany him as he resumes his daily round, and thereafter his enforced departure upon the tasks of the day need evoke no sigh of regret.

As Ibn al-Farid (AD 1182-1235) reveals in this *Tayiyya* (p. 180), there is the power of lifting oneself into the sphere of the infinite and eternal, whereby the daily task becomes transformed, "all breathing human passion far above."

In these days, mass production of all kinds and in great cities—in those days, individual craftsmanship and artistry in secluded places; in these days, the organization of modern medicine for wholesale achievement in all is departments; team workers and the rush of the highways with a certain scorn for the isolated; in those days, a placid and leisurely solitude, in which could be attained a quiet seership of life.

In thought, we of this day may step aside from the rush of the highways and lanes and in our wayfaring find ourselves back in those times, meeting with a solitary and forgotten seer, stay quietly awhile with him, and through him gain a glimpse of Something which nothing else can reveal, Whose very truth is abiding and irresistible.

3 *Symptoms*: the word includes our modern "signs" and "symptoms." *Principles of being*: this is the topic of scholastic metaphysics. *Only through a knowledge of causes*: compare the following: "It is impossible to know a thing perfectly unless we know its operation since from the mode and species of its operation we gauge the measure and quality of its power, while the power of a thing shows forth its nature because a thing has naturally an aptitude for work according as it actually has such and such a nature.

"Now the operation of a thing is twofold as the Philosopher says: "one that abides in the very worker and is a perfection of the worker himself, such as to sense, to understand, and to will and another that passes into an outward thing and is a perfection of the thing made, that results from it, such as to heat, to cut and to build" St. Thomas Aquinas, *Summa Contra Gentiles*, ii. I; 9 Metaph., D.8, viii. 9.

4 The Latin annotator of *The Canon* (1608 CE ed.), Costaeus in his *Contra Gentiles*, speaks of health as a "harmony of the composite, the formal cause of the human body." Galen also defined temperament as the formal cause of the human body. Some traditional theologians define the formal cause of the human being to be what is called the rational soul. St. Thomas Aquinas refuted this by saying: "Harmony cannot move a body or govern it nor can a temperament. A harmony and a temperament also admit of degrees. The notion of harmony rather befits qualities of the body than the soul. Thus health is a harmony of the humors. Strength is a harmony of muscles and bones. Beauty is a harmony of limb and color. Harmony may mean either the composition itself or the principle of composition. Now the soul is not a composition

because then every part of the soul would have to be the composition of the parts of the body. . . ." St. Thomas Aquinas, *Summa Theologica*, lxiii, I. p. 166.

Just as the medieval physicians fell into the rationalistic error so ably and thoroughly exposed throughout the *Contra Gentiles*, when they "freed" themselves from the stereotyped teaching, so with modern teaching. The physical and chemical facts which were discovered in the 19th century appeared finally to controvert both the statements of *The Canon* and those of the scholastic metaphysicians, but it is gradually becoming clear to more and more thinkers that this is not the case.

5 In regard to the last sentence note, "It is not the concern of physical science [including medicine] to study this first origin of all things. That study belongs to the metaphysician who deals with being in general and realities apart from motion" (*Contra Gentiles*, ii, c, xxxvii).

In reference to the same, note also the following passage by S. J. Rickaby, *Of God and His Creatures*, p. 103: "motions, molar and molecular, vibrations and transferences chemical, biological, mechanical or cosmic—are the subject-matter of the professor of physical science; but the Creator and the creative act are above motion . . . the range of physical science is narrower and lower than that of literature . . . . When a physicist pronounces on a religious question either for or against religion, he has overshot his subject. Of course he ought to overshoot his subject. . . . Wherever physical science becomes the staple of education, to the setting aside of Latin and Greek, it will be found necessary . . . in the interests of religion to insist upon a parallel course of metaphysics, psychology and ethics . . . trained on physical science without literature and philosophy, the mind suffers atrophy of the religious faculties, a disease which some seem anxious to induce upon mankind—a painful disease, nevertheless, productive of much restlessness and irritability."

Lecture 2: The Elements

1 Elements: equivalents would be cosmic elements; imponderable elements; primordial essences; first-principles; elementary principles; grades of radiance. It is important to note that these elements are *not* "matter," but have only a virtual existence as explained more fully below (see notes to Lecture 2: Considered Dynamically-Change and §749).

St. Thomas Aquinas commented: "By the words earth and water (in Genesis i), primary matter itself is signified. . . .The power possessed by water or earth of producing all animals resides not in the earth and water themselves, but in the power originally given to the elements of producing them from elemental matter" (St. Thomas Aquinas, *Summa Theologica*, Dominican translation, 1923).

Rumi said in the *Divan-i Shams-i Tabriz* (R. A. Nicholson, *Selected Poems from the Divan-i Shams-i Tabriz*, 235, 5, p. 220).

I am in water, and earth, and fire, and air.
These four around me, yet of these four I am not.

A difference must therefore be observed between them and the literal earth, water, air and fire. Each of the latter, it must be noted, contains all four elements, imponderable elements, the correspondingly named element being merely preponderant (see Lecture 7, endnote 1).

Simple bodies: That is, simple in the scholastic sense; indivisible. "Simplicity is that quality by virtue of which a substance has neither constitutive nor quantitative parts" (Cardinal Mercier, *Manual of Modern Scholastic Philosophy*, ii, p. 523.

2 There are five elements in Chinese, Buddhist and Ayurveda philosophy. In theosophy also, a fifth, named "ether," is given. The alchemists gave three. Aristotle discussed a fifth saying, "The heaven is not of the nature of the four elements, but is itself a fifth body, existing over and above these" (St Thomas Aquinas, *Summa Theologica*, vol. 1, p. 218). These various statements are not actually mutually contradictory (see Introduction: The Doctrine of "The Elements").

Light—equivalents: weak, male (because conferring or inceptive), positive, active. Heaven.

Heavy— equivalents: strong, female (because recipient), negative, passive. Earth.

Rumi says,

Heaven is man and earth woman, in character;
Whatever heaven sends, earth cherishes.
When earth lacks heat, heaven sends heat;
When it lacks moisture and dew, heaven sends them (Jalal al-Din Rumi, *Mathnawi*, translated by E. H. Whinefield, p. 41).

3 The elements come from the world between the moon and the earth, the horizon between matter and spirit in the macrocosm. The sublunary world is called "the world of growth and decay." The element closest to the moon is the igneous sphere (fire), then the aerial sphere (air), the aqueous sphere (water) and finally the terrestrial sphere (earth).

Rumi says: "The earth is the warp and weft of your body" (Jalal al-din Rumi, *Mathnawi*, translated by E. H. Whinefield, p. 41). Earth is understood in respect of its principal property of dryness (St. Thomas Aquinas, *Summa Theologica*, vol. i. p. 234).

4 The Quran says: "*Verily the likeness of the present life is no other than as water which We send down from heaven and wherewith the produce of the earth is mixed, of which men eat, and cattle also, until the earth has received its vesture and is adorned. The inhabitants thereof imagine that they had power over*

the same, but Our command comes unto it by night or by day, and We render it mown, as though yesterday it had not abounded with fruits." (10:24)

In other verses, the Quran says that water enters into plants "*only as long as it is there do they live.*" "*The parable of the life of this world: like water which We send down from the cloud so the herbage of the earth becomes luxuriant on account of it*" or "*water is the channel of life.*"

"Water has especially a life-giving power since many animals originated in water and the seed of all animals is liquid. Also the life of the soul is given by the water of baptisms" (*ibid.*, 74, iii, p. 273). "Augustine holds 'water' to mean 'formless water.'"

Water can be understood as "radical moisture" (Paracelsus), which is absolutely essential to life. H_20 being thus as it were an instrument or substrate. The plant cannot shoot out leaves, flowers and fruit without it so the human being cannot thrive without this radical moisture or innate moisture. Moreover, in this view, the moisture is conserved by a medium which has "material" humidity—a concept which brings us to the domain of chemistry.

The watery nature may be called "fluid nature"; pliability; living character. Inayat Khan, *In an Eastern Rose-garden.*

So in the Chinese conception (Forke, *The World-Conception of the Chinese*, p. 271) explains that the fluid of water is yang and its substance yin. The fluid of earth is yang and its substance yin whereas the fluid of fire is yin and its substance yang. Yin is here understood in a procreative sense, yang in a destructive sense.

5 "The element of air entering into the vital forces (breaths, spirits) is that which enables us to stretch and contract and also makes possible the involuntary movements throughout the body," Inayat Khan, *Various Writings.*

6 The difference between the "element" fire and fire as usually understood is shown in describing flame, for instance, as material fire, and vesicants like cantharides, urtica, as essential fire. Or as stated under air there is a fluid of fire and a substance of fire, just as water is radical or substantial or material.

7 "*Elementa subtiliora predominatur in mixto, secundum virtue; sed grossiora secundum quantitatem*" (St. Thomas Aquinas, *Summa Theologica*, Dominican translation, 71, I, 2m; 91, I, c. 3m).

Fire, Air, Ether; the nourishing flame which imparts heat, life, sense and intelligence (*Catholic Encyclopedia*, xiv. 153).

It is the form that is the motor and not the breath. In this sentence is contained the crux of the whole subject. "Form" used in the scholastic sense has a subtly specific meaning when applied to the human being. This will be explained in further notes. Briefly, the form when associated with the solid, fluid, and gaseous components (earth, water, air) of the body" is called a "living human being," and it accounts for the continual movement of the "breaths" (life-principle) which manifests to the onlooker that the human being really is living.

Position in nature. If the names of the elements are taken as synonymous with the corresponding words describing mundane nature, it is evident that earth (land) is higher than "water;" and that "air" is above both. The fire (solar heat) is above all, but mystically speaking there is such a relation apart from the geographical one.

In the following scheme the classification of "worlds" is set out according to the various schools of thought (Quranic, Persian, Ptolemaic, etc) prevailing in the Middle Ages. The literal discrepancies are simply due to the standpoint having been taken differently—sometimes theological, sometimes philosophical, sometimes scientific—by the several schools of thought.

Scheme of the Position of the Several "Worlds" As Conceived by the Ancients

The Vacuum. *al-Khala; la khala wa la mala.* "Neither vacuum nor plenum" (Nizami, *Chahar Maqala*, p. 118).

Eleventh Heaven. The Empyrean. The seventh heaven of St. Thomas, "wholly luminous." (St. Thomas, *Summa Theologica*, Dominican translation, 68, p. 228).

Tenth Heaven. The Primum mobile (because it originates the motions of the lower spheres). The Plain. The starless Heaven. *al-Falak al-atlas*. Ptolemy's *Empyrean*. (Nizami makes this the ninth heaven).

Ninth Heaven. The Crystalline. The sixth heaven of St. Thomas or "Aqueous"; "wholly transparent." The celestial sphere. The Highest Heaven. *Arsh* (Mahmud Shabistari, *Gulshan i-raz*, p. 22). The movements in this accounts for the irregularities of movement in the fixed stars.

Eighth Heaven. The Zodiacal Sphere. The Throne, *al-Arsh* (Quran). The fixed stars. The zodiacal heaven is the confine of the material universe. The fifth Heaven of St. Thomas: the starry heaven with eight spheres, the first being that of the fixed stars.

Seventh Heaven to First Heaven: "The sphere of the planets."

"Into seven heavens did He fashion it" (*ibid*, p. 22).

"*He made them complete seven heavens*" (Quran, 2:29). "Every *sama* (whirling) is a heaven in relation to what is beneath it and earth in relation to what is above it." Raghib quoted in Woking's translation of the Quran.

"There are seven corporeal heavens in all, in the opinion of Rabanus" (St. Thomas, *Summa Theologica* Dominican translation, 68, 4, p. 228).

Seventh. Saturn: Black. The first to be created.

Sixth. Jupiter: Blue. Presided over by Michael. Formed from the light of spiritual strength (*himma*).

Fifth. Mars: Blood-red. Presided over by Azrael. Formed from the light of inspiration (*wahm*).

Fourth. The Sun: Presided over by Israfil. Formed from the light of the heart (*qalb*).

Third. Venus. Yellow, the world of similitudes. Formed from imagination (*khayal*).

Second. Mercury. Grey. Formed from reflection (*fikr*).

First. Moon. White then silver. Made from Ether. "The heaven of the moon" (R. A. Nicholson, *Studies in Islamic Mysticism*, quoting Jili, p. 122). "Here comes the horizon between matter and spirit" (St. Thomas, *Sunna Contra Gentiles*).

Sublunary world: The '"world of growth and decay" (Nizami, *Chahar maqala*).

Fourth Interspace (*furja* according to Nizami, *Chahar maqala*). The Human Kingdom.
Fourth Elemental Sphere. Igneous sphere. Fire. Divided by Rabanus into an upper region, the ethereal heaven, and a lower, the aerial heaven.
Third Interspace. The Animal Kingdom.
Third Elemental Sphere. Aerial sphere. Air. Divided by Rabanus into an upper region, the ethereal heaven, and a lower, the aerial heaven.
Second Interspace. The Vegetable Kingdom.
Second Elemental Sphere. Aqueous sphere. Water.
First Interspace. The Inorganic World (chiefly East and West; aided by Air and Fire).
First Elemental Sphere. Terrestrial sphere. Earth. Jili refers to seven limbos of the earth (R. A. Nicholson, *Studies in Islamic Mysticism*, p. 124).

Explanatory Extension of Lecture 2: The Elements

I Preliminary remarks.
II The doctrine of matter and form:
(A) considered statically;
(B) considered dynamically.
III Application of the doctrine to biochemistry, histology, etiology, etc.

I. Preliminary Remarks

Lecture 2 is the foundation of the whole *The Canon*, but so entirely has the doctrine and world view of Avicenna been superseded by modern scientific teaching that the whole of his work may be said to fall with it.

The fact that for millions of intelligent people this world view (scheme of things, theory of life, *Weltanschung*) is an intense reality in their daily lives (A. Forke, *The World-conception of the Chinese*, p. 239) is not taken into consideration by modern science and yet even a training in Western universities does not dispose them to abandon it.

So too, the daily-recited Breviary still contains the *Benedicite opera omnia*, in which the four "elements" sing their praise just as for St. Francis in his *Song of the Sun* they were an instruction for us to do likewise.

Their immediate dependence for existence upon the continuously exercised will of the Creator is spoken for both by St. Thomas Aquinas in the West and by the Persian Sage in the East. "Even air, water, earth, and fire draw their sustenance from Him, both winter and summer" (*Mathnawi*). As the mighty servants of God) "to us they seem lifeless, but to God living," *Mathnawi*, p. 15) they offer Him praise (Quran) and service (*Mathnawi*).

The modern world view sets out that the universe is composed of chemical elements grouped into compounds, aggregated into masses varying from the size of vast nebulae to the smaller but still vast "suns" down to the fragments of dust beneath our feet; whereas the modern scholastic philosophy sees in our space-time world only a fringe (Cf. Job xxvi, 14) and allows that the ancient idea of "heaven beyond the blue" evidenced understanding and not superstition. In short, the doctrine underlying Avicenna is capable of justification.

The Doctrine of "Matter" and "Form"
A. Considered Statically

Lifeless or inanimate matter, in a state of rest, is the result of two principles which exist simultaneously: the principle of inertia or passivity and the principle of activity. That inanimate matter which is passive or inert is called primary matter by Muslim scholars as well as by the scholastics of Middle Ages Europe. It is the material cause of a thing. It is represented by *m*. The second or principle of activity is called form or formal cause represented by *f*. It is non-material. Li Ki (translated by S. J. S. Couvreur, *Ho Kien Fou*, vii.3.I) says: "The human being is the result of the combined operation of heaven and earth, of the union of two principles."

Every object has a form (*f*), an activity, but every activity or action is not part of a material object.While some activities or actions are intrinsically dependent on a material object, others can exist apart from it.

The passive form, *m*, the primary matter, remains indifferent and undetermined. It will take an infinite number of activities or forms (*f*), but as soon as a passive object, a primary matter, is given a form, it ceases to be indifferent and undetermined because it has become an animate matter or matter-form, passive-active (*mf*). That is, when a passive form receives activity, it becomes a physical object. The activity (*f*) is said to be "in-form" matter. It is then called "substantial form" (*mf*) as opposed to primary matter. Therefore, the activity or action or form (*f*) is called the formal cause of a thing or the "determining principle" of a thing. The activity or action "perfects" or "completes" that which was passive, inert, inanimate primary matter (*m*). When the passive, inert, inanimate primary matter (*m*) receives an action or activity (*f*), the action is also called "essential form" which it is said gives rise to the active matter, the "essence" (*mf*). Activity or action (*f*) gives a distinctive nature to the primary matter (*m*) and fixes the character and properties and activities resulting from the union. Activity or action (*f*) provides the "deep intrinsic reason" for the now active matter (*mf*). The repetition of this process of action upon the object represents as many different objects, living or non-living.

Activated matter (*mf*), then, stands for the following concepts: (i) physical substance, "physical" or "corporeal" because it is evident to our senses. "Substance" because viewed in its "static" state, it is inactive, stationary. Every chemical substance is a different matter-form, passive-active possibility. (ii) "Nature." Viewed as "nature," it is viewed in its powers of activity. (iii) "Essence." This is when we describe what it is and say what distinguishes one passive-active state (*mf*) from another (*mf*), from all other passive-active states. In other words, it has "transcendental properties": being, essence, unity, distinction from other beings, truth, and good. Every object is a being. Every object is a "creature." Every object perceptible by our senses is a material being. (iv) "Constitution." When we study the passive-active states (*mf*) from the point of view of how it came into being, we are discussing "constitution."

Every object has three causes for its existence: material, formal, and efficient. That which brings about the union of the passive state *m* (material cause) with the active possibility *f* (formal cause) is called the efficient cause. Then there is the final cause, the reason for its existence, the reason for its creation.

As soon as the passive-active state (*mf*) exists, certain qualities become manifest to our senses with which we are able to form a mental image of the object, over and above the "transcendental properties" referred to above. These qualities are called "accidents" represented by (*a*). A concrete object is therefore represented more accurately by the symbol *mf.a*, the dot showing that *mf* forms one essence. To be more exact, then, the different objects around us would be represented by the formula *mf.a*, *mf.'a'*, *mf."a"*, *mf.'"a'"*.

A further scholastic term is introduced if we say that "when *mf* (potentiality) becomes actuality, it is *mfa*. That is another way of saying that until a substance actually exists it has no "accidents" or "qualities."

The same symbol—*mf.a*—stands equally for a chemical atom, a chemical compound—inorganic or organic—however complex; for a whole mineral; for a histological "cell," (microbe, protozoan, cell-colony, simple or complex), for a whole plant or animal, or for a human being as a whole. Any object in the universe—water, stone, tree, mountain, herb, sun—can be represented by this same symbol. Every object is a "creature" in the Thomistic sense. Every object is "in-formed" matter. The differences between them all depend on the *f*.

Human nature is in-formed matter, bearing certain properties or marks and endowed with existence. Each organ in the body is in-formed matter. Every tissue is in-formed matter. The blood, the lymph, the urine, etc, are each of them in-formed matter. Every microscopic cell of which the tissues are composed is merely in-formed matter. So also is every chemical entity which composes the cells, and the whole person also is just in-formed matter.

In the case of a living human being there is this complication that each particle of matter of which he is composed is represented by *mf.a*, and the body itself, as a whole, is representable by *mf.a*. To picture the whole person more satisfactorily we should employ a capital letter—say *M*—to stand for the actual matter of the body and the human form would be representable by another capital letter *F*, for the human form differs from all other forms. Hence the human being is symbolized by *MF*, rather than by *mf.f'* or *mf+f'*—both of which would be inaccurate. *M=n.mf.a*. When death occurs, *MF* become *M* and *F*; *M* becomes *n.mfa* again—simply a collection of chemical inanimate substances. *MF* stands for a human soul. *F* is not soul. *F* does not exist without *M* in the first instance, but after death it does exist without *M*. However, the great and important fact is that at the time of death *F* is no more like *F* at birth; being different it is correct to symbolize it as *F'*.

The object of life is not to alter one's character, but to *control* it so that the passions never come to light. It is not for us to try and "add a cubit to our stature" (Mt. 6, 27) but to direct our unchangeable "character" into the very highest altruistic direction. The object of life is to prevent the character from determining the form of one's actions. See Lecture 8, endnote 11).

Many of the laws operating in the non-living substance *mf.a* also occur in *MF*, although every separate *MF* follows its own laws. The laws peculiar to the chemical substances of which the body is composed necessarily apply in *MF*, as well as those pertaining to his being a particular *MF*. The mere fact of *MF* being altogether more elaborate than its component *n.mf.a*'s (which together make *M*) does not abrogate the applications belonging to those component *mf*'s—a fact which is often overlooked. Rationalism, for instance, assumes that because the lower are still present, the higher must simply be a variety of them.

"In the living conscious being, this qualitative determining factor (the germinal principle) takes a still higher form, its range of activity is wider, its power of applying, directing and disposing of the energy stored in the organism is more varied and more flexible, but it cannot alter the quantity of the capital funded in the self-moving machine. If, then, it be the quality of the forces distributed in the nervous system which the directive power of the soul immediately determines, the liberation and control of a person's physical activity by his thoughts and volitions need not necessarily conflict with even the most rigid fulfillment of the law, of the constancy of the quantity of energy" (P. Couailhac, *La Liberte et la conservation de l'energie, livre* iv, quoted by Maher, *Psychology*, p. 523).

"If an angel or a demon set a barrel rolling down a hill by even a slight push, the action of such a spirit would involve the invasion of the system of the material universe by a foreign energy. But this is not the way the soul acts according to the philosophy of St. Thomas and Aristotle. Here the soul is part of the living being, a component principle capable of liberating and guiding the transformation of energies (it selects and stores up) in the constitution of the material organism which along with its compounds goes to form a single complete individual being" (Michael Maher, *Psychology*, p. 428).

Again, not by virtue of its rationality is the *forma animale*, but through the vegetative and sentient faculties (Aristotle, quoted in *Catholic Encyclopedia*, ix, p. 239).

There is an important passage on matter in the *Summa Theologica* (Q. 85, Art. I, p. 185-6) which brings out the distinction between the ponderable and the imponderable; the interested reader should really study the whole section of the *Summa* on Understanding. "Matter is twofold, common and *signate* or individual; common such as flesh and bone; and individual as this flesh and these bones. The intellect therefore abstracts the species of a natural thing from the individual sensible matter, but not from the common sensible matter .... Mathematical species, however, can be abstracted by the intellect from sensible matter, not only from individual, but also from common matter; not from common intelligible matter, but only from individual matter. For sensible matter is corporeal matter as subject to sensible qualities such as being cold or hot, hard or soft, and the life while intelligible matter is substance as subject to quantity. Now it is manifest that quantity is in substance before other sensible qualities are. Hence quantities such as number, dimension and figures, which are the terminations of quantity, can be considered apart from sensible qualities; and this is to abstract them from sensible matter. . . . But some things can be abstracted even from common intelligible matter as much as *being, unity, power, act*, and the life. All these can exist without matter as it plain regarding immaterial things."

B. Considered Dynamically—Change

Rumi says: "The kettle is silent although it is boiling all the while" (*Mathnawi*, p. 261).

First we tend to naturally consider the material world as being static, stationary. But actually it all undergoes change from the highest to the lowest. There is movement either in the object itself or at the instance of some other object. Therefore we now consider the dynamic changes in *mf.a.*, *MF*.

Changes are of two kinds: "substantial change" or "accidental change." The example of "substantial change" is the chemical change occurring in the course of chemical reactions. "Accidental change" is when water becomes steam, when a person or plant grows, when a person becomes emaciated or an object shrinks in size.

The nature of substantial change is most important in regard to physiology and pathology. The first step is associated with a disappearance of the old *f*, the process called corruption by the scholastics; in modern words, disintegration. There is then a new *f'*—the new form whose appearance is called generation ("God is an Abaser and an Exalter. Without these two processes nothing comes into being," *Mathnawi*, p. 300).

If we look at this from the point of view of causes, there are three steps: a material cause or external agent, a receptive function whereby the previous material receives a new action, activity or form (*f'*) and the efficient cause (*f'*) which brings the action or activity into union with the material (*m*).

In the view of modern science, of course, the properties of "water," for instance, appear at the moment when the H_2 and O meet and unite. The appearance of NaCl and H_20, again, is adequately explained simply from the union of NaOH and HCl in appropriate proportions. But Thomistic science perceives the need of something further. The water-molecule or complex of molecules is something more than the two H atoms linked to oxygen and this something is the inert principle of matter m which releases the old f and accepts the new *f'*. As Rahilly explains, a molecule or a complex of molecules such as an organism, presents not only "colligative or summational properties, but also indiscerptible specific qualities of the whole which cannot be distinctively predicated of or portioned out among the parts." "We must therefore conceive—not imagine!—a spatially complex and disparate aggregate as being in some fundamental sense one being (Rahilly, appendix to Cardinal Mercier, *Manual of Modern Scholastic Philosophy.* In *animalibus quae movement seipsa est magis quaedam colligatio partium quam perfecta continuatio*, St. Thomas, *In VIII. Physic*, I. 7).

The causes of substantial change (the efficient causes) in inanimate "beings" are the well-known familiar extrinsic "forces of nature." But in the case of living beings, the efficient causes are the intrinsic "instinctive drives" which they possess. Some of the latter account for changes of substance while others have to do with a change of position—movement; and others again excite a movement in the mind.

In the human being, the immediate efficient cause of an outwardly visible act consists of the muscles and nerves. Behind that is the more remote efficient cause—the sensuous appetition or desire and behind that is the sensuous cognition which is an integral property of the human passive-active state (*MF*), a passive act, itself a faculty." Behind that, peculiar to the human being, is the all-important final cause. This is described in philosophy as "the means by which perfection of life is reached" whether that "perfection" be relative or absolute, whether the interests of the physical body are served or the intellectual life or whether the highest perfection (that is, of soul) is the goal in view, where matter-form (*MF*) uses matter (*M*) as the "innocent creature of God," in order to attain true perfection.

3. The Doctrine of Imponderable Elements

A. Considered Statically

(1) Relation of the imponderable elements to "matter" and "form"—Do the elements belong to "primary matter" or to "form?"

This problem was discussed in so masterly a fashion by St. Thomas that his words are still applicable and unsurpassable. His perfect understanding of the nature of matter is combined with a precision of explanation which should satisfy every student. The following quotations may be made: "By the words earth and water (in Gen. i), primary matter itself is signified" (St. Thomas Aquinas, *Summa Theologica*. Dominican translation, 66, I, quoting Augustine, p. 194). "The ancient material philosophers maintained that primary matter was some corporeal thing in act as fire, air, water or some intermediate substance (St. Thomas, *ibid*, p. 192). Corporeal matter was impressed with the substantial form of water and with the substantial form of earth (*ibid*., p. 231) The power possessed by water or earth of producing all animals resides not in the earth and water themselves, but in the power originally given to the element s of producing them from elemental matter (*ibid*., 71, i. p. 251)."

The four elements cannot be assigned to literal matter but they cannot be assigned to form either as they have no being until literal matter has itself come into being. Therefore, while the chemical elements are matter-form (*mf*), the imponderable elements are neither matter (*m*) nor form (*f*) for they are inseparable form matter-form (*mf*) and the primary qualities of a thing do not appear until it exists. That is, until matter (*m*) and form (*f*) have become matter-form (*mf*). "The two exist because of the one, but hold not even to this one" (Seng-ts'an in D. T. Susuki, *Essays in Zen Buddhism*, p. 184—words used in another connection but equally applicable).

Paracelsus (quoted by St. Thomas Aquinas, *Summa Theologica*, Rome edition, p. 264) says: "Humidity is not an element of water or burning an element of fire. An element is not to be defined according to body, substance, or quality. What is visible to the eyes is only the subject or receptacle." Fire which burns is not the element of fire, but in another shape. Whatever is fixed is of the element of earth. Whatever nourishes is from the element of air, and whatever consumes is from the element of water. Growth belongs to the element of fire (see lecture 7, endnote 1). Where that element fails, there is no increment. Except the element of earth supplied it there would be no end to growth. This fixes it. That is to say, it supplies a terminus for the element of fire. So also, unless the element of air were to act, no nutrition could be brought about (cf. oxygen) By the air alone all things are nourished. Again, nothing can be dissolved or consumed unless the element of water be the cause. By it all things are mortified, and reduced to nothing (St. Thomas, *ibid*, p. 266). The invisible elements need to be sustained, nourished and increased by some visible thing and at length they perish with them." In other words, the elements only exist as long as there is matter-form (*mf*). "Both are interdependent and related though their activity goes on without waste or loss. . . Each invisible attracts to itself its own. Stones come forth from the strong spirit of the earth" (St. Thomas, *ibid*, p. 279).

Such passages, often supposed to be meaningless, become intelligible in the light of Thomistic philosophy, though according to biographers, Paracelsus would not have wished to appear to subscribe to that.

The imponderable elements must not, however, be confused with accidents (*a*). "*Primae quatuor qualitates non sunt habitus elementorum*" (St. Thomas Aquinas, *ibid.*, 49, 4, I). These primary qualities form the link between the object and our own consciousness, for our knowledge of the universe is really simply a knowledge of those qualities (heat, cold, moist, dry) with that of secondary qualities (subtility, thickness, lightness, heaviness, rarity, density, translucence, opacity, brilliance, dullness, etc.). "Sensible matter is corporeal matter as subject to sensible qualities, such as being cold or hot, hard or soft, and the like" (St. Thomas Aquinas, *Summa Theologica*, Dominican translation, 85, i, p. 186).

So all the concrete objects of this world—from the granite mountain to the microscopic protozoon—are related to one another by virtue of the imponderables. And by virtue of the same, they are related to extra-mundane objects (sun, moon, stars). "The matter of the heavenly bodies and of the elements agree in the character of potentiality" (*ibid.*, 66, 2, p. 199). Since matter cannot exist without them, the human body also manifests them.

(2) In the analogy between the four elements and vibration-rate, the earth

element may be compared with a slow vibration-rate, the water element with a more rapid rate and the remaining elements with still quicker vibration rates. The slower rates are "coarser," and the more rapid ones are "finer." Therefore, as Avicenna says, the earth and water are heavy and the others are more light. The meaning of the imponderable elements is made more intelligible through the idiom of modern science. But in making such an analogy we must avoid the common error of equating things capable of being analogized with the same thing. To compare the elements with vibration-rate is to compare them with light. Soul, radiance, spirit, breath have all been compared with light. But to pass on to identify them in any sense with *lux perpetua* and then with Universal Intellect is indefensible yet even modern thought is not immune from the fallacy. Paracelsus (F. Hartmann, the *Life of Paracelsus*, ii, 264) explains "element" as "spirit (meaning form no doubt) which lives and flourishes in the visible objects of nature as the soul in the body, not indeed, he explains. That it is of precisely the same essence as a soul but it corresponds with a certain degree of resemblance. There is a difference between the elemental and eternal soul. For the first matter of the elements is nothing else than life, which all created creatures possess. The soul of the elements is the life of all created things" (*ibid.*, ii. 264). Averroes said, "of all things the soul is most like light."

The perfect reasoning in dealing with these errors which is given by Thomas Aquinas in *Contra Gentiles* should be studied by all who are inclined to award the last word to scientific theories.

(3) Applications of the doctrine. The application of the doctrine to the subject-matter of medicine is simple when the elements are represented by their corresponding tendencies. A few of the relations are shown in tabular form by way of illustration. Thus, as the following chart shows:

ELEMENT	TENDENCY	CORRESPONDING SYSTEM	EXCRETION	SPECIAL SENSE	OPERATION IN BODY	TYPE OF MIND	CORRESPONDING MENTAL STATE
Earth	Spreading	Skeletal	Feces	Touch	Gives shape	Mental torpor	Obstinacy Fear
Water	Drooping Downward	Muscular	Urine	Taste	Nutrition	Lymphatic	Submissive Affectionate
Fire	Rising	Liver, Blood	Sweat	Smell	Digestion Physical movements	Optimistic	Anger; irate; vexation; and weeping
Air	To & Fro	Vascular Cutaneous	Saliva	Hearing	Respiration	Cheer	Humor
Ether	Stillness	Nervous	Semen	Vision	Reasoning	Reflective	Sadness

The correspondence between body and mind, by virtue of the pervasion of the whole being by the elements is specially elaborated in a particularly interesting manner by Chu Hsi (J. P. Bruce, *Chu Hsi and His Masters*, p. 214) where the five elements are taken as the physical counterparts of five ethical principles (love, righteousness, reverence, wisdom, sincerity) which are present in all beings just as are the elements.

The Buddhist exposition of the human being as composed of five elements: matter, sensation, thought, action and consciousness (*Honen the Buddhist Saint*, translated by Coates and Ishizuka, p. 314) though raising another question—shows how generally the establishing of an intimacy of relation between body and mind is sought after in all periods of history.

Through the doctrine of the elements the existence of a subtle indispensable link between tissues, organs, fluids, and mental attributes become intelligible. The methods of reasoning of peculiar to different peoples and individuals, their changes of mood, their personal behaviors are all to be worked out on this basis, as in his succeeding chapters, Avicenna works out the nature of temperament, humors, and constitution.

"The ether in the constitution of the creature differs in the degree of its clearness and translucence. When the ether with which the individual is endowed is clear and translucent, but neither pure nor complete, some entanglement with creaturely desire is unavoidable; but it can be overcome and gotten rid of and then we have the wise man. When the ether with which the individual is endowed is blurred and turbid, there is the beclouding with creaturely desire to such an extent that it cannot be shaken off and we have the foolish and degenerate" (J. P. Bruce, *Chu Hsi: Philosophy of Human Nature*, i. 117).

(4) Associated factors: Since the primary qualities belong to the elements, the laws of action and passion apply. Various aspects of this law are described by the terms: strength-weakness, *jalal-jamal*, *qadar-qadr*. These determine the phenomena of human life and therefore call for consideration under the dynamic aspects of the doctrine. Statically they are significant to the physician because they reveal themselves in variations of functional capacity of organs. With the dominance of the several elements we may expect corresponding vigour of the several systems of the body—i.e. the nutritive faculty and the liver-function; renal functions, etc. The emotional make-up, character, and even talents for art, crafts, literature, politics, etc., attitude towards life in general—all these are colored by the dominant element. The study of the patient's features, gestures, voice, posture, hands acquires an added meaning, as informing about the strength or weakness of the several systems and faculties to a degree which is not so very inferior to the information afforded by the expensive instruments of modern clinical research. (See Lecture 3, endnote 9 and endnote 12).

"Strength is the manifestation of the positive ether and weakness of the negative. Each of these again is either positive and then good or negative and then evil. Strength when good is righteous, straightforward, resolute, majestic, firm when evil, harsh, proud, soft, irresolute and false. The mean (ideal) is the maintenance of these principles in equilibrium." (J. P. Bruce, Chu Hsi, *ibid.*, p. 11).

Rumi says:

The earthy sign of the Zodiac surrounds the terrestrial earth,

The water sign (Aquarius) sends moisture to it.
The windy sign sends the clouds to it,
To draw off unwholesome exhalations.
The fiery sign (Leo) sends forth the heat of the sun,
Like a dish heated red-hot in front and behind.
The heaven is busily toiling through the ages,
Just as men labor to provide food for women.
And the earth does the woman's work and toils
In bearing offspring and suckling them (*Mathnawi*).

The movement of the elements is mutually opposite (St. Thomas Aquinas, *Summa Theologica*, Dominican translation, 66, p. 197). Change is continually taking place within the human being. This change is either cyclical or progressive. The former characterizes the ordinary phenomena of physiology and the latter manifest as growth. The cyclical changes of physiology (in its biochemical aspect) may be described in terms both of the chemical elements and of the imponderable elements. To do so by the pictorial title of "the dance of the elements" is at once to bring up the atmosphere of the East and the very scenery of Avicenna's mind:

All the four elements are seething in this caldron (the world),
None is at rest, neither earth nor fire nor water nor air.
Now earth takes the form of grass, on account of desire,
Now water becomes air, for the sake of this affinity.
By way of unity, water becomes fire.
Fire also becomes air in this expanse by reason of love.
The elements wander from place to place like a pawn,
For the sake of the king's love, not, like you, for pastime."
(Jalal al-Din Rumi, *Shams-i Tabriz*, p. 338).

The changes are the important things; not the things in themselves, for matter, after all, only exists in virtue of the ceaselessly acting creative power of God. Did He withhold the power, at that instant the matter would cease; it has no reality apart from His intention. It would not be a case of the world being "destroyed," but one of "ceasing to be." We are apt to be deceived by "matter," and devote our thoughts to this instead of to the changes and perhaps the "moment of nascence" (Lecture 2, "Application of the Doctrine") is even more important than the changes themselves. The greatness of the ancient Book of Changes (Yi King) is due to the recognition of this principle.

The advantage of this simile is that it brings out not only movement of a certain orderly kind, but also rhythm and motif; the thought being of such primitive native dances in which the action requires only two dancers (male and female, of course) who are in the presence of many spectators. Each dancer performs entirely different movements, and the two never come into actual contact. The movements are harmonized by the music, which is itself as characteristic and essential as either of the performers

Further, it will be clear that the feelings of the dancers themselves do not concern the watchers; behind their emotions there is the real meaning of the dance, and whether the dancers discern that or not, the observer should strive to discern it. There may be special affinities or attractions between the dancers of the minuet; but neither their pleasure, their displeasure, their steps, nor the music, are the basic reality.

Moreover, the skill of the dancers is not always of the same degree. Artistic genius may produce greater pleasure in the watchers, but there is something greater even than skill.

The phenomena of physiology and pathology may be viewed as a series of changes of analogous character, the cycle of changes in chemical elements, tissue-cells, and other rhythmic phenomena being studied without neglecting the conception of the imponderable elements.

From the doctrine of matter and form it is clear that with the changes from one chemical compound to another in the course of the cyclical phenomena, there is a dropping of the " form " Also, the imponderable elements rearrange, and blend into new modes at the same time. As the author of *Gulshan-i-raz* (Mahmud Shabistari, lines 250-255 and endnote) says:

The elements, water, air, fire and earth,
Have taken their station below the heavens
Each serving diligently in its own appointed place,
Before or behind which it never sets its foot.
Though all four are contrary in their nature and position,
Still one may see them ever united together.
Inimical are they to each other in essence and form,
Yet united into single bodies by fiat of necessity.
From them is born the three-fold kingdom of nature.

To present a simple example, for illustration-glucose) for instance, would be described as WA2F4, each letter representing the corresponding imponderable element. When this substance is broken up into alcohol and CO2, by the dispersal of the "cohesive force between the three elements (e.g., by the influence of an opposite": the yeast-ferment), two portions of WF2 result, the "air" having escaped, and the "fire-water" of the aborigines being left behind.

The germination of seeds may be described in similar terms. Thus, it would be said that the ethereal undulations from the sun penetrate the loosened earth round the seeds, and by their successive shocks affect the particles of matter composing the germinal center of the seed. The readjustments of atoms and compounds with oxygen result in the generation of vital energy. The " earth" (mineral substances, and remnants of animal and vegetable matter) mingled with "water" (moisture) forms the factor of "heavy elements" (§26). The "air" (its oxygen content), "fire" (solar heat), and "ether" (sunlight) make up the factor of "light elements." The two series together affect the starch in the seed, bring about its change into glucose, whereby the seed swells until the plumule emerges, and the rootlets begin to penetrate the soil in search of "water" and "earth," while the leaves expand to take in the "air," and "ether" by the aid of "fire."

Expressed in another way, there has been a change of vibration-rate. Or we might regard the imponderable elements as compulsorily riding upon the chemical elements during their metabolic interchanges, although the fire, water, earth or air cannot be thought of as retaining a sort of identity throughout. It would be better to use another idiom: the noumenal is coterminous with the phenomenal. Or, comparing it with wave-motion, it is as if there were two superimposed curves. When the two curves tally, every dip of one meets a dip in the other. The imponderable dips down, as it were, into the world of matter, illuminating the "ocean of physical matter" a according to the mode (intensity of vibration) in which it touches the lower curve. At each rise of the wave, the former returns into the metaphysical "ocean," and in doing so, the physical matter returns to (momentary) inactivity.

The breaking down and building up of substance, in the course of metabolism, is the same as the scholastic "corruption" (disintegration), and "generation" (reconstruction); and is concurrent with the changes in the imponderable elements. In Avicenna the process is thought of in their terms, whereas to the physiologist the process is worked out in terms of the material chemical elements.

So, in Chinese philosophy, we are introduced to the alternating opening and closing operations of nature, which are controlled by the "law, as the pivot controls: the opening and closing of a door" (p. 134). (Cf. with *uruj-nasul* in Sufi philosophy).

Therefore we find that Thesis III is working out the dynamic consideration of the imponderables, under the title of "temperament." It is the action and passion between the opposites which results in temperament. This conception carried through all aspects of man provides the explanation of the diversity which characterizes the unity-one human being.

Mentioned by Whinefield is the *Akhlaq-i jalali* says: "In truth there is one and the same principle, which, if prevailing in the attempered elementary particles is equipoise of temperament, if produced in musical tones is excellent and delightful intervals if apparent in the gestures is grace, if found in language is eloquence, if produced in the human limbs is beauty (*'though their beauty charm thee,'* Quran, Sura 33:52), if in the qualities of the soul equity. Of this principle the soul is enamored and in search, whatever form it may take, whatever dress assume" (Verses 625-630 of *Gulshan-i-raz*; many other passages in this poem are equally applicable).

Application of the Doctrine

(a) To biochemistry.

Starting with the conception of matter so far detailed, both statically and dynamically, and applying the dynamic aspects of the imponderable elements designated as a "dance," we may proceed to trace the chemical elements and compounds through the body, entering as they do in the form of solid and fluid articles of diet, or by means of respiration. The chemical elements are seen to be in a form which is sometimes fixed or bound (combined, sometimes free. They pass into the tissues, and linger there for a longer or shorter time before passing out again. During practically the whole of this time they are combined, but at the actual moments of chemical interchange they become free or nascent-the moments when f becomes f'.

It may be said that that moment of nascence is the focus, or the whole purpose, of the cycle of changes which occur in the body-anabolic and katabolic. That one moment is the opportunity for vital actions to actualize. That moment finds its location in this or that histological unit or tissue-element, which itself is, in a certain real sense, itself the actualization of that moment! This moment achieved, they become bound once more and steadily descend the ladder of metabolism until they are found once more outside the body. To quote from as deep thinker of the early Victorian age: "Nitrogen, like a half-reclaimed gipsy from the wild, is ever seeking to be free again, and, not content with its own freedom, is ever tempting others not of gipsy blood to escape from-their thraldom" (G. Wilson, *Religio Chemici*, p. 149).

At this same vital moment of the cycle, there is a change of the pivot of function in the substances concerned. All the substances with which the subject of metabolism deals belong to the carbon compounds, whose structure is well known to be described with the terms straight chain, double-chain, ring-compounds, etc. With these forms of "skeleton" are associated the various "side chains" which are to the others as the limbs to the body. All the familiar groups of biochemistry (paraffins, primary and secondary alcohols, aldehydes, acids, amides, ketones, ethers, sulphonic acids, albumoses, leucins, purins, diaminoacids, sugars, etc.) may be thought of as presenting a sort of individuality which depends more on the side-chains than on the skeletons, and yet the radicals of which these side-chains are composed owe their character more to stereo-chemical position or other relations than to the elements which belong to them. With change of formula there is no doubt a change of physical state (colloid, crystalloid), of electrical reaction and so forth. But the fact of change (see endnotes to Lecture 3: The Doctrine of Imponderable Elements) is still more important, even than the change of personality or individuality (so to speak). The pivot of function changes from one element-carbon, i.e., to another (nitrogen, sulphur, phosphorus, i.e.). The important thing is that from being carbon-centric, the physiological processes are nitrogen-centric, sulpho-centric, phospho-centric. Or, uni-centricity gives place to duo-centricity (i.e., sulpho-ferro-centric), or perhaps multi-centricity (e.g. in albumen), because the function cannot pass on to a new pivot unless two or more other elements have come into special association.

For instance, in oxy-centricity, a compound constructed on the straight-chain skeleton (-C-C-C-C-) may become oxy-centric, because the new basis is -C-O-C- (formation of anhydrides, esters, etc.). Here the important thing is that the center of function is -O- and no longer -C-. In nitro-centricity, the change is associated with the appearance of -C-N-C-, the center of function being now -N-, which is important. In sulpho-centricity, a compound with a group -C-S-O_3H (thio-ethers, allyls, etc.) may arise; this is quasi-pathological for the human body, and however insignificant the -S- may be to the chemist maybe it is evident to the senses in virtue of a distinctive odor. Such compounds as sulpho-cyanides, taurocholates, indoxylsulphates, melanin, various mucins, lardaceous substances, hair, and the horny skin have an importance of their own, and some of them form the links between nitro-centric and sulpho-centric compounds. In phospho-centricity, the dominance of the phosphorus atom is the culmination of the purpose of the metabolic change. So the author of *Religio Chemici* (G. Wilson, p. 149) said "phosphorus is in the active condition at the centers of vital action and in the passive (allotropic) state at the outlying points." In the case of lecithin, there are variations of centricity. Its nitrogen, phosphorus, or hydroxyl may be dominant according to the metabolic circumstances, and the subsequent linkages and fate of each successive derivative is according to those circumstances.

Other elements may come to form important pivots of function, under more or less exceptional conditions (i.e., arsenic, silicon, etc.).

It is clear then, that we can watch the metabolic processes from the chemical side as a sort of pageant or procession. But if we view it as the chemist does, according to syntheses and analyses, oxidations and reductions, and according to the intermediate products which he discovers when he arrests that pageant, as one might stop a dance in order to be sure that a certain individual was present or not, we may easily come to conclusions quite at variance with the living truth. Stop the dance, and the illusion is destroyed. The life has gone! The living cell does not necessarily follow the program of the laboratory. Indeed it might be doubted whether any substances as such ever appear except at the end. The actual process might well be like a shuffling of cards, whereby the order of the cards is altered and the order or relative position- is the important thing. On the anabolic side there is always the face; on the katabolic side there is always the back. Between the two there are always the same atomic personalities which remain as it were in the same room but change about to receive different ranks with respect to one another.

Each element may be traced through its various phases, through compound after compound, its behavior being modified by the side chains, and its importance altered, so that now it has a regal position, with the others as its slaves, and now is reduced to slavery, subservient to another element which has now assumed the royal position. Each in turn receives homage from its fellows; each enjoys a brief reign upon the throne.

Such is the chemistry of life, viewed mystically. It is an incessant movement. Interchanges proceed continually, and not only in one substance at a time, but in a thousand at a time; not one element only (C, H, N, O, S, P) but all of them simultaneously—not necessarily one ruler, but sometimes co-rulers, in the various substrates of action; not all at the same rate, but at different rates and with different rhythms.

In histology. These pictures o f biochemical processes must be linked up with what we actually see with the naked eye and with the microscope. Morphological changes are all manifestations of the unseen or invisible biochemical cycles. Not "structure first, then function." Not "function first, then structure.'" The two are inseparable both in time and place. Therefore, however exact his histological knowledge, the physician must hold clearly before him the activities which only the mind can hold and piece together and watch. The histological appearance shows us the processes arrested at a particular moment when some group is dominant and another recessive. Its very appearance is artificial, the produce of reagents acting upon a dead fixed protoplasm; a reaction between-complex dyes and the chemical substances produced by the fixatives. That which appears to be the permanent substrate for functions, a definite scaffolding, is quite otherwise. In the picture given of the dance of the elements in the body, the skeleton seems a base from which side-chains arise and give purchase-for the dancing element; but as a matter of fact the skeleton, the side-chain, and the element are mutually necessary. The whole structure is altering the whole time. So with the tissue. The change of chemical substances entails a change from solid to colloid, colloid to fluid, fluid to gas or back to colloid; and while-so doing they become perceptible under the microscope as cell-substance, cell-fluid, cell juice, tissue juice; fluids aggregate and condense into cells (colloid phase); cells constantly dissolve or splay out into fluid, or undergo partition from larger and larger particles into submicroscopic and finally into visible microscopic particles, or else undergo partition into supernatant fluids of simpler chemical composition. In the course of these changes solids and the like separate out; and these last are usually but faultily regarded as products of metabolism comparable to the goods manufactured in a factory. The appearance of granules rather than fluid, or precipitate rather than solution in the tissue, depends on the kind of elements concerned (mineral atoms, ordinary atom-groups), and the direction of interchange. See Lecture 4, endnote 8.

Some examples of the steps of the cycle towards visibility:

Fluid Phase	Colloid Phase	Submicroscopic Character	Microscopic Appearance	Fate
Homogeneous humor	Cell-substance	Spongioplasm	Tissue Cell as a Whole	Excretable substance and protein derivatives
Abnormal humor	Atrabilious humor	Less collodial	Coarse particles (insoluble)	Inexcretable without medicine aid
Tissue-fluid	Serum-protein	Amino acids	Bioplasm; occasional crystalline deposit	Urea, etc.
Sulphur	Colloid sulphur potentially excretable phase	Larger particles of sulphur	Cell-granules cell-wall	Sulphur derivatives; sulphonic acids, etc.

It is not possible to prepare a fully exact correlation between the carbon, nitrogen, phosphorus, and sulphur series and structure seen under the microscope. Broadly speaking, the carbon series is related to the cell-substance; the nitrogen and phosphorus series are associated with the nuclear structure. Certain kinds of cells are associated more with some elements than with others.

Moreover one must always bear in mind that the movement is all through the cell, all through the whole histological unit. The fulfillment of the functions of such a unit implies the simultaneous movement of all the elements concerned, and each cycle proceeds at a different rate.

It is less easy still to present a picture of the movement in a whole tissue in these terms. Only here and there does some product emerge which is identifiable by the physiologist and biochemist.

Endless intermediate steps and changes find their concrete expression in the one product which we perceive as some detail of cell-structure under the microscope. We may trace various isolated substances in certain parts of certain cells of the body, and yet are not able to dogmatize about them, because in the process of life in the tissue there is a constant flow of matters the visible becoming invisible, and then again visible. That is, the visible food material taken in, the invisible changes and interchanges of elements and atom groups (the metabolism) and their changing pivots of function; and the finally visible product of excretion. If there be a range of variation from a normal in the steps of this dance: there is at least no doubt that ill-health comes of a change of rhythm when the foot falls are out of time, or some of the " steps omitted.

It is clear that if the changes in the imponderable elements should chance to fail to run concurrently with the breaking down and building-up of substance (the scholastic corruption or disintegration and generation or reconstruction), this would also mean a break in the rhythm; the wave-motion would not be symmetrical, to use the previous simile; and the body would be ill. But it may be added, in passing, that the varying dispositions exhibited by people are the manifestations of lack of perfect symmetry and synchronism; perfect symmetry would show among other things as a cheerful disposition.

The histology of an organ is the visible sum total of chemical units, with the atom groups of ponderable elements successively formed in the cells and tissues. These constitute the stage and scenery of the metaphysical dance-that of the imponderable elements which interweave and complete the picture of the living processes. But to understand the picture itself, and see its meaning, brings us to questions which must be deferred at this point.

The wonderful insight into the processes taking place in the human body which is afforded by the conception of macrocosm and microcosm used by the alchemists of old, and still rightly used by many thinkers, is sufficient justification. In nature we see, for instance, a crowd of human beings, composed of hundreds of units which have aggregated for a relatively few moments. We may call it simply a crowd, or we may specify and say what kind of a crowd. As one watches its people come up to it; others leave; others walk by without deviating their steps. Perhaps in five minutes it has all dispersed.

What of it? What was its purpose? What was its effect? Here or perhaps elsewhere? Perhaps it is subversive of order, anarchical, pathological; perhaps it is simply mechanical, obstructive, congestive.

Such may be observed under the microscope, but we call the components cells or perhaps excretory products or foreign bodies. To some, such analogizing is fanciful and useless. But that Avicenna found this method of enquiry vastly productive and helpful there is no doubt. As a faithful Muslim, too, he would realize the voice of the Quran, saying: "*These things are to you for a sign.*" Words belonging not only to the moral law, but also to the law of nature in all its ramifications for the Artificer and the Lawgiver are one.

By the time we have grasped these several aspects arid associated them with the chemical aspect of life, we have formed a nearer approximation to the true picture of life at that moment of fire. But it has already passed on to something different! However, there is no way of keeping pace with that except by understanding the cycle of changes in each and every case. Cycles of incipience, of growth, of maturation, of decay. The reason, or causes of the change, is to be understood before one can keep pace.

The causes at work in the dance of the imponderable elements. The mutual attraction and repulsion which underlies all change is to be found inherent in the imponderable elements, as it were by definition. The active and passive qualities of the separate elements come into play when they are compounded) and (because they necessarily occur in the same geographical spot, and are only separable by mental analysis) they have to do even with physical state (solid, fluid, colloid, gaseous) and form (granular, amorphous, crystalline) and physical property (solubility and insolubility; positive or negative electrical charge). Hence they may be said to affect the direction of movement, whether to less colloid state, or more colloid, to differentiation or de-differentiation, clearness or sharpness of reaction, or to confused state.

This doctrine may be brought beside the Chinese principle of yang and yin. To the yang principle belong the ideas: anterior, south, rising, fecundating expanding, growth, advancing, strength, order, heat, motion, cheerfulness,-life. To the yin principle belong: posterior, north, falling, breeding, contracting, decay, retarding, weakness, confusion, cold, rest, anger, death.

In relation to the body: yang belongs to the breath, the head, the speech, the eyesight, exhaling; the shape of the body. Yin belongs to the blood, the feet the vital force, silence, inhaling; the body itself.

Yang is active, flowing, fullness, straightness, music. Yin is passive, tending to inertia, emptiness, crookedness of form, ceremonial.

There are relations between yang and yin, and hardness or softness, and the organs of the body. (Forke, *The World-conception of the Chinese*, 216). "When the ether has the proportions of the yin, and the yang correct and harmonious, there is perfection of the ether, and it is equally permeable by all five elements, as in the case of man. When the proportions are unequal, there is imperfection of the ether, the manifestation of the elements is unequal, as in the case of animals" (J. P. Bruce, *Chu Hsi: Philosophy of Human Nature*, endnote, i. 115).

The idea of yang and yin swinging as a pendulum may add to our conception of life. The rocking of the cradle has the subtle purpose of throwing the yang and yin into rhythm, and the movement of the infant's breath into rhythm, which, once started, will continue for at least an hour or two (See Avicenna 698).

Uruj—nasul (Inayat Khan), rise and fall. The anabolic process belongs to the former; the katabolic (formation of effete substances, their removal from tissues and organs-whether by deposition in tissues, as atheroma, or by discharge from the body) belong to the latter. These terms in Persian mysticism emphasize the fact of changes and movements running in cycles. Each individual has his own characteristic cycle of changes; the movement of the breath goes by cycles. The life as a whole shows its cycle, being sometimes seventy-five years, sometimes more, more often much less. In addition, there are the smaller cycles—waxing and waning of vital force in a certain rhythm peculiar to the person, and carrying with it susceptibility or resistance to infection, and the like.

Other principles: these would be expressed as laws, which can be classified into various groups-those belonging to nature in general; those belonging to human nature; those belonging to our conceptions of life, health and disease. Law of *qada* and *qadr*; construction and destruction; of distribution; of interdependence; of intention; of compulsory visibility (discontinuous functions, etc); of desires. See Lecture 2, "The Doctrine of Imponderable Elements."

Cause of synchronism: namely between the two dancers in the simile; these dancers being the material element and the imponderables respectively. This lies in the conception of breath or life-principle, with its cycles.

(d) Extra mundane and extra corporeal influences on the human body in virtue of the common content of the four elements.

That there are definite extra corporeal influences on the metabolic workings of the human body should now be intelligible. The effect of heat, cold, wet climate, dry climate is well enough known, but is widely ignored, as evidenced by elaborate researches into chronic articular rheumatism being apparently made in every direction but this.

To go further, and agree with the ancients that epidemics and the like had relation to planetary influences, is not necessary; nor is it necessary to dismiss their possibility off-hand. It is not safe to argue that there is no relation between the planets and stars and life on this earth simply because some relation once thought to be true is now discredited. If the whole universe is one organic whole, there cannot but be some relation.

The relation between seasonal irregularities and the interactions of the "elements" is referred to by Forke (*World-conception of the Chinese*, p. 298, end-note), in showing how the Chinese associated each season with the dominance of a given element.

According to the influences prevailing at the time of birth, so is the endowment of the person born with such an ether. "If toward the disposition is bright and good . . . if untoward, not." *Chu Hsi: Philosophy of Human Nature*, p. 85). In time, and with constant self-culture, "the inequality of ethereal endowment will of itself disappear" (*ibid*., p. 86).

Lecture 3: The Temperaments

1 "The temperament is something set up by contrary qualities as a kind of mean between them" (St. Thomas Aquinas, *Summa Contra Gentiles*, Dominican translation, lxiii, p. 165 where "complexio" is rendered temperament as it is throughout the present work).

How strange that the elements should be so contrary,
And yet be forced to live together (Mahmud Shabistari, *Gulshan-i-raz*, p. 26).

2 "*Elementum aliquod oportet predominari in omni mixto*" (St. Thomas Aquinas, *Summa Theologica*, Rome, 1894, 49, 6, i, m, 79, 2, 2m). "This is a drawn battle" (Costaeus, *Annotations to Avicenna*).

3 "One or the other proves victorious" (Costaeus). "Fire, water, earth, and air, the four elements of which bodies are compounded, lose their individual qualities in the compound bodies and equipoise (equity) is what unites them into homogeneous compounds" (Mahmud Shabistari, *Gulshan-i-raz*, p. 61). "When . . . the elements attain equilibrium the beams of the spirit world fall upon them" (*ibid.*, couplet 615). "When it is said that the nature of a man or thing is hot and of another is cold, such statements include both the physical element and the immaterial principle with which they are endowed" (Chu Hsi in J. P. Bruce, *Chu Hsi: Philosophy of Human Nature*, p. 94).

The idea of "balance" may be applied to a variety of phenomena in health and disease—both of body and mind. Lack of balance brings sickness and explains death. Examples: atony; hypertonicity; hyperacidity; excessive trichosis; the various phenomena nowadays ascribed to loss of balance in the domain of endocrine secretions and hormones. The body may be too cold (subnormal temperature); the mind may be "cool"; the heart may be too "warm." There may be inadequate repose after mental activity leading to loss of mental balance. There is dynamic balance as well as static balance.

4 The fact that temperament is concerned with the primary qualities and not with secondary ones should enable one to avoid the idea of weight (pondus) in regard to the subject. In the annotation of the 1608 edition there is a reference to Averroes as agreeing with this point. However, if one realizes that the "elements" are "imponderables," it becomes self-evident that Avicenna's dissertation is correct and that he himself quite realized the attitude claimed for him in this treatise.

5 See also Lecture 3, endnote 9 and the quotations given which insist on the fundamental difference between man and animals.

6 Fire "feeds on" air. So innate heat consumes the innate moisture (Costaeus, *Annotations to Avicenna*).

7 "The more the organ of touch is reduced to an equable complexion, the more sensitive will be the touch" (St. Thomas Aquinas, *Summa Theologica*, Dominican translation, 76, 5; p. 44).

8. "An artificer produces diverse works of art" (St. Thomas, *Summa*

Theologica, Dominican translation, 65, p. 186). "Every creature exists for its own proper art and perfection" (*ibid.*, p. 184).

9 "The human body is the most noble of all lower bodies and by the equability of its temperament is most like the heaven which is free from all contrariety" (St. Thomas Aquinas, *Summa Contra Gentiles*, Dominican translation, i, 70, p. 178). "He gave each thing its limits and all things their disposition" (*ibid*, ii, 26, p. 49). "God makes man after one type and a horse after another; the types of things are manifold in the divine mind" (*ibid*, i, 54, 118). "Lord, Thou hast ordered all things in number, weight and measure" (*Wisd.* xi, 21). "There is diversity and inequality in things created—not by chance, not as a result of diversity of matter, not on account of certain causes or merits intervening, but from God's own intention; in that He willed to give the creature such perfection as it was possible for it to have" (*ibid*, ii, xiv, p. 108).

We may also quote from the Chinese: "All beings possess the five imponderables, but only the human being has them in perfect balance as the constitution of his nature." "That which differentiates the human being from the brute is his possession of the mean or equilibrium, that perfect balance of the elements in the constitution of his nature of which Tzu-Ssu teaches in his famous classic—the doctrine of the mean" (Chu Hsi, in J. P. Bruce, *Chu Hsi and His Masters*, pp. 214, 217). "In the life of men and other creatures, the nature with which they are endowed differs from the very beginning in the degree of its perfection. But even within the differing degrees of perfection there is the further variation in respect of clearness and translucence" (Chu Hsi quoted by J. P. Bruce, *Chu Hsi: Philosophy of Human Nature*, i, p. 57). When the ether received is limited, the immaterial principle received is also correspondingly limited. Thus, the physical constitution of dogs and horses being as it is, their functions are correspondingly limited in their range" (*ibid.*, p. 60). "Man receives the ether in its perfection and the ethical principle permeates it completely and without impediment while in the case of other creatures in which it is imperfect, the ethical principle is impeded and unintelligent. He receives the ether of the universe in its perfection and therefore possesses moral and intellectual faculties" (*ibid.*, p. 67). "In birds and animals, although they possess the nature, it is restricted by the corporeal element which creates an impenetrable barrier" (Chu Hsi in J. P. Bruce, *Chu Hsi and His Masters*, p. 61).

10 In general, organs rich in blood are of hot temperament; those poor in blood are of cold temperament (Aegineta).

11 Link between soul, passions, and temperament. St Thomas Aquinas writes (Summa Theologica, Dominican translation, ii, 63, p. 166): "The soul rules the body and curbs the passions that result from the temperament. For by temperament some are more prone than others to desire or anger and yet refrain more from these things."

12 "*All things have We created after a fixed decree*" (Quran 54:49).

The four elements are as birds tied together by the feet;
Death, sickness and disease loose their feet asunder.

The moment their feet are loosed from the others,
The bird of each element flies off by itself.
The repulsion of each of these principles and causes
Inflicts every moment a fresh pang on our bodies.
That it may dissolve these composite bodies of ours,
The bird of each part tries to fly away to its origin;
But the wisdom of God prevents this speedy end,
And preserves their union until the appointed day (Jalal al-Din Rumi, *Mathnawi*, translated by E. H. Whinefield, p. 162).

The "death of nature" may also be explained on the basis of uruj and nasul (see Lecture 2, following the chart of the cycle towards visibility and Lecture 7, endnote 1) because when the positive and negative phases in the cycle of the elements and of the breath clash—that is, enter the phase of *kamal* (completion), the bodily functions all cease. The *kamal* phase may be reached long before the allotted span.

The presence of this phase and its probable duration before death actually occurs may be discerned in practice if the law be understood. This fact throws a significant light on the statements in the Chinese work on the pulse (Wan K'an T'ang, *Complete Guide to the Human Pulse*) where the time of death is foretold from the study of the pulse and other factors—assigning not a number of hours or days but a particular period in the lunar cycle. Chu Hsi (*Chu Hsi and His Masters*) in ascribing the varying fortunes of individuals during their life to differences of endowment of ether (*Chu Hsi and His Masters*, p. 217) betrays a knowledge of the cyclical changes pertaining to body and mind as well as to the outer world at large.

It would be fallacious to argue from this that skillful prognostication of this kind would render medical treatment superfluous. The value of realizing these phases lies in the understanding with which measures are applied in order to tide over the patient during the dangerous period of inertia of vitality, breath, or other factors.

This would not dispense with the constant sense of "*fiat voluntas Tua*," both on the part of the lay and of the profession.

Quotations from the Chinese, for instance, in whom the conception of belief in fate is vivid and almost dominant, brings no conviction to those many who claim to have no belief in fate whatsoever. Nevertheless a few proverbs may be quoted as expressing the conception usefully: "there is a day to be born and a time to die"; "before life has been, death has been appointed." "In the beginning it was decided whether one should have long or short life; whether one should have honor or poverty." "The swallow living in the hall does not know the great building is about to be burned." "A physician may cure disease but he cannot heal fate." "The lucky physician sees the patient at the end of the disease; the unlucky physician sees the patient at the beginning of the disease” (C. H. Plopper, *Chinese Religion Seen Through the Proverb*, chapter xi).

No doubt where a possibility of “destiny” is to be admitted for one form of circumstance, the application of the same principle to many details of human life is not so readily conceded. That it is allowable for much more than is customarily accepted will be credible when the existence of occult and inscrutable chains of causes or attractions operating together is realized.

Fate is supposed by some to be blind by others to be the decree of a far-off potentate. It is neither. It is the manifestation of a series of combinations of conditions which by “natural” courses of sequences operate in the individual human life. Everyone shares in the weaving of his own web. The web is a by-product in some great scheme which we need not question. Fate ceases to signify for such a rise into the scheme itself. For to them their life is as the throwing of the stone unerringly into the bull’s-eye; the intervening events, the debris, what of them?

Rather than criticize severely the idea of the length of individual human lives being preordained, Mahmud Shabistari (*Gulshan i-raz*, p. 54) rightly asks:

> If destiny be not the arbiter of mundane affairs,
> Wherefore are men’s states contrary to their wishes?

“Who, then can say, ‘I am an individual, independent and free. I can think what I wish and I can do what I wish?’ You are not doing what you wish . . . thinking what you wish! There are various thoughts around you in the form of mean and animals who influence your mind and feeling and thought; you cannot escape them . . . . There is always some person stronger than you and always someone weaker than yourself . . . .Our lives are tied together and there is a link in which we can see one current running through all” (Inayat Khan, *Various Writings*, p. 52).

No doubt “destiny” is often supposed to negate “free will” which is so much insisted on as man’s prerogative. Destiny belongs to the body, freewill to the soul. Or, to be more accurate, it is our will which is important and not the body or its length of life. Or, to be still more accurate, by employing the algebraic symbols already fixed on—we are born *MF’* from that moment with each further reception of feeding on sights and sounds or other sense-impressions, we become *MF”*. But the purpose of human life has been shown to rise quite beyond this and our goal is to become MF” before we die. In each case *M* goes into corruption but the position of *F’* and *F”* is vastly different.

“The voices of nature are the mother of the soul.” *F”* is the outcome of a consistent usage of “freewill” by the will in a certain direction—namely supernatural, combined also with a “feeding” (to use the same term as above) on supernatural impressions.

To quote from theology in which domain we are brought, “supernatural” does not refer to superstitions, evil practices and hypothetical experiences; it is a term used in the sense of "supernatural grace." The ordinary human being is body plus rational soul in the natural order; but it has been intended that he shall be body plus rational soul in the natural order plus soul in the supernatural order (Irenaeus). "There should be no clash between the natural order and the supernatural for the Author of both is God (Vassal-Phillips, The Supernatural Life, p. 31, 31). Wherein lies the importance for a proper attitude by the physician towards his patient in regard to the serious moments of life among others, when deceit, equivocation and concealment of the gravity of the malady are to be deprecated.

13 Earth says to the earth of the body: return to thy root (Jalal al-Din Rumi, *Mathnawi*, p. 162).

Lecture 4: The Humors

1 Humors: Fluids of the body. The word "humor" does not now bear the sense which formerly made it an exact equivalent of humor. The term "sanguineous" or simply, "blood" is not to be regarded as identical with the fluid drawn, for example, by venesection, and studied before or after clotting. Phlegm is not properly represented either by "phlegm," "mucus," or "lymph," although having some resemblances to each. "Serous humor" is preferred to the older phlegmatic humor. Similarly "yellow bile" in *The Canon* may not be restricted to the fluid in a normal gallbladder and "black bile" cannot be made synonymous with black pathological gallbladder contents.

Furthermore, it should be said that the "humors" are quasi-material. In many passages of *The Canon* it would seem that when "matter" is spoken of, in connection with disease, "humor" is often meant and particularly a morbid humor. But it is also clear that behind the humor there is what Paracelsus would call an "essence," or "radical humor," which itself governs the nature of the humor and whether or not it is going to become morbid. Health depends on the maintenance of the essential humor in a state of purity in such a view.

Again we may say that the blood is the "salt principle" of the body, the serous humor the "sweet principle," the bilious humor the "bitter principle," and the atrabilious humor the "sour principle of the body. According as one or other of these is predominant in a person, so is his constitution or temperament. In addition to this, the view of the nature of a humor may be extended by suggesting, for instance, that fatty acid is an essential of choleric humor, whereas, neutral fat is an essential of sanguineous humor; that sulpho-centric substances are an essential of atrabilious humor.

The idea belonging to the doctrine of the humors is not affected by biochemistry or cytology, any more than the theory of "four elements" is really affected by modern chemistry. To retain the idea is to claim a practical value in drawing a distinction between "humors" and the body-fluids. In §111 speaks of the blood as a product of the liver, the material for its manufacture being derived almost directly from the food itself. As to the blood-cells, had he known of them he might justly still regard them as incidentals; as forces accresed for a time, and always changing in substance. After all, they are importations into the blood; whatever tissue be their real source, whether their origin is local or widespread, they are not the real trouble in anemia. Remedies will increase their numbers, but do not touch the real disorder. From Avicenna's point of view it might be said that the glamour of the revelations of the microscope has only diverted attention from the real "sanguineous humor" and its ultimate sources and similar subtleties, thereby leading treatment away to attacks on the red and white cell forming organs. For the blood is itself living, not a mere chemical conglomerate. Hence in this field there is a need for reverting to the old paths. The constant endeavor also to reduce everything to terms of cellular individualities as opposed to one single complex, the human being, inevitably carries errors in its train. When St. Thomas wrote, "Health is a harmony of the humors (*Sanitas est quaedam harmonia humorum*)," (*Summa Contra Gentiles*, Dominican translation, ii, 64, p. 166), he was so near the truth as to maintain his place even in these days of excessively refined details of knowledge.

2 From the above definition it is clear that body-fluid is not synonymous with humor. Urine, too, though a fluid, is not a humor. In a sense, body fluids are the meeting-places between various opposed forces or elements and their chemical composition is the mode in which such forces or elements are expressed. In this sense, the term body fluid does not conform to the wording of the above paragraph.

3 The familiar phrases "good-humored," "bad-humored" of modern conversation may not have the same significance to the speakers as they had in Shakespeare's day, but retain their value.

4 Blood may well be regarded as comprising: sanguineous humor, corpuscles, the canalicular system of the whole body, and the tissue-elements abutting thereon; that is, as including the lymphatic channels and their floating cellular population. In addition, there are the blood-forming centers which are the meeting point of two vitalities—the livingness of the blood and the livingness of the tissues. The hemopoietic centers are foci disseminating "vital force," as also are the endocrines, the abdominal ganglia, etc. The energies so well-known as chemical, physical, osmotic, etc., are not primary, but conversions from the living force of these centers. When the blood changes, or its cell-formula changes, it is because the vital force is changing its mode. Instead of radiating in one way, it is disintegrating in other ways and it involves some one organ more than usual. The balance of action on organs and the balance in interchange now ceases to be "just," and the organ or organs concerned therein are then apt to receive the brunt of the physician's attention.

5 Table of Forms of Serous Humor

i. Normal

Sweet

ii. Abnormal.

A. Arranged According to the Taste

No.	Description	Remarks	Temperament
1	Sweet	(i) Outcome of action of the vegetative drives	Hot and moist
2	Salt	(ii) Due to admixture with blood. Due to admixture with bile, "bilious serous humor"	Hot and dry
3	Acid or Sour	(i) Intrinsic in origin (ii) Due to admixture with acrid atrabilious humor	Cold and dry
4	Bitter	(i) From undue infrigidation (ii) From admixture with atrabilious humor	
5	Insipid	Attenuated serous humor	Cold and moist

B. Arranged According to Essential Nature

No.	Description	Remarks
6	Watery	Attenuated serous humor. This may be salty if there arise in it some sort of putrescence.
7	Excrementitious	A superfluity of foreign nature and evident as such to the senses as a mucilaginous material.
8	Crude	This is a sub variety of the preceding; to the senses it appears to be the same as the preceding, but actually is different.
9	Vitreous	Glass-like in texture; taste sometimes sour, sometimes absent.
10	Calcareous	Opaque white. Denser than the crude form. The attenuated part has been dispersed; that which is denser than all the others therefore lingers too long in the foramina and joints.

Note: This table is constructed from the statements in the text in conjunction with the table devised by Joannitius (Hunayn ibn Ishaq al-Ibadi, *Some Writings* included in the Latin Venetian edition of *The Canon*. The additional matter does not therefore follow the same order as the Latin text although including all the information therein.

6 Types of Bilious Humor

Type	Variety	No.	Description.	Site	Origin	Quality
A	Normal.		Clear and pure	Liver, blood	Foam of blood.	Hot
B	Abnormal by admixture with alien substance.	1	Citron-yellow	Liver	The alien substance- is attenuated with- serous humor, added to normal	Less hot
		2	Vitelline-yellow- color of egg yolk.	Liver	Dense (coagulated- serous humor added to normal	Less hot
		3	Oxidized bile, type b. It is ruddy-yellow not transparent, resembles blood, but is tenuous. Various other colors may appear in it.	Liver, blood	Simple admixture with atrabilious humor.	More deleterious than 4
		4	Oxidized bile, type a.	Gallbladder	Spontaneous oxidation of bile= attenuated part + ash. But this ash	More deleterious than 3.

					does not separate out.	
C	Abnormal by internal change of substance.	5	Hepatic form.	Liver	Oxidation of attenuated part of blood. The denser part of the blood separates out as atrabilious humor.	Moderately toxic.
		6	Leek green bile Gastric type a.	Stomach	Oxidation of vitelline bile.	Less toxic.
		7	Mildew or verdigris green bile Gastric type b	Stomach	Intense degree of oxidation of vitelline bile until all moisture is lost	Very hot, extremely toxic

No. 7 is possibly derived from No. 6 by an increase in the degree of oxidation whereby all the moisture is dried up. The fact of becoming too dry accounts for the whitish color. For we know that when heat is applied to a moist substance, it first turns black until all the moisture has vanished and after that the blackness changes into whiteness. When the moisture is less than half and half, whiteness begins to be visible. Thus, wood is first charred and finally becomes a white ash. Heat applied to a moist body makes it black; applied to a dry body it makes it white. Cold applied to a moist body makes it white and applied to a dry body makes it black. Such is our opinion about the leek green and verdigris-green bile.

Verdigris-green form of bile is both hotter and more depraved and more deadly than all other kinds of bile. It must therefore be classed as one of the toxic substances.

7 The abnormal atrabilious humor is hotter and lighter than the natural form and it has in itself a strong penetrative power of moving from the upper parts to the lower and also a destructive action (Joannitius).

8 Tentatively to draw up correlations between modern biochemical data and the humors as above described would not be quite a useless exercise. From the description, it is clear that any given sample of blood contains: (1) all four normal humors; (2) a certain proportion of immature humors—that is, under-oxidized digestive products; (3) excrementitious humors—the tissue-wastes or effete substances; the by-products of complete oxidation. In diseased states it may also contain (4) certain depraved humors, including: (a) over-oxidized products; (b) putrefactive substances of various kinds.

To (1) belong: as regards the sanguineous humor—serum-globulins and serum-albumen, neutral fat, glucose, and the salts concerned in maintaining the acid-base equilibrium; as regards the bilious humor: big-pigments, cholesterine, and perhaps lecithin and volatile fatty actids; to atrabilious humor; neutral sulphur, nitrogen compounds when in colloidal form, certain mucoids.

To (2) belong: glycogen, animal gum, soaps, various states.

To (3) belong: the non-protein nitrogen group (urea, ammonia, cretinin, etc.).

To (4) belong: the products of bacterial growth, various auto-intoxications, diamines, etc.

To complete the correlations, some idea should be formed as to the morphological place to which the substances are severally to be assigned as doubtless the humors occupy blood-corpuscles and other particulate components of the blood.

9 Table of Causes of Humors

Name of Cause	Sanguenous	Bilious	Serous	Atrabilious
Material Cause	Those parts of the solid and fluid aliment which are of equable temperament	The attenuated hot, sweet, oily, and sharp by-product of aliment	The dense humid, viscid, cold by-product of the aliments	The very dense by-product of the aliments, very deficient in moisture and exceeding in heat
Formal Cause	Exact and good digestion	Digestion verging on excess	Imperfect digestion	Precipitative tendency, preventing the flow or dispersal
Efficient Cause	Attempered heat	Attempered heat for normal bilious humor (foam). Undue heat for abnormal bilious humor. Site: liver	Feeble heat	Medium heat, i.e. a heat of oxidation which surpasses the limits of equipoise
Final Cause	To nourish the body	Primary: nutrition; attenuation of blood. Secondary cleansing bowel wall; desire for stool	Primary and secondary purposes	Primary and secondary purposes: nutrition inspissation of blood; nourishment of spleen; tone to stomach; aid to appetite

10 This is a truth worth noting. The tissue-foods carried by the blood and the tissue wastes discharged into it, undergo treatment within it which is only efficient if certain salts and acid bases re present; otherwise conversation of such substances into available form fails to occur; and deposit it in various tissues, fasciae, and joints and even in the vessel-walls (i.e., atheroma) and nerve-sheaths occur with ill-effect. These deleterious substances may be thought of as composed of particles too large to permeate the invisible pores of the tissue-boundaries referred to and the pathological condition of obstructions which looms so largely in *The Canon* here finds its *raison d'etre*.

11 "Anger, joy and passions of a like nature are accompanied by a change in the body" (St. Thomas Aquinas, *Summa Theologica*, 75, 3; p. 11, trans.).

The temper of a cow frequently determines the quantity of the milk it yields, if it gives milk at all. But under the influence of such passions as anger, rage, fury, the milk changes in quality and develops noxious or poisonous properties. Even the flesh may become poisonous if the animal suffered intensely or protractedly, either mentally or physically. Over-driven cattle may thus yield meat which contains toxic substances injurious to the human consumer (W. Lauder Lindsay, *Mind in the Lower Animals*, 11, 270, etc.).

Effects of colors on bodily functions. Red and yellow are injurious to the eye. Blue light soothes the movement of the blood while red light stimulates it. Morning light aids nutrition. Colors vary in their effect according to their intensity. Conversely darkness benefits various conditions. It helps to induce inactivity and sleep (Pareira, *Materia Medica*; E. D. Babbit, *Principles of Light and Color*).

Light in another sense has an effect on the emotions: for instance, the light of intelligence converts fear (earth element) into caution, affection (water element) into benevolence.

LECTURE 5: ANATOMY

1 Table of Organs

Auxiliary Organ Afferent	Sense Organs Attractive Drive	Lung	Stomach and Intestine Veins	Constituents of Humors
Principal Organ	BRAIN (Animal Breath)	HEART (Vital Breath)	LIVER (Natural Breath) Expulsive Drive	REPRODUCTIVE GLAND
Immediate Auxiliary Organ Efferent	Nerves	Arteries	Gallbladder Spleen, Kidney	Ducts and Genital Adnexa
Remote Auxiliary Organ (Elementary Tissues)	Bones, Cartilages Ligaments, Muscles, Fasciae, Tendons, Membranes	Flesh Fat	Intestinal Tract	

2 As the text states, it will equally read "to all parts of the body." As we know, the belief was that the blood left the heart through both the arteries to all parts of the body and also left through the veins. The arteries carried the breath while the veins carried the digested material. The heart, therefore, drove blood away from it on both sides. The distribution into tiny capillaries was known for both the vessels of the arteries and the veins. But it did not seem to occur to anyone that the two flows were in opposite directions and that as much went out of the heart as came into it. The conviction that the two qualities were not equal was the real reason for not going on to the truth of the literal circulation. At bottom it was the equality of the two quantities which Harvey had to prove in order to establish circulation.

3 We know today that the viscera are only sensitive to touch and pain via their peritoneal covering.

4 "There are the minds of the cells of the liver and the liver-mind—the mind that regulates the activities of the liver-cells. Above the liver-mind and above the stomach-mind and the heart-mind is the general physical mind and above that general physical mind and also above the intellectual mind is a higher mind still. There is a hierarchy and kingdom within us" (Eustace Miles, *Self-health as a Habit*, p. 92).

5

Preparative Member	Member Subserved	Auxiliary Member
Lung	Heart	Aorta
Stomach	Liver	Veins
Liver with other nutrient members and the guardians of the breath.	Brain	Nerves
Testis or ovary	Generative organs	Penis and erectile tissues and ducts. Female organs carrying the semen to the site of conception. Uterus as perfector of the virtue of the semen.

6 "*We made the life-germ a clot*," (Quran 23:74). The word sperm is more exact than semen because semen is equivalent to something + sperm. Therefore it is to incorrect to speak of a female sperm. Note that only a portion of the spermatozoon enters into the new human being and not all the ovum. Paracelsus wrote that the sperm is not the visible seminal fluid of man, but rather a semi-material principle contained therein or an "*aura seminalis*," to which the semen serves as a vehicle. (*De generatio hominis*, F. Hartmann, *The Life of Paracelsus*, p. 72). In another place, Paracelsus says: "The matrix attracts the seed of both persons, mixed with the semen, and afterwards expels the semen, but retains the sperm. Thus the seed comes into the matrix. The matrix does not merely mean the womb of a woman; the whole body of the woman is a mother, a matrix" (*De morbo. matric*).

7 Note this proof that Avicenna knew the arteries contain blood.

8 The next four subsections of the text are omitted [in the Gruner translation, but added to the text here to complete the English translation of the first volume of *The Canon* from the Shah translation]. They deal with the anatomy of the bones, muscles, nerves and blood-vessels, and are naturally inadequate in comparison with modern anatomy.

Ancient anatomy has been criticized for allowing as a basis the dissections of monkeys and other animals, apparently overlooking the important factor of circumstance, in order to give the impression of lack of acumen in those days. But in our days, ability and acumen being taken for granted, it is considered allowable to base conclusions in the domain of physiology and pathology upon laboratory reactions obtained from the same kinds of animals. Some workers are alive to the possible insufficiency of data so obtained, but make a virtue of necessity. This may also be claimed for Avicenna.

Avicenna was seeking to express a certain truth in these subsections as well as in other parts of *The Canon* and it is profitable to abstract it and develop it further in the light of "modern" knowledge. The following are some of the considerations in mind.

The variations of anatomical structure which are observed throughout the animal kingdom are the expression of the differing nature and requirements of the respective animal-types. But in dealing with comparative anatomy it is usual to regard evolution as the essential factor, and a false meaning to the phenomena is thereby instilled. We speak of animals as "higher" and "lower" for convenience, but strictly all are equal, because "each creature has such perfection as it was possible for it to have" (St. Thomas, *Summa Theologica*, Dominican translation, p. 108) and its place is in accordance with the 'end' for which it was brought into being, the word 'end' bearing the scholastic sense. . . To raise either to the dignity of 'truth' necessitates an overlooking of the fundamental properties of the nature of being.

Deformities. These may be explained on an evolutionary basis using the ideas of "reversion," "atavism," etc. When the individual is studied in regard to his "end" (in the scholastic sense) a different conception comes to light. But as this brings in the question of events belonging to the category of morals ("to the third and fourth generation"), the problem is at once evaded. Such a conception would not be vitiated by the existence of deformities among animals.

The intimate structure of the body is always changing although the anatomical structures appear to remain unchanged. Hence it is possible to see in these structures merely a locus for the various faculties and functions pertaining to the physical, mental and emotional life of the individual. Compared with his existence in the scheme of things, the anatomical details are mere 'moments musicales.'

To take a special example, one might regard the blood-forming centers as the momentary point of meeting of two vitalities (Lecture 7, endnote 1).

Relation between structure and function. This formed the subject of a classic in medical literature—that in which Galen regards anatomy as the expression of the *nous*. Such a teleological view is not in favor today and, indeed mistakes (as Galen did) the root principle emphasized in these pages. To use the symbolism given Lecture 2, endnote "Explanatory Extension of Lecture 2: The Elements, ff., *M* is not the expression of *F*. In associating structure with function this must always be remembered. The examples available for Avicenna, striking as they seemed to him, are surpassed by those possible through modern knowledge. Thus, harmonious succession of events, both in time and place, is to be discerned throughout the body. The output of bile, for instance, is fitful—sometimes a delicate trickle, sometimes in spurts, sometimes in larger quantities; and this in coordination with the activity of the muscular bundles beneath the membranes which secrete the digestive fluids—in which both nervous and vascular variations play an intimate part. Out of many other instances, the following may be given. The adrenal vein joins the inferior vena cava at a given point in order to secure that the adrenal secretion shall enter the blood in time to receive the activating substances supplied for it by the liver before it becomes exposed to the oxygen contributed by the respiration; for otherwise the activation would be nullified."

It is view of the transcendence of organs, fluids and the like beyond anatomical boundaries that elevates this view of medicine to the wholistic view of the human being. considering both the quantitative and qualitative aspects. Thus (a) 'heart' includes the arterial system and something more; 'liver' includes the venous system and something more; 'brain' similarly goes beyond the organ within the cranium to the cutaneous nerve-endings. This is why a 'function text' for a given organ is never satisfactory. (b) Vascular channels and tissue spaces are simply demarcations of fluids from adjoining tissues. The river exists because there is water to flow and incidentally is an 'anatomical feature' of the country, serving various purposes. Its presence is the indication of, and continues only as long as, certain incessant changes occur in nature at large. To use other words, the vascular channels are the materialization of the stream of blood; or, the current of 'life' made the blood-vessels become demarcated. (c) The humors of the body circulate also in the subtle fashion suggested thus: the sanguineous humor is not only in the blood vessels but also in lymph channels; the serous humor moves in the connective-tissue spaces as well as in anatomical lymphatics, and appears also in the form of the '*eau de constitution*' (Vallery-Radot, *Precis de Pathologie Medicali*) of the tissues: the bilious humor may be followed in the track of cholesterine (and other constituents). The constant loss of hair, nails, teeth, should also be recognized as being part of the constant separation of 'superfluities.' (Cf. F. Hartmann, *The Life of Paracelsus*). (d) If we realize that tissue-spaces and cavernous tissues are forms of channels, it will be clear that the whole body is really an aggregate of 'tubes' of some sort. It may then be said further that disease always starts from the tubes—namely with their lumina are blocked or when their 'walls' become semipermeable or quite impervious.

Anatomical structures depend for their existence on chemical structure. Water, for instance, may be said to come into visibility in the form of an anatomical structure. Conversely, other substances are only visible as long as they are not yet an integral part of the living substance of the body, and others are visible because they have ceased to be such.

As soon as microscopic visibility is attained, the visible thing has ceased to be "living." Stability of form entails the stagnation of certain substances, and also implies that they have been rejected from the cycle of life in order to provide the substrate or platform or *points d'appui* for the actual living substance (i.e., the life-principle) to manifest its faculties during a certain (often limited) period of time (Lecture 4, endnote 8).

Histology (microscopic anatomy) and function. From the preceding consideration, when a tissue is observed through the microscope, the thought should be "that is the spot where this or that substance has emerged into visibility at this moment." This conception is specially applicable to the case of the blood-cells (cf. Lecture 2, endnote "Application of the Doctrine").

Anatomy as the expression of strengths and weaknesses. It is clear that the relevant development of different parts of the body from "head to foot" show its physical strengths and weaknesses. Where one part is weak, another is strong. It is, he points out, less obvious that anatomical conformations are also related to and associated with mental and moral make-up. The root concept of *jalal* (majesty) and *jamal* (beauty) (see Lecture 2, endnote "The Doctrine of

Imponderable Elements") is relevant throughout and in a multitude of directions. Mental and moral capacities and activities affect the vegetative processes just as do the emotions for their influence lasts throughout life. St. Thomas Aquinas says: (a) "Every operation of the sensitive soul belongs to the composite (*Summa Theologica*, Dominican translation, 75, 3, p. 10). . . . (b) "There are certain operations common to the soul and the body, such as fear, anger, sensation and so forth; for these happen by reason of a certain transmutation in a determinate part of the body, which proves that they are operations of the soul and body together" (*Contra Gentiles*, ii, 57, p. 139) . . . . "We find in the intellective appetite, which is the will, operations specifically similar to those of the sensitive appetite, differing in this, that in the sensitive appetite they are passions because of its connection with a bodily organ, whereas in the intellective appetite they are pure operations. For just as by the passion of fear which, in the sensitive appetite, one shuns a future evil, so without passion, the intellective appetite has a like operation" (*ibid.*, 90, p. 190).

From all this it is clear that much is to be learned from external anatomy (head, face, hands, joints, skin markings, etc.) as to the strength and weakness, not only of the body as a whole, but of the several organs in particular. Were the study of internal anatomy combined with the external, the associations should be more appreciated. The 'case' is not really finished when a 'handful' of viscera has been studied in the autopsy room or even in the laboratories attached thereto. The remaining 'shell' passes on into oblivion bearing its wonderful secrets with it, for its language is such that however loudly it 'speak,' there are few with ears to hear and perhaps none with ability to interpret.

Lecture 6: General Physiology

1 "Life appears through various operations in different degrees of living things" (St. Thomas Aquinas, *Summa Theologica*, Dominican translation, q. 76, art. 1)

2 Instinctive drive or faculty is the name of a property whereby the phenomenon of life is manifested. Function is the actualized potentiality. Instinctive drive or faculty=power=potentiality. Instinctive drive is not force, it is potential power. It is static. Power is the instinctive drive in a state of activity. It is dynamic. The complete ensemble of instinctive drives is the soul while the complete ensemble of functions is life. Weakness of instinctive drive corresponds to hypofunction. Excess (plethora) of instinctive drive corresponds to hyper function.

3 These three terms, derived from the Latin version, only properly express the meaning of the Arabic if they are taken in their original sense. The third term is rendered "psychical" by some translators (Max Meyerhof, *The Book of the Ten Treatises on the Eye Ascribed to Hunayn ibn Ishaq*) but is open to objection because its modern usage does not sufficiently correspond to the idea of *nafsaniat*.

Other words are preferred in the course of the present translation. The familiar "vitality" is convenient for the first term. The words "vegetative," and "sensitive," employed in the Dominican translation of the *Summa* are satisfactory renderings for the other two terms, and are to be understood strictly in the Thomistic sense. The term "natural" is reverted to in §1137 for reasons there given.

The variations in scope exhibited by these and allied terms are conveniently indicated in the following table.

Analysis of Certain Terms Applied to Living Things: Beings Endowed with Life

Term	Drive	A Vegetable	B Animal	C Human
I. Distinctive Quality[1] Modern Language	Vital[2]	Vegetative Organic Powers	Sentient Lower Mental	Rational Intellectual, Higher Mental Life, Psychic Powers
Platonic Term		Nutritive	Appetitive	Rational
Avicenna[3]		Natural[4]	Animal[5]	Ratiocinative
Scholasticism		Vegetative (Life or Soul)	Sensitive (Life or Soul) Sensuous (Necessarily implies appetition)[6]	Rational (Life or Soul)
II. These terms are based on: (a) drives pertaining to each:				
(i) Pre-modern thought	Breath[7]	Plants have only nutrition, growth, reproduction	Animals have also sensation and movement	Human beings have also intellect or intelligence
(ii) Modern		But modern research shows sensory and motor powers	But some animals exhibit intellectual-powers often supposed to be purely human.	But this is not so for some races of men and in come cases of disease of the brain.
(iii) In terms of consciousness.		Unconscious life.	Subconscious life and lower conscious	Fully conscious
(b) On essential manifestations (3. Avicenna).		As "nature"	As sensation, movement and cogitative power.[8]	As capacity for abstract concepts.
(c) On fundamental causes (4. Scholastic basis).		Effected by means of a corporeal organ by virtue of a corporeal quality.	Effected by means of a corporeal organ but not by virtue of a quality. Deals with particulars.	Is effected apart from a corporeal organ or quality. Deals with universals.[9]
(d) On theological considerations.		Mortal	Mortal	Immortal: (a) absolutely (Scholastic view); (b) conditionally (some creeds).
III. Chief organ concerned.				
1. In modern thought		All vegetative organs equally im-	Nervous system (automatic and	Brain (grey matter of cortex).

	portant (biochemical central) processes in general.		
2 Platonic	Liver	Heart[10]	Brain
3 Avicenna	Liver and gonads	Brain	
4 Scholastic	All viscera. No special organ because "life" belongs to all.	Nervous system, but also the whole "being."	No material organ.

Notes to Chart:

1 Boundaries of the Three Kingdoms: These are admirably set out in *Chahar Maqala* (E. G. Browne, translator): "When the vegetable kingdom was produced, God gave it the four forces and the three instinctive drives. When the animal kingdom was produced, God added two more instinctive drives—that of perception (with five external senses and five internal senses) and of movement. When the human kingdom was produced, God added a capacity for abstract concepts (intelligence)."

2 Vital faculty. This is not specifically mentioned by St. Thomas Aquinas because implied in the word "life." He refers to it thus: "The vital operation . . . whereby something is shown to be living" (St. Thomas Aquinas, *Summa Theologica*, Dominican translation, liv. 2. p. 44). "Life-principle" has a wider scope than implied in "vital instinctive drive" is the 'foam' or determining principle of the living being. Coalescing with the material factor it constitutes the living being. It unifies the material elements into one individual. It holds them together . . . as a mass of chemical compounds, many of them most complex and in very unstable equilibrium, constantly undergoing change and tending to dissolution into simpler and more stable compounds. When life ceases, the process of disintegration sets in with great rapidity. The function, then, of this active informing principle is that of a unifying, conserving, restraining character, holding back, as it were, and sustaining the potential energies of the organism in their unstable condition" (Michael Maher, *Psychology*, p. 427).

3 Avicenna's division: this is determined by medical requirements.

4 Natural faculty, i.e. "pertaining to the 'nature'. That is (a) the mere fact of living at all, (b) powers in common with laws of nature in general. Compare the term 'natural science,' 'natural philosophy' (used before the present era) applied to the modern chemistry, physics and their subdivisions. The ancients recognized that physiological phenomena in regard to the 'natural' life were kin to those of our chemistry and physics.

Note also the meaning of 'nature' in: 'the natural appetite is that inclination which each thing has of its own nature for something. Wherefore by its natural appetite each power desires something suitable to itself" (St. Thomas Aquinas, *Summa Theologica*, Dominican translation, p. 78).

5 Animal instinctive drive. The word "animal" really denotes simply "a thing with an anima." Therefore the human being is an animal. But different people among all nations use the word (in their own language) entirely vaguely and thus give rise to perennial confusion of thought when applying it in daily life. The following meanings are assigned to it:

(i) Generally or collectively, it refers to the presence of life. That is, anima-te; in-animat-te.

(ii) Specifically or particularly. (a) indefinitely as (a') "soul" (a") "mind" (a"') "spirit" (*quaecumque substantia invisibilis*) (St. Thomas Aquinas, *Summa Theologica*, Rome, i, 41, 3, 4). (b) More definitely "lower soul" as opposed to animus, the higher soul whose seat is the heart, the center of cognitive and emotional life (*ibid*., xiv. 153).

6 St. Thomas Aquinas, *Summa Theologica*, Rome, 78, i. p. 78.

7 Manifestations as "breath" or by means of the breath. See Gruner 161. Breath = spiritus which is denied by St. Thomas as "an instrument of the soul, *tenue, lucidum, calidum, ex puriore sanguine*" (i. 41. 3. 4). Cf preceding note under "spirit."

8 St Thomas Aquinas recognized such powers in animals. "Cogitative and memorative powers are not distinct, but the same, yet more perfect in the human being than in other animals." (St. Thomas Aquinas, *Summa Theologica*, Dominican translation, 78. i. p. 90).

9 *Ibid*., 78, i. p. 78.

10 The heart. In the Platonic view it is the chief organ of the appetitive soul; in Avicenna it is that of the breath. See Lecture 7, endnote 1. But this would make the appetitive soul equivalent to the vital drive which it is not. Another objection to the Platonic view is explained by St.

Thomas (*ibid*., p. 145).

"Only three powers or parts of the soul are commonly assigned—namely, the vegetable soul, the sensitive soul, and the rational soul . . . . There are five genera of powers of the soul—the vegetative, the sensitive, the appetitive, the locomotive, and the intellectual. Of these three are called souls and four are called modes of living." . . . The reason for this diversity lies in the various souls being distinguished accordingly as the operation of the soul transcends the operation of the corporeal nature in various ways because the whole corporeal nature is subject to the soul and is related to it as its matter and instrument. There exists, therefore, an operation of the soul which so far exceeds the corporeal nature that it is not even performed by any corporeal organ; and such is the operation of the rational soul. Below this, there is another operation of the soul, which is indeed performed through a corporeal organ, but not through a corporeal quality, and this is the operation of the sensitive soul; because though hot and cold, wet and dry, and other such corporeal qualities are required for the work of the senses, yet they are not required for the work of the senses, yet they are not required in such a way that the operation of the senses takes place by virtue of such qualities: *but only for the proper disposition of the organ*. The lowest of the operations of the soul is that which is performed by a corporeal organ and by virtue of a corporeal quality. Yet this transcends the operation of the corporeal nature because the movements of bodies are caused by an extrinsic principle while these operations are from an intrinsic principle for this is common to all operations of the soul since every animate thing, in some way, moves itself. Such is the operation of the vegetative soul because digestion and what follows is caused instrumentally by the action of heat as the Philosopher says" (St. Thomas Aquinas, *Summa Theologica*, Q. 78, art. I, Dominican translation, p. 75, 76).

4 Hippocrates said: "There is in the body no one beginning, but all parts are alike, beginning and ending, for a circle has no beginning."

5 Classification of the Natural Instinctive Drives: General Purpose of the Individual:

Dominant Drive	Subservient Drive	Synonyms	Qualities	Element	Corresponding Mental Process
Nutritive	Attractive	Apposition	Hot/Dry Present Prosthesis	Fire	Perception
		Retentive	Cold/Dry agglutina; adhesion; prosphysis.	Earth-	Memory
		Alterative	Hot/Moist transformative;	Air	Cogitation

	Expulsive	assimilative poietic (haemopoietic). Propulsive; expeditive	Cold/Moist	Water	Expression
Augmentative	Plastic; incremental				Acquistion of knowledge
Generative	Masculine factor			Ether	Creative and inventive drives
(i) in the strict sense (ii) primary transformative drive					
Informative	Plastic operates in utero. The feminine factor.		Constructive drives		

6 From the annotations by Costaeus: “Reproduction implies a plastic drive and that implies transformative power and that depends on the four qualities. Growth cannot occur without nutrition; nutrition cannot occur without agglutination or assimilation; agglutination cannot occur without apposition; assimilation cannot occur without transformation; transformation cannot occur without retention; and retention cannot occur without affinity. Each successive step entails the removal and excretion of the products and by-products of the preceding steps for these are hindrances to reproduction, nutrition and growth.” (Marginal notes in Latin translation.)

7 The word “attraction” in the original is primarily concerned with the thought of the attraction of (female) beauty and has a particularly appropriate application as a consequence.

8 Summary of Points Made

	Duration of muscular contraction	Amount of longitudinal movement achieved
Attractive Drive	Quite short	Marked
Retentive Drive	Long; continued	Moderate
Alternative Drive	Continued	None
Expulsive Drive	Momentary	Considerable but super-added from without

9 Thus the attractive drive is not equal in degree in all organs. Heat is stronger in the liver than in the stomach and intestines, in arteries than in veins. The liver at one time is hotter (and therefore the attractive drive is greater) than at another. So also in the case of the stomach. Therefore, if the stomach is empty and the liver is hot, the stomach will draw out the

serous humor and bile from the liver. Just as a strong person can take something out of the hands of a weak person if he wants to, while on another day, the other person is the stronger (Daremberg, *Oeuvres de Galen*, ii, p. 307).

"The operation of the vegetative principle is performed by means of heat, the property of which is to consume humidity" (St. Thomas Aquinas, *Summa Theologica*, 75, p. 81).

See I tung cheng mo (circa AD 1056) on page 25 of the subdivision "Mo Chueh Chih Chang" referring to the changing dominance of the types of "breath" in the various organs, perceptible by a study of the pulse.

Vital drive, *virtus vitalis*, vitality, innate heat, "spirits" (corporeal, vital, natural, animal)=breath (which is its manifestation)=Spirit=refined form of bodily substance or fluid believed to act as a medium between mind and the grosser matter of the body (*Catholic Encyclopedia*, xv, p. 220) = "a kind of very subtle body which penetrates all parts of the material body and infuses them like the essence of a rose, oil in sesame, better in milk" (Carra de Vaux).

In part it corresponds to "life principle," and also in part to "substantial form," but it is not the "soul." It is one of the powers of the soul. The soul is a bundle of life, a bundle of drives and powers which complete the material body. Soul: body:: vibration: atom.

10 Scholastic argument against such a conclusion: "If the human being is to be understood as three or two (souls) using a body, it follows that the human being is not one thing, but two or three, for he is three souls or at least two. And if this be understood of the intellective soul only, so that the sensitive soul be understood to be the body's form, and the intellective soul, using the animated and sensified body, to be a human being, this would again involve absurdities, namely that a human being is not an animal, but uses an animal; and that a human being does not sense but uses a sentient thing. And since these statements are inadmissible, it is impossible that there be in us three souls differing in substance, the intellective, the sensitive and the nutritive" (St. Thomas, *Summa Theologica*, Rome, p. 144).

If the primary temperament helps the breath to receive the primary or instinctive drive, then the vital powers, the breath and the faculties are its perfection. The primary vital faculty is not sufficient by itself to enable the breath to respond to the other faculties, but needs an appropriate temperament first. The physicians also claim that this faculty, besides paving the way for "life," itself initiates the movement of the attenuated spiritual substance (that is the breath) towards the various members (organs), and is the agent which brings about the contraction and expansion of respiration and pulse. In that it assists life it is "passion," and in that it assists the activity and functions of mind and pulse, it is "action."

11 Expressed in another form:

PHILOSOPHICAL TERM	CORPOREAL SOUL (lower reason)	NATURAL FACULTY	ANIMAL FACULTY
Medical Term	Animal Faculty	(Higher) Natural Faculty	Natural Faculty
Scope of Term	Seat of movement action, operations	Seat of Passions and starting point of 'apprehension'	Vegetative Functions

LECTURE 7: THE BREATH: ITS ORIGIN, FORMS, SOURCES AND RELATION TO BEING

1 Explanatory Extension of the Subject of the Breath

Synonyms. "The breath of life" (Gen. 2:7, Quran 32:9); *souffle de vie*; *ruach* (Heb.); *ruh* (Persian, Arabic); *hu* (Sufi); *ch'i* (Chinese); *prana* (Hindu); [The Hindu system of physiology recognizes five breaths as supporting the body. They are: *prana* (the air inhaled), *apana* (has a downward course), *samana* (essential to digestion), *udana* (has an upward course, or passes into the head), *vyana* (pervades the whole body and moves in various directions, transverse and otherwise; therefore, equivalent to the "breath" of the present section.) But *prana* includes the rest, ordinarily speaking.-E. A. C., Kaviratna, Chakara Sarnhita, ii. 20]; *hauch* (German); Spirit (as a translation of "*spiritus*," for which " breath " is the better equivalent: see Lecture 6, endnote 3, and Lecture 6, endnote 9; *spiritus* is the Latin translation of the Arabic *nafs*).

Primordial aura (J. P. Bruce, *Chu Hsi: Philosophy of Nature*, p. 101); "ether"; vivifying principle; vital fluid; vital (cosmic) force.

Definition: that which binds the vegetative and sensitive life into one connected whole. It is common to, and like in, aid living things.

"That which centers in the cardio-pulmonary center."(Baraduc, *Les Vibrations de la vitalite humaine*). "It is a subtle vapor which rises from the blood, diffuses itself to the remotest arteries, and resembles the sun in luminosity, (*Chahar maqala*, p.8)

Negative definition. "Breath" is not "respiration," "breathing," drawing in breath. Therefore it is not the equivalent of *anhelitus, nafas, anfas, Atem*.

The expression "he breathed his last" actually describes the departure of the "breath," but there are two events taking place simultaneously, and the literal respiration is only one of them.

It is not "soul" (*anima*). The latter is the Latin translation of the Arabic ruh in various passages.

It is not "vitality," for this is the manifestation of breath.

Vitality stands for the vegetative soul. Thus, enfeebled vitality means lessening of the ability of the vegetative soul to accomplish some or all of its instinctive drives. Therefore, it is not "life." ("Allah made life to be in breath." *1001 Nights*, Lady Burton, v., p. 422). It is not the "vital air" of the 18th century chemists. It is not even " vital drive." It is not amenable to either physical or chemical methods of investigation. It is not a force at all, and, therefore, not analogous to electricity, magnetism, heat, etc. though in the course of its activity it manifests all such phenomena.

Breath Is Not "Individuality"

Description by analogy—being immaterial, and representing a notion foreign to Western thought, breath is almost indefinable, whereas to the Eastern mind there seems little difficulty in the conception. Analogies such as to flame, a pendulum, a ladder or lift to a higher plane of being, a chain linking the three aspects of the soul to light, to vibrations, and so on, are necessarily misleading.

By picturing the breath as a sort of aura pervading the body, with a polarity correspondent with the cosmic ether (its source, whence it individualized into the human being), the conception of orientation (in time and space) becomes feasible. The angle of incidence is then to be considered, both in regard to every direction of space and to the time of day. Thus an infinite variety of constitution in these respects becomes obvious.

The substance of the breath—this is mentioned in several passages in *The Canon*. Though immaterial, the breath needs a material basis or substrate. The substance is described as twofold: (a) an aqueous vapor, in the case of healthy breath, as occurs when the humors—the source of the substance of the breath (see §487) are healthy; (b) a fuliginous vapor, like the mist of the early morning landscape, if the breath be unhealthy—namely because superfluities are present in the humors.

A more tangible idea of the substance of the breath is furnished by taking it as partly consisting of oxygen, for the functions of oxygen in the body are the same as those attributed to the breath which it carries. Thus to quote L. S. Beale, "Oxygen is necessary to disintegrate the soft formed material and combine with some of its constituents" (*Bioplasm*). That is, breath=*mf*, where *m* is oxygen.

In the Hindu system, there are ten substrates for the life-breaths, but these are anatomical (Chakara, i. 402).

The "primordial substance" of Chinese philosophy, the ground of all phenomena, physical and psychical, fulfills the theory of the breath. It is invisible and intangible, but manifests as matter (solid, fluid, gaseous), as psychic existence, and as spiritual existence. This substance agrees with "breath" in showing cyclical changes, passing from energy to inertia, from activity to passivity, incorporeality to corporeality. The incorporeal is "the rule of existence implanted in every living being"; and "Li" is the nature implanted by the decree This principle of activity appears in modernist philosophy as mind. (Cf. Bruce, *Chu Hsi and His Masters*, p. 109.)

The constant activity of the breath—were the breath not in constant activity, the body would be "dead." The activity consists of: (1) changes in quality; and (2) movement from place to place. Actually, both occur simultaneously, but description would be impossible without taking each form separately.

(1) Changes in quality—this is a rhythmic waxing and waning in intensity; a change from a strong phase to a weak one, and back to a strong one; a change from positive to negative; an ebb and flow; a condensation or concentration ("inspissation") and an expansion or rarefaction ("attenuation"). In the one phase, there is attraction of energy from without symbolized by inhaling air; in the other, there is repelling of energy from within symbolized by exhaling air.

These phases of movement are represented by the terms *jalal, jamal* (Persian); *jalal, jamal* (Arabic); *shiva, shakti* (Urdu); yin, yang (Chinese); masculine, feminine; active, passive; etc. The rise is called *uruj* in Persian terminology, and the fall, *nasul*; it is a rise from no intensity (incipience) to great intensity; there is a period of maximum intensity (maturation) and a fall from thence to no intensity (decay, defervescence, decline).

This cycle of the breath is continuous, but varies in rate hourly (every two hours), twice-daily, daily, weekly, monthly, seasonal. According to its changes, so does the feeling of well-being of the person change; according to its changes, so are there differences of bodily vigor in one and the same person. Every family, every race has its type of "breath." Wherever we turn in living nature we can see the traces or signs of this "pulse of life"—in vegetable life, in animal life, even the greater range of human history itself; the rise and fall of nations; the rise and fall of pandemics; the solar and planetary cycles—all show the traces of this activity, though no doubt many would consider the connection with "breath" very intangible in these instances.

The explanation of this activity—this is to be found in the fact of the cyclical changes in the imponderable elements, for the two phenomena, as already suggested, are part and parcel of the same phenomenon. Thus, breath conceived as a vibration rate, is now slow, now quick; now coarse, now fine. The range and changes of vibration from "earth" (slow, coarse) to ether " (quick, fine), and back, as has been intimated, are associated with changes of activity of the breath. These elements are, as it were, the *points d'appui* of the breath and they constitute an "immaterial" circulatory system.

Relation of breath to temperament and the emotional character—so close is the relation between "breath," "imponderable elements," and "temperament" that description of the one readily lends itself to being a description of one or both the others. If we trace changes in "earth," "water," etc., we are at the same time tracing changes in the activity of the "breath," and we use words which apply to both "temperament" in the old sense, and emotional character as spoken of today. Dominance of "water" is as much as to say "the breath" remains in the "water" phase over a longer period of time than in other phases in this person. It also goes with "jamal" type of character, the exact form of manifestation varying according to other factors in the "make up," i.e., quiet endurance, silent submission to pain, ardor of aesthetic emotion, keen sense of beauty, love of certain kinds of music, certain colors, flowers, etc. (Note, then, how intimate this idea of "constitution" becomes).

Relation of quality of breath to will power—the will power should dominate the breath. But it cannot do so consciously if the individual is ignorant of the existence of "breath." Persons of vigorous will power will dominate it unconsciously. It would be easy to see that dominance of will power by the breath should be very common, with the corollary that actions supposed to the initiated by the personality are really quasi-automatic

Will power may be used to "develop the breath"; that is, the way the breath flows through the body, through the various (nerve) centers.

Relation to " innate heat"–the subject of innate heat is very prominent in the pages of *The Canon*; it is closely linked with "vitality" (popular sense of the word like i.e., "enfeebled vitality," "has very little vitality"; "full of vim). The close relation to breath is expressed by saying that as the breath wanes (*nasul* phase), the innate heat lessens; as the innate heat is restored in the course of nutritive processes, so the breath "waxes" (*uruj* phase). The rate of waxing and waning of the innate heat varies with the individual and shows a relation with the similar phases of activity of the breath. Innate heat is expended simultaneously with "breath," and at the same time comes that indefinable phenomenon—real enough nevertheless—called "atmosphere," "personality," "radiance," "aura."

This subject bears on the theory regarding the appearance of pathological changes in the humors. Normally, the innate heat is the agent which separates normal effete matters from healthy humors. But in disease—that is, when the cycle of the breath is not in harmony with the process of formation of the humors—injurious effete matters (acrid, corrosive, etc.) appear as by-products of the abnormal humoral state, the latter being the result either of a change in the innate heat or of a conflict between this and "foreign heat" (i.e., bacterial products, see §1030, Gruner's Introduction, "The Guides to the Diagnosis of the State of the Patient").

(3) Relation to metabolic changes spoken of (Lecture 2, endnote "Considered Dynamically-Change") under the picturesque title "dance of the elements." The picture of imponderable elements dipping down into the world of ponderable elements (or, to be precise, the individual human being), and entering into the changes of metabolism expressed as changes of pivot of function from C to O or H, or N, or S, or P in compound after compound, and breakdown into CO_2 or H_20, etc. or as formation of tissue cells and their subsequent necrobiosis, etc.—all this is completed by the view of the breath, passing from phase to phase, from strong to weak, not merely in one organ, but in every particle of the whole being. With the ascending phase of the breath come the formation of increasingly complex substances, "generation"; with the descending phase, goes the disintegration into simpler substances, "corruption." Viewed as life-principle, we may think of the breath as controlling the vegetative faculties of the soul, which are associated by an intimate mutual rela-

tionship.

In this connection, the observation may be here noted that change of electric potential arising from the metabolism of the salts is necessary to the formation of active (as opposed to inert) fat in the body.

Hence physiological action—that is, anatomy in motion—is not merely a question of the behavior of C, H, O, N, S, P, in the various side-chains, etc. It is a sum of potentialities possessed by the separate imponderables and by their varying combinations in a particular individual at any given time. The common denominator or collective formula which represents this sum adequately is necessarily very complex, and yet it is really essential that it be elucidated before one could be said truly to grasp the real basis of a person's ill-health, or intelligently work out the fundamental bases of prognosis.

(2) The activity of movement—the second mode of activity of the breath consists of a cyclical movement, a movement in place, a movement comparable with a. circulation. During the course of this movement, the breath comes successively into relation with the several tissues and organs, one after the other until it reappears at the starting-point.

The movement may be anti-clockwise: as well as clockwise in the various parts of the body.

But there are two paradoxes here. Firstly, there is no period of time when the breath can be said to have passed a given point. It is not like an object going round and round, like an imaginary drop of blood. The breath is all through the body all the time. It is more as if there were a series of lights in an electric circuit, and they burning the whole time, but the intensity is changing successively from point to point. The breath is always in the great centers of the body (the *chakra*s, *prana*s but it is brightest in the liver at one moment and the brain at the next and so on, yet following a certain order. [This was realized also by the Chinese physicians as shown in the classic on the pulse (vol. lxxx, p. 28)].

Secondly, the circulation has no anatomical boundaries. [Possibly this idea underlies the seemingly impossible Chinese statement: the blood is inside the vessels, the spirits outside.] Not only this, but it is flowing left-sidedly or right-sidedly. This is transparently non-anatomical. Many would reject the possibility and even an attempt at proof would be unsatisfying. The justification for the statement that the breath is now left-sided now right- sided, flowing down each side separately, depends on-subtle observations which are beyond the scope proposed for this work. It will suffice to suggest just this: the peculiar attitudes adopted by all creatures (animals as well as human beings) during sleep; when standing or sitting; when exercising or at repose; also the different moods shown by a given individual—these and similar phenomena, carefully watched, furnish adequate indications of the truth of the statement. There is also a circulation along such intangible channels as the temperaments of the organs.

However, there is an actual relation to anatomical organs as well. There is no ambiguity about this. The passage of the breath from liver to brain, from heart to tissues is orderly and deliberately specified not only in *The Canon* but in the *De viribus cordis*, lest the unwary should be misled by the faulty ideas of Avicenna's predecessors and contemporaries. The heart as the center of life, and the seat of formation of the breath, is no mere fancy. To speak of the flow of the breath through the major organs awakening each center in turn (cerebral, thoracic, digestive, and genital) and then necessarily reaching the lesser organs (including the tissues and cellular elements) is to give a true picture of life. To insist also that in meeting the centers, the breath is altered; that it receives and then proceeds in that altered or renewed form to the lesser tissues, is to fulfill the great law—the law of giving and receiving; both together; simultaneous; balanced in degree. Both are true. To omit one is to speak inaccurately because one represents only in part.

Application to physiological histology—as has been suggested, physiological histology is microscopic anatomy in motion. It is the blackboard on which can be demonstrated the reality of the truths of the scholastic conceptions. So, in studying the tissues microscopically we must remember to introduce the conception of the flow of the breath through the tissue-spaces, the juice-canals, which are also the channels of the breath. Synchronous with this flow there is an attenuation of cell-substance into fluids; and a disintegration of complex chemical substances into simpler ones. At the same time, one must say the change in the breath is attenuation and aggregation of such substances.

Substances pass from the colloid to the fluid state; from the colloid to the crystalloid state: from complex to simple, and vice versa. They pass by aggregation from fluids into cell-substance (assimilation). It is all one single process. That which we see is with the aid of the microscope is the visible manifestation of cyclical changes in atom-groups, of carbon, hydrogen, oxygen, nitrogen, sulphur, phosphorus, etc. The excrescence which we cannot see on the nuclear contour of the leucocytes: for instance, is this subdominance of the several chemical elements—whether the change be the outcome of "attenuation" or of "aggregation." Not only this, but the excrescence of the nucleus is also the effect of the change in the breath which at different times belongs to different chemical elements, and so to different morphological histological appearances.

The conception of the blood-forming centers as the meeting point of two vitalities has already been suggested (Lecture 4, endnote 8).

Application of the conception to pathology: (a) disease as the result of interference with the freedom of flow of breath, not only round the body, but also away from the body altogether. It is clear that an actual obstruction in a tissue (whether it can be seen with the naked eye, or felt with the hand, or whether it is in so minute a channel that the microscope is needed to demonstrate it) prevents the flow of tissue-fluids and is the forerunner of a morbid condition-a disease. But it exerts this effect primarily because the flow of the breath is obstructed and its rhythm degraded. Could the two series of events occur independently, the fact is that the former, the material of obstruction, would not suffice tog set up such a morbid condition.

The following are useful, concrete examples of diseases produced in this way. The dire effects produced by hysterectomy in young persons, once in much vogue for instance for severe dysmenorrhea; and the persistent ill-health which appears when it is done in older persons round the prime of (child-bearing) life. The explanation is to be found in the destruction of the "channels" of the breath—the severance of non-medullated nerve-fibers and even the actual removal of important nerve ganglia. This indefinable vital component of the being. which must "circulate," goes so far, and then finds a void, and its activity is turned back on itself; there is a revulsion; and the patient is aware of a great distress which nothing will (or can) relieve or jejunal ulcer following gastro-enterostomy, or excision of gastric ulcer.

(b) Disease as a result of disturbance in the rhythm of the breath. A change of rhythm, or an ataxy of the breath would suffice to initiate a loss of immunity to bacterial agents. Since there must also be an outflow of breath, any associated interference with its current would have the effect of holding back any of the isolated microorganisms which are always to be found in the tissues.

In this way the organisms would have time to develop into active colonies. Structural organic changes then appear in the body. When Paracelsus said that " life-principle may decompose and become a strong poison furnishing life to innumerable, invisible (i.e., microscopic) existences, by which infectious diseases are caused," he was not speaking foolishly (F. Hartmann, *The Life of Paracelsus*, p. I55).

(c) Loss of balance between the normal qualities of the breath and the functions of the body may initiate disease.

(d) The relation between the intracorporeal cycles of the breath and the cycles in the outer world is a factor for consideration in regard to the study of bacterial cycles in nature, outside the bodies of animals and other human beings.

(e) Sudden recovery from incurable diseases should be intelligible in view of the nature of the breath. Remembering the existence of polarity, and a point of penetration into the corporeal being, and considering the fact that in disease there is a distortion of the "shape" of the breath, it is not difficult to conceive that some outer force or power breaks through and restores the polarity to normal, in which event the sick person would be once more in proper relation to his terrestrial conditions, and be freed from the interference (analogous to the interference of light which has previously occurred in the activity of the breath. The event of such a revulsion occurring at all, whether the subsequent physical recovery be instant or only reached by gradual stages; would bring the case within the category of miraculous cure.

Changes of quality of activity of the breath are simultaneous with its movement from place to place within the body. The two aspects of the activity of the breath must be considered simultaneously, for they are not actually separate. Thus, to sum up, we picture the breath circulating from nutritive organs to those of the sensitive life, awakening as it does so the lower passions (the nutritive=appetite; the reproductive=desire (see Lecture 8, endnote 11, "Details Regarding the Emotions"); and then the higher (the emotions, the atmosphere, the inspiration). The faculties of each organ are activated as the breath traverses them; their vitality augments, and the breath itself concurrently receives something from each center. The natural breath is the phase, then, when the breath is considered in regard to the natural or vegetative processes of the body, is located in the liver, and is associated with venous blood. The vital breath is the phase when it is located in the heart, and is associated with arterial blood. The animal (or sensitive) breath is associated with the nerve-fibers. Yet there are not three breaths, but one breath—"not three souls, but one soul." And the breath is not the "soul."

The changing activities of breath are associated with changes in the composition in regard to the cosmic elements; with changes in chemical composition. Movement of quality (type, rate, primary quality) goes with movement in regard to place.

The expressions "a matter-of-fact person," an "emotional person"; a "neurotic person," in the light of the considerations presented at such lengths are seen to be capable of interpretation in terms of corresponding types of "breath," which are dominant in the given individual (Lecture 7, endnote 1).

All these changes have been analogized with a "dance." The breath is the controller of both aspects of the dance. It is the music of the dance which holds the dancers together. When the music ceases the dance ceases, or degrades into a meaningless disorder. And the ceasing of the dance is "death"; and the degradation is the subsequent decomposition processes.

The player of the music, and the movements of the two dancers should blend harmoniously to make the perfect dance. What if there be inattention on the player's part? What if he should not correspond to the capacities and capabilities of the dancers? What if the giving and receiving between the music and the dancers should fail at any moment? Surely, then there is disease. Whatever modern medicine has to say about etiology, this fact remains at the root of the phenomena of all disease. In health, the dancers depend on the player, and their dance is so perfect that they always respond to his tune. But there comes the time when the (hidden!) Improvisor of the music cries out "Halt!"

The following repetition of some of the important facts so far discussed is justifiable for still greater precision.

Abbreviations: *a*, animal, *b*, breath; *B*, body as a whole, *C*, vital centers (heart, liver, brain, gonad); *f*, faculty; *h*, heart; *j*, vegetative; *l*, "life"; *L*, life-principle; *m*, mind; *n*, natural; *r*, rational; *s*, sensitive or sentient, or sensuous; *S*, soul in the Platonic sense; *sp*., spirit, *v*, vital.

(A) General Statements :_

L exhibits *jf, sf, rf*, and *vf*.

But *L* is not the same as *jf, sf, rf*, and vf; or the same as (*j.s.*)*l*.

L is not = *jf* + *sf* + *rf* + *vf*

L is not the same as *S*.

S is not the same as *L*; or *m*; or *sp*.

S includes *L, b, jl, sl, rl, vf*.

b is not *l*, or *L*, though almost equivalent to *l*.

l implies *b*.

af (Avicenna) belongs within the domain of *sf* and *rf* (scholastic).

jl (scholastic) comprises *vf* and *nf* together (Avicenna).

sl (scholastic) comprises *vf, nf*, and *some af* (Avicenna).

sl (scholastic) is equivalent to *nf, vf*, (*af-rf*) (Avicenna).

rl (scholastic) comprises *vf, nf, af* (Avicenna).

rl (scholastic) includes *jl* and *sl* (scholastic).

(B) Special Statements

(i) The three chief views of the nature of a "person" are:

Modernists or scientific or rational	*B*+*m*
Popular or Platonic	*S* and *B* or *S* + *B*,
Aristotelian	*S.B.*, or *S* x *B*

(ii) The scholastic view may be thus expressed -

\- "Nature" is *L.B.*; the "vegetable nature" is *jl.B*; the "animal nature" is *jl. sl. B*; "human nature" is *jl. sl. rl. B*.

(iii) Comparing the description given by Avicenna, with that given by St. Thomas, we have:

Avicenna	(*b, nf, af*), B (C)
St. Thomas	*L.B.*; or (*jl, sl, rl*) *B*

2 It may be noted that corporeal bodies receive life when they enter into the composition of living matter, whether of protozoa or the like, or of highly organized animals and lants. The author does not say that all corporeal bodies are "forms of life," as some have assumed. The distinction between matter and form already discussed (see Lecture 2, endnote "Explanatioory Extension of Lecture 2: The Elements") makes clear that which is expressed slightly differently in the preceding passage. It should be borne in mind that the first principles are really neither "matter" nor "form;" the discussion in the text is relevant only because the listener is supposed to have failed to realize this. Although the first-principles are coterminous with the "infinity" of the universe, they have not either mass or volume. The comparison between a "point" and a "world" is characteristically medieval.

3 Differences Between Potentiality and Disposition

Potentiality	Disposition
1. Pertains equally to both contraries.	Does not.
2. One and the same person can be glad and sad.	Optimism and pessimism can only exist in distinct persons
3 Is perfected into a disposition.	Is perfection of potentiality towards one or other contrary.
4 To pass one's life with a breath of sad or potentiality is one thing.	To pass one's life with a breath of sad or glad disposition is another..
5 Glad or sad potentiality can harmonize	Glad or sad disposition does not.
6 Potentiality for both contraries is inseparably inherent in the breath from the very first.	Disposition towards a contrary (emotion) is not inseparably inherent in the breath from the outset may appear under the influence of supervening agents.

4 'Delight is a perfection of operation," *Summa Contra Gentiles*, xc, p. 190;; "joy and delight differ in aspect. For delight is caused by a good conjoined in reality, while joy does not require this conjunction because the mere repose of the will in the thing willed suffices for the notion of joy. Therefore, delight is only in a conjoined good if it be taken in its proper sense whereas joy is in a separate good" (*ibid*, p. 191).

5 Cf. The Theory of Pain, §929.

6 This passage is characteristically Sufic. The reference being to the effect of purification of the "breath" in the exercises culminating in "shah hal"; the personal success and accuracy of the physician in his dealing with the sick being progressively enhanced the more the purification of his "breath" is secured. The rarefaction of the breath, and the replacement of coarseness by fineness are desirable in all, but come from experience and not from study.

7 Disposition of Mind and Corresponding Character of Breath

Disposition of Mind	Corresponding Character of Breath	When Met With
Cheerful	Quantity: plentiful Temperament: balanced. Substance of breath: brilliant, full of light	
Gloomy	Quantity: scanty	In convalescence In prolonged illness In old age
	Temperament: unbalanced	In disease
	Substance: dense and gross	In old age; melancholy
	Substance: attenuated	In women during convalescence
	Substance: confused	In melancholy

8 Compare the following: "all the passions of the irascible appetite rise from the passions of the concupiscible appetite and terminate in them; for instance, anger rises from sadness, and having wrought vengeance, ter-

minates in joy," (St. Thomas Aquinas, Summa Theologica, Dominican translation, 81, a. 2; p. 130).

9 Cf Ps. 118:32; 2 Cor. 6:11.

10 Relations Between the Various Blood-states and the Several Emotions

Blood	Effect on Breath	Effect on Emotional State
Plentiful, bright, hot	Oxidative processes active; movement swift	Tendency to anger
Plentiful, bright, attempered	Abundance of clear breath of laudable substance and attempered.	Tendency to delight
Bright, watery, cool, tenuous	Oxidative processes slow; breath heavy; moves centrifugally; less is formed; more is dispersed.	Tendency to fear; neither joy nor anger; heart tends to be weak.
Thick, turbid, over hot	Breath turbid as the blood tends to "inflame," the breath thickens, and fails to cool properly.	Tendency to sadness and even continual vexation. Therefore the emotion persists.
Rarefied; bilious humor increased	Breath of intense heat and rarefied.	Anger which comes and goes.
Ditto but also bright and clear		Joy
Thick but not turbid (rarely met with)	Thick but not turbid.	Not sad but strong and bold. Very little anger because joy neutralizes this.*
Thick, not turbid, cold	Thick, cold, not turbid	Timid, dull, upright.
Thick, turbid, cold		Gloomy, solitary; a person of rancor and resentment; anger arises only at great provocation.**

* Joy easily overcomes the emotion of anger. It is sadness that fosters anger because anger is an impulse to expel. Happy things harmonize with pleasure and pleasure entails a tendency to attract or gather in. Therefore, it will need a bid thing to make such a person angry; and as a very concentrated breath will result, there can be very little fear.

** The anger will not last as long as it would in hot-blooded people (in whom other like conditions are associated), but longer than it does in persons whose blood is rarefied. Therefore, he comes to be a man of resentment, because the disposition to hate implies the persistence of hurtful images in the imagination.

Lecture 8: Psychology

1 The *Chahar maqala* says, "Now the perceptive drive (*mudrika*) is subdivided into ten branches, five of which are called the external senses and five the internal senses. The former are touch, taste, sight, hearing and smell" (E. G. Browne, translator). The drives may also be designated drives of the lower mind or lower reason. Augustine says, "The higher reason is that which is intent on the contemplation and consultation of things eternal . . . but he calls the lower reason that which is intent on the disposal of temporal things. Now these two—namely, eternal and temporal—are related to our knowledge in this way that one of them is the means of

knowing the other" (St. Thomas Aquinas, *Summa Theologica*, Dominican translation, p. 112).

2 These senses are not further discussed in *The Canon*. The following quotation from *Chahar Maqala* (E. G. Browne's translation) may be therefore added: "Hearing is a sense located in the nerve which is distributed about the auditory meatus so that it detects any sound which is discharged against it by undulations of the air compressed between two impinging bodies, that is to say, two bodies striking against one another, by the impact of which the air is thrown into waves and becomes the cause of sound, in that it imparts movement to the air which is stationary in the auditory meatus, come into contact with it, reaches this nerve, and gives rise to the sensation of hearing. Sight is a faculty located in the optic nerve which discerns images projected on the crystalline humor, whether of figures or sold bodies, variously colored, through the medium of a translucent substance which extends from it to the surfaces of reflecting bodies. Smell is a drive located in a protuberance situated in the fore part of the brain, and resembling the nipple of the female breast which apprehends what the air inhaled brings to it of doors mingled with the vapors wafted by air-currents or impressed upon it by diffusion from the odorific body. It is really a very delicate kind of taste. The sense of taste detects soluble nutrients in those objects which come in contact with the tongue, discriminating between sweet, bitter, sharp, sour, etc. The sense of touch is distributed throughout the skin and flesh of the animal, the nerves thereby perceiving and discerning anything which comes in contact with them—such as the four primary qualities: dryness, moisture, heat and cold; and the secondary qualities of roughness, smoothness, harshness, softness."

The five sounds, the five tastes, the five colors are simply manifestations of the five elements (A. Fowke, *The World-conception of the Chinese*, p. 238), "Your taste, your seeing, your hearing, etc.—these are the elements so say not they exist not!"

3 The sensations of sight, smell, touch, afforded by an object are conjoined, and the qualities perceived by the different senses become gathered into one single percept. This faculty exists by virtue of the fact that all sensation and muscular action are two aspects of one process. With the exercise of every sense-organ there goes an exercise of muscular action and the latter cannot occur without at the same time arousing muscular sensations because sense-organs for muscular senses are everywhere present along the fibers of which the muscles are composed.

4 Regarded from the scholastic point of view, the imagination may be distinguished into (a) sensuous, (b) rational or intellectual. The former is equivalent to Avicenna's term for it concerns itself with natural objects. The second form is concerned with ideas, is creative or productive, and manifested as "invention" (artistic, mechanical, scientific, etc), whereas

sensuous imagination is simply reproductive. But in both cases the drive is defined as "the power of forming mental images or representations of material objects apart from the presence of the latter." (Maher, *Psychology*, p. 163).

Source of the images: (1) the sensations, emotions and actions of the body; (2) trains of thought which are chiefly on the higher plane of rational life; (3) the intellect; (4) other external influences such as other minds, whether human or angelic.

The difference from "common sense" is that the latter only deals with objects while present.

5 Imagination combines or separates as the mind selects those particular percepts which are stored in the imagination. It is more clear to place the cogitative drive into the higher plane of rational life. It really belongs partly to the intellectual imagination ad partly to the rational drive, the understanding.

6 Clearly the apprehensive drive of the text covers both lower reason and reason as ordinarily understood. The former is also called instinct. The difference between the two is easily defined in theory but difficult to apply in practice. Instinct is the sense of what makes for the well-being of the individual. "Concrete relations are perceived without an abstract conception being formed. Instinct therefore differs from reason in the absence of abstract universal knowledge. At either end of the scale the external manifestations are clear and absolute.

Instinctive actions may be described as highly complex reflexes, the movements being spread over a variably long time-period and appearing after a variably long interval. Thus we have: (1) sensory stimulus to lower nerve-centers to immediate reflex movement; and (2) the stimulus of a perception to higher nerve-centers to a series of complex movements. With (1) there is no need to reach consciousness and (2) goes on without a consciousness of the general (not particular) end or purpose of the movements.

While the subject of instinct is always discussed in regard to the actions of animals, it should be admitted that nine-tenths of our daily actions really belong exactly to the same plane or order. The use of the expression "lower reason" enables a vast number of particular instances of animal behavior to be classified along with many similar actions performed by the human being perhaps especially during childhood.

Much of the difficulty about instinct versus reason in animals is avoided in this way. It is also to be noted that while speech and language exist in various orders of creatures, articulate speech occurs in man alone (Bock, *Das Buch vom gesunden und kranken Menschen*). Animals can express their own emotions to one another and can understand our speech in that it conveys emotion. But that is different from the reasoning processes which scholastic philosophy limits to the human being.

7 The philosopher discusses whether apprehension and memory are to be taken together or separately. Is apprehension merely a treasury of reflection? To the physician this problem is irrelevant because the same noxa, be it an intemperament or a depraved constitution, would affect both and in either case the seat of disease would be in the same region of the brain.

The apprehensive faculty: memory:: common sense: imagination. But the composite sense preserves forms and memory preserves ideas—the ideas discovered by judgment (*wahm*). (See E. G. Browne, translator, *Chahar Maqala*).

In scholastic philosophy, the memory is two-fold: sensuous and rational. Sensuous memory is the power of retaining, reproducing and recognizing the representations of past experiences, and of referring an event to its place in time. The concrete objects of memory under this category are: memory of size, form, position, weight, sounds, rhythm, scent, color, faces, persons, and of certain events. The degree of capacity for memory in regard to each of these varies widely, producing various "types," such as auditory, visual, motor, etc. The memory of emotional states is called "affective" memory. Rational memory, the power of recollection, reminiscence, the power of active recall, volitional memory is restricted to the human being (Maher, *Psychology*, p. 180).

The differences in the Shah translation from the Urdu translation with the Arabic and notes from Gruner translated from the Latin is interesting to note. This is how Shah translated this section:

Thinking or ideation.

Physicians call this process thinking. Those who try to be precise call it variously ideation or thinking. It is termed ideation when it functions spontaneously or in subservience to intuition. It is termed thinking when it is employed by the rational mind. Both processes differ from perception. Whether the perception functions collectively or singly, it receives and retains only sensory impressions. Ideation on the other hand, rearranges the impressions with some addition and substraction. Hence, ideation not only produces images derived from perception, but may occasionally add some of its own which may be contrary to all perception, that is, the flight of a human being in the air or the seeing of an emerald mountain. Imagination on the other hand, presents only those images which had been received earlier from perception. This process is located in the mid-ventricle of the brain.

Intuition

Intuitive thinking is a sub-variety of ideation and is similar to the internal sensibility of the animals. Intuition is the process which informs animals that the wolf is their enemy and that they have to take care of their young ones and that the shepherd is a friend who need not be shunned. As these ideas are not dictated by the intellect and as it is obvious that love and hate are matters not of the external senses and are not perceived but felt by the animals, there must be a separate process dictating such actions. It may not be the intellect, but it is certainly a process of some kind. This process is sometimes used also by the human beings who in this regard are like the animals.

Intuition differs from imagination in that the latter keeps the percepts as they are, while intuition adds a meaning to it which had not been communicated by any sense organ. Intuition also differs from intellect in that the latter, unlike intuition, presents the percepts in complex forms but without any cognitive effect. Intellect provides an integrative direction to the sensory percepts, while intuition gives a cognitive effect to that which has no perceptual basis.

Just as perception controls the sensory impressions, intuition directs the supersenous ideas which are independent of perception. Some people as a matter of convenience call intuition 'instinct'. They are at liberty to do so as long as they keep in view the correct significance of these terms.

Physicians seldom take the trouble of understanding 'intuition'. This is because disorders of this process are generally due to disturbances of the preliminary processes of perception, ideation and memory which will be described shortly. Physicians are interested only in a process whose disturbance produces some disease. If the disturbance of a instinctive drive is due to some other condition, such as a temperamental or structural abnormality, the functional disturbance has to be noted, but the physician must diagnose the underlying temperamental imbalance or structural abnormality for the prevention and cure of the disease. It is not necessary to diagnose the condition of the instinctive drive affected secondarily.

Memory and Recall

Strictly speaking, the third process described by the physicians is in reality the fourth or fifth in this order and is known as memory and recall, which are a storehouse for instinctive ideas, but not for the percepts held by the imagination. Its seat is in the posterior ventricle of the brain. It would be interesting from a purely philosophical point of view to speculate if the memory and recall which bring back stored images are both one and the same process or two different processes. This is, however, not important from the physician's point of view, as in both processes the disturbances are due to temperamental or structural abnormalities of the posterior part of the brain.

Intelligence

The fourth process of internal sensibility is the human intelligence whose endowment has raised the human being to the highest position amongst all beings. It is this process which gives the human being the power of logic and discrimination.

Physicians do not take notice of intuition for the above mentioned reason and are naturally indifferent to the working of this process. They are generally content with the study of only the first three processes. (End of Shah translation)

8 Charts have been devised in order to co-ordinate various terminologies applied to the sensitive and rational faculties.

I. Avicenna	II. Arabic (Nt. 449)
	Higher Drives
5. Ratiocinative Drive	5. Thinking
4. Memory	4. Memory
3. Cogitative Drive	3. Perception
	Lower Drives
3. Apprehension	
2. Imagination	2. Imagination
1. Common Sense	1. Common Sense

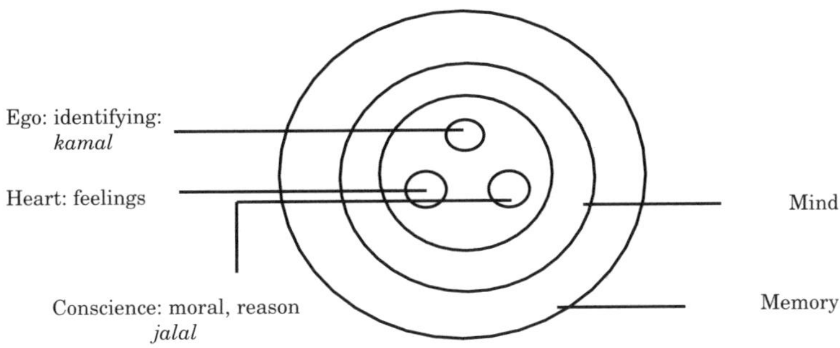

III. Modern Sufi (Inayat Khan, *In an Eastern Rose Garden*)

IV. Jili (R. A. Nicholson, translator, *Studies in Islamic Mysticism*)	V. Modern (Psychiatric) (Stoddart, *The Mind and Its Disorders*)
	Conscious
Thought (of God)	Reasoning
Heart (*sirr, qalb, ruh*)	Insight
Intelligence (*aql*)	Concentrating Power
Reason: logical drive, the blamer	Volition
Judgment, the watcher (*wahm*)	Conduct
Reflection, cogitative drive (*fikr*)	Ideation
Intuition	Association of Ideas
	Subconscious
Higher will, attention (*hamm*)	Sense-memory, instinct, emotion
Perception (*mudrika*)	Perception
Fantasy (*khayal*)	Stereognosis
Imagination (*musawwira*)	
Memory of ideas (*dhakira*)	VI
Memory (*hafiza*)	
Lower will (*nafs*)	

VI. SCHOLASTIC (Michael Maher, *Psychology*)

Human
Understanding
Intellect
Power of Thought
Supra sensuous
Reason

Animal
Imagination
Memory
Sensuous
Instinct
Common Sense
Perception

Note: These and innumerable other views regarding the drives of the "mind" are partly accounted for by difference of purpose in view. In ancient medicine, everything was related to the cosmic elements. In modern medicine, anatomy is all-important. In regard to mental diseases, cortical structure (strata of types of nerve-cell) is naturally a basis of interpretation. Many modern textbooks of psychology consider principles of education of the young. Moral philosophy has another object in view. Eastern mystics regarded the matter in terms of the problem of attaining elevation of the soul to God. Standard modern Catholic teaching envisages all such aspects without making clear the links between "theoretical" drives and the actual microscopic anatomy and histological physiology of the human body. But these links are the essential interest in this treatise and are outlined in the special chart described and discussed in Gruner 157 sqq.

9 That the soul is endowed with a locomotive drive is simply an ultimate fact. Our life-long experience assures us that mind and body do interact, but how we cannot tell. The skeletal system is the instrument of animal life. Movement occurs in plants but so slowly that it was not positively discerned until recent years and is not a locomotion.

10 Gruner, in notes, further explains the correlation of the various instinctive drives.

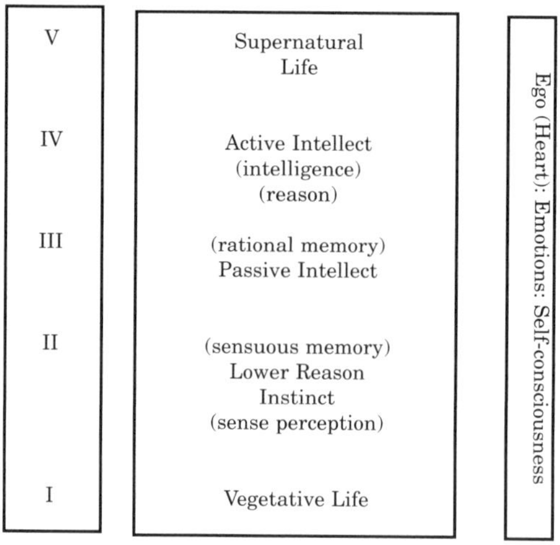

V	Supernatural Life	Ego (Heart): Emotions: Self-consciousness
IV	Active Intellect (intelligence) (reason)	
III	(rational memory) Passive Intellect	
II	(sensuous memory) Lower Reason Instinct (sense perception)	
I	Vegetative Life	

THE CORRELATION OF THE VARIOUS FACULTIES

The correlation between the various faculties with the inter-connections between the visible bodily organs is usefully indicated by means of a suitable map or chart.

The following considerations are 'necessary in studying the accompanying diagram. (1) There are no actual boundaries between the drives, even in the case of the discrete viscera. The internal senses are "merely diverse aspects or phases of a single sensuous faculty" (Michael Maher, *Psychology*, p. 96) as Aristotle perceived. To name "departments" of the mind, it must therefore be constantly remembered, is simply to help the memory, and assist analysis of the various mental operations. (2) Subdivision of drives into "animal" and "human" is to be avoided. (3) The enumeration of mental drives given by phrenology is not vitiated by the fact that phrenological charts are not anatomically correct. (4) Since the strength of one drive involves a corresponding weakness of some other, even the very existence of the drive may be virtual.

BRIEF DESCRIPTION OF THE CHART

Six discrete "planes" are represented, and are named according to certain terms selected from those used in various classifications. The vertically placed plane serves to indicate a close relation between this and each of the horizontal ones.

Plane I. This refers to the vegetative life, and shows the various organs and their inter-connections, as well as their relations to the superposed planes. Connection with the lower extremity of the vertical plane indicates the existence of "unconscious appetition" in this sphere of life. This, the so-called " natural appetite," is defined as " the inclination towards a thing which is in concord with its nature, without any knowledge of the reason why such a thing is appetible" (*Catholic Encyclopedia*, I, 656). It is inherent in the nature of "being" on this plane.

Appetite is: (1) natural (hunger, thirst, sleep, exercise, sex); (2) sensitive (reflex, instinctive); (3) rational. The two former depend on organic conditions, which are not regulated by reason. The sensitive appetite is under the control of the will, and can be strengthened or checked thereby (*ibid*, I, 656). Appetite, in the sense of sinful desire, belongs to another aspect of the subject.

Plane II. This refers to the sensitive life. Sensitive life comprises the "power to know" (that is, the instinctive drive already discussed in *The Canon* §557 sqq., and shown in the charts in Lecture 8, endnote 8, and the "power to love" (= "appetition"="the power of loving that which is the good for the individual"=appetitive faculty=desire). The power to know is represented by Plane II and the power to love is represented by the lower part of the vertical plane. Both find their realization in organs depicted on Plane I.

"Lower" is used as equivalent to "animal" (as opposed to human).

Scholastically it is the antonym of " higher." "Reason," again, is made equivalent to " instinct" because popularly the latter word is taken to be the same thing as automatism. In scholastic philosophy the phenomenon of instinct is appraised properly. Hence " lower reason" comes to be applicable for a certain series of phenomena, for that which scholastically is called instinct is that which in modern life is called "lower reason." The word reason should however be applied strictly to those higher operations which scholastics define with masterly precision.

Coincident with the mental representation of the thing—whether it be good or evil for the individual—there is an agreeable or disagreeable passive state of consciousness, and this is called an "emotion." Emotions are subdivided into "concupiscible" and "irascible." The former imply attraction and are: love, desire, delight and are oriented towards preservation of the species. The latter concern repulsion and are: hatred, abhorrence, sadness all oriented towards self-preservation. They are: hope of acquiring an object which it is difficult or dangerous to obtain; despair of so doing; fear of a threatening evil or danger, with impulse to flee; courage, when there is an impulse to remain; anger.

The objects of each of these emotions are: concrete objects, whether inanimate or living; muscular activity; experience (excitement, adventure) or emotion itself. For example, there may be fear of hunger, cold, lack of necessaries of life; (clothing, etc.); of illness; of death; of punishment, of reproaches, of tears; of loss of prestige or reputation, of being misjudged or considered eccentric; fear of failure.

Planes III and IV together refer to the rational life. They appear separated in order to bring out the idea of active and passive intellect. They stand for: the "power to think." The vertical plane belongs with these two planes as representing "the power to will."

The power to think or understanding, is regarded as two-fold—speculative and practical. The former, under the influence of the will produces the act of contemplation, the object in question being purely ideal (poetry, music, art, refinement, taste). It sees resemblances, sees the "simplicity" of creation, and makes even the most thorough difference seem quite secondary and insignificant. It includes foresight, research, "wisdom." The practical understanding, under the influence of the will, and by the use of the physical body, accomplishes constructive work.

The power to will, or "rational appetite," precedes voluntary movement. The inclusion of the terms "attention," "consciousness," "heart," "ego," on the vertical plane, is for convenience and does not imply synonymity in every respect.

Plane V, as representing the "supernatural" life, is only introduced for completeness, and its relation with the "lower" planes, though intimate, is purposely not specified. Its necessity was perceived by Jili (taken as a representative of Islamic mysticism by R. A. Nicholson, *Studies in Islamic Mysticism*) when he discusses the "perfect" or "ideal" human being, and some of its features appear in the chart representing his views (Lec ture 8, endnote 8).

Details Regarding the Emotions

(1) It will be seen that there is no separate account of the emotions in *The Canon*. They are only referred to incidentally, except in the chapter on the Pulse (§1227) which describes the effect of five particular emotional states on the pulse.

(2) While classification of the emotions is unsatisfactory, as Michael Maher points out, the short list given by Avicenna is convenient in practice, because every patient may be regarded as fundamentally governed by one or other, the others being relatively unimportant.

In this section such emotions as aesthetic and moral feeling are not considered. The self-regarding emotions are referred to under "Ego" (see Lecture 8, endnote 11).

Emotions and Their Correlations

	I.	**II.**	**III.**	**IV.**	**V.**
Latin Name	Gaudium	Laetitia	Tristitia	Ira	Timor
Arabic Name	Surur	Lazzat	Gham	Ghadab	Faz
Chinese Name	Hsi	Ai[1]	Ai	Nu	Chu
Translation	Joy	Delight Concupiscence[1]	Sorrow	Anger Repulsion[1]	Fear
Corresponding Element					
Sufi	Ether	Air	Earth	Fire	Water
Chinese[2]	Fire	Earth	Metal	Wood	Water
Corresponding Phase of Breath[3]	*Jalal*	*Jamal*	*Jamal*	*Jalal*	*Jamal*
Dominant Humor Corresponding	Sanguineous	Sanguineous	Atrabilious	Bilious	Serous

1 The Chinese speak of seven chief emotions, concupiscence and irascible being the two additional ones. Instead of delight, liveliness and love are equivalents of "ai."

2 Su-Wen (A. Forke and L. Wieger, *History of Religious Beliefs*, p. 167).

3. In theosophical language this relation is expressed by saying that emotions belong to the "astral" plane.

(4) Relation between the emotions and the "elements"—there is not a strict relation between individual emotions and individual elements, as has been explained, all the elements occur together, though one may be said to be

more frequently dominant than another.

The same applies to the phases of the "breath"—the degree of vitality. Every emotion goes through three phases of activity—rising, acme, falling,-as do the types of breath. Hence different words are required to describe each emotion according as it is weak, strong, balanced, pure or mixed. (See Lecture 8, endnote 11).

This complexity is illustrated by the following instance—the relation between "anger" and "fire." Fire varies from dull smoldering to a red-heat, and so to flame-flicker, lambent, gentle, pale, lurid, sudden flare, continued light of different degrees of intensity, fierce burning, ferocious fire. The phrases: one's blood boils, he flared up, and so on, are graphic enough. Actually, the vessels engorge, the muscular power is intercepted, the mind becomes confused; the bile is set in motion, and may be expelled from the gall-bladder, leading to relief (bodily as well as mentally), or enters the blood more freely, engendering heat and increasing both the acid and the bitter throughout the body. Whether a person is irascible, or is difficult to rouse to anger, whether the passion will smolder (and hence show as a resentment, and spirit of vengeance) will depend on whether the humors are mixed or whether one or other is definitely preponderant in the resting state.

An angry person gives out a definite atmosphere, a feeling of being "on edge." The effect on bystanders depends on their dominant emotional state; in some it provokes quarrelsomeness; in others perplexity owing to the discovery that the person is unapproachable. Silence and appropriate interior exercises are indicated. Angry words produce mental "sores"; they may heal, or they may be kept going, or they may be reopened, or become incurable.

An outburst of anger may be provoked by a clash of interests. These vary widely. Thus, two wills may clash; the function of one organ may clash with that of another (e.g. menstrual irritability or outbursts of temper); clash of duty with self-will. The intensity of the outburst is according to the principle of *jalal-jamal*.

Anger may be manifested as a liver-storm (variable duration), storms from stagnation in connective-tissue spaces (longer duration), nerve-storms (short duration), mind-storms (leading to criminal acts). These phenomena may come on unawares.

(5) Physical effects of emotional disturbance—the effect of anger on bodily functions has been referred to. Fear may manifest as gastric trouble, indigestion, constipation. Panic-fear may provoke diarrhea, and polyuria. The blood becomes flooded with toxins, and the kidneys are taxed in consequence. The blood-state is altered during the sway of emotions. The blood-cell formula may also alter.

The humoral formula changes during emotional phases, but there is no rigid relation to be assigned. Those given in the table are not absolute.

Analysis of a total emotional process—viewed as a complex process, the following components must be considered in regard to a total emotional process: (i) A cognitive state associated with a nervous change in the cerebral centers (a), (ii) a conscious appetency or impulse excited by (a) associated with a diffused outgoing process along motor nerves (b), (iii) bodily commotion caused by ii + b; this reaches consciousness through sensory nerves (c). Psychically, the emotion is made up of i + ii + iii; physically it comprises a + b + c. (after Michael Maher, *Psychology*, p. 446).

Details Concerning Some of the Drives and Phenomena Pertaining to Rational Life

The term "mind" is variously defined. It is taken as synonymous with: (1) intellect; (2) intelligence; (3) consciousness, conscious intelligence; (4) the nervous system; (5) the brain (thus, behaviorists employ "mind" for "brain" from a dislike of the materialistic sound of that word (S. McGonagh, *Dominicana*, p. 299), (6) the entire psychical being. It is defined as (1) a sum-total of the mental processes (Howell's physiology); (2) that which thinks, feels and wills; (3) "the terminus of an evolutionary progress from reflex and tropism by way of memory and imagination to intellect and reason"; (4) "mind is to be interpreted in biological terms, as an organism, an organ of adjustment, a structural fabric" (purposive school of psychology, see *ibid.*, S. McGonagh). "Mind" is analogized with a room in which the soul lives; with a mirror which reflects every thought coming into it. The purpose of this analogy is to illustrate differences between individuals just as there are different kinds of rooms, styles of decoration or colored windows.

The scholastic definition of the mind is that it is the proximate principle of understanding and designates rational life as opposed to sense-knowledge. Mind is not a special power over and above the memory, intelligence, and will, but is a potential whole comprising these three. It includes all those powers which in their operation are entirely removed from matter and from material conditions. (St. Thomas, *Quaestiones Disputatae, De Veritate*, x. 1 and 12; *Summa Theologica*, 77, a. 5)

Activity of mind—this may be considered in three aspects: mobile, rhythmic, and chaotic. The former is shown in gentleness, generosity, gratitude, goodwill, easy-going disposition. Rhythmic activity is shown in reason and logic; in business-like character; moderation in love and hate, likes and dislikes. Chaotic activity is shown in intolerance, suspicion, imprudence.

The Intellect (Plane III, IV)—the active intellect is defined as the power of abstracting, whereby the object obtained by the senses (the image stored in the imagination) is disengaged from its individual conditions and rendered intelligible. It abstracts from the representations of concrete things or qualities, the typical ideal essential elements, leaving behind the material and particular (*Catholic Encyclopedia*, I. 74), "manipulating them like algebra without immediate reference to the concrete." It considers things apart from quantity, quality, place, and time.

Relation of intellect to corporeal organs—intellect is a function of the mind alone; it is not exerted by means of any organ (Michael Maher, *Psychology*, p. 239, 240). Intellectual activity depends extrinsically, or per accidents, on the organic faculties, as the school men said (*ibid.*, p. 241). Intellect is a spiritual faculty.

Whereas sensations of touch, or phantasms of color are possible only to "a soul that informs a body, and can only be elicited by modification of an animated system of nerves, intellectual judgments are not the results of a stimulus of a sense- organ, but are products of purely spiritual action." The inferior mode of mental life is awakened by the irritation of sentient nerves, the superior activity is due to a higher reaction from the unexhausted nature of the mind itself; and the ground for this reaction lies in the fact that the same indivisible soul is the root of both orders of faculties" (Maher, *ibid.*, p. 242).

B. Perception, imagination—these are shown on both the II and the III plane. (see Lecture 8, endnote 8).

C. Concepts v. images—the formation of concepts must be distinguished from that of fantasies, or images. The concept is a representation of objects of a class; the image pictures only one particular color, shape, size, etc. The concept is fixed, immutable, and has no relation to time. The image is unstable, contingent, and fluctuates. The concept represents the nature or essence in an abstract condition, "ignoring or rescinding all accidental individualizing conditions." "The image reproduces the object clothed with these concrete determinations" (Maher, *ibid.*, p.237).

D. Thought—this cannot be called a "sensation," as shown by the question raised by Balmez (quoted in Michael Maher, *Psychology*, p. 243): "Is the perception of the difference of the smell of the rose and that of the pink a sensation? If we answer that it is not, we infer that the judgment is not the sensation transformed, for it is not even a sensation.

The mechanism of thought—"the external objects stimulate the senses and effect a modification of the sensuous faculties." "The result is a sensuous percipient act." A sensuous phantasm arises in the imagination. The intellect now acts and abstracts the essence, thereby generating the concept which expresses the essence of the object. This abstract concept is then viewed by 'reflection' as capable of representing any member of the class. A formally universal idea is now constituted" (Hirschberg and Lippert, *Die Augenheilkunde des Ibn Sina*, p. 311). "By comparison, reflection and generalization, the idea is elaborated until we attain to the distinct and precise concepts or ideas which accurate science demands" (Michael Maher, *Psychology*, vii. 633).

B. Reasoning—this is defined as a process in which a succession of cognitive acts representing-the various "notes" of a thing are unified, through relations being established between them. It is the opposite process to intuition. By intuition, one single act conveys all that can be known of a thing. The instinctive drive or faculty of reason seeks new and differential characteristics. The most minute differences are essential. It includes: discerning power, sense of discrimination, classifying power, sense of proportion: observing power for (a) things, to see analogies and resemblances between them; (b) persons, e.g., character reading; (c) ideas which link this faculty to that of the intellect. It also includes the attributes of orderliness; method; sense of absurdity and therefore merriment, humor, wit, sarcasm, ridicule; curiosity, mimicry, character interpretation as by actors; arguing, and reasoning power pure and simple.

F. Intuition or intuitive knowledge–this term is variously used. In the present volume it is intended to refer to a particular kind of knowledge obtained through the use of the intellect, as applied to many of the topics of medicine.

That which is called esoteric knowledge, or "wisdom," may be included under this heading. Foresight, so-called mystical interpretation, insight are obtained by the use of the intellect influenced by mature experience. "The spirit of faith is the habit of seeing everything in God, and God in everything." (Fr. Pius.)

From the scholastic point of view, the following are proper propositions:

(1) All knowledge begins in the data furnished by sense-experience.

(2) Primary principles are known by intuition.

(3) Abstraction and discursive reasoning are the instruments wherewith we discern the nature of the data of sense-experience, their laws and causes. Through these two servants of intuition the mind gains a scientific and philosophical knowledge of things (*Summa Theologica*, i. 58, a. 3; II-IIa. 49; a. 5, ad 2m.). Through the same two servants of intuition we arrive at the notion of immaterial beings and of God Himself. (St. Thomas Aquinas, *Summa Contra Gentiles*, Dominican translation, i. 12), (St. Thomas Aquinas, *Summa Theologica*, Dominican translation, I, 84-88).

(4) "Concepts and reasoning, therefore, are in themselves inferior to intuition; but they are the normal" (i.e., usual, or most widespread) "processes of human knowledge."

"For the school men, the intuitive act of intellectual knowledge is by its nature the most perfect act of knowledge, since it is an immediate apprehension of and contact with reality in its concrete existence, and our supreme reward in the supernatural order will consist in the intuitive apprehension of God by our intelligence: the beatific vision. But in our present conditions of earthly life our knowledge must of necessity (the lives of saints, however, show that for them at any rate there was very often not such "necessity") make use of concepts and reasoning" (*Catholic Encyclopedia*, Sauvage, vii, p. 83).

OCCULT PHENOMENA AND POWERS

1. Common usage applies the terms "occult" to such phenomena as psychic power, healing power, thought-reading, telepathy, clairvoyance, crystal-gazing, fortune-telling, discernment of the future, interpretation of dreams and visions, medium-ship, character-delineation (e.g palmistry), divination, magic, sorcery, hypnotism, obsession, wining another who is at a distance to perform some desired personal service. Such phenomena are studied in theosophy, hermetic science, astrology (and medical astrology), spiritualism, Christian science, and also figure in new-thought movements and many other revivals and elaborations of ancient pagan pursuits (*Catholic Encyclopedia*, ii. 19; xi. 199).

Whereas in all these cases there is the suspicion of trickery, deception, fraud, and charlatanry, the term "occultism" is quite properly applied in an entirely different manner, namely, to the investigation, by the use of reason and logic, of the occult (i.e., hidden, not self-evident) causes and effects operative in ordinary human affairs. The events of one's own daily life, and those of one's fellows, are all natural sequences of previous behavior. This is not realized, and wrong conclusions are apt to be drawn—such as ascribing good or ill fortune to " fate," or an extra mundane agency, or "to the deliberate ill-will of others." Better knowledge of such a subject would enable one to avoid misjudging others, and to help them better, by realizing that every soul has his own way to go and his own manner of proceeding on that way, toward the one final goal of all.

II. Occult phenomena and powers—meanings of the term—are: (a) true, or (b) false. The latter are achieved by deception, or illusion, charlatanry, or may be evidence of self-deception, or of disease (hysteria, neurasthenia, mental disorder, insanity). The former belong to two categories: (i) impersonal: that is, explicable according to physical laws, though at present only imperfectly understood. Such phenomena manifest sometimes in inanimate objects, sometimes in organized beings—animal or human (by virtue of their possession of a receptive nervous system). (2) Personal. (i) Natural. That is, manifested in human "nature" (a) actively in the case of phenomena of the kind referred to in Lecture 8, endnote 11; (b) passively—in which case the phenomena manifested in one person originate in another or in numerous others (e.g. crowd-psychology), or in "supernatural") beings. (ii) Supernatural agencies: (a) so called disembodied spirits; (b) angelic beings—good and beneficent or bad and malevolent, evil, satanic; (c) the Supreme Being.

III. The word "supernatural" has another application which is properly and accurately explained only in traditional philosophy (see Cuthbert, *Catholic Encyclopedia*, p. 28, sqq.; Poulain, *The Graces of Interior Prayer*, chap vi; Vassall-Phillips, etc.). Ordinarily, the human being lives a "natural" life, however cultured, unselfish, altruistic, pious, virtuous. He may live a "supernatural" life, by entering a "state of grace," so that the human nature is transcended (*super*), as indicated by Plane V in the Chart. While living such a life, phenomena may become manifest (e.g. visions, revelations) which must not be confused with those called "occult."

IV. Emotional states as a basis of occult phenomena—strong emotional states may impress places and things sufficiently to, affect other persons in the absence of the original impresser. Obsessions and haunted places are accounted for in this way. " A place or thing such as a weapon or article of furniture, almost anything in fact which has played a part in events that aroused very intense emotional activity on the part of those who enacted them becomes itself saturated as it were with the emotions involved. So much so that it can influence people of exceptional sympathetic powers and enable them to observe the original events more or less perfectly as if they were enacted before them. Thus in some cases the person will see the occurrence as if taking place before his eyes" (R. Pater, *Mystic Voices*; cf. Mgr. R. H. Benson, *Light Invisible and Other Writings*).

V. Occult powers natural to human beings—some of the powers enumerated in the previous section are inherent in the human organization. They remain latent, or they develop more or less unwittingly as life advances, or they are developed by suitable training. In a few persons they are naturally: so decided as to constitute a special talent which may have been inherited.

The possession of psychic powers (clairvoyance, telepathy, thought-reading etc.) is sometimes looked on as evidence of special favor, or "spirituality," or of superiority, being a "very advanced soul" to be emulated. Such powers are taken as evidence of sainthood in Islam and among Buddhists. In the case of Christian saints, such phenomena are regarded as incidental, and not a criterion of sanctity. Not only is there no relation between the presence or absence of such powers and the virtue of the individual, they are attainable apart therefrom.

VI. The basis in the human constitution upon which such powers depend is fivefold:

(1) The vital faculty	Vegetative Life
(2) Instinct	Sensitive Faculty
(3) The emotional makeup (J. P. Bruce, Chu Hsi, *Philosophy of Human Nature*) (The scholastic concupiscible and irascible phenomena)	Sensitive Faculty
(4) The imagination	Sensitive Life
(5) The reasoning powers: deductive logic	Rational Life

The following powers are specially pertinent to medicine: (1) ability to read character. Fundamentally, this is the instinctive discernment of friend from foe. It exists from infancy, and is to be observed among domestic animals. With the development of reason, the consciousness becomes more and more aware of the attractions and repulsions produced by another individual, whether actually present or only thought of. As life proceeds the contact with relations, friends, acquaintances, and strangers, leads to better knowledge of character, though perhaps nothing more than a form of "worldly wisdom." The reasoning power may be deliberately brought to bear, since delineation of character is amenable to rule, and can be studied, and taught to others (the Chinese sought to establish a relation between character and physique as long ago as 450 B.C. (See L. Wieger, *History of Religious Beliefs*).

As in business, so in medicine it is a subject worthy of attention. Indeed it is always imprudent to neglect it.

(2) Telepathy: thought-reading—these depend on the first three of the above-named powers, and not on reason. They cannot be learned from books, and the experience cannot be taught to others. The most striking examples of genuine powers of this kind are furnished between (a) parent and offspring, when there is intense mother love; (b) persons between whom there is special friendship; (c) husband and wife, when there have been years of unbroken mutual understanding.

Since they are powers inherent in human nature, they may be developed gradually by concentration—and will power, exerted—not over others, but over oneself. (Cf. P'u Sung-Ling, *Seltsame Geschichten*).

(iii) Healing power: (a) involuntary—success or failure in the handling of many cases in ordinary practice is usually ascribed to the concrete methods employed or the appliances used. Yet it is often thought that the personality; of the doctor (whether he be specialist or not) has at any rate something to do with the efficacy of the treatment.

The following factors contribute: inspiring confidence, the bodily state being influenced through the emotions; possession of great vitality, which favorably influences a debilitated state through the vegetative powers, even apart from actual personal contact; will-power even if used unconsciously has a bracing effect on the patient; psychic power, even when the owner is unaware of it, may directly influence endocrine and harmonic activities beneficially, and the vegetative life in general. A disharmonious person will actually drain vitality from a weak person. The mother's touch takes away the bodily pain of her little boy.

(b) Voluntary—among the laity there is sometimes a deliberate attempt made to develop so-called specific psychic healing powers, through healing circles, and the like (theosophy, Christian science, etc).

The fact that such practice is at the expense of exact anatomical and physiological knowledge and is exalted above medical training, cannot but arouse condemnation. Medicine itself is not a little responsible for the rising up of "healers," in its lack of appreciation of the insistent reality to many patients of the sufferings which it cannot explain or find a physical basis for. On the other hand, if the psychics possessed genuine powers, they would not lose them by going through the proper doors of the medical curriculum, and their patients would be the gainers.

Miraculous healing—by this term is meant supernatural intervention apart from human instrumentality. Of this it might be said that medicine would not suffer by candidly acknowledging its occurrence through her leading voices. Not to do so exposes her to disrepute in the minds of those who have experienced the cures, or have personally met with such cases. Though ignorance in various forms (prejudice, intolerance, party spirit) is inevitably in her ranks, it should not be chargeable to medicine.

"The sectarian thinks that he has the sea ladled into his private pond" (Tagore, *Fireflies*, p. 209).

LISTS OF TERMS APPLICABLE TO MENTAL FACULTIES AND AFFECTIONS

Individuals may be described in terms of a series of "notes" (physique, the emotional make-up, the temperament, or disposition, the character, and the talents or intellectual capacities. These together make up the "individuality)."

The following lists under each "note" do not attempt completeness, and some of the descriptive words might be placed equally under other headings than those given.

I. PHYSIQUE: (i) general, robust, spare, wiry; strong or delicate ("constitution") good or deficient. (ii) Special—classified according to the nine systems of Maude Abbot's *Descriptive Catalog of the Medical Museum of McGill University*, Part IV, Sec. 1 or classification not according to such types as these (M. O. Stanton, *An Encyclopedia of Face and Form Reading*)—vegetative, thoracic, glandular, muscular, osseous, nervous, etc. Basis: features of the face; size and shape of head, hands, fingers, feet, etc. Throughout, it is necessary also to specify the qualities of strength and weakness in their degrees: 1 slight or minimal; 2 moderate; 3 normal, average, mean, or "equable"; 4 well-marked; 5 very well-marked or excessive.

II. EMOTIONAL MAKE-UP—classification according to the five headings of the table in Lec ture 8, endnote 11. Basis: the character and phase of the breath; the degree of vitality; the dominant imponderable element; the dominant humor. To draw up a formula to represent the emotional make-up conveniently for clinical work, the initial letters of the (Latin) names of the emotions may be used, the dominant emotion being expressed by a capital letter. Degrees of intensity are indicated by index figures drawn up as in the preceding paragraph. For example, a "*timor*" person might be represented by the formula g^2 1^2 tr^1 i^1 T^5: an "*ira*"—person might be represented by g^1 l^3 tr^1 I^5 t^1.

List of Words Descriptive of the Several Emotions: these are arranged alphabetically, and not according to order of severity. In some cases the words apply also to mental states or attributes sometimes associated with the given emotional-type.

Joy: blissful, buoyant, ecstatic, enraptured, enthusiastic, entranced, exalted, excited, gleeful.

Delight: affectionate, amorose, cheerful, contented, eager, excited, gay, inquisitive, lively, love of (a) objects (collecting spirit), (b); wealth in various forms; (c) opposite sex; pleasure; sentimentality; sympathetic. (Some of these convey ideas associated with this emotion).

Sorrow: afflicted, anguished, anxious, bitter, broken-hearted, chagrined, cheerless, dejected, depressed, despondent, discontented, displeased, disquieted, distressed, fretting, gloomy, having heartache, infelicitous, languishing, low-spirited, miserable, mournful, sense of (a) desolation, (b) disgust, (c) dryness or aridity, (d) repugnance, (e) uselessness, solicitude, sorrow, stricken, tepidity tribulation, troubled, unhappy, unquiet, weak, wretched.

Anger: acrimonious, aggressive, ambitious, bellicose, bitter, boiling, bold, bristling, cantankerous, capricious, captious, caustic, choleric, churlish, contentious, contrary, cross, cynical, daring, desperate, displeased, easily offended, exasperated, exceptions, excitable, fierce, fiery, fractious, fuming, furious, hasty, having hatred, impetuous, indignant, infuriate, irate, irritable, irritated, jealous, passionate, peevish, petted, petulant, pugnacious, quarrelsome, querulous, rabid, raging, relentless, resentful, severe, shrewish, sore, storming, sulky, sullen, suspicious, tart, testy, vengeful, vexed, vindictive, violent, virulent, wrathful.

Fear: afraid, aghast, alarmed, anxious, apprehensive, astounded, browbeaten, cowardly, cowed, coy, craven, daunted, despairing, despondent, diffident, discouraged, dismayed, disquieted, dreading, envious, faint-hearted, faltering, fearful, fidgety, flinching, flurried, frightened, fussy, gentle, harassed, hesitating, horrified, horror-struck, irresolute, irritable, jealous, mistrusting, nervous, panic stricken, penitent, perturbed, pious, pusillanimous, quailing, quaking, quavering, repentant, restless, scared, scrupulous, shrinking, shuddering, shy, skulking, sly, solicitous, startled, suspicious, temperate, terrified, terror-struck, timid, timorous, trembling, trepidation, unmannered, weak-hearted, whining, worrying.

Moods. Moodiness. Disposition. "Moods are the waves rising in your heart." They are due to the changes in the breath from hour to hour or day to day. The rate of change varies in different persons. When the change is comparatively frequent, the person may be described as "moody," changeable. This character may occur more at some periods of life than others, in the same person, Thus, it is more frequent at puberty and during youth. It is possible to rise above the cycle of moods by the exercise of self-restraint. Moods change with surroundings (places and people).

III. Temperamental type or disposition—basis: the humoral formula. This is expressed outwardly in differences of: (a) texture—varying solidity of the tissues of the body; (b) development of the various parts of the body; (c) rate of activity of (i) vegetative processes—nutrition, waste, formation of germinal cells, etc., (ii) expenditure of nervous energy; (d) tonicity of muscles and nerves.

The words descriptive of temperament often apply also to II. Examples: aggressive, amiable, austere, buoyant, capricious, cheerful, chilling, churlish, complacent, conservative, courageous, depressed, despondent, discontented, energetic, enthusiastic, excitable, fastidious, forbearing, fretful, forward, gushing, harassed, impetuous, indolent, intolerant, irascible, irritable, jealous, malicious, moody, obstinate, petulant, querulous, rebellious, reckless, remorseful, ruffled, secretive, spiteful, stubborn submissive, suspicious, taciturn, tranquil, tyrannical, uncompromising, unforgiving, verbose, vindictive, zealous.

Many of these terms also apply to the description of II and IV.

It is worth noting that among these types there are many which are supposed to be evidence of high human aspirations, and yet strictly belong to the "lower mind." Hence it has been very truly said: "Those sweet affections which incline the heart to God . . . come from the sensitive temperament, or bodily disposition, rather than from the solid piety of reason, and are carnal rather than spiritual" (F. X. Lasance, *Thoughts on the Religious Life*). Things that are apparently of the highest order in knowledge, art and sentiment are not things of the spirit, but things of the senses alike in the philosophy of Thomas Aquinas and in the modern researches in the domain of the brain." (Dom Anscar Vonier, *Life of the World to Come*).

IV. CHARACTER—this is really a collective term, since all the other "notes" contribute to it. The terms which describe character may be grouped under sensuous, intellectual, moral, and esthetic groups, or under the five sub-divisions of mind in Sufi terminology (ego, memory, mind, heart, conscience). Many terms have more than one component, and therefore do not belong strictly to one group alone.

Ego: Positive: acquisitive, amative, approbative, artful, artless, avaricious, arrogant, boastful, churlish, domineering, gluttonous, grasping, grouching, inquisitive, jealous, lewd, licentious, loud, obdurate, obstinate, pugnacious, quarrelsome, sociable, superstitious, vain, voluptuous, worldly. Negative: Abstemious, apathetic, hasty, indolent, indulgent, miserly, shy, timid, unselfish, weak.

Heart: Positive: accessible, adaptable, affable, altruistic, ardent, benevolent, contemplative, emotional, charming, compassionate, facetious, fascinating, frivolous, gay, harmonious, hospitable, lively, peaceable, philanthropic, sincere, simple, tranquil. Negative: tepid, meek, lenient.

Conscience: Positive: acetic, austere, blameless, brave, conscientious, conservative, courageous, diligent, exacting, fastidious, humble, industrious, persevering, scrupulous, sensitive, strong-willed, thorough, truthful, well-balanced. Negative: deceitful, defiant, flippant, impetuous, impulsive, imprudent, malicious, pusillanimous, resentful, slow, treacherous, unforgiving, ungrateful, unsociable, untruthful, vindictive (the moral sense may be absent).

Mind. Agnostic, ambitious, brusque, censorious, cunning, enterprising, foreseeing, intellectual, loquacious, methodical opinionated, orderly, plausible, practical, prejudiced, refined, reticent, satirical, skeptic, serious, stilted, subtle, superstitious, uncompromising.

It should be noted that character is (1) native and unalterable (whatever some educationists say); (2) capable of being fashioned by the will of the person himself or by that of the persons amongst whom he lives. To have a "strong character" is considered the highest ideal by many; (2) is therefore much advocated. But this idea is not necessarily true. Animals have character in that different kinds of ego are as it were personified in them (cf. F. Hartmann, *The Life of Paracelsus*, p. 209).

Character is necessarily intimately related to physique, emotional type and temperamental type. Hence character delineation is possible from a close study of those aspects.

The skeletal system (bones, joints, ligaments, muscles, etc.) is the expression of the character of the cerebral nervous system. The viscera are the expression of the character of the vegetative system. Hence it happens that the usual autopsy discusses the least important part of the case (see Lecture 4, endnote 8).

Interests—personal interests: the preservation of one's life and health and general welfare; interests of the family; of the social circle, etc. Interests manifested in the use of the various talents.

V. Talents—these are best classified according to the subject-matter to which the mind is directed though they may be classified according to the faculty concerned.

Mechanical—constructiveness; architecture, etc.; technology.

Scientific—all branches of learning; mathematics, sciences, logic, analytical talents; calculating powers. Domestic science. Administration.

Intellectual—all branches of knowledge. Philosophy, history, sciences.

Aesthetic—arts and crafts, music, sculpture, designing, painting, poetry, literary art, dramatic art; wit; women's crafts of all kinds; poise.

Imaginative—originality; inventiveness.

Moral—perseverance, concentrating-power, law.

Other talents—language; intuitive perception; foresight; pedagogy; rhetoric; vocal.

Social—domestic interests; love of children, of home.

Political—military, sport (athletics, acrobatic art, adventuresomeness).

Commercial life—agriculture, animal husbandry.

Much overlapping is necessary present in preparing such a list. It might be extended to include all the subjects taught in universities, and schools of all kinds, for persons of all ages.

Interactions Between the Various Aspects of the Soul

I. Intellect. Acts on vegetative life via emotions. (Effect of emotions on bodily functions: see Lecture 7, endnote 1).

Is acted on by:

(1) Vegetative life: physical desires, sense-impressions, especially in dream states and the like.

(2) Sensitive life: psychical desires, either in oneself or from others. The imagination influences it in hypnosis.

(3) The will: compelling attention or forcibly diverting attention.

(4) Other wills: ditto, includes angelic intelligences as well as human.

II. Reason—acts on vegetative life via the emotions, with their desires and fears.

Is acted on by sensitive life—emotions strongly affect the reason in of certain dispositions.

III. Will—acts on vegetative life-effecting exterior actions.

Acts on sensitive life—through sensuous cognition it acts on the emotions; feeds or starves or fails to starve the sensitive appetite, and so acts in the same three ways on the emotional states, aided by reason.

Acts on the practical understanding—with the aid of bodily mechanism it leads to the performance of useful or artistic work.

Acts on the speculative understanding—produces acts of judgment, or worship or contemplation.

Acts on the intellect—concentration.

Acts on the memory—"recollection," "watchfulness."

Acts on itself—brings perseverance in the performance of a design conceived and elaborated by the intellect.

Actions upon the will.

Intellect—as when this propounds to the will what is the greatest good; conveys sense-impressions to the will.

Emotions—anger is very powerful in nullifying will to good, and increasing will to evil. So also, fear of another person, fear of an idea, fear of a thing. Passions a hinder the judgment, and so affect the will.

Emotions can be sublimated by interaction with Plane V.

Sensitive appetite—a sensitive appetite: this acts directly on the will. If the objects of both appetite and will coincide, the will is strengthened; otherwise it is weakened. The passions modify the organic conditions and this influences all cognitive faculties, and their intensity may prevent the mind from applying itself to the higher operations of the intellect and will

Vegetative life—the corporeal state affects the will.

Environment—circumstances of life, personal atmosphere of neighbors etc; presence of persons of strong will, all interfere with or modify the actions of the (patient's) will.

Diseases of the will—inconstancy, irresolution (lack of energy), impulsiveness (excess of energy; excitability), and "mortal sin." Domain of moral philosophy).

IV. Practical Application—the fact that feelings, imaginations and thoughts influence the character is of the greatest practical importance, but by using the will-power to control them all, one becomes also master of one's life and "fate." Each emotional "note" has its own effect on the body and mind, and can be overruled by the will. The influence of the imagination is implied in the phrases "looking on the bright (or dark) side of things." Cheerful, gloomy, constructive, destructive, upright, deceitful thoughts all affect the sum total of the conduct, the attitude of the mind towards others, and can all be over ruled by the will. "If the endowment is great in one direction, it is at the expense of some corresponding defect in another direction, as when tender hearted men are lacking in judicial faculty, while men in whom the judicial faculty is prominent tend to be tyrannical" (J. P. Bruce, *Chu Hsi: Philosophy of Human Nature*, p. 59).

The study of all such interactions as are suggested by the lists of synonyms above given affords a better idea of what constitutes ideal "balance" in regard to the various components of the human being. A more graphic and tangible idea is at the same time obtainable in this way of much of the subject-matter of ethical and moral philosophy. To assign a distinct place for it in the domain of medicine is not to disown the precedence of religion.

Notes to Part Two

Lecture 9: A Discussion of the Cause of Disease, and Symptoms

1 Costaeus says: "It is to be noted that the term 'cause' does not refer to 'efficient' cause, for disease, not being a definite entity, does not require an efficient cause. In other words, disease is not in-formed matter. This applies equally in modern thought. If the changes of disease are modified biochemical reactions, they cannot be considered in terms of matter and form. But formal causes and substantial causes as well as the differences between qualities and dispositions, tendencies, passive and active states, and fixed morbid conditions, are all better understood under the precise thought of modern scholastic philosophy. A cause may be understood as anything which effects or assists or maintains or imparts a morbid function whether actively or passively—morbid, because this part of *The Canon* is concerned with disease.

Human body—not an animal body. The teaching to be presented does not necessarily apply to veterinary medicine.

Fixity of state—not that some state as are labile and others are stable or fixed. Labile states are more or less easily curable, but fixed states are very difficult to resolve or cure.

State—we must distinguish carefully between cause, disposition, state, habit, symptoms.

2 It may be noted that in this view, the state is primary and the disease secondary. To the modern view, the disease comes first and the state is its result. The state is "the reaction to the causal noxious agent." Such a state is (a) detrimental to the body by an "aggressive" action upon the tissues by the agent or an unfortunate by-effect, producing degenerations of various kinds and degrees—sometimes mechanically (pressure on parts, interference with vascular supply)—sometimes incidentally in the form of late toxic actions of the microbic poisons or beneficial to the body—through indirectly since it is certainly damaged in the process—as tending to destroy the invading organisms or at least neutralizing the poisonous products.

In Avicenna's view, however, both agent and state are equally important. One cannot speak of a "reaction," any more than one would say (for instance) that sodium carbonate is a reaction to hydrocholric acid. Unless both substances are there, there is no reaction. So, without an abnormal state, there is no malady. Note also that "poisoning" ("intoxication") is not a disease.

The following classification of words often used indifferently for "disease," as if they were really synonymous will help to develop a more precise usage.

A. Terms bearing primarily a general sense include the following.

Ill-health: not used specifically; there may or may not be a diagnosable disease.

Illness: the state of being ill; sickness. Vaguely used for anything from slight disability to a fatal condition. More definite in meaning than ill-health.

Malady: (lit. ill condition; male habitus). A synonym for an illness appearing in polite literature for conditions not necessarily organic or for conditions which have not been diagnosed and yet may prove fatal.

Ailment: this may be some definite morbid condition or simply imply discomfort (possibly short of actual pain). Literally is synonymous with a sickness, an illness.

Disorders: in general. This term is used still more specifically as a rule. See under B.

Disease (*morbus. marad*): in general, this word is technical whereas the other words have a more popular application.

B. Terms bearing a special sense whether used in that manner or not.

(i) Disease: any condition in which an organic lesion—some macroscopic change in the body is present.

Sickness implies a more or less serious disturbance and even suggests the risk of death. The lesions present often determine the distinctive name of each separate disease. Where the etiology is still unknown, the disease may be provisionally named sickness.

(ii) Conditions in which there is not necessarily any organic lesion or where such a lesion has not been detected. These conditions do not receive distinctive names; are not necessarily serious; are probably not fatal. The name of each condition originally bore a distinct meaning.

(a) Arising out of the temperament: distemper (in the scholastic sense).

(b) Arising out of the disposition or state: now means simply not fit or vaguely ill-health: indisposition.

(c) Implies involvement of bodily functions: may be sub-classified according to the system involved or vaguely means simply something is out of order: disorder.

(d) Implies involvement of the nerves or nervous system (i.e. almost equivalent to functional as opposed to organic): implies a certain amount of pain: affection.

(e) A condition in which pain is the chief feature whether general or in some special region, but the pain is presumably not very severe: subclassification according to the region or organ: complaint.

3 A lengthy discussion about what is to be regarded as a symptom is given by Costaeus. He shows that the word "symptom" was derived from the Greek to indicate something which occurs simultaneously with the disease producing it. He also discusses the exact meanings of the terms: weakness, impaired function, loss of function, abolition of function, affections, preternatural excretions and retentions. The question is also raised as to whether a given symptom is directly due to the disease or is indirect or is collateral or is in no real relation to the disease.

Avicenna's brief statement really covers all these points. As regards our modern ways of thinking, one gathers together all the phenomena which are ever found to occur in a case of a given disease and we simply arrange them as far as possible into the immediate effects, the remote effects, and those phenomena whose nature is not absolutely certain—they may be caused by the disease; they may be sequels; or they may be concurrent because some other morbid condition is, or happens to be, simultaneously present.

Example of a Cause	Example of its Corresponding Malady	Example of the Corresponding Symptom
Decay; putrescence	Fever	Thirst, headache
Fullness of lacrymal sacs from developmental error	Obstruction of uvea	Loss of Vision
Acrid flux	Ulcer in lung	Flushed cheeks; curved nails

4 It is asked: are symptoms to disease as shadow is to object? The answer is that the two are associated but are not inseparable. In other words, the symptom in a scholastic symbolism and not matter-form. The term "symptom" refers to many phenomena, some of which are really the direct consequence of the disease, while others are only indirectly its result. This question would never arise were it not for the custom of supposing "diseases" are entities of some kind.

5 Costaeus says: "To the patient, "colic" is "pain." The distension is the

cause of the pain. The pain interferes with or even arrests the vitality of the part, and in that sense produces the syncope. Pain is: the contact of disordered disorganized function upon the consciousness. It is a form of "touch." The consciousness "touches" the impaired function. "Paralysis" is "loss of the drives of movement and sensation." "Convulsions" = "depravity" of the drives of movement and sensation. There is, therefore, a certain literal truth in the general statement.

6 Costaeus adds: "Pain interferes with the 'breath' and may even arrest it. In consequence, a 'refrigeration of the heart' takes place. That is, the temperament of the heart becomes below normal in regard to 'cold.' But this is a disease. This change of temperament accounts for the syncope. Descent of matter (inflamm. exudate) as a cause of pain. The acridity and similar qualities of the exudate do actually irritate the nerve endings and therefore produce pain in addition to that due to tension."

7 Costaeus adds: "Pain such as headache may simply be a symptom, that is, evidence of an 'intemperamental state,' or 'solution of continuity.' But to the patient it is the thing; it is the malady. Little does it concern the patient that there is an underlying cause to be treated if the practitioner proves unable to relieve his pain. Further, persistent pain impairs vitality. In this sense a pain is a disease.

Symptoms are still confused with diseases in our textbooks. Thus "jaundice" appears amongst the diseases instead of being placed separately along with a number of other characteristic symptoms, like asascites, which is not taken as a specific disease even by the lay. Originally, symptoms were explained in terms of changes of quality and the like. This theoretical explanation was abandoned owing to a degradation of metaphysical knowledge. The symptoms then became diseases. The diseases were then investigated and found to be more numerous than the symptoms (which was already understood).

8 Errors of Development

Group	Subvarieties	Examples
1. Errors in form. Here the form is changed from its natural grace to an extent which impairs its utility.	Deviation from a natural straightness.	Head broad and round with ossified sutures to an extent hindering mental power.
	Straightness of a naturally curved line.	Curved shinbones; *genu valgum*; clubfoot.
	Squareness where there should be roundness.	Pupils congenitally elongate or slit-like or small.
	Rotundity where there should be squareness.	
2. Errors in passages.	Too wide.	Wide pupils; varices; aneurysms; the dilated blood-vessels in pannus.
	Too narrow.	Small pupils; narrowed eyes; stricture of trachea or bronchi; stricture of oesophagus.
	Occlusion.	Of venous orifices, i.e. in liver.

3. Errors in cavities or sacs.	Too large (distended).	Scrotum.
	Too small (contracted).	Contracted stomach; contracted cerebral ventricles in epilepsy.
	Emptied.	Cardiac cavities emptied of blood by reason of excessive joy or extreme pain.
4. Errors of surfaces.	The normal roughness replaced by smoothness.	At the orifice of the stomach; also in lienteric diarrhea.
	The normal smoothness becomes rough.	Trachea; fauces (hoarseness).

9 Decline: the term refers to a condition in which the body seems to wither or fade away without obvious reason or in spite of taking food. The term refers primarily to the causeless losing of flesh by horses, whereby they come to be in an ill-conditioned state. The same word would apply to the wilting of cut flowers or the whithering of plants from lack of water or from reduction of their vitality to such a point that they will not imbibe water any more; that is, they cannot be re-vived. Such a condition in man is noted by the laity but is only referred to in medicine when its pathological basis is visualized; as for instance in wasting from *tabes mesenterica* or *tabes dorsalis*.

10 Swelling = *waram* = apostema = tumor (used in a general sense); any "lump" or excrescence or protuberance. Intumescence, tumefaction, new-growth, nodositics—these are special kinds of swelling. In most passages an inflammatory swelling or mass is meant; waram or apostema is translated accordingly. It may be noted that an apostema is more likely to be colored and to feel warm to the touch whereas a swelling which can be called a tumefaction is colorless and does not feel warm; that is, it is a cold swelling.

11 Cancer appears in *The Canon* as a disease associated with change in the atrabilious humor. Therefore one condition for the production of this disease is the entry of it into the metabolic cycle in a pathological manner.

12 Puffiness. This stands for *tahabbuj* (swelling) or *tahayyuj*; cachexia, excitement, agitation = tumefaction. The Latin glossary explains that it is meant specially as that which results from liver disorder; when it appears in the limbs it has a different origin. The puffiness of the eyes from lack of sleep or from too much sleep is also different.

13 Therefore some cases of induration may have been what is now called scirrhus.

14 "Excessive corpulence and excessive leanness are especially worthy of condemnation" (*Chakara-Samhita* translated by K. A. C. Kaviratna).

15 Latent disease belongs here; occult as compared with the other three stages which are declared, visibilia.

16 This classification of the types of disease still holds good today. The nomenclature is rather different because it is now made more definitely in accord with pathological findings.

Some confusion as to the scope of the various terms still exists even in the minds of those who are no longer students. Clinical and pathological conceptions do not agree in scope. On the one hand, there is an underlying endeavor to specify diseases and to separate out new entities in accordance with variations in the clinical manifestations. In pathology, the distinction between general and special is more clearly adhered to and the latter is described as much as possible according to the former which is proper.

In regard to an actual case before us, however, the pathology cannot be elucidated at once; the clinical manifestations therefore receive the chief consideration. But such manifestations are limited in range, are of general character (universal, not particular), and should rank with *genera* in natural history; the pathological character or process would furnish the specific name. Clinically, diseases naturally comprise swellings, deformities, discolorations, displacements, ulcerations, various solutions of continuity, aches and pains, and the like. Pathologically there are only four main groups of lesions—inflammations, new-growths, nutritional changes (degenerations and hypertrophies), and errors of development. (The short list presented by Avicenna is not a real fault when considered from such a point of view). If such a system cannot be allowed either by academic medicine or the laity (who insist on a name for a disease) it has at least the advantage of enabling one to visualize from the first what is important to the patient and to concentrate on it.

The opposite procedure—that which rules the day—is that of describing diseases in all their forms and types, typhoid fever being awarded the crown. The literature is always receiving reports on new types of disease. This method has the advantage of being capable of unlimited extension for the number of types is (as should be obvious) exactly the same as the number of individuals affected thereby. In other words, all these types are simply the expressions of the individual's make-up and have nothing whatever to do with the infective organism except in so far as it varies in virulence (i.e., in the composition of its excreta).

The idea that treatment cannot be correct unless the disease is correctly named is also very widely spread and has the same effect—that of blinding the mind to the real simplicity of truth. The unknowing abhors simplicity; he ever seeks to improve—that is, to introduce more and more complexity.

Notes to Lecture 10: Causes of Illness (Etiology)

1 Correlation, adverse or absent or excessive, between time, mental faculties, and objects of the senses, constitute in brief the threefold causes of disease affecting either the body or mind. (*Chakara-Samhita*, i. 5). If the activity of the life-principle takes place in a harmonious and regular manner, unimpeded by any obstacles, such a state is called 'health.' If its activity is impeded by some cause and if it acts abnormally or irregularly, such a state is called disease (F. Hartmann, *The Life of Paracelsus*, p. 181).

2 Other examples: privation of food, shelter, covering; environment (monotony, solitude, restraint, neglect, subjection and their opposites). These are predisposing causes.

3 The above groupings of causes are the expression of a mode of thought now foreign to us. We seek more practical statements and rightly. But when he things of causes, Avicenna goes back to fundamentals. This patient is before him and the illness owes its origin to external factors which the patient cannot escape—the atmosphere, the weather, the climate, the drinking-water, the soil over which he lives and works; or to factors operating within the body, producing aberrations in the physiological processes.

The external factors naturally fall under the categories of the four elements (five, if we include ether represented by sunlight), and the memory is securely aided by thinking of each in turn. The internal factors are classified according to the qualities—heat, cold, moisture, dryness. These also serve as aids to memory since many aberrations in physiological processes amount to disturbances in these several qualities in the different parts of the body.

Changes of vitality as causes of disease are not here specified because they are secondary to the other causes. It is true that disease is evidence of loss of vitality, of loss of radiance of the breath, but this is the effect of antecedent causes—repletion with humors; depletion of humors; and these again can be traced back to interactions of qualities and changes in the proportions of the elements.

The following table is added for clarity:

Name of Cause	Nature	Relation to bodily state	Examples
1. Primitive	Non-corporeal	May be direct or may only be through an intermediate state.	Solar heat Violent exercise Heating articles of food (i.e., garlic) Sadness Wakefulness. Blows. Cataract. Fever.
2. Antecedent	(1) Corporeal (i.e. humor)	Is indirect via an intermediate state	Suffusion of the orbits. Lachrymation.
	(2) Temperamental (3) Compositional		Repletion with fever.
3. Conjoined	Corporeal	Direct; immediate	Blockage of an aperture by a humor. Blindness from obstruction of the optic nerve. Sepsis with fever.

4 An essential cause is one which alters the nature. That is, that on which the primary qualities of the body (heat, cold, moisture, dryness) depend.

5 The time factor: the time occupied before a given agent can produce its effect varies with different individuals just as some persons have a long digestive time-factor and others a short one. This was spoken of very long ago (*Chakara-Samhita*, ii, 793), the lesson being, in the case of digestion, that the

number of meals per day should depend on the time-factor and not on popular custom.

6 It appears that the idea of gaseous interchange within the lung was not grasped. What we know as residual air comes to be what Avicenna speaks of as breath (*ruh*). Hence the description in the text is right in idea but lacking in exactitude.

7 This chapter is taken by Andreas de Alpago Bellunensis as the proof that Avicenna was a native of Persia.

8 The fancy or jest that summer-heat and winter-cold are the result of the greatness of the boiling of hell (i.e. the interior of the earth) makes a breathing twice a year, expiring in summer and inspiring in winter (*1001 Nights*, Burton, 487).

9 The changes which the seasons produce on the human body are ascribed in this chapter at least in part to the changes which the seasons produce in the ground itself. We are introduced to the idea of ground-air, ground-water, ground-fire (that is, ground temperature). That which *The Canon* here hints at is found to be entirely accurate in the light of modern investigations.

Movement of ground-air—in the interstices of the soil there is an abundance of "vapor" which moves in and out of the earth into the atmosphere, as the ground-water moves up and down. We may rightly picture the earth as a huge lung. It exhales ground-air into the air we breathe and if the former is humid, owing to a high ground-water level, the exhaled air will be "damp"; if the temperature of the earth be low, the exhaled air will be cold. If the ground-air be polluted the air we breathe will become fouled. The conception of the earth as a lung is given in almost those very words by Avicenna (§670).

Movement of groundwater—the groundwater may move merely up and down, or it may travel horizontally great distances. Its height varies with the rains, the season, the nature of the rock beneath, the character of the subsoil, and the presence of vegetation (crops, undergrowth, woodland, forestland). The movement up and down may be compared with tidal movements. The "waters upon the earth" move, as do the seas. Clearly, then, floods and droughts, swamp land and gravelly land, all have wide effects. The interference with vegetation also alters natural conditions, whether beneficially or detrimentally to human welfare. Lane-Notter (*Encyclopedia Britannica*, 25, p. 348) states that it has been estimated that an acre of cabbages will absorb and transpire from their leaves more than ten tons of water per day when the weather is fine from the land. The destruction of trees arrests the upward movement of ground-water which previously was carried high up into the air as if by so many chimneys and so affects other places at considerable distances.

Practical bearing of these facts—innumerable living things pass the whole or part of their lives in the groundwater. They are carried along with it both to the surface and horizontally underground, possibly to great distances.

The following groups may be specified: (1) Bacteria: these are derived from: (a) the earth's surface from refuse in the neighborhood of habitations, from excreta, trade-effluents, slaughter-houses; (b) deeper strata: cesspools, which do not necessarily filter off the organisms; (2) protozoa; (3) moulds and spore-bearing organisms generally; and (4) invertebrates of many orders.

These all flourish according to the presence of putrefactive matters in the soil (vegetable or animal), according to the ground-temperature, and according to degrees of anerobic state (which has to do with cycles of development).

"The earth is a great stomach in which everything is dissolved, digested and transformed and each being draws its nutriment from the earth; and each living being is a stomach that serves as a tomb for other forms and from which new forms spring into existence" (F. Hartmann, *The Life of Paracelsus*, "Paramirum," p. 205).

Organisms gain access to the human body: (a) directly from the surface soil, from the drinking water, from insufficiently cleansed vegetable foods, in partly decayed vegetables or vegetables which have become stale in the markets, from the inhalation of infected dust (especially the dust of earth pulverized by being parched in times of drought); (b) indirectly, by contamination of food by insects whose larvae infest the soil to an extraordinary extent; and by use of vegetables infected by invertebrates which themselves harbor pathogenic organisms.

Diseases associated with ground-water—damp soil favors putrefaction with ultimate pollution of the air. Phthisis is favored in such localities. When the soil is actually wet, from the rising of the ground-water, typhoid epidemics have been noted. Fleas or rats which burrow into soil polluted by plague-infected ground-water become infected themselves.

Diseases associated with variations of earth temperature–cold soil favors bronchitis and other chest complaints. Warm soil favors the multiplication of certain organisms—those which flourish best at certain temperatures and anerobically. (Favored by admixture of the soil with manure).

The subject is therefore plainly of importance both in regard to the study of pandemics, epidemics and endemic diseases and in regard to the daily condition of the individual patient, the progress of his disease, and even the exact form which a disease takes in his case. As Avicenna says, the practitioner would benefit by noting the successions of weather-changes, the type of the season and the seasonal cycles, especially interpreted in terms of movements of the water, air, and fire in the earth.

10 Harmonious, as in conformity with the laws of nature–in this case the season is considered as the variable and the human temperament, the constant. But it may be noted that the whole of our life is a matter of conformity with the laws of nature from highest to lowest. If the government conforms in all respects, thus exhibiting the great conformity—requiring master minds and master wills—and if each individual, in turn, conforms, the society would

become the ideal state. The application in regard to the incidence of disease in the individual being is very wide and this section of *The Canon* becomes suggestive to a most interesting extent when the classic just quoted is considered in association with it.

11 Taking human nature as the variable and laws of nature as the constant.

12 See also the chapter of the Pulse where the effect of the seasons on the pulse is discussed.

13 One may also add: germ-laden dust or particles of saliva and exhaled particles of moisture charged with possibly pathogenic microbes. Note that exhaled air contains 0.5 percent of organic impurities which are much more a source of disease than the carbon dioxide gas produced by respiration.

14 The effects of the different climates (hot, cold, damp, dry) on the body and the diseases associated with each are given by various traditional writers but the statements are often at variance with one another. It is sufficient to consider the possibility that, apart from infective agents, the temperature and humidity of a region affects the nutrition of the body, the vigor of the body, and is accompanied by liability of certain organs to disease (gastric, pulmonary, cerebral, cardiac).

The humidity of the air has been studied in modern times in its relation to liability to induce disease. The average normal relative humidity is 75%; excess of moisture makes the air feel chilly. Mists are detrimental because they absorb the warming rays of the sun.

Stagnant air produces stuffiness in rooms. This is due to the air heated by the skin remaining close to the skin and preventing the latter from cooling. The surface circulation fails to receive its proper stimulus in consequence (*Harmsword Home Docto*r, p. 120).

The following passage in the Su-wen is of interest: "Huang Ti asked in what manner cold and heat, dryness and moisture, wind and fire operated on the human being and how they produced the transformation of all things. Chi Po replied, 'The five fluids come forward in turn, and each of them takes precedence once. When they do not keep in their proper spheres, there is disaster; when they do, everything is well ordered'" (A. Forke, *The World-conception of the Chinese*, pp. 250-252).

15 In summer the ground temperature is highest (up to 63 degrees F. at the end of August or in September in northern latitudes).

16 That the frequency of disease in hot weather is to be partly ascribed to the multiplication of flies under the favoring influence of the ground heat and warm air was, of course, not known in Avicenna's time. On the other hand, the cause of souring of milk in hot weather is still not understood and the incidence of some febrile conditions is parallel.

17 Cf. the corresponding disease in spring, in this case due to serous humor. The reason of the difference of humor in the two forms lies in the fact

that the season preceding in each case favored the prevalence of that humor and it is this that constitutes the "soil" upon which the anginal infection thrives.

18 There are charts available which show the seasonal variations in the character of the blood (red cell content; hemoglobin) as made out by modern investigations.

19 Abnormal quality of the seasons—this idea is developed in an interesting manner in the Chinese classic *Li Ki* (translated by S. Couvreur) as showing the consequences in terms of weather (storms, floods, droughts, hurricanes, etc.), and in regard to the prospects in the crops (maturing too soon, maturing too late to yield any produce, diseases of crops, or infections by various larvae or insects), as well as the possibility of pestilential outbreaks, or the prevalence of such diseases as bronchitis, rheumatism, skin diseases, general ill-health (debility); flourishing of certain objectionable weeds among the grain or cereals.

Seasonal cycles have to do with the sequences of development noted among the very low forms of life in nature, i.e., the growth of various orders of fungus (saprophytic, parasitic, non-pathogenic, sub-pathogenic, and pathogenic) in various types of soil or landscape, depends on the existence of cold, cold and wet, warmth, warmth and wet, warmth and dryness, as they are traced through their various cycles (basidium, with basiodiospores, mycelium with gametes, and acidiospores, uredospores and teleutospores). The cyclical changes which result in the apparent transformation of one "specific" micro-organism into another "specific" schizomycete require investigation in the open field of nature. Bacteriology may be said to have been imprisoned in the doctrine of immutability of species, which is only upheld within the limitations of artificial culture-media and inoculation experiments in warm-blooded animals. Many of the types so familiar in human bacteriology may be looked on as terminal phases of cycles, capable of being maintained at the same rank for almost indefinite periods. The remaining nine-tenths of the cycle are unknown, from inability to cause the types to re-enter it artificially.

20 Solar, planetary and stellar influences on man and their relation to disease. The subject may be summarized as follows: (1) genuine influence: (a) solar—the observation of sun-spots shows that there is a relation to the character of the weather in certain regions, a relation to the development of earthquakes and also a relation to mental states. H. W. Newton (*Quarterly Journal Royal Meteorological Society*) traces an eleven-year cycle of change both in the earth's magnetic changes and in the sun-spot cycle. The sun-spots are described as tornadoes of white hot gas and affect both ultra-violet ray activity and electric radiations. He also suggests that there may be another cause concerned which controls both solar storms and terrestrial magnetic storms.

The relation may be made more tangible by suggesting that after all there are actual flames of fire emerging from the sun and extending in a tenuous and yet real form right across space into our own atmosphere with inevitable effects both in inorganic and organized worlds. Hence to suggest a relation between sickness, suicide, and crime and solar storms or even planetary disturbances is not new and cannot be lightly set aside.

(b) Solar and lunar—everyday experience shows that the atmospheric conditions vary according to the time of day and night. The bearing of this on health has therefore been seen from the earliest times (*Ayurvedic*, 1924, August, p. 53).

(c) Planetary rise and setting, lunar phases, positions of stars and constellations are all data for the study of the progress of the seasons. Hence two kinds of cycles come to notice: the cycle of climactic changes with an apparent relation to health and disease both in cattle and human beings and the cycle of extraterrestrial changes. Naturally the observers of ancient times who were so convinced of the unity of the visible universe sought to reduce to rule certain coincidences in these cycles. Even if their association is irregular or only discernible from generation to generation the subject would invite study. Even nowadays it is unsafe to decide that there is nothing at all to study in it.

Fictitious relations: (a) symbolical, permissible, but superfluous. (i) Stars may be spoken of as healthy or unhealthy, propitious or unpropitious (*Costaeus Annotations to Avicenna*), as a convenient abbreviation for a more or less complex group of concomitant climactic conditions. (ii) The names of planets or constellations may be used to represent combativeness (fiery temper), ambition and pride, love and desire, melancholy, dreaminess, intelligence and wisdom. These are seven types assigned to the as many planets. Again, the term astral may be claimed appropriate because they are common to the stars and the astral form of man. The same idea occurs in Paracelsus (F. Hartmann, *The Life of Paracelsus*, "Hermetic writings," ii, p. 291), where he speaks of the senses and intelligence and wisdom of the offspring being its "sidereal body," and derived "from the stars." Such usage of names implies that there is some specially "deep" learning being propounded which is denied to the ordinary student, who has not been initiated into the inner circle of some group—hermetic, rosicrucian, theosophical, and the like. The fact is, however, that the phenomena of the so-called "astral plane" are those of the "sensitive life" of scholastic psychology; careful and thorough study of this will show that the other obscurities are superfluous. (b) Fallacious. Those who take the symbology of (ii) to be literally correct are "*of the erring people*" (Quran 6:78).

But in these days it is easier to fall into the error of supposing that there is no relation whatsoever between this world and sun, moon, and stars than to mistake purely terrestrial relations for the transcendent.

21 This statement contains an important truth. Certain spas and health resorts (Carlsbad, Bath, Droitwich, Baden, Bourbonne-les Bains, Nancy, Wiesbaden) owe their virtue not merely to the chemical composition of the

water which is taken by the patients, but also to the locality itself. The radiations which pass outward at those parts of the earth produce a beneficent influence upon them as they walk over the ground.

The inorganic elements in plants are really very finely powdered stones (limestone, iron-stone, magnesium stone, potash stone, etc.) which have entered a condition of food substance under the influence of light, heat and life.

22 Though we now know that "pestilential" air is so because it is germ-laden, the general principle remains the same. At the present day it is assumed that the air is always contaminated from without—from the dust, i.e. on the ground that sunlight destroys germ-life. However, facts speak otherwise in open nature.

In regard to climate and modern day considerations like: the earth heat, the radiant energy of the sun, the cooling power of the air, altitude, ventilation of the dwelling should be added: prevalent winds, proximity to the sea, scenery, nature of the ground—whether rocky (cold and dry), fertile (hot and moist), muddy (cold and moist); whether porous or impermeable; water-holding or not; actual chemical composition.

23 This carries the reader back to §25 sqq. and the comments there. The writings of the Chinese philosophers on the one hand and of European alchemists on the other may be interpreted accordingly as Avicenna would have done. Examples of earth: soil, metals, naked creatures, water, spring water, rain water, ditch-water, lake water, the sea, millet, shellfish, fire, wood, oil, stones, lightning, the glow-worm, will o the wisp trees, flowers, beans, feathered creatures. Seemingly there is very little in common. Forke (*The World-conception of the Chinese*, pp. 275-276) refers to the subject at the same time referring to writings by Agrippa von Nettesheim.

24 A dry climate with warm soil where the sun power is good and the cooling power is moderate (that is, places with pine forests and sheltered valleys) is beneficial for chest cases. Dry uplands in places where there are not periods of unsettled weather and not near the sea are beneficial for rheumatic cases.

Choice of food according to climate. For hot climates: no meat, use vegetable oils instead of animal fats. For cold climates: meat, animal fats. For dry climates: fruits are needed. For wet climates: sugar is needed (*Harmsworth Home Doctor*, p. 1076).

Note that the weather affects animals as well as humans. Cold, hot, damp, dry weather, thunderstorms, affect domestic animals (W. Lauder Lindsay, *Mind in the Lower Animals*, ii. 307).

25 High altitude are beneficial for nerve cases but unfavorable for heart cases.

26 Maritime places are beneficial for nerve cases.

27 Type of house. The importance of this is well-known but not as often

practically attended to. Overcrowding of houses is well-known to be a source of continual illness and loss of working capacity, yet is only very slowly being remedied. It is not sufficiently realized that the befouling of the air through lack of air space between the houses is as dangerous as close contact with the organic emanations from the human body. Such emanations cling to walls, floors, furniture, fomites, and foster the multiplication of infective organisms.

28 There are three kinds of movement: (1) local: successive and continuous reception of new positions in space. Here belong exercise, gymnastics, bathing; (2) in quality (alteration): this consists in the reception of new qualities; (3) in quantity (increase or diminution). A certain amount of matter is acquired or lost.

29

Factor Associated During the Time of Sleep	Effect on the Body
Profuse sweating	Accumulation of nutrients
Gastric contents digestible	Completion of digestion and blood-formation: formation of innate heat
Hot bilious humor	Cooled; heat is dispersed
Indigestible humor	Cooled; expansion of heat

30 During the waking state the body becomes hot exteriorly, cold and dry interiorly (Joannitius).

Aetius adds: "Among the good effects of sleep are: forgetfulness of mental sufferings, rectification of the distracted powers of reason; relaxation of contracted tissues. The best time for sleep is after a meal; it should end when the food is digested (shown by percussion over the stomach), after which the bowels should be emptied. The best time for sleep during the twenty-four hours is the night because the humidity and drowsy stillness of the night contributes to perfect digestion. The worst time is the day because in that case one does not sleep long enough to enable the digestion of the food to be completed. The result is acidity, flatulence, gurgling in the bowels.

31

Movement of the Breath	Direction	Associated Emotion
Sudden and forcible: Expansion	Outward	Anger
Gentle and gradual: Expansion	Outward	Delight and moderate joy
Sudden and forcible: Contraction	Inward	Fear, terror
Gentle and gradual: Contraction	Inward	Gloom (contracted heart); mental depression

32 See Abnormalities in bulk, decline.

33 Superficially, the suggestion that conception is synchronous with coition would seem an instance of medieval ignorance. Costaeus, in annotating on the passage, accepts the opinion that a strong desire on the part of either partner to see self or partner repeated and reproduced is capable of securing that the conception shall yield a child in whom the desire is ultimately realized. Favorable patency of the internal ducts (cervix) whether anatomically or emotionally in association with voluntary control of supposedly purely involuntary muscular tissue, are cooperative factors whereby the

above suggestion is not error but sometimes fact. The law of *jalal* and *jamal* plays an important part which is ultimately in due time manifested by the sex of the product of conception. Thus when the male is *jalal*, the product is female and vice versa. The *jalal* or *jamal* relating not only to physical affection but to anguish of love and the physiological cycles in the two organism have also to do with the chances of conception.

The belief that maternal mental states affect the growing embryo, both physically and psychically, is natural though rejected by some physicians. It is a valuable saying that "we can control the attributes and thoughts of the offspring and give it a far more valuable inheritance thereby than by any material fortune. It applies as an admonition to both parents.

"The woman produces an offspring like that being upon whom her thoughts dwell at the time of conceiving" (*Chakara-Samhita*, ii, 704).

By contemplating beautiful scenes of nature, beautiful pictures, pious persons, etc., the mother contributes to her make her child beautiful and virtuous and possessed of other desirable qualities (*ibid*, p. 745).

34 Another classification would be (a) medicines which produce change without destruction of function or tissue; (b) those which actually destroy function or tissue. In each case there are two degrees—one imperceptible to the senses, the other plainly evident. This is Galen's grouping. The grouping into four degrees still survives in the classification of burns.

Substances which are definitely poisonous may be classified into four groups as follows:

(1) Corrosives: these produce immediate and violent irritation. Example: mineral acids, alkalis, corrosive sublimate.

(2) Irritants: (a) metallic, such as lead, copper, arsenic, phosphorus; (b) vegetable such as drastic purgatives (aloes, colocynth, croton oil); (c) animal such as cantharides. This group produces effects which simulate natural disease such as gastric and intestinal disease, peritonitis, abdominal catastrophe.

(3) Neurotics: Examples: hydrocyanic acid and the cyanides, opium, strychnine, aconite, belladonna.

(4) Gaseous: (a) irritant: halogens, ammonia; (b) anesthetics; (c) coal-gas, carbon monoxide, etc.

There is another group classifiable under §825, 1 and 2, exemplified by common salt which is injurious or even toxic in cases of kidney disease (Vallery-Radot, *Precis de Pathologie Medicale*, p. 390); and by those foods against which some persons have idiosyncrasies or "protein sensitiveness" (shellfish, fruits, etc.).

35 Fate of medicines taken into the body:

A. They are changed by the body (passive change).

(i) The body itself is not changed nor restored to health.

(a) Medicine changed into the likeness of the body: pure

nutriment.
(b) Medicine changed, but not into the likeness of the body: attempered medicine.
(ii) The body itself is also changed (active action)
(a) change in medicine produces change in body and interferes with or even arrests function
(1) The change is into the likeness of the body: medicinal food
(2) not into the likeness of the body: pure medicine
(b) the change in the body continues until life is destroyed: venomous medicine
B. They are not changed at all by the body, but they produce a deleterious change in the body (active action on the body): pure poison

In saying a medicine is "not changed by our body" we do not mean that it does not induce a formation of heat in the body by affecting the innate heat for as a matter of fact, most poisons only act on the body in that way thereby producing warmth. We mean that its "form" is not changed and that in consequence its power continues to influence the body until the latter has destroyed the "form." For instance, if the nature of the medicine be hot, its nature reinforces its property of dispersing the breath. Examples: viper venom; aconite. Again, if the medicine be cold, its nature reinforces its property by congealing or enfeebling the breath. Example: scorpion venom, hyoscyamus (or hellebore).

Anything that is nutritious will eventually change the temperament of the body and in a natural manner. It warms the body because when it becomes blood that is the natural effect; and the body becomes warmer. Lettuce and gourds warm in this way. So in saying "warm" we do not mean "warm, the 'form,'" but "warm, that which arises out of its own intrinsic quality—the 'species' remaining."

Medicines which are foods are altered by the body first in quality and later in "substance" This change in quality may be in respect of heat so that the medicine warms (i.e. garlic); or it may be in respect of cold, so that the body becomes cold (i.e. lettuce). Afterwards, when the digestion and conversion into good blood has been completed, the medicine produces warmth to the same extent to which it has added to the volume of the blood, thereby increasing the "substance" of innate heat. How could it do otherwise than furnish heat when it has itself been made hot, and its coldness thereby abstracted?

But even after the medicine has been changed in substance there still remains some of its innate quality (some hot, some cold). There is some of the coldness of lettuce left in the blood which as been made from the lettuce and there is some of the heat of the garlic left in the blood which the garlic has given rise to. This holds good for a certain period of time.

36 Classification of Food-stuffs

Texture of nutriment	Nutritious quality	Name of Aliment	Notes
Attenuated (i.e. produce attenuated blood)	Rich	Meat juice, wine. Eggs raw or lightly cooked. Pottage	These are considered rich in nutriment because most of their substance is utilized by the body.
	Poor	Potherbs Juleb Fruits (matian, pomegranates, and the like)	These are attempered in substance and quality.
Dense (i.e. thicken the blood)	Rich	Hard-boiled eggs; veal	
	Poor	Cheese, salted meat, eggplant and the like.	These are considered poor in nutriment because only a small portion of them becomes blood.

37 Arranged according to quality of chyme: making good chyme: egg-yolk, wine, meat-juice are highly nutritious. They are attenuated. Lettuce and pomegranate are very nutritious. These are attenuated. Boiled eggs, year-old lamb are highly nutritious. These are dense in texture.

Making bad chyme: newly-killed meat of pheasant, partridge, lung. These are highly nutritious and attenuated. Radish, mustard and many other kitchen-herbs are nutritious and attenuated. Veal, duck, horseflesh are highly nutritious and dense in texture. Salt meat is feebly nutritious and dense in texture.

The study of food should include the following aspects: (1) Digestibility. This depends on the density or tenuity of texture of the food-stuff as well as on the materials with which it is associated. Thus the more fat-content, or fat-addition (from foods combined with it), the less digestible, because the less permeable. Again, digestibility may be completely removed by so simple a procedure as taking certain liquids (among them, pure water) at an unsuitable time after digestion has begun or liquids which are incompatible with certain foods before digestion or in a state of partial digestion. Avicenna's conception of the gastric contents as a "broth" or "emulsion" is legitimate and if these contents are "torn off" the mucosa by foods or fluids taken after the digestion of the meal has got under way, the whole process may stop beyond the power of renewal. The same holds good for the process in the small intestine. This idea, ruling in *The Canon*, can be verified by anyone in his daily experience. Palatability has to do with digestibility.

(2) Assimilability: This depends on the kind of chyme which will result.

(3) Nutritive value: This, according to *The Canon*, will depend on the kind of humor which the food yields, how much residue its leaves (therefore, whether constipating or relaxing). Thus we have the classification of foods according as they (i) enrich the blood: cereals, dairy produce such as soft boiled eggs, milk, flesh meat, fowl, certain vegetables; (ii) enrich the serous humor: mutton, one-year lamb, the potherbs atriplex and purslane; (iii) increase the amount of bile made or excite a flow of bile: chicken, fish with few

scales and agile in habits, the potherbs garlic, mustard, nasturtium; (iv) increase the amount of atrabilious humor: like goat flesh, freshly killed meat, cabbage, lentils. In each class there would be subdivisions according to the digestibility—whether digestible within two hours or four hours or later.

(4) Physiological value: This is a more general aspect in that the other aspects contribute to its assessment. The old division of foods into proteins, carbohydrates, fats, salts, water is not necessarily to be rejected in favor of the modern division of foods according to energy-values, heat values and "accessory factors." Chemical analysis of foods suffers from the fallacy that the substances so found do not exist as much in the food—a statement based on the same principle as will be discussed more carefully under the subject of "drugs." Moreover, were these substances present as such, they certainly do not circulate in the body or function in the tissue cells in the chemical form found under artificial conditions. Physiological values may be assessed according to whether an ash is left in the tissues after oxidation or not. Thus, body-building foods leave an ash, heat generating foods do not. The important matter is the formation of ash because of the risk of this lingering in the body or even becoming firmly imprisoned in its tissues. Foods may also be studied in regard to their deputative properties according to their alkalinity or acidity, etc.

Thus there are other considerations than the popular ones of work-production and the practical objects which rule properly only in the management of domestic animals.

38 There is much to be said as to the part played by water in the economy. Through apparently simple, its chemical structure is complex. It is a mixture of units of varying molecular complexity, each unit being called a "hydrone." The number of molecules of hydrone and polyhydrones constantly varies even at steady temperatures so that equilibrium regarding them is easily disturbed. The foreign matter always present in the water of nature is essential to life, assimilation being only possible by virtue of such constituents. Apart from this, water is essential to metabolism—absorption, digestion (enzyme action depends on it), osmosis, temperature regulation, the maintenance of the salt concentration of the blood at a constant level. The necessary reservoir of water in the tissues is furnished by the muscular tissues and their depletion has serious consequences (§1067, Gruner, Introduction, "The Notion of the Nature of Disease") and their repletion entails important interference with the physiological functions. It may be noted however that the idea that plentiful consumption of water "flushes" organisms out of the body is not reliable (Hemmeter, Med. Rec., May 22, 1920).

39 The characteristics of pure water, therefore, are (1) aspect: limpid, clear, pellucid, diaphana; (2) taste: tasteless or sweet, pleasant to drink and refreshing; (3) odor: none; (4) touch: soft or gentle, cool; (5) other properties: weight, vegetables boil quickly in it; the place from which it is obtained is nei-

ther too hot nor too cold; fertilizing and calm; passes out of the body quickly.

40 The Oxus River (modern Amu Darya) is one of the great rivers of Central Asia. It runs through the province of Khorasan between Samarqand and the country called Bactria as stated in the Glossary to the Venice edition of *The Canon*. Arising in the enormous glaciers of the mountainous ranges between East Turkestan and Afghanistan and receiving important tributaries from the northern slopes of the Hindu Kush, it emerges into open country, being here bounded by Bukhara on the north. It varies from 1000 yards to a mile in width in this region and the stream flows from 2 1/2 to 5 miles an hour. It empties into the Aral Sea. So great a river would naturally be prized by the Persians who regarded it as the equal of the Nile. The fact that the great trade route of Central Asia from Khorasan to China crossed this river in the above-mentioned region made it well-known to Avicenna although virtually unknown to Europe unto 200 years later when Marco Polo and his companions entered this country.

41 River water was preferred before others by Rhazes while other ancient physicians preferred the Nile water to all others. Spring water: the qualities vary according to whether the water comes from the north, south, east or west according to Hippocrates.

42 See repletion and depletion.

43 Venery—coitus: Galen placed this in the first rank among the obligatory causes of disease, but most physicians group it partly under "exercise" and partly under "evacuations" (excretions). It causes dryness of the body, weakens the vegetative drives, infrigidates and sometimes the concomitant emotional excitement entails a heating effect.

44 Points relative to water-baths: (1) the bath room itself: temperature of the air in the different rooms (temperate, warm, hot, cool); mural decorations; (2) the person serving in the bath; (3) the bath itself: quantity of water (full to immersion, partial, sitz, etc); temperature of water (hot, tepid, cold); duration of stay in the bath (long, short, medium); kinds of water employed; intrinsic quality (cooling, moistening, etc.); (4) the person bathing: relation to food (fasting or hungry, immediately after a meal, soon after a meal, at the end of the first stage of digestion); state of skin (dry, moist, dropsical); state of the humors and their quality (cold, immatured); frequency of bathing; season for open-air bathing; effects of the bath: on respiration, on pulse, on innate heat, on the strength (relaxing effects, syncope, impotence); on the humors (helping maturation, drawing to surface, diverting superfluities to different parts); on the quality of the body (dry, cold, moist); on the general nutrition (making the body thin, stout, or weak); (5) special purposes of the bath (treatment of hectic fevers for affections of the stomach and spleen).

46 Cold bath: when taken while fasting imparts warmth and moisture. If taken after a meal, it will make the body cold and remove moisture.

Hot bath: when taken while fasting, it is attenuant and refrigerant and does not impart moisture. If taken after a meal, the bath is heating and moistens the body according to Hippocrates.

Warm bath: this relieves lassitude, is soothing and has a warming and softening effect. it dispels plethora and removes flatulence from wherever it may have lodged. It favors sleep and promotes digestion (Haly Abbas). It opens the pores. It induces plumpness of the body. it is beneficial for all—men, women, young. old, rich, poor. The best time for it is before food and after exercise.

47 Add a fifth part of heated oil to the water. Such a bath is highly anodyne. It relieves lassitude and nervous pains. Uses: for prolonged fevers, convulsions, retention of urine.

48 Douching with emollient herbs.

49 Agents which alter the several qualities of the body include: calefacients, refrigerants, humectants, desiccants, agents causing changes of form, agents causing obstructions of channels, agents which open up the channels, agents causing roughness, mollificants, agents causing displacements of parts, agents preventing apposition of parts, agents preventing expansion of parts, agents causing abnormal movements, causes of numerical increase, causes of numerical decrease, causes of loss of continuity, causes of ulceration, causes of inflammatory swellings, the subject of pain, agents producing retentions or evacuations, causes of over-repletion, causes of debility, asthenia, and lack of vigor in members.

Sclerosis: this refers to the thickening of the skin which occurs after long exposure to the weather. It becomes harsh, coarse, and presumably less pervious.

Steam: horses steam when they have been hard-worked. The exhaled air appears like steam. This steam is the substance of the breath so that it is permissible to translate the word accordingly. This steam which pervades organs, tissues and tissue spaces and cavities is the visible manifestation of the breath. It is natural to think, then, that if the skin is so hardened that it will not let this vapor out, the latter will accumulate in the body and make it hot as happens after severe exercise until the body cools down. It is also natural to reason that if the vapor is able to expand owing to laxity of the connective tissues, it will impart a sense of glow to the body for everyone has experienced it.

Rarefaction: when this term is applied to the skin it refers to a condition opposite to sclerosis. The skin is unduly soft, supple, and is evidently relaxed instead of tight.

These considerations apply to sub-heading 5 of §907.

In modern language, the warmth of the body depends on the relation between heat loss and heat gain. Heat enters the body from: (a) the external air or surroundings: warm air of summer, artificially warmed air in winter baths; (b) heat derived from: (i) food and drink; (ii) exercise; (iii) toxic action of foreign matter (sepsis, drugs); (c) heat fostered by preventing heat loss:

clothing, sleep; (d) local heat (fomentations, etc.); (e) emotional influence.

Heat is lost from the body by: (a) excreta: urine, feces, skin action, exhalation by the air expired; (b) external conditions: cold, wet.

Note that baths vary in their effect. An ordinary hot bath renders the body warm; a brief immersion has a different effect; a long continued immersion is depressant.

50 Humors.

51 General discussion of the causes of pain include: general discussion of the causes of pain, theory of the nature of pain, list of the types of pain and the explanation of each, agents which alleviate pain, the effect of pain on the body, the causes of pleasurable sensations, how movement brings on pain, how depraved humors evoke pain, and how gaseous substances produce pain.

52 In regard to the kinds of pain, it is of interest here to recall the eight kinds of pain inherent in human life given in the *Nirvana Sutra:* (1) birth pangs; (2) pains of age; (3) pains of disease; (4) the pain of death; (5) the pain of parting with loved ones or things; (6) the pain of meeting with what one dislikes; (7) the pain of not obtaining what one seeks; (8) the pain of the five elements: that is, the body itself produces pain (Ishizuka's notes to *Honen the Buddhist Saint*, p. 446).

Re-arranged alphabetically, the fifteen kinds of pain are: boring; compressing; corrosive; dull; fatigue-pain; heavy pain; incisive; irritant' itching' pricking' relaxing; stabbing; tearing; tension; and throbbing.

53 Plethora: "passive congestion" is over-repletion with blood. It is associated with stasis. "Active congestion" is the equivalent of apostema (*waram*). Oedema is over-repletion with lymph (*serous humor*). It is associated with stasis in the lymphatic channels or serous cavities. The practical result is that the channels cannot drain or empty within the available time. Hypertension is a form of plethora. Corpulence is over-repletion with fat, namely, in the connective-tissue spaces. One practical result of this is that supervening disease produces greater affliction than otherwise as was written in the *Chakara*. Plethora of the connective tissue spaces with a mucoid change in the fluid may produce the appearance of obesity. This peculiar change is met with in the female sex. It fluctuates in degree from time to time and may appear or disappear within a few days. Intestinal stasis is over-repletion of the large intestine. It may be noted that the effect of stasis anywhere is to interfere with that flow of breath which is essential to health or even life. The breath is "choked" or "strangled." The faculties are also at a disadvantage for their free operation is conditional on free flow of breath through all parts of the body. In modern terms, oxidative processes are retarded or arrested.

54 Retributive or Expiative Causes of Disease:

The idea that illnesses were a form of "judgment" or punishment, or retribution for misdeeds, was formerly widespread, but is not regarded seriously in modern medicine. In the case of all peoples who hold the Buddhist belief in *karma*, this ancient idea holds good because every event, good or bad, in individual life is believed to be the outcome of events in a past life—whether in this particular existence or in a previous incarnation. Whenever the theosophical teachings hold, the same view would be held. Moreover, in Islam there is no difficulty in the idea because "there is no second cause," and as is written in the *Mathnawi*, in speaking of Israil, the angel of death, God is said to "operate by disease and sickness and men will not look for any cause beyond these diseases" by virtue of the truth of the text, "*He is nearer to you than you are yet you see Him not*" (Quran 56:84).

Ghazzali in his *Alchemy of Happiness* says: "Illness is, so to speak, a cord of love by which God draws to Himself the saints concerning whom He has said, 'I was sick and you visited Me not.' Illness itself is one of those forms of experience by which the human being arrives at the knowledge of God. As He says, 'Sicknessness themselves are My servants and are attached to My chosen.'"

During medieval Christian times pandemics were regarded as the manifestations of divine wrath and the incidence of illnesses is sometimes still explained in similar terms in modern Christianity, the microbic and other tangible causes of disease being taken simply as the instruments whereby the event is achieved (Lecture 3, endnote 12).

As in the case of the idea of "fate" and "destiny," the subject is apt to be viewed incorrectly. Illnesses are sometimes evident warnings; sometimes they belong to the category of expiation, whether in relation to others or to the victim himself. In any case, diseases may be regarded as in some way connected with that experience of life which the sufferer has himself to undergo. In Thomistic terms, such would be the "final cause" of disease.

In the life of St. Lydwine of Shiedam (J. K. Huysman, *St. Lydwine de Schiedam*) we read how a celebrated physician, Godfried de Haga, endorsed and deferred to "the divine law" that every malady is an expiation; that if God does not regard the expiation as satisfied, the course of the illness cannot be altered by the art of medicine. Cure cannot result from his treatment unless his intervention coincides with the completion of the expiation which has been imposed on the patient by his Lord." (It was subsequent to the named physician's life-time that Paracelsus wrote the words actually quoted adding "when the time for redemption has come, the patient will then find the physician through whom God will send him relief." Paracelsus classified the causes of disease under five headings: those arising in morbid states of the body; those belonging to the category of poisons (intoxications); those arising from "astral" origins; spiritual causes (passions, disordered thoughts, morbid imagination); and retributive [F. Hartmann, *The Life of Paracelsus*, pp. 199, 221]).

In modern times this belief is manifested as a conviction in the pastoral instructions to the Catholic medical man that he is not entitled to continue his ministrations on a patient gravely ill unless his Catholic patient has fulfilled his spiritual duties within a certain number of days of the onset of the severe symptoms.

"*Hay muchos decretos eclesiasticos que prohiben a los medicos visitar mas de tres veces, si el enfermo no se ha confesado*" (Vilarino, 142, p. 645).

The following advice to the patient himself is less harsh to appearance: "first when thou feelest any indisposition, accept it as a dispensation of the love of My Heart. . . . Afterwards, unite thy sufferings with Mine. . . . If thy affirmity increases offer to Me thy body as a living victim. . . ." (Arnold, xvi).

This teaching leaves no room for doubt about the true answer to the oft-aired question, "Should the doctor tell his patient that his illness is likely to prove mortal?"

Part Three

Lecture 11: The Signs and Symptoms (Diagnosis): General Remarks

1 The science of the diagnosis of disease by internal symptoms is founded upon six canons: (1) the patient's actions; (2) the waste of the body; (3) the nature of the pain; (4) the site of the pain; (5) swelling; (6) the effluvia given off by his person.

2 Joannitius gives a rather different classification of symptoms and signs, though summarizing from the same text. It may be said that every classification is a matter of personal convenience. There is not necessarily any principle involved, for the subject comprises so great a variety that a strictly logical classification serves no special purpose. In some cases symptoms are characteristic of a cause, in others of an error of function, in others of a special disease. To adhere consistently to one rule of classification necessarily entails the relegation of some symptoms which are important in actual practice to a subsidiary or insignificant position in the list. Therefore, it may be said that Avicenna's classification will hold good as well as any. The student obtains his knowledge from his own experience and not from memorizing a given list.

The following list of simple ailments or evidence of disease may be offered at this point: (1) Pain. the first evidence of disease or ill-health. Its localization is very significant and charts depicting its possible sites and their meaning are of great use. Thus headache is very commonly simply a sign of indigestion (gastric or intestinal) or constipation. The type of pain is most important. Thus pain in the abdomen relieved by pressure suggests gaseous distension due to abnormal fermentation of food whereas pain increased by pressure suggests inflammation. (2) Abnormal discharges. Abnormal in quantity (increased or diminished), such as diarrhea, polyuria. Abnormal in quality such as nose-bleeding, hemoptysis, expectoration, nasal discharge, salivation. Abnormal in manner, such as incontinence. (3) Abnormal acts. Vomiting, coughing, hiccup, eructations, yawning, sighing, shivering, sleepiness, insomnia, altered gait, altered posture (from palsy, exhaustion, collapse), tremors, twitchings, convulsions, etc. (4) Abnormal subjective sensations. In special senses: floating specks before the eyes in dyspepsia, ringing in the ears in cases of nervous debility, or after certain drugs or from wax; bitter taste in dyspepsia, dizziness arising from nerve derangement or circulatory errors. In general: nausea, palpitation, throbbing, labored breathing, altered appetite, thirst, sense of lassitude or asthenia, irritability, loss of memory. (5) Outward signs. Discolored or "heavy" eyes. Offensive breath in indigestion and constipation. Wasting or obesity. Hot and dry skin in fevers or states of mental excitement or from excess of salt in the diet. Cold sweating from exhaustion, etc. Altered color of skin. Edema of skin; skin-eruptions; signs derived from examination of the mouth. Pale tongue and gums from blood-deficiency, bleeding gums from excess of salt in diet and other causes; colored line on gums in metallic poisonings, coated tongue in digestive disturbances, loosened teeth from errors of diet or the use of adulterated foods, etc.

3 Color of the Hair

Color	Corresponding Temperament	Remarks
Black	Hot	In such cases oxidative processes are in excess of the mean (Joannitius).
Brown	Cold	
Tawny/red	Equable	There is an excess of "unburned heat" so that the hair always grow red (Joannitius). Therefore the proneness to anger (a form of "heat").
Very fair	Cold and very moist	Note how plants lose their dark or green color when
Grey	Cold and very dry	dried, and become red or white. In the human being, this change is produced towards the close of desiccant diseases

The following details are from Joannitius:

Black: due to: smallness of crystalline lens; setting of the crystalline lens too far back; abundance of aqueous humor; turbidity thereof; uvea redundant; peculiarity of the visible "breath" (scanty or confused).

Brown: due to the contraries of the above—crystalline lens large or further forward; paucity of albugineous humor; clearness of this; deficient quality of uvea; the visible breath plentiful or clear.

Intermediate colors (black and brown mixed). The visible breath varies in amount and clarity.

Grey: visible breath less plentiful.

4 Joannitius ascribed it to decomposition changes in the serous humor occurring in old age; greyness, he says, means excess of atrabilious humor.

5 See chart above.

6 Joannitius adds: fleshiness (excess of heat and moisture in the temperament); fatness (excess of moisture and intense coldness); leanness (hot temperament and intense dryness); delicate build: cold and very dry; massive build: cold and very moist or very cold and very moist; justness of form: well-balanced humors.

7 This passage is evidently an attempt to explain the nature of bacterial action and infection without the knowledge of the actual bacteria themselves. The description is so ingenious that it requires little change to modernize it.

The following may be applied accordingly: (1) the meaning of innate heat; (2) the nature of "foreign heat" and "foreign cold"; (3) the meaning of the term "hot poison"; (4) the meaning of hot and cold as relative terms.

(1) Innate heat. This term, particularly in this passage, is equivalent to "vitality." This word describes a complex concept. Though regarded as vague and quite unsatisfactory today, it may be said to be amenable to reduction to a formula—and a formula into which several factors enter. The condemnation of the term is due to the non-recognition of this fact and non-recognition that many well-known and freely-accepted data belong to it.

(2) The nature of "foreign heat" and "foreign cold." These refer to material agents now known as pathogenic micro-organisms. The material substance which is stated by Avicenna to be oxidized by "innate heat," is the bacterial substance which as we know undergoes lysis in the course of the immunizing processes of the body. The "heat" refers to what we know as the bacterial toxins which act upon the thermogenic centers and produce numerous other effects on the tissues. The word "heat" thus comprises two things: the pyrexia produced by bacterial invasion may be theoretically distinguished from the innate heat, but practically speaking, the rise of temperature is generally admitted to be part of the so-called defensive mechanism against infections. The destruction of the bacteria, and of their products by anti-substances—these events are comprised in the words "dispersing the foreign heat." After all, both bacteria and products are "dispersed." We are only being told the same fact in different language.

In the case of foreign cold, here the organisms and products differ. But if the temperature becomes subnormal, the immunizing process is not ascribed to the lowered temperature. Recovery from the infection still depends on the "innate heat" or "vitality" that is, a series of processes of immunization which take place, whether the patient develops fever or not.

Avicenna considers that the formation of septic products is more likely if there is not much pyrexia on the ground that in such a case the bacteria, as we should say, meet with less resistance, and are enabled to produce those decompositions of the body fluids which we know to take place readily as soon as the vitality of a part is lowered.

(3) The meaning of the term "hot poisons." Clearly the word poison must be understood as covering both bacterial agents and their products. The toxic products may produce rise of temperature and are, therefore, reasonably called "hot." Others do not have this effect.

(4) The meaning of hot and cold as relative terms. In this passage a thing is hot or cold according to its effect on the bodily sensations or its effect on the heat centers of the body. Taken in its literal or surface meaning of hot temperature, cold temperature, the passage is of course pedantic and useless. It should be evident that the words "hot" and "cold" cannot possibly have meant literal heat and cold.

8 A strong inclination to sleep denotes debility—a loss of tone of the muscular power. Histologically, sleep depends on a break in the ideation-zone of the cerebral cortex. If there is a break in the layer below that, the sleep will be that of stupor or coma. The break in this situation is marked in amentia and dementia. Wakefulness or insomnia denotes poisons circulating n the blood, powerful sensory impulses (pain) or powerful emotions.

9 Functions may be weakened, exalted, depraved, obstructed in their action or abolished.

10

SIGNS DERIVED FROM THE STATES OF THE MIND DURING ACTION AND PASSION

EVIDENCE	NAME OF TEMPERAMENT	CORRESPONDING
EMOTIONAL ASPECT	HOT	DRY
Concupiscible	1 Shameless[1] 2 Excitable 3 Lively, vivacious	Infatuation: love, passion
Irascible	1 Hopefulness 2 Courage; temerity[2] 3 Easily provoked to anger	Brooding Anger lasts some time
Duration	Short	Long[1]
Mental Capacity		
Intellectual power	Good	Imaginative
Power of observation	Good	
Capability, talent	Good, conspicuous	Memory good
Moral Aspects	Stern Virility of morals and manners Diligence Much flexibility of opinion[2]	Gentle
Ego Instinctive Drive	Love of good opinion Not easily perturbed or downcast	Takes things to heart
Movements and Gestures	Rapid	
Dreams	Of warming oneself at a fire; sitting in the hot sun[3]	

1 In the case of the moist temperament, the duration of emotional disturbance is short.

2 These represent negative or weak aspects.

3 In the case of a cold temperament, the dreams are of being in the cold, out in the snow or of being immersed in cold water. In short, the character of the visual images in the dream is related to the character of the dominant humor, partly because the dream varies with the state of the "breath" at the time.

11

EVIDENCE OF THE FOUR PRIMARY INTEMPERAMENTS

EVIDENCE	HOT	COLD	MOIST	DRY
Morbid states to which there is a tendency.	Inflammatory conditions becoming febrile	Fevers related to the serous humor Rheumatism	Same as Cold	
	Loss of vigor		Lassitude	
Functional power	Deficient energy	Deficient digestive power	Difficult digestion	
Subjective sensations	Bitter taste in the mouth		Mucoid salivation	
	Excessive thirst	Lack of desire for fluids.		

	Sense of burning at cardiac orifice		Sleepiness	Insomnia, wakefulness
Physical signs	Pulse extremely quick and frequent; approaching the weak type met with in lassitude	Flaccid joints	Diarrhea Swollen eyelids	Rough skin Spare habit (acquired, not inborn)
Foods and medicines	Calefacients are all harmful, Infrigidants benefit	Infrigidants are all harmful Calefacients benefit	Moist articles of diet harmful	Dry regimen harmful Humectants beneficial[1]
Relation to weather	Worse in summer	Worse in winter		Bad in autumn

1 Hot water, rarefied oils are beneficial to the dry temperament and are avidly taken up.

12 Sleep quiet, uninterrupted, and followed, on waking, by cheerfulness, and a contented mind.

13 Therefore no conscious feeling of digestion or discomfort of any kind. Micturition painless, the urine not feeling hot, having an odor neither sweet nor sour, amber-colored and forming no deposit. Defecation without soiling the skin, the feces firm, but not hard. The appetite according to genuine hunger and for natural foods, thirst only for water. Mouth closed when breathing. Adaptability to climate and season (*Chahar maqala*).

14 The modern term "hypertension" is covered by the old term of plethora or repletion. The correspondence is verified by some of its symptoms. Thus hemorrhagic phenomena occur—in the nose, retina, cerebrum, meninges, labyrinth, the skin and as hematuria and hemetemesis simulating organic disease. Hypertension causes fatigue of the heart shown by: dyspnea, palpitation, quick pulse, anginal attacks, nocturnal pseudo-asthma, brut de galop.

15 One or two of the data given (under general physique: on the hair; the surface veins) are from Rhazes. Note the patient at rest (in repose) and in activity (gestures, attitude). Note that the signs of his temperament are accentuated when he is ill. The type of reaction to infection is determined by his temperament.

16

EVIDENCE WHICH SHOW WHICH OF THE HUMORS IS DOMINANT

EVIDENCE	SANGUINEOUS	SEROUS	CHOLERIC	ATRABILIOUS
Aspect: General physique	Good	Effeminate; bones slender; joints well-covered.	Lean; joints large.	Emaciated.
Color	Ruddy	Unduly pale.	Yellow tinge in and conjunctiva.	Dusky; whole body seems dark, hairy.
Feel of body	Flesh firm	Soft and cool		Flesh hard
State of skin	Reddens on rubbing; furuncles			Skin rough; liable to dark eruptions; intractable ulcers.
Hair		Absent on truck.	Hairy.	Hairy.
Surface veins	Full	Constricted	Thick and hard	
Vegetative Drives				
Mouth	Liability to pustules.	Abundant sticky saliva	Bitter taste	Sense of burning at mouth of stomach
Tongue	Red		Rough, dry	
Nostrils			Rough, dry	

Pulse		Soft, tends to be slow, infrequent	Rapid	
Urine		White		Dark colored or black; dense
Feces				
Sensitive Drives				
Special senses: taste	Unusual sweetness in mouth, senses dull		Bitter taste	Sense of burning at mouth of stomach.
Appetite for food			Poor	Depraved
Appetite for fluid		Absent unless salt is taken esp. for elderly	Thirsty	
Muscular tone	Weariness not accounted for by exertion.	Flaccidity of limbs		
Dreams	Sees red things; blood coming out of body; of swimming in blood, etc.	Sees waters, rivers, snow, rain, cold, thunder.	Sees fires, yellow flags; objects not yellow appear yellow; a conflagration; hot bath; hot sun. etc.	Fear of darkness; of pain; terrifying black things.
Movements (gestures)	Yawning, stretching			
Rational Drives	Reaction time slow. Continual drowsiness.	Somnolence, laziness, tiredness.	Hebetude.	Sense of anxiety; wakefulness.
Abnormal Phenomena				
Nausea	Present		Present	
Vomiting			Yellow-green bile, acrid flux.	
Goose flesh			Needle pricks	
Headache	Sense of weight in back of eyes and temples.			
Others	Blood flows our readily from nose, anus, gums.	Weak digestion and acid eructations.	Severe diarrhea	Splenic disorders often occur, also morphoea; evil ulcers.
Preceding Factors	Note	Note	Note	Note
Diet				
Occupations				
Locality living in				
Habits				
Season of year				
Date of last venesection				
Previous temperament				

17 The subject of obstructions is capable of great expansion. The symptoms differ: (1) With each of the humors: (i) Thus serous humor obstructions are manifested as oedema of the glottis, odema of the lung, nasopharyngeal hypersecretion, odema of the kidney tissue, of the blood itself, vomiting, diarrhea, headache (too much cerebro-spinal fluid), convulsions, delirium, coma, Cheyne-Stokes respiration, amaurosis. (ii) With the different substances, thus

in nephritis, obstruction of the channels in the skin prevents the wastes leaving the body by that route with consequent manifestation as arthritis, anginas, otitis, etc. (iii) With the atom groups, thus obstruction to the outlet of nitrogen (azotemia) manifests as hypertension, vomiting, diarrhea, sialorrhea, stomatitis, parotitis, retinitis, anemia of plasmatic type, arthralgia, fibrillar tremors, coma, loss of appetite for meats. Viewing diseases in this way, the important thing is to find both site of obstruction and substance or atom-groups concerned. (2) The symptoms may be monosyndromic or polysyndromic. (3) There may be obstruction to the flow of "breath." (4) The pores which may become obstructed vary in size from that of the orifices of the body down to the smallest channels, whether visible to the naked eye or only with the microscope or whether sub-microscopic or ultra-microscopic. The pores vary in shape and consistence, resilience, elasticity, distensibility. Fluids may traverse them in both directions, but when there is obstruction, they may be able to pass only in one direction or not at all.

Lecture 12: The Signs and Symptoms (Diagnosis): The Pulse

1 It is necessary to inquire diligently into the properties of the pulse, for diagnosis and for the use of drugs. Every important variety of pulse revealed by the sphygmograph was recognized, described, and named, before the Christian era. We count the beats and note their force and volume to ascertain the strength of the sufferer and the effect upon him of the disease. . . . Many of the indications obtained from the pulse do not depend on a knowledge of the circulation at all (the following section on sphygmology is therefore not obsolete, but of real value to the modern practitioner.).

2 In modern language it is the change of shape from the flattered condition impressed on the vessel by the finger which the artery assumes under the distending force of the blood within it which constitutes for us the pulse.

3 This reason is important in the East where the doctor may not expose a female patient in any way. This interdiction accounts for the extraordinary erudition attained in the art of feeling the pulse, for instance in China. "The old Chinese doctors are remarkably good diagnosticians. Although the study of the patient is restricted to the examination of the two radial pulses, and noting the state of the eyes and tongue, the diagnosis is disconcertingly accurate" (F. Hartmann, *Chinesische Heilmethoden*).

William of Rubruk, a Franciscan friar (1253 AD) recorded: "The Cathayans . . . are first-rate artists in every kind and their physicians have a thorough knowledge of the virtues of herbs and an admirable skill in diagnosis by the pulse" *Encyclopedia Britannica*, vi, 189 by Prof. Giles who also says: "The variations of the pulse have been classified and allocated with a minuteness hardly credible" *(ibid*, p. 228). Eusebius Renaudot (*Ancient Account of India and China*, p. 209), in 1733, wrote:, "They are so sure of the disease that they tell all the precedent symptoms to a nicety."

The heart and arteries all pulsate with the same rhythm so that any artery can be used for feeling the pulse. But most arteries are embedded in flesh and cannot be distinctly felt. The order of clearness is: wrist, soles, behind ears, along arms.

Arteries within bones cannot of course be felt; nor can arteries be made use of which have other bodies in front of them except in emaciated persons where for instance the aorta or limb arteries to become palpable for the first time.

4 If the patient be a male, use the left hand; if a female, the right. This ancient Chinese idea, that the pulse of one side has a different significance to that of the other, is also met with, in a different form, in recent literature. Thus, Eli Jones (*Medical Times*) states that the pulse at the right wrist informs of the state of the constitution, or vitality, and that of the left wrist informs of the local disease, and the real and true condition of the patient. He further states that when both pulses are fully strong and regular, after an illness, the patient is nearly well.—Baraduc (*Les Vibrations de la vitalite humaine*) on the basis of biometric observations of an elaborate kind, asserts that reactions obtained with the right hand belong to changes in the physical or material vitality of the body, whereas those obtained with the left hand belong to the psychic vitality. These statements are of interest in relation to the ancient Chinese idea.

The position of the observer's hand. This must be adapted according to the position of the patient. The middle finger must be placed exactly at the junction of carpus with lower end of radius. The other two fingers are allowed to rest upon the artery, one on either side (*ibid.*). The index finger should be nearest the heart. (Broadbent, *The Pulse*, p. 39).

Emotional state of the patient—the pulse should be felt at a time when the patient is not in a state of excitement or anger, or affected by exertion, or under the influence of the emotions, or in a state of satiety (which renders the pulse heavy), or of hunger; nor must it be a time when usual habits are neglected or new ones are being formed.

The state of the observer—the observer must be in a calm state of mind. He must be very attentive and free from the least distraction of thought. The body must be tranquil, and the at ease. The respirations should thus be unimpeded and regular. His own state of health should be good (Duhalde, *Description of China*).

Other instructions given in the Chinese system of sphygmology—the instructions for feeling the pulse include the following: first apply the fingers gently, touching the skin very lightly at the three places corresponding to the three fingers—named C (for cubitus, or lower end of radius), G for "gate," and W (for wrist), the successive fingerpulps being in contact with those three places. The character of the pulse is now noted in reference to the vital organs.

The next step is to apply the fingers a little harder, but not hard enough to feel the bone. The attention should now be directed to the state of the pulse at G. The third step consists in applying pressure till the bone can be felt, and then making tests with a view to deciding on the state of each of the five main organs.

If the wrist be long, the fingers need not be readjusted; but if short, re-adjustment of the fingers must be made several times, moving to juxtapositions each time.

The attention must not be allowed to wander from the search in question the five vital organs and the six viscera. The sensation imparted to each finger is noted for the purpose. Great exactitude must be observed. The observation will evidently occupy a considerable period of time.

"Fine though these distinctions are, the sedulous physician will perceive and remember them."

A copy of one of the numerous diagrams in the work quoted is here appended, substituting a translation for the actual accompanying text. (For guidance in the translation of this passage and many parts of the work quoted, grateful thanks may be here expressed to Prof. J. P. Bruce and Mr. Li).

Table of Terminology
A. General Terms
(Arranged in Pairs of Opposites)

Group No.	§ in this Translation	Term Used in English	Term in Latin Latin Text	Term in Bulaq Text	Term in Chinese Text
1	521	Long-Short Broad-Slender Deep-Elevated	Longus-Curtus Latus-Strictus Profundus-Elevatus	tawil-qasir arid-dayyiq munkhaffad-mushrif	ch'ang-tuan ch'eng-fu
	522	Large-Small Thick-Slender	Magnus-Parvus Grossus-Subtilis	azim-saghir ghaliz-daqiq	ta-hsiao
(2)	523	Strong-Weak	Fortis-Debilis Vehemens*-Imbecillus Validus*-Languidus	qawi-daif	li-jao hung
(3)	524	Swift-Slow (Rapid-Sluggish)	Velox-Tardus	sari-bati	k'uai-ch'ih
(4)	525	Hard-Soft (Compressible-Incompressible)	Durus-Mollis Lenis*	salb-layyin	shih-juan (Ke)
(5)	526	Full-Empty	Plenus-Vacuus	mumtali-khali	man-kung (hsu)
(6)	527	Hot-Cold	Calidus-Frigidus	harr-barid	
(7)	528	Hurried--Infrequent Brisk-Sluggish Sense-Rare	Frequens-Rarus Continens-Resolutus Spissus***Lassus	mutawatir-mutafawut mutadarik-kmutakhalkhil mutakaif-mutarakhi	chieh(?)-huan (?) mi (chin)-san
(8)	529	Equal-Unequal (Regular-Irregular)	Aequalis-Diversus	mustawi-ikhtilaf (mukhtaf)**	jun-k'ou
(9)	530	Orderly-Disorderly	Ordinatus-Inordinatus	muntazim-mukhtalif	
(10)	533	Rhythmic-Arhythmic	Pondus-Arrythmus	wazn-ardal-wazn	ting-tai

* Synonymous words occuring in older Latin editions.

** These synonyms all appear together in the Bulaq text.

***In the Latin, the term "spissus" is often used as the opposite of "rarus." In the Arabic, the latter is mutafawut to which mutawatir is the opposite. In the passages in which spissus is used, the Arabic is often mutawatir and not mutakaif. There is actually a slight difference between frequens and spissus, for the former has the thought of an abrupt rise in the pulse-beat according to group-number 2, where spissus conveys the idea of beats very close together. Rarus may be taken as the counterpart of either thought: if it means a leisurely rise, it is in accordance with group number 3; if it means "spaced," this is also the idea in mutafawut. The Arabic distinguishes the two ideas of rarus by using mutarakhi for sluggishness.

The words rapid, hurried, brisk—slow, sluggish, leisurely, rare, and the words frequens, spissus, velox—rarus, tardus, languidus, are apt to be misleading, and it is difficult to avoid inconsistency, both in the Latin and the English, for in some cases, one work conveys a better idea of a shade of meaning, and in others, another, whichever Arabic term is employed.

B. Distinctive Terms

(Arranged Alphabetically)

Term Used	§	English Synonym Translation	Term in Latin Text	Term in Bulaq Text	Term in Chinese Text***
Bounding	540, 571	Undulatory	Undosus, fluctuosus	al-mawja*	hung (?)
Chord-like	549		Chordosus	mutawattir	hsien
Continuous	538	Unbroken	Continuus	muttasil	
Creeping	541, 572	Vermicular	Vermicularis	al-dudi	
Dicrotic	546, 568		Bispulsans; dicrotus	dzuwa-qaraina	
Failing	547, 568	Fading, Falling	Cadens in medio	al-waqi fil wasat	wei
Flickering	545	Recurrent	Reciprocus; mesalius; pulsus inclinatus (Rhazes) pulsus innuens (Haly Abbas)	musalli**	
Formicant	542, 572		Formicans	al-namli	
Harsh	543, 565	Serrate, Sawing	Serrinus; serratus	minshariy	se
Intermittent	538	Interrupted	Intersectus	munqata	chan hsieh
Jerking	539	Gazelle	Dorcadissans; gazellans	al-ghazali	ts'u
Mouse-tail	544, 567	Decurtate	Cauda soricina; murus innuens	zanabul l-far	fu
Recurrent	538		Reditivus	aid	
Spasmodic	548, 569	Tense	Spasmosus	mutashannuj	chin
Swooning	567, 600	Recurrent mouse-tail	Cauda reditiva	ghashiya	fu, jao, tai (?)
Thrilling	548, 570	Trembling	Tremulus	murtaish	tung (?)
Wiry	548	Twisted	Retortus	multawi	hsi

* Literally, a fast-going she-camel whose girth slips through the inequality of the motion of the fore and hind feet.

** Literally, the thrid horse in a race.

*** Some of the Chinese equivalents here given are free of ambiguity, whereas others are only approximately correct. This is because the basis of Chinese sphygmology is different. Dual terms also exist which may prove to be more exactly representative of the types given in part B of the Table. It is of interest that the "water-hammer pulse" is described in the Chinese work (tan, she, or yen tau), but does not appear to be represented in *The Canon*.

Some noteworthy theoretical considerations arising out of the Chinese work may be added as applicable to [Islamic] conceptions, without attempting to outline their full system.

We must study the subtler aspects of the nature of the human being by invading the domain of "occult" science (by some considered to be forbidden), if we are to understand the real position not only of the great Chinese work; but also that of *The Canon* itself. With such a key, many of the passages acquire an entirely new aspect and value. The expansion and retraction of "the breath"—so important in regard to the subject of the nature of the pulse, respiration and other periodic movements—are part and parcel with diurnal and other changes in what is called the "cosmic ether." By working out the formulae embodying the behavior of the human vibrations, using biometric methods, Baraduc makes concrete that which is usually passed over as unauthenticated and apocryphal.

The interpretation of the pulse depends on the interpretation of the body itself. The latter follows: "world-conception" rather than concrete anatomy. The natural phenomena of the patient harmonize with those of nature in general; and the two must be taken conjointly.

According to the classical style—"the two ideas"—"urge" and "change"—how important they are! They provide the key to physiological processes, and also to the understanding of the pulse. They represent something deeper than our modern idea "forces of nature"; they are over and above the ordinary course of nature, as expressed in the Latin "*praeternaturalis*." These two ideas provide the purpose of study as the physician sits with his hand on the pulse and his mind stilled for no small period of time. The relation between the root factors of life and those of the patient is to be elucidated; and they find their expression in terms of functional activity of the several organs of the body. Thence this science of sphygmology pays regard to the seasonal variations, the age, the sex, the personal constitution, the dominant "element," its phase (rise or fall), and especially the character of the vital force—active, passive, negative, positive. It aims at forming an opinion as to whether the illness is slight or deep-seated, easily curable or incurable, fatal or not, and if fatal in how long a time.

The permutations and combinations—the five *tsang* pulses, the six *fu* pulses, the seven *pyau* pulses, the eight *li* pulses and the nine *tau* pulses—all these afford ample scope towards a system which may encounter ridicule but is too rich in minutia to be lightly put aside.

For, quoting Broadbent again: "It is impossible to examine with attention a large number of pulses, whether among the healthy or the sick, without being struck by the extraordinary diversity of frequency, size, character, tension, and force met with. This diversity prevails quite independently of disease in both sexes and with all ages, especially in regard to diameter of vessel and tension and force of pulse. . . . Taking everything into account, there must, when we compare the small, short compressible pulse of one man with the large, firm and long pulse of another be great differences in the velocity and energy of the movement of blood through the capillaries in different individuals and clearly there are great differences in the circulation of the same person at different times. The fact that such differences are compatible with health and vigor is conclusive evidence that nutrition and functional efficiency, even of the nerve centers, are not in such close relation with and intimate dependence upon the blood-supply as we are sometimes apt to suppose."

The endless diversity in the pulse is not an incident, it is fundamental; the ancients sought to reduce it to a science because they (rightly) believed there was a law underlying this diversity. This goes with the fact that the various organs of the body actually vary greatly from the standards adopted by the pathological anatomist. The amount of blood discharged from the heart at each beat is very different in various persons. The state of health is as it were something over and above the ordinary physiological mechanisms so fully expounded in modern textbooks. The attempt to reduce nutrition to mechanical laws is an attempt to bind to mechanics that which is beyond mechanics.

Therefore, the study of the Chinese system, and of their world conception affords additional justification, not only for contending that the corporeal form, corporeal phenomena, and mental phenomena features, contours, build, mannerisms, talents—all belong together and are mutually illuminative, but also for proceeding to the formulation of these associations and inter-relations.

If in so doing, a medicine is built up in which disease takes a very minor place, and "soil" (a rather tiresome, though expressive word) a first place, which it is the object of the physician to elucidate and a continuously realize, It will at least be a guide to something approaching universality of application, and cease to attempt multi-specific therapy.

The idea that different sensations can be imparted to adjoining fingers by one and the same pulse may be discussed briefly here. It must be assumed that there are potential waves of different lengths passing along the artery at the same time. Long waves reach one finger, but not another. The long sweep of an artery can actually be seen in thin subjects. The waves usually thought of are the short ones induced by the force of the impact of the heart wall on the blood. Long waves consist of changes of tension in a spiral direction, and careful concentrative observation will allow such an accession to be felt.

The relation between pulse and special organs is not to be regarded as fanciful, when one obvious instance alone will justify it—the influence upon cardiacs: activity and force of beat which the state of the stomach exerts.

The frequency of missed beats, and the number of misses compared with number of respirations, exemplifies another very widely neglected aspect of the study.

The names given to pulses are of interest, but it is difficult to assign Chinese terms to particular Arabic or Latin names. It will suffice to present the following comparisons of-pulse-types with natural objects, and human actions:

(a) Natural objects: blade of small onion, solid within; stone bullet shot out of a crossbow; drop of water; down; drum-head; grate in a passage; hole in a flute filament of hair, scattered leaves, a pestle; pills; a silk thread, the handle of a staff or spear; untwisted string; worn-out cloth.

(b) Actions seen in nature: a bird pecking; a bubbling spring; the branches of a willow tree in a gentle zephyr in spring; drops of water dripping through a crack in the roof; frisking fish; feathers agitated by the wind; a bird flying low; liquid being constantly—gulped down; rolling of thunder; scattered leaves, swimming on the surface of water; the pace-of a toad embarrassed by weeds; water simmering in a kettle over a fire; waves running into one another.

(c) Human actions: throwing earth over an object; going by stealth; the strokes of a knife-point; a knife scraping bamboo; puffing and blowing in going upstairs; turning back.

(d) Ayurvedic sphygmology: Sarangadhara gives eight or nine verses showing how to examine the pulse, and gives the characteristics belonging to derangements of Vayu, Pitta and Kapha singly or in combinations. But this interesting subject is necessarily not dealt with here.

5 Additional points: frequency, or number of beats per minute; number of beats to each respiratory movement (inspiration plus expiration; mode of rise and mode of fall, and kind of pause at C, G, and W as one tests from skin to bone and back; the number of beats which occur before there is an intermission (an intermission is almost certain to occur in everyone), the comparison of the patient's pulse with one's own, or with that of a person of definitely equable temperament; the comparison of the pulse with that which should be present at a given season.

6 Broadbent remarks that the classification of pulses according to length, breadth and thickness is superfluous. "Deserting the path of observation, Galen did not see that a cylindrical tube would expand equally in all directions, and that there could not be any difference between its breadth and depth. . . . The permutations and combinations of large, moderate and small pulses, to the number of twenty-seven varieties of pulse—an over-refinement on purely theoretical or transcendental grounds, which led to extreme confusion."

A careful consideration of the text of *The Canon*, in conjunction with the Chinese writings, suggests that something more was in mind. One is dealing with waves, not with cylindrical tubes merely. There is a subtle distinction between breadth and thickness. Every tiny portion of an artery is fluctuating continuously both in health and disease by virtue of its vasomoter endowment; and it is this that is sought. Here as in so many matters in regard to the living being, the simple mechanistic conception leads to error (and to skepticism about the existence of unthought of detail). It is possible in the physiological laboratory to reduce the experimental animal into something very nearly a mechanism or actually into a mechanism and in that way secure results which triumphantly prove the contentions offered; but the living human being with the full possession of all his faculties constitutes a very different "proposition." Moreover, observations on the more subtle vibrations as by biometric study, go to suggest that there may be reason in the ideas in question (see Baraduc, *Les Vibrations de la vitalite humaine*).

7 Short pulse: impact sudden; acme momentary; subsidence of wave abrupt; dicrotic wave present; artery large; tension low.

Long pulse: impact deliberate; acme persisting; subsidence of wave gradual; artery contracted.

Normal pulse: impact sudden, acme moderately high; subsidence of wave gentle; tension moderate.

8 A small pulse may seem to be a large one in a wasted subject; hence, the pulse may be palpable in arteries in which it is not usually felt. The aorta may be felt. A pulse may seem small because carelessly felt in a person with a thick waist.

9 Strong or violent pulse. Impact strong; acme high; artery incompressible. Occurs temporarily in emotional states or after the bath. It is habitual in persons of passionate nature. Weak or feeble pulse. Impact faint; acme low; artery between beats is compressible.

10 Empty pulse: the artery feels as if it contained bubbles of air so that the fingers seem to fall on an empty place. Chinese simile: "The hole in the flute."

11 Equal pulse: this is always regular.

Unequal pulse is not altogether irregular. Supposing it to have no equality, and yet to preserve a certain period, such, i.e., as to extent of diastole, if there are two great and one small, then again two great and one small, and so on, such a pulse is unequal but regular. If it not only had no equality, but also no order in its inequality, such a pulse would be not only unequal, but also irregular. So, too, with the other kinds.

Irregular pulse: sometimes there is altogether an irregularity, observing no periods whatever. Sometimes there is regularity as to periods, but, having no continued order, they may in this respect be called irregular. However, in so far as they observe a certain period regularly, they are regular as to their periods, i.e., two great, two small, three great, three small, and so on (Aegineta after Galen).

12 The analogy between pulse and musical time is found in the Chinese work as well as in Avicenna. The fact that they compare certain beats with those produced on particular musical (stringed) instruments shows that they had something in mind like that suggested above. The *kin* pulse is so named after a musical instrument of that name; another pulse is compared with the vibration of the thirteen stringed instrument named *tseng*.

13 Relation between beats to musical time may be equally exemplified from Arabic poetry, for the richness of the poetic meters gives a simple and

ample parallel. Cadences, pauses (corresponding to intermissions of beat) of various lengths produced by the words and phrases and intonations belonging to emotional expression being natural sequences with evident relations to physiological variations. A short passage of poetry may sometimes be sufficient basis for a correct—impression of the whole, but it is better to hear the whole. So, in feeling—the pulse, much may be learned from the observation of the beats for a minute or two, and yet it is better to study a long series of beats in order to be sure there is no intermission at all. This thought is applied in Chinese sphygmology.

Rhythmical successions of words—musical rhythm—effects on emotional state and on physiological processes: the effect of words uttered in rhythm resembles that of musical successions of sounds. The different forms of rhythm which are adopted in different kinds of poetry have each their own effect on the emotional state, and tend to produce in the brain all the concomitants of the emotional state which they themselves belong to. Therefore the reciter is able to produce specific effects on the minds of his hearers. For this reason, the idea of rhythm and cadence can be pursued both in Arabian poetry and in Arabian music; and it can be pursued with respect to both aspects of esthetics in any country or language, though some languages are more potent in their influence, according as they are intrinsically more, or less, musical.

We may note that as the rhythm, whether of words or musical notes, evokes an influence on the pulse-rate in the course of their effect on the ear itself—both internal ear and the ear of the mind—so the emotional effect will be produced even though the hearers are not purposely or specially receptive. This emotional effect may be inevitable, or it may be deliberate. To quote from numerous passages in the touched with it a masterly touch, at once exciting to sadness and changing sorrow to gladness . . . went on to sing . . . to many and various modes, till our senses were bewitched, and the very room danced with excess of delight and surprise (Max Meyerhof, *The Book of the Ten Treatises on the Eye Ascribed to Hunain ibn Ishaq*); meseemed the doors and the walls and all that was in the house answered and sang with him"; "played a measure which made all hearts yearn (Richard Burton, *Thousand and One Hearts*, ii. 291; IV. 322; 1. 337).

When the effect is deliberately sought, it is stronger the more thoroughly worked out the principle is—which explains why some composers meet with more response than others, and why some compositions are considered more perfect or attractive than others. Yet a great composer may still be in ignorance of why that particular music should meet the need, he may be guided by the effect which the thought of the particular music has on his own organization; or he may even work according to stereotyped lines elaborated by theoretical developments and studies without having even "intuitive" feelings of his own. (Cf. Frederick Corder, *Modern Musical Composition*, p. 7).

Music, the composer, the listener—all three show the same possible aspects: the purely artistic; the emotional, the scientific or intellectual; and, more rarely, the inspirational and the celestial. The number of listeners: whom he will attract depends on the type of music which the composer employs. In this way, for some the pleasure is in the stirring-up of desire to accompany the music with the bodily movements of various dances; for others the pleasure is through the feelings; for others it is through the intellect (i.e., the fugue); for others it is through some glimpse of the abstract Truth which such music renders' possible, even though they understand not what it is doing. But the last named does not need of which it has been said, "The music of God is everywhere for those whose hearts are open to hear it."

We may also note that it is not only the pulse-rate and the manner of the pulse beat which is influenced by the musical rhythm; the effect pervades the body (bearing on this is a recent paper by Swale Vincent and J. H. Thompson: "the effects of music upon the human blood pressure" (*Lancet*, March 9, 1929, p. 534), because all the vibrations which belong to the secretions and excretions, and to the nervous system throughout are affected, and tend to harmonize, each in their own was the successive waves becoming set so that all reach the same phase at some same moment which recurs every so often. The movements belonging, for instance, to the emergence of secretory granules from a salivary or peptic cells or an adrenal cell, alter in rhythm during the time the music lasts—and possibly for some time after. That these movements are essential in the vital phenomena is easily verified by studying such cells, e.g., in invertebrate with the ultramicroscope, or even by studying saliva itself.

Additional remarks on rhythm. Let *a* and *c* represent the heart-sounds, and *b*, *d* the pauses. The ratio *b/d* is remarkably constant, whatever the number of beats per minute. Exercise, excitement, fever, etc. increase the rate, yet do not alter this ratio.

The normal rhythm is *ab/c/d*; that is, "triple time."

Double-time is *ab/cd*; where the sound is "tick-tack," *b* is the same length as *d* (for instance, owing to shortening of *d*). Such is what occurs in palpitation or tachycardia.

If, however, *b* becomes long, it shows that the peripheral resistance is greater. If a is stronger, *b* is longer. If the time is still triple, it necessarily implies that the pulse-rate is slower. But if this rhythm now becomes double-time, it shows that the resistance is too great for the heart, and that the heart is dilating or dilated. This happens for instance in chronic renal disease, or acute renal dropsy associated with myocardial change.

Four-time. (1) *ab/c/d/d*. The contraction is quick, the resistance is low. This occurs in fever or in excitement. This rhythm tends to return to triple by shortening of *c* to: *ab/d/d/*. The pulse is short.

Such a pulse may follow on a double-time pulse for instance in chronic renal disease. The prognosis is then grave.

A similar effect is produced if the cardiac contraction is not completed either because the muscle is too weak or the resistance too high. To find such a pulse forewarns the physician of cardiac asthenia forty-eight hours beforehand.

(2) *aa/b/c/d*. This is met with where the systemic and the pulmonary pressure are not equal. The former may be too high from renal disease, the latter may be too high from pulmonary or bronchial disease. Where the heart is hypertrophied, such a rhythm denotes failing heart.

The second "*a*" is not usually loud, but it may be as loud as the first "*a*." In such a case one could feel both ventricles beating separately over the apical region. *ab/c/c/d* may appear simply by holding the breath. It may also appear in mitral stenosis, in bronchitis with emphysema, in pericarditis, in pleural effusion and in cases of cerebral tumor.

Five-time: *a/b/c/c/d*; *a/b/c/c/d*; *a/b/c/c*^{1}*/d*; or *a/b/c*^{1}*/c/d*, These are all variants of "*bruit de galop*." The problem to solve in each patient is: which is the source of the second c? Is it the pulmonary valve? The causes are the same as of the preceding. *Pulsus bigeminus*: *ab/c*^{1}*d//ab/cd//ab/cd*, etc., in the case of the heart, but ab /cd /ab /cd / /ab /cd / etc., in the pulse at the same time. This type is found in mitral stenosis under treatment. Another form: *ab/cd//ab/cd//ab/cd//* etc. in the case of the heart and *ab/cd/d/d//ab/cd/d/d/* in the case of the pulse. This type is found in more advanced cases, and in cases of epileptiform attacks. It simulates alternate action by the two ventricles. Pulsus trigeminus; *ab/cd/d/d//ab/cd/d/d//*.

Some heart beats are too weak to reach the wrist or, in some cases, too little blood enters the heart. The pulse may therefore be irregular though the heart is regular or the pulse may be more irregular than the heart.

14 Intermitting pulse: a smaller beat occurs after one or more great pulsations: sometimes even the smaller beat is wanting. Inter current pulse: this is the opposite. When we are expecting an interval of rest, a supernumerary pulsation occurs (Aegenita).

15 "When the radial artery is completely closed by one or more fingers until the direct pulse is arrested, a feeble and retarded beat can be felt in the distal part of the vessel. This is because the blood-pressure is-low, the arteries are relaxed, and the force of the heart strong" (T. L. Bullock, *Progressive Exercises in the Chinese Written Language*, p. 52).

16 Variations in rate of expansion: Sudden deliberate; second expansion quick; or slow; first sudden and then tardy, or vice versa.

Rate of fall or contraction of the vessel: abrupt, or gradual and gentle.

Variations of degree of expansion: large, small, moderate; forceful or feeble; alike in every beat or unlike.

Variations of duration of expansion: first short, then long, or vice versa; momentary; persisting; or mean.

Variations of duration of pause: first short, then long, or vice versa. Pause when there should be a beat; beat when there should be a pause.

Variations of size of successive beats or between the beats: first diminished and then increased; first increased, then diminished. The size of the artery between the beats informs of the constant pressure in the artery. To ascertain it, roll the artery transversely between the beats; it should not be-palpable between the beats unless the skin is soft and flexible and thin.

Inability to feel the pulse between the beats means low tension; if easy to feel, the tension is high.

Variations in successive beats: the fourth beat may be irregular in one or other respect, or the fifth or the sixth or the seventh. Every beat may be different (irregular disorderliness).

17 Just before the wave begins to subside a second heat is felt (Broadbent)—"a swifter spring than before" (Aegenita)—the two phases of the one beat are unequal.

Cause: febrile heat. If the commencement of the diastole is feeble, and there is an increase in velocity towards the end and beginning of the systole, this shows that putrefaction is prevailing, nature hastening on the discharge of the fuliginous superfluities. But if, on the other hand, the commencement of the systole is feebler and the speed is towards the diastole, this means that heat is prevailing.

In fever cases, such a pulse is accompanied by density, and sometimes by largeness, if the artery is not too rigid (Aegenita). This pulse is characteristic of pericarditis.

18 Aegineta says: "The whole artery is not expanded at once, but first under the first finger, then under the second and so on; like a series of waves. The wave may be carried on straight or obliquely; it may be high but short, low but long, broad or narrow, unequal in speed and force." Rhazes says: "It is one which in breadth takes up much space of the finger; with this it is soft and full, but there is not touch rise or fall; one rise seems to join to another until it resembles waves, one following the other."

19 The feel is that of a worm wriggling. It is a weak form of the undulatory pulse. The size of the artery is not of the same inequality at all times. There are waves of pulsation, the whole artery not being distended at the same timed (Broadbent).

20 The artery, says Aegineta, feels swollen to the index finger, and very slender to the last finger. He speaks of a "failing" or "swooning" myurus, where the smallness of the last beat is maintained; and of a recurrent myurus, where the pulse resumes its original amplitude.

21 "Your first finger feels it small, your middle finger feels it large and swelled, and your little finger feels it small; the expansion is only slight" (Aegineta).

Cause: weakness of arterial wall, and wasting of the tissues round the artery. Significance: extreme debility; wasting from unresolved inflammation or any other cause.

22 As regards the dicrotic pulse, some have regarded it as a wave reflected from the periphery, but it is really the elastic recoil of the aorta that accounts for it. It is most distinct if the peripheral resistance is low. The semilunar valves form the fulcrum of the rebound (Broadbent, *The Pulse*, p. 26).

The first beat of the pulse is large, the artery rising strongly to the finger; then it stops and recedes; the second beat is small. The artery is as if repelled at the first beat and then trembles a little, and then quickly resumes its beat but less strongly, and at too short an interval.

23 The spasmodic (or "tense") pulse suggests that the artery is being stretched and dragged and pulled by its extremities like a cord (Aegineta). The "thrilling" (modern term), or tremulous pulse is hard, quick and frequent. It suggests the quivering of arrows thrown with great force (Aegineta).

24 The pulse is *visible* under the following circumstances: whence the radial artery follows an abnormal course, immediately under the skin; when the patient is spare, and the skin is thin; when the tension is very high, and the blood-vessels are enlarged and tortuous; and (entirely pathologically) in aortic regurgitation—where the artery is empty and collapsed between the beats, and the blood rushes in with extreme suddenness and violence, especially if the hand in raised. Such a pulse may be audible as well, and at the same time there is conspicuous throbbing of the carotids and temples and facial artery. The tension is here very low indeed. Visibility is not mentioned in *The Canon*; and whether the "empty" pulse is comparable at all with the "Corrigan" or not, is not clear. It seems hardly likely that so striking a pulse should not have been observed, even though they did not know its explanation.

Hectic pulse occurs in marasmus and phthisis. The components do not vary greatly. The pulse suggests "being entangled, and never getting free," because the state of disease is actually diffused throughout the body. This pulse therefore agrees with the Chinese type named "like a toad embarrassed a by weeds." This may be simply a form of the "thrilling" pulse.

Pulse-rate (Broadbent, *The Pulse*, etc.).

Increased pulse-rate: lowered resistance quickens the pulse rate. Diurnal a variations: the pulse-rate is greater in the evening, and slower in the early morning. The fact of the latter explains the following: morning headache; tendency to depression of spirits; to awake tired; the tendency to asthmatic attacks and epileptic fits (the blood-pressure is now minimal).

Posture: the erect posture adds eight beats to the minute.

Emotions: the rate is increased by fear (the force is feeble), and anger (force violent); the explanation is that the tension is increased by the emotions.

Exercise: at first the rate is increased as well as the force and the: pulse becomes "vehement." The explanation is threefold (a) nervous factors; (b) muscular action drives more blood to the heart and fills up the right side; the heart has to beat quickly and strongly to get it through the lungs; (c) accumulation of blood in the lungs produces breathlessness and panting.

Food: the rate is increased after food, and the vessels are relaxed.

Drugs, etc: stimulants increase the rate and cause greater relaxation of the vessels; alcohol and ether belong to this category. They lower the peripheral resistance by acting on the central nervous system, and also stimulate the heart directly; nitrites increase pulse-rate, and at the same time cause great relaxation of the artery. Pungent essential oils and ammonia increase the rate and through the peripheral nerves relax the vessels. Belladonna and atropin also increase the rate.

External warmth: slight increase of rate and slight relaxation of the vessels.

Respiratory movements: cause irregularities.

Increased pulse-rate in relation to morbid stages: these diseases in which the rate is increased, show the same rate, even in repose, but exertion makes the rate increase inordinately, out of all proportions. Emotional disturbance has the same effect.

In pyrexia: the rate rises according to the degree of fever, but chiefly according to the effects on the system and according to the patient's reaction to the disease. The peripheral resistance falls. The force may be increased (sthenic fever: pulse frequent, sudden, vehement, large, short, dicrotous) or diminished (pulse weaker, less sudden, less large, dicrotous). Towards the end of the illness, the weaker the patient, the greater the rate; even a few beats are per minute are serious. In septic fevers (septiczemia: modern term) a quick rate forewarns of shock, and a fatal issue (in puerperal cases). A "racing" pulse is a danger sign.

Among special fevers: scarlet fever is characterized by a very quick pulse-rate.

Specially quick pulse-rates. In young people: over strain from athletics; the "irritable heart" (the blood-pressure is high). In older people: sudden single acts of excessive exertion (sudden dilatation of the heart). Special cases: paroxysmal tachycardia: due to flatulence, emotions, gout; gastric trouble.

The pulse is frequent, short, variable in fullness and strength, not vehement, occasionally irregular. The heart-sounds are confused and short, and cannot be analyzed. May arise suddenly from a fright or sudden noise, or violent emotion.

In this condition the motion of the blood has not accelerated. It is a vibratory alternation of pressure with little onward movement. The left ventricle is not dilated. It may be that the ventricle is not expanding properly. Cf. Auricular fibrillation; auricular flutter. This form of pulse must be among those described by the Chinese, but certain identity has not been reached.

The quick pulse of "Graves' disease" might be included here.

Middle-aged and elderly women: here the occurrence of throbbing aorta may be referred to, though it is not a true "quick pulse"; it arises from lack of tone in the aortic wall.

Decreased pulse-rate. Increased resistance slows down the pulse. Habitually low pulse-rate (bradycardia) forewarns of the risk of cramp when swimming. In this category belong—the slower rate of jaundice; of fatty degeneration of the heart (not often met with here); the special pulses: *pulsus bigeminus* and *pulsus trigeminus*: heart-block.

Intermissions. Irregularity. On the one hand there is a variation of force between successive beats. On the other hand there is a drop of a beat, or an interposition of a beat.

Intermissions may be habitual or constant, the person being unconscious of it except during exercise or excitement It is accentuated when the body is fatigued or the disposition is nervous. The patient is conscious of it during prexia.

Occasional intermissions are produced in shock, in hypochondriasis after the use of tobacco; in fatty degeneration of the heart. In these cases the heart itself is beating, though hurriedly and imperfectly.

Irregularity is habitual in mitral regurgitation, where it is produced by the variations of pressure dependent on breathing. Inspiration forces blood into the left ventricle, expiration sucks it out of the left auricle. A similar occurrence is found when the heart is dilated, and under nervous conditions.

Irregularity is occasional as a result of flatulence of the colon, or stomach, which disturbs the action of the diaphragm; as a result of tobacco.

Irregularity is usually more serious than intermission.

Rules in regard to intermission in Chinese textbooks: omission of one beat after forty shows a lack in one of the five "noble" organs: "death will follow in four years, in spring." If there are no intermissions within fifty beats, the health is perfect. But if there is an intermission then, it has a similar significance to the preceding and shows "death will follow-five years later."

Other rules cannot be presented without also discussing the theory of the relation between pulse-type and physiological value of the several organs. Thus an intermission of one in 12, or 19, or 26 (and: so on), beats differs in significance according as the pulse-type is "heart," "lung," "liver," "kidney," and so on. After all, such a classification is justified, and it should be easily understood that intermissions under such circumstances might have distinct significances.

Relation of pulse-rate to respirator rate—in the Chinese works this form of observation replaces our own habit of estimating the number of beats per minute, and also the number of respirations per minute. In health there should be four beats to one respiration; five beats in the same period is allowable as consistent with health. But over five is pathological, and eight beats is a bad prognostic-sign. A reduction to three or two is pathological and a reduction to two is a bad sign. When death is imminent there may be only one beat to two respirations. Full details are stated to be given in *The Book of Eighty-One Difficulties*.

25 It maybe noted that the close resemblance between the Latin version and the corresponding passage in Galen makes it seem as if Avicenna had simply introduced a translation into Arabic from Galen. But in the Greek the natural pulse is simply a mean between extremes; and is so called presumably because usual in health; whereas with Avicenna this is not so: he speaks of a distinct kind of pulse, and is truly consistent in his usage of the term "nature"—"the body is a unity"—throughout his physiology, pathology, and sphygmology.

This rendering brings out the real meaning of the word "natural" (*tabi*). It is not synonymous with "normal," but refers strictly to "the nature," i.e., the state of the vegetative soul, when in health.

In short, a pulse which is "*mutadil*" is not therefore necessarily "normal"; still less is it necessarily "natural."

A pulse may be (a) natural and normal, (b) not natural, yet not abnormal, (c) not natural and also abnormal.

26 The last-named is, in Avicenna, taken to be a question of the degree of innate heat, and its relation to heat-loss; not a question of peripheral resistance as a factor in producing blood-pressure.

The influence of the three factors varies with the non-essential factors which may be associated with them at the given time.

27 Variants of large pulse, and their causes (Aeg.):—

Large and also soft: hot baths.

Large and also hard: hot intemperament, especially if there is dryness of the system.

Large and mean between hard and soft: massage; exercise.

Large and vehement: wine; anger.

Large and unequal: concealing anger: deceiving the doctor in regard to definite questions, as to possibility of heating factors.

Large and also a hasty contraction: putrefactive changes in humors.

Large and also quick and dense increase of heat in the heart from various.

Large only in appearance: emaciated state of the tissues at the wrist.

28 Causes of broad pulse redundancy of humidity from natural causes or from external causes, such as a soft artery (Aeg).

29 Cause of change from feeble pulse to strong pulse: (a) when the vitality becomes strong again, after being enfeebled from lack of food, wakefulness, immoderate evacuations, grief, cares, syncope, or any cause of intemperament. (b) When humors are matured: when noxious substances are excreted, when there is passion, when an intemperament is rectified; also, after use of

certain foods, of wines; after exercise (Aeg.)].

30 Hard pulse must be distinguished from a strong pulse. The latter is usually also large, swells up and strikes the finger forcibly. A hard pulse cannot be large, for the artery is unyielding; a hard pulse is also small, quick, and sometimes dense. (Aeg,).

Causes of hard pulse: hardness of artery; this is due to immoderate cold, dryness, or tension of inflammation, or spasm. (Aeg.)

Cause of strong pulse: the force of natural vitality, associated with hardness of the artery (Aeg.).

31 Other causes (Aeg.): humid state of artery due to (a) preternatural causes: coma, lethargy, dropsy, affections related to the serous humor. (b) Non-preternatural causes: more liquid food, much sleep, a more abundant diet, immoderate baths, hilarity.

32 If the harshness be slight, it shows that the inflammation is mild; if more marked, it means that the case is severe and dangerous, with a danger of of empyema or tuberculous change (Aeg).

33 Recurrent mousetail means: (1) failing vital powers, with a greater or less degree of prostration; (2) weak power, which is still struggling on in face of the odds (Aeg.).

34 Significance: inflammatory changes at the nerve-origins (meningitis; acute epilepsy). It can be felt after death has taken place, while the body is still warm (Aeg.).

35 It denotes inflammation in fibro-muscular tissues which are well supplied with nerves. A strong expansion is required, with adequate vital power. The hardness of the artery prevents adequate expansion.

36 The beats are indistinct; the dicrotic waves blend. At the same time the first cardiac sound disappears. Significance: crisis approaching by sweat (Rhazes, Haly Abbas), or by bowels; humid affections like sudden dropsy, lethargy, peripneumonia (Aeg.); typhoid fever; and malaria; extreme cardiac asthenia (Broadbent, *The Pulse*).

37 Significance: sudden loss of vital power due to excessive hemorrhage, diarrhea, cholera, etc. Failing life (Galen). In the formicant pulse the powers of life are at a still lower ebb than in the case of the vermicular pulse (Aegineta). Chinese simile: a silk thread.

38 The duration of the pause is lessened in old age. Equality between expansion and pause denotes a normal temperament of the body. It occurs in early life. If the pause is greater in duration than the expansion, the temperament is hot (that is, adult). If the pause is less than the expansion, it shows that the temperaments is cold (that is, the aged). Change of rhythm changes the rate and frequency of the pulse (Aegineta).

39 Full pulse is produced by plethora from food or wine; or any mere abundance of fluid-intake; empty pulse is produced by lack of nourishment, or undue discharges. The pulse feels warm: (1) if there is great heat in the

heart—the rest of the body being cold; (2) if the artery is in a sort of spasmodic state; (3) in catalepsy, and in persons who are becoming comatose. (Aegineta, quoting Archigenes).

The influence of low resistance upon the pulse—there is a sudden impact; the acme is brief; the subsidence rapid and the dicrotic wave is present. As it subsides quickly under the fingers it is called hurried. If at the same time the heart beat is forcible, the pulse is "full and bounding"—large, sudden impact, vehement; artery easily flattened. If the heart is beating feebly, the artery is—narrow; the pulse is small, easily compressed: the impact is not sharp, and therefore the fingers must be applied very lightly in order to be able to feel the pulse. An extreme degree of this kind of pulse constitutes the "running" pulse. Sphygmographic variants are: hyperdicrotic and "anacrotic" (which is a form of "gazelle").

Clinical causes of low resistance: (a) congenital; (b) transient—after bath, in fatigue, in exhaustion; after a meal, especially a hot meal; lack of nitrogenous aliments; alcohol; (c) emotional: anxiety, depression; (d) morbid states: obesity, fever; flatulence; constipation; sleeplessness; headache; nervous conditions; chlorosis; fatty degeneration of heart.

Other facts—a low resistance occurring in a person with a high tension is a bad sign; a person suffering from habitual constipation, and having a low blood pressure, should not be given purgation, much less mercurial purgation.

The influence of high resistance (high tension) on the pulse. This depends on the force of the heart. The pulse is full between the beats; the artery feels like a tendon or the *vas deferens*; or is even visible under the skin. The artery is large or small. It may be thrown into a curve; there may be nodosities along the artery. The wave is gradual; lasts too long; subsides too slowly; seems weak, but is more plain when one presses harder. There is no dicrotism.

A variant, called "virtual tension," is where the artery is large and full between the beats; moderate pressure does not make the pulse seem stronger, it is not compressible; the impact is sudden, the acme is short, and the subsidence is sadden. Such a pulse shows that the heart is unable to cope with the resistance.

Clinical causes: excitement; exertion; external cold (which drives the blood from the surface); migraine; early meningitis: early acute nephritis (the water cannot get out through the kidney); plethora; presence of certain waste products; in the blood which cause the small vessels to contract.

Types of Pulse and Various Conditions (Modern)

Sleeplessness—two types of pulse: (1) Impact gradual; acme long; may subside suddenly; artery large or small; full between beats, and usually not easily; compressible. It may be weak and yielding. The condition in this respect depends on the state of the heart; (2) Impact sudden; acme short; artery full between the beats; low tension. A sleepless person with such a pulse will be able to sleep readily in the daytime; he may be able to sleep sitting up though unable to do so lying down. The pulse is unstable.

Emotional excitement—impact strong; rate increased.

Fevers.

Catarrhal: the pulse varies according to the degree of obstruction to the pulmonary circulation (bronchitis, i. e.).

Pneumonia: pulse frequent large, vehement, dicrotic, not short, not compressible. The pulse can be felt with the third finger after pressing hard with the index finger, because the pulsation goes round the radial arch. When the lungs become engorged more and more, the artery is small, the beat is weak, but the heart itself is very forcible, working hard to get the blood round the lungs. Violent heart action and weak pulse!—venesection indicated!

Diphtheria: at first the pulse is weak and small especially if the heart is affected. The heart rhythm is *ab/c/d/d* or *ab/c/d/d/d/d*.

Erysipelas: large, soft, very dicrotic ; tends to become undulating

Septicemia: artery small; pulse-rate 140-200, beat sharp; compressible-tick-tack heart. The pulse varies much in different cases.

Pyemia: pulse frequent, and sharp apart from the degree of pyrexia. The pulse is that of shock.

Acute rheumatism: the character of the pulse varies with the degree of inflammation in the joints, etc.

Inflammation of serous membranes: first, small, long, frequent, hard, full between beats; not easily compressible. Later—shock: very small, weak, compressible; “wiry” or “thready” pulse due to the filling up of the abdominal vessels.

These characters are more noticeable with peritonitis than with pleurisy.

Cerebral conditions.

Tumor: rate slow; artery full-between beats. Later on the impact is very weak, and the acme short; the artery: small; the artery empty between beats denoting feeble heart and relaxed arteries).

Coma: the pulse varies with the state of the heart.

Convulsions: impact strong; rate increased; tension lowered; the blood pressure is sometimes increased, sometimes low.

Epilepsy: low tension is a bad sign; if a high pressure is present and continues, the case is tractable. The tension is always high in senile cases.

Meningitis: early cases show the “hesitating” pulse, the force is not quite constant; the time is not quite regular. The impact is deliberate, the acme long; the artery is contracted. The rate is slow. Later on, the rate becomes quick; there is no tension (owing to compression of the brain).

40 From the Chinese—in the male sex, the pulse should be more brisk than at C; in the female sex it should be more brisk at C than at W. From deviations of normal character of the pulse in women one may become aware of menstrual errors; of the presence or not of pregnancy, and the size of the pregnancy. The C pulse is noted for these purposes, and the right arm is used.—The exact details required for diagnosis require the application of the special

nomenclature of pulses which is richer in variety and subtlety than that of the list of

Age: bloom of life: pulse firm and full; persons of nurture may show a slow thin, even: soft, pulse, uniform at C, W, and G; if not uniform, such a pulse is a sign of shortness of life.

Old age: the pulse is slow and weak. Some old men have the pulse of long life—strong, firm, fairly swift, not skipping. (The presence of a skipping or hesitating character would show that the strength of the person is outward, 'and that life would not reach an extreme length.)

41 The following details from the Chinese work are tabulated for convenient survey:

Month and Season		Dominant Element (Chinese name)	Type of Pulse
First	Spring	mu	Tremulous: long
Second	Spring	mu	Remulous: long
Third	Fifth	t'u	Moderately slow, strong, hard
Fourth	Summer	huo	Superficial: strong, scattered
Fifth	Summer	huo	Superficial: strong, scattered
Sixth	Fifth	t'u	Moderately slow, strong, hard
Seventh	Autumn	chin	Superficial, short, brisk
Eighth	Autum	chin	Superficial, short, brisk
Ninth	Fifth	t'u	Moderately slow, strong, hard
Tenth	Winter	shiu	Deep, soft, slippery
Eleventh	Winter	shiu	Deep, soft, slippery
Twelfth	Fifth	t'u	Moderately slow, strong, hard

If the pulse proper to one season is met with during a different season, this is usually to be regarded as morbid, and may betoken a long or a short or a fatal illness according to the particular inversion. The autumn type in spring; the winter type in summer; the summer type in autumn, are grave signs.

It is to be noted that the third, sixth, ninth, and twelfth months form a fifth season and are not counted under the corresponding season. These months therefore correspond to those named in Avicenna "period between the seasons." The pulse changes are definitely specified in the above table, though only spoken of generally in *The Canon*.

42 That is, into the abdominal viscera, in whose veins the blood has now collected.

43 The thought underlying this passage may be expressed as follows: the person is supposed to have gone to sleep shortly after completing his meal. The body heat is now concentrated round the digestive organs in order to render digestion possible. The surface of the body becomes cold. Later when the first digestion is accomplished, the products are distributed to the various parts of the body. The heat now leaves the interior parts (i.e. the splanchnic system), and may be pictured as passing to the surface again, whence it had come so as to be ready to receive these digestive products. Once more does it preside or brood over them so as to render possible the further (third and fourth) digestion which they are about to undergo in this new situation.

The pulse is strengthened by two factors: (a) the access of body-heat which has now left the abdomen; (b) the food-products. The latter affect the pulse in two ways: (i) indirectly by making the temperament more hot; (ii) directly by making the arterial wall soft.

The person, it will be borne in mind, is supposed to be still sleeping. If he continues to sleep, the pulse will change in the manner next to be described;

if he awakes, the conditions also change, and the pulse alters as described below.

44 The word "exercise" includes (1) athletic sports of all kinds: running endurance tests, sprinting, gymnastics of all kinds, military exercises, laborious manual or physical work; (2) to work in the fields; (3) necessary exercise and walking exercise taken for health's sake and recreation; (4) mental.

45 The pulse is frequent, strong and the artery is moderately contracted.

46 Violent, but not excessive exercise, renders the pulse frequent, strong, sudden, vehement, large, short, dicrotous.

47 Exhaustion produces a frequent, sudden, short, not vehement, very dicrotous pulse. It is large unless the heart is very weak. Fatigue makes the pulse slightly slow; the force is diminished, the arteries are relaxed.)

48 The Chinese say: a pulse at C which is constantly superficial (or swimming) or deep in an otherwise healthy woman, with amenorrhea, betokens pregnancy; so also a high strong C pulse; a "slippery" pulse at C is a certain sign. An overflowing and high or deep and full pulse at the left C goes with a male pregnancy; a superficial and high pulse at the right C betokens a female pregnancy,

A number of other rules are given, the changes in the character of the pulse during the successive months of pregnancy being specified. Thus, first month: W pulse small, C pulse brisk. Third month: pressure with the finger makes the pulse seem to disperse. Sixth month: pressure does not alter the typical character. Seventh-eighth month: full, hard, strong pulse betokens a good labor. A deep and slender pulse forewarns of difficult labor.

Death of the foetus makes the pulse long and tremulous.

If the C pulse is continually small, weak, and sharp, and the nature is cold, with a tendency to shiverings, pregnancy will never be possible.

49 In sthenic fever, the pulse is frequent, sudden, vehement, large, short, dicrotous. In asthenic fever it is frequent, sudden, not vehement, large (unless the heart is weak), short, and very dicrotous. In peritonitis, the arteries are extremely contracted. (Broadbent.)

50 *Nafsaniat*. See sec 160, iii and iv and 174 sqq.

51 Excitement apart from anger.—The pulse is frequent, strong, and the artery is moderately contracted.—Note also the modern observation that "excitement always increases the blood-concentration, sometimes by as much as 10 per cent." (Barbour and Hamilton, *Journal American Medical Association*, 1927, pa 91).

52 Love: "now the lover's pulse is variable and irregular, especially when he sees the object of his affections, or hears her name, or gets tidings of her. In this way one can discover, in the case of the one who conceals his love and the name of his beloved, who is the object of his passion. . . " (*Dhakhira-i-Khwarazm-shahi*, Book vi. *Guftar* i, *Juz* 21, ch. 3; E. G. Browne's translation, *Chahar Maqala*, p. 89).

53 Pulse in convalescence from acute disease: the rate is normal or slightly slow; the force of the heart is diminished and the arteries are relaxed. The force of the heart and the arterial tone increase as convalescence advances.

(Broadbent, p. 51).

The "renal pulse": the frequency is normal or slightly diminished. force of the heart beat is increased. The arteriolas are contracted (*ibid.*).

LECTURE 13: THE SIGNS AND SYMPTOMS (DIAGNOSIS): URINE AND FECES

1 Because digestion, whose efficacy the urinoscopy determines, will have had time to be completed in a normal person.

2 The patient must have slept through the night.

3 The name *tafsira* is given to "inspection" because it "explains" (*yufassir*) and makes manifest to the physician; it is an indication or guide (*dalil*) to the patient's condition. See *Dictionary of the Technical Terms used in the Sciences of the Mussulmans* and E. J. Browne, translator, *Chahar Maqala*, p. 142) carried out with due observance of the above mentioned conditions provides valuable indications of health and disease.

4 Variants of (1). If the urine is plentiful also, it shows that a crude humor is being excreted by the urine. If there is also a sediment which is white, smooth, equable and plentiful, it shows that the digestion is good. If thicker and a sediment is present, it shows that the digestion is not altogether bad. If gritty, scaly, furfuraceous, with black, livid, green or fetid sediment, this shows entire lack of digestive function.

5

VARIETY OF WHITENESS	SIGNIFICANCE
(a) Mucilaginous	Excess of serous humor and crude humor
(b) Wax like	Liquefaction of adipose tissue
(c) Greasy, soapy	Liquefaction of serous humor; or it may denote diabetes, active or latent
(d) Musty whiteness:	
(i) Tinted with blood and pus	Ulcers discharging into the urinary passages
(ii) Not tinted with blood	Great excess of crude non-matured matter; vesical calculus
(e) Semen-like	
(i) Critical in form	Crisis in an inflammation arising in serous humor Diseases associated with vitreous serous humor Seminal emission
(ii) Not critical in form and no inflammation	Forewarns of apoplexy and palsy
(iii) Continuous throughout a fever	The fever will soon become quartan
(f) Lead-white, no sediment	Bad
(g) Milk-white in acute diseases	Ominous
(h) Previously colored in acute fevers	This shows that bilious humor has descended to some member about to develop an inflammation (i.e., the abdomen or which is worse, the head)
(i) Sudden change from red to white in the course of a fever.	The patient will become delirious.
(j) Whiteness persisting in a person apparently healthy	Absence of digestion (esp. in the venous system: *Chahar Maqala*) and in diabetes
(k) Whiteness like buttermilk in acute fevers	Fatal issue or wasting

6 Brilliant—Arabic *mushriq*; Latin: *clarus*. This term describes the color-

effect produced in urine by the presence of bile-pigment (as shown by its use in the next paragraph, where it is evidently equivalent to our "dichroic"). Other equivalents are bright, shining, refulgent, lustrous, luminous. In this passage at Avicenna seeks to warn the reader that a urine is not necessarily free of "bilious humor" because it happens to be very pale (white).

Brilliance, however, may be taken as evidence of health, for when metabolism proceeds quite normally, the urine assumes a peculiar clear shining color when viewed in the light. In this case, we may think of the various stages of catabolism proceeding without the formation of irregular intermediate substances, or by products and the moments of nascence are "sharp" throughout.

7 Unusual coloration of the urine, produced by eating saffron or cassia fistula must be borne in mind; tricksters may alter their urine thus (Alsaharavius).

8 The density here spoken of is not the equivalent of "specific gravity," through may of the statements in the text would apply equally even in the modern sense. The difference in specific gravity shown by the morning and evening urine was not discernible with unaided senses, but the general rule still holds that a persistently dense urine indicates a need for deputative foods (greens, acid fruits).

9 A very dense urine sometimes denotes that digestion is unduly excessive (*Chahar Maqala*).

10 In modern language we would say that urine which is clear when passed, but is turbid on standing; if acid, the deposit is (a) urates, which are not soluble in the cold; or (b) bacterial decomposition, stellar and triple phosphates separating out. We should heat the specimen. Also, a cloud in an acid urine would be albumen. Urine which is turbid when passed or becomes turbid on standing; if alkaline, the deposit is earthy phosphates (magnesium and calcium). It is met with after a rich protein meal or vegetable meal. Such a urine may become cloudy on heating, from the deposition of (calcium) phosphates, which are soluble again if acetic acid be added.

11 A moderately fetid urine denotes defective digestion: Haly Abbas

Offensive odor may be ammoniacal, as in alkaline fermentation Sweet; odor may be "fruity or like new-mown hay" in diabetes. Specific odors result from the use of certain drugs (modern).

12 The general significance of a sediment is that there is an excess of soluble or insoluble toxic substances in the blood.

13 The mineral constituents which are attached to the organic substances in the urine are: (1) perfectly oxidized; (2) partly oxidized and partly unoxidized; (3) entirely unoxidized.

14 The quantity of night urine (9 pm to 7 am) should equal that passed in two hours during the day. If greater, it denotes arterial disease. Vallery-Radot states that the day urine is normally thrice the night urine (*Precis de Pathologie Medicale*).

15

Tabular Summary of the Preceding Section

	Aspect	Color	Deposit
1 First stage of digestion			
Good	Urine plentiful, rather opaque	White	Homogeneous
Moderately good	Moderately fetor		Round contour, red
Absent	Watery, limpid	Pale or Yellowish (bilious humor)	Gritty, scaly, black, green or livid
Excessive	Very thick		
2 Maturation stage			
Normal	Opaque first then clear	White	White, homogeneous, delicate, sinks to bottom
Difficult	Clear first then opaque	Tends to be dusky	Discrete particles, sinks slowly
Quite absent	Opaque		
3 Completed	Clear; more dense	Color appears	Rapid, proportional to completeness of digestion
Digestion of Humors			
1 Immaturity in general	Turbid		Mucoid
2 Serous humor	Opaque or dense; foam persists		
3 Vitreous serous humor	Plentiful	White	Powdery, compact, not homogeneous
4 Viteline bilious humor	Dense	Foam persists yellow	
Oxidation of Humors			
1 Sanguineous		Tends to red	Coarse particles like barley flour
2 Serous	Limpid	Mucoid	Scale-like bodies float in it; cineritious
Gross humors maturing	Thick, opaque		
Cold humors putrefying	Offensive odor		
Fasting State	Very acrid	High	Red
Intemperaments			
1 Hot	Dark, offensive	White, if heat due to dominance of bilious humor	
2 Cold	White, turbid, limpid	Red if serous humor is obstructing bile ducts	
	No odor	Other colors	
3 Dry	Limpid		
Vitality			
Deficient because of cold intemperament	Turbid		
Weak	Oliguria		
Innate heat too great	Color deepens to red-yellow Odoriferous		
Innate heat increasing	Color deepens to flame yellow		
Innate heat subsiding	The urine clarifies		
Innate heat extinguished	Urine dark or black; in acute diseases it becomes colorless		
Functional Activity of Organs			
Liver inflammation	Turbid, red urine; sediment orobeal or tare-like or dusky read or hirudiniform		
Splenic disease	Sediment hirudiniform		
Renal inflammation	Red urine; ;no deposit if grave; otherwise orobeal or fleshy and yellowish		
Venous congestion	Limpid urine		
Stone in bladder	Dark		
Special Diseases			
Obesity	Urine abundant		

Puerperal convulsions	Urine dark
Fevers just before crisis	Urine may become thin and transparent
Fevers at other times	Opaque urine; depends on which humor is responsible and on outcome of illness
At the crisis	Polyuria; dark or black

Corresponding Table from a Modern Textbook (J. K. Watson, p. 156):

Disease	Quantity	Color	Odor	Deposit	Additional Modern Facts
Acute gout	Diminished	High		Urates abundant	
Acute nephritis	Diminished or absent	Blood-stained		Blood casts urates occ.	Urea diminished Albumin
Chronic cystitis	No change	Turbid	Offensive	Mucoid pus	Alkaline
Chronic nephritis	Increased	Pale		Scanty	Albumin varies tube-casts
Diabetes mell.	Increased	Pale	Sweet		Urea incr.; glucose; diacetic acid
Fevers, general and special	Diminished	High Turbid		Urates	Urea incr. Albumin, blood, tube-casts
Gastric catarrh	Normal	High		Urates, oxalates or phosphates	
Heart and lung disease	Diminished	Dark		Urates	Albumin
Jaundice	Normal	Frothy, greenish-brown		Varies	Bile present

Considerations arising out of this section. For the detection of changes in the composition of the urine, the ancients were restricted to the evidence afforded by its color, odor, and what may be called its "texture" (though this term applies usually to solid substances). The evidence was apt to be fallacious because wide differences of composition may produce similar appearances, etc., and differences of appearance do not always denote noteworthy changes of composition.

On the other hand, the limitations in the utility of these simple observations were balanced by the relatively vague conception of the bodily functions. The whole outlook on disease was lacking in detail without being basically incorrect. Thus, many diseased states were ascribed to defective digestive processes, a fact often overlooked today in the counter-attraction afforded by the study of diseased conditions which are not so ascribable. To say that the whole body is concerned in digestion is, broadly speaking, correct, especially if we realize that the term digestion covers what we call metabolism. In *The Canon*, digestion is viewed in two aspects: (1) that which begins in the alimentary canal and ends in the liver: (2) that which is called "maturation," which concerns the digestive products in their course through the body and ending in the tissues. If such maturation is not completed, surplus substances appear, and may undergo sedimentation. The phenomena of disease are attributable to this defective maturation. Consequently, the business of diagnosis and prognosis comes to be a matter of assessing the efficiency or otherwise of maturation.

The study of the urine is therefore directed to this assessment, its different physical properties being noted, both in health and under various unhealthy conditions. Translucence, opacity, separation out into visibility of various substances, the appearance of gaseous matter (in foam), and changes in odor—all these are interpreted in the light of the two-fold division of digestion above referred to: that culminating in the liver, and that culminating in the tissues.

This basis of study is reasonable, and it is not right that they should have been superseded as is the case in modern times. We are armed with a knowledge of innumerable chemical details about the substances met with in metabolism and nutrition in general. We have within our reach the very answers, in vastly improved detail and accuracy, to the self same questions which were paramount to Avicenna. But this technical laboratory knowledge tends to be sterile. Urinalysis informs us of the presence of abnormal substances, and of the amount both of these and of normal urinary constituents. By their means we reach conclusions about the functional capacity of various organs, and decide whether organic renal disease is present or not. But this is insufficient.

In the first place, these organs belong really only to one system—the nutritive; and in the second place, the illness has proceeded to another phase before the information from the analysis is available.

Moreover, the clinician has already taken up his tale before the laboratory work can possibly reach completion, so that those whom he instructs naturally receive the impression that such work is parenthetical, if not purely ritualistic. The clinical aspect of the case is discussed on its own merits, as might be done with a museum specimen which is possibly unusual, or with some topic for a connoisseur. The pathological aspect of the case, again, has a different, and separate interest.

It is not enough to combine these different aspects. Functional activities, morbid states, and clinical manifestations must centralize in the patient, and they do so, not because he happens to exhibit them all—but because they are one unity—himself. The organs whose capacity has been assessed are the gateways of entrance and departure; the crafts of the body—its real life—proceed in the tissues, which are the analogues of streets, houses, shops, plazas and bazaars. There are also the gateways of the senses, and these are directed routes into the audience-chamber of the presiding sultan himself. But he is not a separate being. He is in every member of the community—organs, tissues, sense-organs. Equity reigns throughout, and must be considered as much as the invaders of his domain.

So if we visualize in a practical form everything that is relevant we must not forget the dynamic aspect of the matter. Changes are going on hour by hour, and the laboratory cannot keep pace with them. Consequently, we shall in the end make use of the self—same data which Avicenna relied on entirely, and we learn from him to scrutinize the urine—not merely to find such things as albumen blood or pus and casts—but deliberately to know: (1) is there any insufficiency in the digestive processes in the pre-hepatic stages; (2) if not, is there any hepatic insufficiency, and in what direction; (3) if so, or if there is trouble in the tissues at large, arising out of ante abnormal condition of one or more of the "humors," which is at fault? In what way is it at fault? Is it entirely morbid or not? What degree as well as kind of defect is there—in modern chemical terms? (4) What is the degree of vitality of the patient (Avicenna) included "innate heat" in this? Is the vitality increasing, or failing, or inactive?—recovery from illness, or its duration, or succumbing top illness is often primarily a matter of vitality. (5) Other questions.

Such fundamental questions the modern practitioner (even in cities) can still answer from the simple data used of old and combine them with the intimate study of the pulse to realize the nature of the processes in the organs and tissues of the sick from day to day, and to feel himself actually armed with that real insight into the state of the particular patient which relatives and friends sometimes incorrectly assume him to have.

Changes in the urine were further studied in those days to decide on the presence or absence of inflammatory states in general, on febrile conditions in general, and to draw a relationship between these changes and certain symptoms, such as headache, pains in various parts of the body, palsies. In such cases, the character of the urine reveals the nature of the pathological changes in the humors, out of which the disease has arisen.

16

The Expectoration (from Aegineta; Haly Abbas)

The expectoration denotes some affection in the organs of respiration.

	Quality	Cause	Disease
Consistence	Thin and scanty	Attenuated humor	Not fully developed
	Moderate; homogenous, white, unctuous	Attenuated humor	Acme of a disease; maturation of morbid substances is complete
	Thick	Density of humor	Is declining
	Indefinite		Failure of maturation
Color	Black or dark	Intense heat	Outlook grave
	Yellow, golden, frothy, thin	Deficient maturation	Outlook not entirely bad
	Intense yellow, golden, frothy		Bad significance
	Green	Presence of green bile	
	Verdigris green		Fatal sign
	White	Serous humor	
	Red	Sanguineous humor	
Odor	Fetid	Putrefaction	Lung: air-passages
Mode of expectoration	Easy		Good sign
	Difficult		Bad sign

Notes:

Any color other than that of blood is a sign of a bad intemperament produced by pathological heat. Admixture with colors is intermittent.

The sputum may be described as an excrementitious humor which is forced out through the capillaries of the lung. It is contributed to by proteins which are imperfectly elaborated (i.e. hemialbumose) because of defective digestion. The mucoid material within it forms a film over the respiratory mucous membrane so that gaseous interchanges are interfered with. This is sometimes shown outwardly as cyanosis, especially when the amount of expectoration becomes very considerable—many ounces a day in some cases.

Menstrual fluid: This may be mentioned as being one of the excretions. Its characters are usually only noted in relation to lochial discharge.

Notes to Part Four

Lecture 15: Upbringing

1 Macrobius (Saturn v. 11) gives the following reasons why the healthy mother should nurse her child: "Just as the strength and nature of the semen goes to fashion the likeness of the body and mind, so the natural dispositions and properties are conveyed by the mother's milk."

2 Some idea of the cradle songs actually used in the days of Avicenna may be formed from the instances recorded by Fod-Strangeways in his work on the *Music of Hindostan* (pp. 62-68).

Baby mine, light of my eyes,
Here in thy cradle bright with flowers
Through sunny hours I bring thee sleep
I rock thee and sing thee to sleep
On the wings of my melodies
Srinangam island rises fair
Where the divided Kaveris meet
I lay thee down there at His feet,
At Sriranga raja's feet
Full sure of His tender care
The golden nails no longer move
On which my baby's cradle swung;
The song is sung; my ship is borne
Safe home, my ship is borne
Safe on the ocean of love.

3 Melilot: a sort of clover.

4 The word exercise includes lulling with music and singing lullabies: exercises are to be followed by gentle rubbing; and after that comes the bath, which must be cold (Aegineta).

5 Aegineta advises rubbing the gums frequently with the finger alone or anointed with fowl-grease while the infant is in the bath. When the teeth are just about to show, anoint the head with sweet oil and drop some into the ears. He recommends the amount of food to be increased and advocates warm baths. For itching of the gums, he says the flesh of an old pickle will relieve.

6 Cf. modern teaching: "Vomiting and diarrhea must always be looked upon as due to some cause other than dentition, particularly to improper feeding" (Elder and Fowler, *Diseases of Children*).

7 To the lay mind, all forms of gastro-intestinal catarrh, skin eruptions

and nervous phenomena (particularly convulsions) are attributed to dentition. Beyond admitting that there is usually some congestion of the gums, with exaggerated salivation, some loss of appetite, restlessness, temporary rise of temperature, and general uneasiness, Elder and Fowler (*ibid.*) teach that these various phenomena depend chiefly on rickets, and nutritional errors. There is however something to be said for the lay view.

After the teeth have appeared, Aegineta recommends the infant to be allowed to bite at a piece of nearly dry decorticated iris root. Butter and honey should also be inuncted.

8 Loss of voice in infants is due to constipation. Give cabbage juice by the mouth or rectum (Aegineta).

For vesicular eruptions, Rhazes advises: (1) decoction of dates and figs with fennel-water; (2) when the rash is fully out, give rose-water baths, myrtle-water baths; and then rub the skin with oil of roses.

Pruritus—forment and anoint with refined oil in which a little wax has been melted (Aegineta). Correct the acrimony of the mother's milk (Alsaharavius). Stop all sweets and salts in the mother's diet because they inflame the blood. Immerse the child in a bath of mallows, pearl barley, fenugreek, gouds, etc. (Rhazes).

Use gymnastic exercise to strengthen the body and prevent indulgence in carnal desires. Wine should be allowed sparingly. Pursue mathematics and being philosophy (Aegineta).

9 Snoring says Aegineta is due to improper food. The stomach becomes loaded with phlegm. A linseed linctus is to be given or honey. If that does not suffice to stop it, vomiting is induced as above.

Laryngismus stridulus may correspond to this and the preceding since the *laryngismus* is apt to occur during sleep and as aggravated by crying whereas stridor may disappear under both these conditions. The question of adenoids would also come to mind.

Lecture 16: The Regimen for the Mature

1 Rumi says:

How happy is he who takes advantage of early days and pays his debt to God.

Those days when he has power, health, energy of heart and strength.

That state of youth, like a verdant and fresh garden, yielding produce and fruit unstintingly.

The springs of strength and eager desire flowing and the soil of the body verdant through them (*Mathnawi*, p. 107).

The real object of conserving the energies of the body likes in the attainment of spiritual development. The actual bodily occupation is itself, if we will it so, the practical means of that attainment. The energy of will to associate this means of worship with the subjugation of the vices inherent in our frailty must be employed during the early years if we are not to find ourselves in old age powerless to advance along the critical stages of the journey to the only true goal. This principle underlies the idea of "right regimen."

The soil of the body and the desires having been consistently tilled and purified and tended, the coming of old age cannot but also reveal spiritual blossoms full of delight for others. Do not then wait, says Rumi till:

The soil becomes barren, dry and poor.
Never do fine plants grow from barren soil.
When the water of energy and the water of eager desire cease,
He derives no benefit from himself or from others;
The eyebrows hanging over like a crupper-strap;
The eyes watery and dim;
The face through old age like the back of a lizard;
The articulation and taste defective and the teeth useless;
The day late, the ass lame, and the road long;
The workshop (i. e., the physical body) gone to ruin.
And the work disorganized,
The roots of a bad nature fixed firmly in him,
And the power to tear them up diminished (*Mathnawi*, p. 107-8).

A picture admirable of the state of affairs in old age and also full of significance in regard to the well-being of the soul.

2 The value of exercise: (1) it hardens the organs and renders them fit for their functions; (2) it results in a better absorption of food, aids assimilation, and, by increasing the innate heat, improves nutrition; (3) it clears the pores of the skin; (4) it removes effete substances through the lungs; (5) it strengthens the physique.

Vigorous exercise invigorates the muscular and nervous system.

3 Equitation "strengthens the body especially the stomach more than any other mode of exercise. It clears the organs of special sense and renders them more acute. But it is most inimical to the chest" (Antyllus). The mental excitement of hunting is good for many diseases.

"Dancing," said Hippocrates, "is beneficial for amenorrhea and has been used for procuring abortion. Swimming in the sea has a warming effect and strengthens the body and renders it thin. It is beneficial for dropsy, skin-eruptions, elephantiasis. But it may be injurious for the head for the head and nerves. The body must be rubbed with oil first" (Oribasius).

4 Reading aloud in a high tone helps to remove redundant humors through the skin. Reading in a moderate tone helps the insensible perspiration throughout the body, attenuates effete matters, and gets rid of saliva,

mucus and phlegm by coughing. Frigid people should read aloud frequently because of its warming effect. This method of exercise requires control and judicious management if the system is full of depraved humors or if the stomach is loaded with crudities, because otherwise noxious gaseous substances are distributed all over the body. Ritual: first empty the bowels then anoint the body, then sponge the face and lower parts with water. The tone of the voice should be moderate at first, and the person should walk about while speaking. Then a louder tone should be used and verses should be repeated several times.

5 The urinary signs of the proper time for undertaking exercise are specified in Aegineta. The urine should be deep yellow, because this shows that the digestion has long since been completed. If the urine is moderately pale, it shows that the digestion has only just been completed. An evacuation of the bowels is here indicated. If the urine be watery, it shows that there is still some undigested chyme in the stomach.

6 Two kinds of leprosy are distinguished by the Arabs: *baras* and *juzam*. The former is "white" and the latter is "black." The latter is leprosy of the joints. Both are ascribed to dietetic errors, especially fish-eating and milk drinking (Burton, iii. 370). The term used in the present passage is *juzam*.

7 Polenta=*sawiq*=ptisane (Lane). This is native frumenty and green grain (mostly barley), toasted, powdered, mixed with dates or sugar, and eaten on journeys when cooking is impracticable. It is carried in a meal-sac (Burton, iv. 491).

8 Soured milk is milk artificially soured. It is eaten with rice and is a component of *salatah*, cucumber salad (Burton, iv. 132; who adds, "All nomads who live on milk never take it fresh."

9 Kabab: this is mutton or lamb cut into small squares and grilled on skewers. It is the equivalent of our roast meat (Burton, iv. 154).

10 Strictly speaking, instructions on diet to the patient should rest upon practical acquaintance with the culinary art as having a prior place over the questions of forbidding and allowing such and such articles of food, food values, and the like. The form in which a given article in the dietary is to be given is of real importance, and the combinations into which the foods enter require notice at least to the same extent as is done with the ingredients of a medicinal prescription. Mutual decompositions occur with foodstuffs either before or after ingestion. Interactions may render the " composite " indigestible, or non-palatable, or actually harmful; the use of too little of one ingredient in a recipe or of too much should be prevented; the temperature to which the mixture is exposed—the rate at which that temperature is reached, whether too quickly or too slowly-whether it is maintained steadily or whether through some mismanagement the "mixture" was allowed to cool noticeably in the midst of the operations—all such details call for consideration both as to a possible explanation of persistent gastro-intestinal trouble, and as to guiding the manage-

ment of any ailment in any system or organ.

The displacement of *materia medica* from its ancient throne is partly to be ascribed to a cessation of attention to detailed knowledge about herbs and the part which horticultural skill and care, as well as climatic conditions and geographical factors play in the production of efficacious remedies; it is also ascribable to entirely insufficient attention to the preparation of the recipes-for these originally were exacting as to manner of compounding; and both these types of indifference rest upon a skepticism as to the possibility of such details being of the least importance. In the absence of knowledge on these points, the decriers of the use of drugs, and of complex prescriptions speak unjustifiably.

So, again, in the matter of the preparation of the invalid's food, or the dietary for the chronic ailment, it is reasonable to plead for that care whose real importance is every day proved by those who, having the means, will desire their meals from some one chef in preference to another.

In the whole of the preceding chapter, Avicenna is referring to a cuisine which is foreign to us. Perhaps of all European countries, Spain offers the nearest approach to his. Those who have been in the East, and have inquired into the practical details in their cookery recipes, not merely such as may be available in written form, but also such as are actually carried out in well-to-do establishments or by the humbler housewife, (for in this country also there is much difference between Beeton and actual practice) are more easily able to follow Avicenna's nomenclature.

Very little research suffices to convince the enquirer of the very great scope of this subject. Interesting as it is, it would, therefore, lead too far to attempt proper discussion in these pages. It must suffice to insist that the names of foods and dishes which Avicenna gives bear a different meaning to those same names with which we are familiar. Confusion would only be prevented by giving the names in the original language. Many of the words are Persian; some of the dishes are Syrian; others are Indian.

The following notes from Lane and Burton will serve to show the type of dishes which may be regarded as characteristically Arabian.

"Among the more common dishes are the following: lamb or mutton cut into small pieces, and stewed with various vegetables, and sometimes with peaches, apricots, or jujubes, and sugar; cucumbers or small gourds, or the fruit of the black or white eggplant, stuffed with rice and minced meat, etc.; vine-leaves or pieces of lettuce-leaf or cabbage-leaf, enclosing a similar composition; small morsels of lamb or mutton roasted on skewers, called kabab. Fowls simply roasted or boiled, or boned, and stuffed with raisins, pistachio nuts, crumbled bread, and parsley; and various kinds of pastry and other sweets.

"The repast is frequently commenced with soup, and is generally ended with boiled rice, mixed with a little butter, and seasoned with salt and pepper;

or, after this, is served a water-melon or other fruit, or a bowl of a sweet drink composed of water with raisins, and sometimes other kinds of fruit, boiled in it, and then sugar, and with a little rose-water added to it when cool. The meat, having generally little fat, is cooked with clarified butter, and is so thoroughly done that it is easily divided with the fingers. A whole lamb, stuffed in the same manner as the fowls above mentioned, is not a very uncommon dish. (Lane,l59 Nights, i. I7I.) -

"They brought him . . . dishes of poultry besides other birds and brewises, fritters and cooling marinades." (Night 415, Burton). . . . "a mess of cooked pomegranate seed." (Night, 712.)

"A very common kind of pastry is a pancake, which is made very thin, and folded over several times like a napkin; it is saturated with butter, and generally sweetened with honey or sugar; as is also another kind which somewhat resembles vermicelli." (Lane.)

adasiyah: soup of yellow lentils, made by boiling them in water till nearly dissolved, and then adding vinegar, coriander, and salt.

faturat: junket: a light food for early breakfast, of which the *fatirah*-cake was a favorite item. (Burton, vi. 160.)

Fruits: almond, almond-apricot apple, apricot, banana, bergamot pears bitter orange, blood-orange, cherry, citron, date, fig, grape, hazelnut, jujube, lemon, lime, lote, mulberry, olive, peach, plum, pomegranate, quince, shaddock, sugar-cane, sweet-orange, sycamore-fig, walnut, water-melon. (Lane, i. 30I; Burton, v. 28I-287)

hisrimiyah: a broth of kid's flesh, lamb, and fowl seasoned with *hisrim*, the juice expressed-from the grape while unripe.

jamar: palm-pith eaten with sugar (Burton, v. 284).

kaak al-id: "cake"; bun; a special sweet cake eaten with dates and sherbets. (Burton, iv. 394.)

kabab .

kunafah: vermicelli cake; a favorite dish of wheaten flour worked somewhat finer than our vermicelli, fried with *samn* (butter melted and clarified) and sweetened with honey or sugar. It may be-sweetened with bees' honey (Night 989) in preference to.the frequently used various syrups. (Burton, vi. I50.)

sawiq: polenta.

sikbaj: acid minced fresh meat, dressed with vinegar and honey, or with acid syrup. Raisins, a few figs and chiches were sometimes added. (Lane, i. 435.)

shurayk: a cake or bun, the size of the palm of the hand, with two long cuts and sundry oblique cross cuts, made of leavened dough, glazed with egg and clarified butter, and flavored with spices (cinnamon, curcuma, artesmisia, prunus mahalab, and sundry aromatic seeds specified by Lane as aniseed, nigella, absinthium (Artemisia arborescens) and camphor, etc. (Nights, v.

509.)

Soured milk.

yakhmi: stew. A complicated broth prepared from rice and meat. (Burton, iv. 387.)

zardah: a rice dish. Rice dressed with honey and saffron (ib. p. 385).

zirbaj: a sour meat dish similar to *sikbaj* (above).

11 Of the total humors of the body, a certain proportion reaches the subcutaneous tissues and may become stagnant in that situation. They require dispersal and the agents used for such purpose are called "discutients." Possibly some of these agents were what are now called diaphoretics. But it must be remembered that the theory supposes the existence of matters which are discharged either in fluid or in gaseous form, the exit being by different "pores" in each case.

Lecture 18: Concerning the Regime of Those Whose Temperament is Abnormal

1 Galen adds: if bile passes down plentifully, good; but if it regurgitates into the stomach, vomiting will become inevitable and tepid water should be taken. Exercises should be done before meals; and they must be slow and gentle in character.

Gymnastics are not required by persons of very hot temperament; walking exercise is enough. The baths may be taken after a meal in such cases.

If the temperament is hot and dry, the regimen should be diluent (succulent) food—bathing—avoid much or strenuous exercise.

During the summer the bath should be taken early and repeated after the main meal. Cold drinks may be allowed.

2 Aegineta adds: "the dry kind is the worst because this is the form characteristic of old age. Warming agents and diluents are needed (namely moderate exercise, moist heating food, heating wines, plenty of sleep). The bowels should be emptied daily. Venery should be avoided.

The moist kind is bad because there is a liability to rheumatic affections. Here avoid bathing and take light exercise often and make use of moderately calefacient inunctions.

If the temperament is dry, avoid tiring exercise, exposure to the sun, prolonged wakeful state, cares, venery.

If the temperament be humid, more exercise is necessary, the digestion in the stomach needs assistance and also the urinary secretion. Rheumatic and plethoric complains are liable to occur. The bath should be taken before meals and twice or three times in the day. Aperients and diuretics should be given before food. Masticatories, cathartics and diuretic wines are allowable.

3 Note that emaciation, leanness, or wasting is here understood as including the condition of a person convalescent after a long illness.

Other causes of lean habit of body: attenuant regime, attenuant medicines; mental anxiety in a person of dry temperament.

A warm temperament also predisposes to leanness. Fat persons are of cold temperament and there therefore benefitted if made warm.

4 Pitching consists in rubbing into the skin a preparation made by melting dried pitch in a little oil, and warming it to a suitable consistency. The skin must be shaved first. The plaster is then removed before it has quite set. it is then warmed again and reapplied. This is repeated several times.

Bituminous and sulphur baths may be used with the advantage.

5 It will be seen that in this regimen, the bath is taken on an empty stomach. It will be noted that the rules regarding bathing state that a person is made thinner if he take his bath after a meal, before th food has digested.

Sleep should be encouraged.

Emotional life: pale persons who are poorly nourished should become stouter if they were aroused to anger and mental excitement (Aeg.).

If only a part of the body is wasted as for instance after fracture, the vital powers must be stimulated; moderate friction will encourage the circulation in the part and warm water is douched over it in small quantities until the skin reddens and swells. Suitable exercises are also carried out. Pitching may be done. If the part feels cold, friction with linen cloths should be done or some mild calefacient applied, like thapsia made up with honey or was (Oribasius).

6 Other details: (Aeg.) meals: only one a day; drinks: take a fragrant draught before a meal. Wines: use thin, white wines. Sleep: must not be protracted. Baths: use natural disphoretic waters. If these are not available add flower of salt to a sea-water bath or add a large quantity of nitre. Sandbaths. Massage: dry rubbing with thick towels; rub with rough salts such a s nitre. Medicinal agents; attenuants that is medicines which attenuate the humors, wild rue seed and tops of macedonian parsley, various strong diuretics with or without pepper and with or without asarabacca and anise. Also the other remedies named in brackets above. Winter favors the formation of flesh and blood.

Lecture 19: Changes in the Atmosphere

1 The Symptoms Premonitory of Diseases

Symptom	Remedy	Danger
Tremor of the heart continuing persistently		Sudden death.
Nightmare and vertigo frequent	Evacuate the gross humor.	Epilepsy; apoplexy
Jerking movements of the whole body	Evacuate the serous humor.	Convulsions; apoplexy
Ditto, persisting long enough to affect vision and bodily movements. Also plethora	Ditto	Ditto
Loss of sensation in the limbs	Ditto	Paralysis
Much twitching of the face	Procure cranial depletion	Trismus
Face becomes very red; tears flow; vision fails; headache	Blood-letting purgation, etc.	Insanity; delirium

Inexplicable sense of gloom and dread	Evacuate the oxidized humor	Melancholy
Face reddens, swells, and darkens and stays		Lepra
Body heavy and relaxed; veins prominent	Bleeding	Rupture of a vessel; apoplexy; sudden death
Face, eyelids and limbs slightly timid	Treat the liver	Dropsy
Great stench from the feces	Treat the putrescence in the vessels	Fever
Offensive urine	Ditto	Ditto
Lassitude and loss of spirits	Ditto	Fever
Loss of appetite; undue appetite		Illness (in general)

2

Description	Morbid Sate Corresponding
Heaviness and stabbing in right side	Liver disease
Heaviness and tightness in sacral and lumbar region; urine abnormal	Kidney disease
Colorless stool	Jaundice
Persistently scalding urine	Vesicle or penile ulcers
Burning pain in anus on defecation	Dysentery
Anorexia, vomiting, distension, pain in legs	Colic
Pruritus ani, not due to worms	Piles
Eruption of many boils and pimples	Internal imposthumes; rupture of an abscess
Serpiginous eczema (ringworm)	Leprosy; black vitilego; white
White morphen	White vitilego

3 Persons of humid and phlegmatic temperament are not liable to develop fever from exposure.

4 Instructions differ according to the season of the year in which the journey is being made. In winter, a purge should be taken before starting. The binder should be longer than above stated. The body is not to be anointed at the stages in the journey. In summer the body must be covered to protect it from the sun. The binder is to be as stated above.

5 Rhazes suggests chewing pickled onions en route to assuage hunger. Note that nighttime is preferred for traveling across deserts or in hot countries generally.

6 Rhazes gives: water with polenta sprinkled on it and a moderate quantity of salt. Or hold cool liquid in the mouth, pour cold water on the hands and feet.

7 At the end of a journey, take a comfortable apartment; do not go near the fire. Rest. Do not go to sleep for an hour. After that, the bath may be taken. Massage is then given until the skin is all ruddy, then the traveler may go to sleep on a soft couch (Rhazes).

8 Persistent sea-sickness: avoid all food. Take a little vinegar and honey with water in which thyme has been infused or pennyroyal water with some fine polenta or take some weak fragrant wine with fine polenta. Take artabilious remedies (Rhazes).

Simple precautionary measures: (1) counteract the disagreeable smell of the ship by sniffing at quinces, thyme or pennyroyal. (2) Do not look at the sea. (3) Beware of drinking wine. (4) Note the diet already mentioned. (5) Have remedies against vermin. Mercury, oil, long birthwort on wearing wool smeared with oil or mercury ensures against lice.

Notes to Part Five

Lecture 20: On the Treatment of Diseases

1 These channels comprise: (1) the ordinary anatomical inlets and outlets of the body; (2) orifices of ducts which open into the alimentary tract, etc., and are not visible externally; (3) channels of microscopic size which would not be included in an ordinary anatomical description; (4) tissue spaces which are not defined by limiting membranes, but are traversed by fluid constituents of the body. The terminal portion of a duct often shows an ampullary dilation which comes under the category of a "receptacle" in the text; (5) expansions of lumen of this kind also occur in the vascular channels; (6) perivascular and peritendinous sheaths.

Lecture 22: The Use of Eliminants: Purgation, Emesis, Cupping, Venesection, Leeches

1 Articles of food which increase the alvine discharge (Aeg.) and purify the blood: mildly aperient foods: soft eggs, potherbs: (beet, mallows, cabbage, sorrel); shellfish soup. More strongly aperient foods: milk whey with salt; herb mercury boiled in water with salt, honey, elder-tree leaves; polypody root (oak fern), two drachms sprinkled on pickle or taken in a ptisan; broth of old cock taken with our without two drachms of bastard saffron; aloes to the amount of three chickpeas taken at supper-time; dodder or thyme in wine taken after a moderate supper. Still stronger: dodder of thyme (one dram) wine, infused in vinegar and honey, taken before breakfast in spring time.

2 Annotations by Costaeus to this chapter refer to sea sickness. In this case, if much bilious humor is being brought up, all food should be stopped or only the merest taste of light food allowed. If the vomitus consist of phlegm, light food may be allowed. The reason is that in the former case there are sure to be remnants of the unhealthy humor left behind in the stomach. If the vomitus consisted of mucus or phlegm, one knows the stomach is empty and one may consider whether one should leave the stomach devoid of food or not. If the emesis is the result of a medicine, food must not be taken unless the stomach is weak in which case one may give a little light food with three glasses of cold water.

3 Annotation by Costaeus: the object underlying some of the above measures is to centralize or concentrate the life-breath in the interior of the body (i.e., round the solar plexus) and prevent it from being disseminated over the

body in which case there would not be enough in the vital centers to maintain life.

4 Enemas are useful to relieve constipation when the stomach is weak and will not tolerate purges. (Aeg.)

5 Materials for making enemas: If the humor in the intestine is seo-mucous: give beet, decoction of dried figs, dill, honey, nitre, root of wild cucumber. If the enema is used to remedy undue dryness: give marshmallows, fenugreek, chamomile, oil, or small quantities of honey—all of which are emollients. A half hemina of oil (a half-pint) may be given. (Aeg.) The addition of honeyed water makes the mixture more efficient than plain water. The mixture must, of course, be tepid. Astringent enema: vervain (Celsus). Acrid enema: sea-water with or without oil, nitre or honey. This kind of enema is very drastic and painful. (Celsus) The patient must resist the first desire to go to stool. (Celsus)

Modern usage is much more simple. Plain water, soap-suds or thin gruel is the usual base and the amount to introduce is from a half to three half-pints of fluid. To either of these bases may be added one ounce of castor oil or glycerin or castor oil with a half-ounce of turpentine. Olive oil is sometimes used (6-10 ounces). Half-ounce injections of glycerin are also popular.

6 Note that douching over the head may be done from a jug or similar vessel or in the form of a spray or shower. The fluid may fall from a height or close to the part. The part treated may be the head or a limb or other part. The fluid employed may be plain water or medicated. If medicated it may be mineral or herbal. If mineral, artificial or natural.

7 The distinction between wet and dry cupping is not very evident. In the medieval drawings referred to below the use of scarifiers with the cupping seems usual. It will be clear that the action of the two measures is quite different, dry cupping leading to the formation of autoemolysins, the wet cupping being more of the nature of a mild evacuation, a less drastic procedure than bleeding from a vein—perhaps largely because the victim did not see the blood and because the quantity of blood withdrawn was necessarily limited in amount.

8 During the Middle Ages in Europe cupping was practiced as part of the ritual of the bath house. The subject is very fully dealt with by Alfred Martin (Jena, 1906) who presents illustrations from contemporary literature. Though the practice has disappeared from our customs, it has done so only comparatively recently and may be still practiced among other peoples. The necessity for several attendants during the course of the ritual determines its restriction to public institutions, only the very wealthy having their own suite for their own families. Both sexes were employed in the service which included most of the operations now confined to the barber: women were chiefly employed for fetching and carrying, men for seeing to the heating apparatus. But the service of cupping and venesection was confined to men, generally the

bath men who specialized in the work.

The rules found in *The Canon* appear to have been conformed to. Thus the association of cupping with bathing is found in the pictures representing the bather in the hot room or calefactorium, sitting on a special bench, with his feet in a hot bath reaching to the knees to make the blood watery while the bath man is engaged in applying the cupping glasses or horns.

The practice of cupping in the ordinary routine of life was an expression of the universal desire for ensuring prophylaxis against disease. Concurrently it was applied for the treatment of declared disease and this use survived the other. Even in these days it is occasionally employed with advantage and the method is deserving of much more attention by both students and practitioners.

9 The leech must not be let go until it has taken proper hold, as one can tell by the sinuous movements of the neck and from the circumstance that the head forms a right angle to the body.

To ensure that they will not crawl into the gullet or nose or anus, one must draw a thread through the tail end from above down, not from side to side, otherwise one would injure the large blood vessels of the animal.

Place chosen for the application. One must not apply leeches to unhealthy skin, or to places where there are subjacent large vessels, or where the skin is very thick (palm of hand; heel), or in a situation where healing would subsequently be interfered with because of pus or septic matter flowing over it from near by.

10 Alum, cobwebs, pitch, gunpowder, hydrates, sesquioxide of iron, or pressing the skin into the folds have been advocated. The cautery has been necessary as a last resource. All such remedies should be at hand.

Do not leave the patient till the bleeding has quite stopped, and if it is a child, watch it the following night as well.

If a leech should have got loose and been swallowed, give saltwater to drink, copiously. If a leech has wandered into the anus, give a salt-water enema.

Do not use leeches again if they have been applied to a case of typhoid fever, cholera, smallpox, or syphilis.

Annotation by Costaeus: Leeches are very effective also for pleurisy and for opening the hemorrhoidal veins.

One may detach them before they are full, because the patient is fainting or develops cramps.

Bibliography

Primary Source

Abu Ali al-Husayn ibn Abd Allah ibn Sina, *al-Qanun fi'l-tibb*. Critical edition prepared under the auspices of the Institute of the History of Medicine and Medical Research in association with VIKAS Publishing House, Pvt., Ltd.

Secondary Sources

Abbott, Maude. *Descriptive Catalogue of the Medical Museum of McGill University*. Part IV, Sec. 1. Oxford: 1915.

Allen, Charles. *Curious Observations About the Teeth*. 1687. London: Bale Danielsson, Ltd., W. 1.

Ameer Ali, Syed, *A Short History of the Saracens*. London: Macmillian and Co., Ltd., 1921.

Ameer Ali, Syed, *The Spirit of Islam*. London: Christophers, 1923; also, "The Life and Teachings of Mohammed." London: Williams and Norgate, 1873.

Ardalan, Nader and Laleh Bakhtiar. *The Sense of Unity: The Sufi Tradition in Persian Architecture*. Chicago: ABC International Group, Inc., 1999.

Aquinas, St. Thomas. *Summa Contra Gentiles*. Dominican translation. London: Burns, Oates and Washbourne, Ltd., 1922.

Aquinas, St. Thomas. *Summa Contra Gentiles*. Rome: 1894.

Aquinas, St. Thomas. *Summa Theologica*, especially Part I, questions 60-102. Rome: 1894.

Aquinas, St. Thomas. *Summa Theologica*. Dominican translation (vol. 4). London: Burns, Oates and Washbourne, Ltd., 1922.

Arnold, Fr. *Imitation of the Sacred Heart*, 1846.

Arnold, Sir Thomas. *Painting in Islam*. Oxford: Oxford University Press, 1928.

Avicenna, *Dahish namah*, quoted by E. G. Browne in *Arabian Medicine*. Cambridge: Cambridge University Press, 1921.

Ayurvedic Writings and Works. Ayurveda Journal. Calcutt.

Ayurvedic, notes on. *British Medical Journal*, 1923, 477-479.

Babbit, E. D. *Principles of Light and Colour*. East Orange, New Jersey, 1896.

Baraduc. *Les Vibrations de la vitalite humaine*. Paris: J. B. Bailliere et Fils, 1904.

Barton and Castle. *British Flora Medica*. Chatto and Windus, 1877.

Bauer, J. Ann. Int. Med., 1928, ii. 127.

Beale, Lionel S. Various Works especially: bioplasm; microscope in medicine, how to use the microscope, the liver. 1878-1880.

Bechold. *Die Kolloide in Biologie u. Medizin*. Dresden: Theodor Steinkopff, 1912.

Benson, Mgr. R. H. *Light Invisible and Other Writings*.

Bier, August. *Gedanken eines Arztes uber die Medicin*. IV. Die Seele, Munch.

Med. Woch., 1927, 684-6Das Buch vom gesunden und kranken Menschen. Leipzig: 1893.

Broadbent. *The Pulse*. London: Cassell and Co., 1890.

Brockelmann, Carl. *Geschichte der arabischen litteratur*. Weimar: 1898.

Browne, E. G. *A History of Persian Literature Under Tartar Dominion*. Cambridge: Cambridge University Press, 1920.

Browne, E. G. *Arabian Medicine*. Cambridge: Cambridge University Press, 1921.

Browne, E. G. *Chahar maqalah*. Translation, E. J. W. Gibb Memorial, xi, 2. London: Luzac, 1921.

Browne, E. G. *Literary History of Persia*. Cambridge: Cambridge University Press, 1902.

Bruce, J. P. *Chu Hsi and His Masters*. London: Probsthain's Oriental Series, 1923.

Bruce, J. P. *Chu Hsi: Philosophy of Nature*. Translation and Commentary. London: Probsthain's Oriental Series, 1922

Bullock, T. L. *Progressive Exercises in the Chinese Written Langauge*. London: Crosby, Lockwood and Son, 1923.

Burton, Lady. Edition of the *1001 Nights*. 6 vols. 1886.

Buzzard, Sir Farquhar. *Lancet*, 1927, 1003.

Campbell, D. *Arabian Medicine and Its Influence on the Middle Ages*. 2 vols. London: Kegan Paul, Trench, Trubner and Co., Ltd., 1926.

Carra de Vaux. *Avicenna* (Les Grands Philosophes). Paris: Felix Alcan, 1900.

Carra de Vaux. *Ghazali*. Paris: Felix Alcan, 1902.

Carus, Paul. *Chinese Thought*. Chicago: Kegan Paul, Trubner Co., 1907.

Catechism of the Council of Trent. Translated by J. McHugh and C. J. Callan. New York: Joseph F. Wagner, Inc., 1923.

Catholic Encyclopedia.

Charaka-Samhita. Translated by K. A. C. Kaviratna. Calcutta, 1896.

Chou, Hung. *I tsung chin ch'ien*. (General Medicine).

Coppens, C., S. J., and Spaulding, J. S. J. *Moral Principles and Medical Practice*. New York: Benziger Bros., 1921.

Corder, Frederick. *Modern Musical Composition*. London: J. Curwen and Sons, Ltd. (no date).

Costeus. *Annotations to Avicenna*. Venetian edition of 1595 or 1608.

Cuthbert, Fr. O. S. F. C. God and the Supernatural. London: Longmans, Green and Co., 1920.

Daremberg. *Oeuvres de Galien*. Paris: J. B. Bailliere, 1854.

Dictionary of Technical Terms Used in the Sciences of the Mussulmans. Calcutta: Bibliotheca Indica, 1862.

Duhalde. *Description of China*. Translated by Hervieu: Section on "The Pulse." 1770.

Dutt. U. Chand. *The Materia Medica of the Hindus*. Compiled from Sanskrit Medical Works. Calcutta: Thacker, Spink and Co., 1877.

Elder and Fowler. *Diseases of Children*. Edinburgh, 1899.

Fernie. *Herbal Simples*. Bristol: John Wright and Sons, 1914.

Flagg, P. J. *The Patient's Point of View*. Milwaukee.

Fonahn, Adolf. *Zur Quellenkunde der Persischen Medizin*. Leipzig: 1910.

Forke, A. *Chinesische Mystik*. Karl Curtius Verlag, Berlin, W.35, 1922.

Forke, A. *The World-Conception of the Chinese*. London: Probsthain's Oriental Series, 1925.

Fox-Strangeways.

Garrod, Sir A. *The Huxley Lecture on Diathesis*. Lancet, 1927, Nov. 26, p. 1113.

Gilani, *Commentary on The Canon*. 1519. MS in India Office Library.

Gilbert, J. W. *The Gospel of Health and Healing in All Ages*. Philadelphia: 1919.

Giles, H. A. *Chuang tzu*. London: Quaritch, Ltd., 1926.

Goodman, L. E. *Avicenna*. New York: Routledge, 1992.

Haeser. *Lehrbuch der geschichte der medizin*. Jena, 1875.

Haly Abbas. Liber Regius. *Kitab al-maliki*. Cairo edition, 1877; Latin translation printed at Lyons in 1523. Also, Kamil us-sinaa.

Harmsworth Home Doctor. 6 vols. Educational Book Co., 1928.

Hartman, F. *The Life of Paracelsus and the Substance of His Teachings*. London: Kegan Paul, Trubner and Co. (no date).

Hartmann. *Chinesische Heilmethoden*. Munch: Med. Woch, 1927, 935.

Hirschberg and Lippert. *Die Augenheilkunde des Ibn Sina*. Leipzig: Veit and Co., 1902.

Holmyard and Mandeville. Avicenna, *Kitab al-shifa*. Paris: Paul Geuthner, 1927.

Honen the Buddhist Saint. Translated by Coates and Izhizuka. Kyoto, Japan: Imperial Request, 1925.

Horne, J. *Many Days in Morocco*. London: Philip Allan and Co., 1879.

Horten, M. *Die Metaphysik Avicennas*. (Das Buch der Geneesung der Seele, eine philosophische Enzyklopedia Avicennas). Leipzid: Rudolf Haupt, 1909.

Howarth, Sir Henry. *History of the Mongols*, 1876-1888.

Hubotter, Fr. *Die chinesische Medizin*. Leipzig: Verlag der Asia Major, 1929.

Hughes, Ed. Lancet, 1920, 63.

Hujwiri, Ali b. Uthman al-Jullabi al-. Translated by Nicholson, R. A. The *Kashf al-mahjub*. London: Gibb Memorial Series. Luzac and Co., 1911.

Huysman, J. K. *St Lydwine de Schiedam*. London: Kegan Paul, 1922.

Hyrtl. *Das arabische und hebraische in der anatomie*. Vienna: 1879.

Iqbal: *The Development of Metaphysics in Persia*. London: 1908.

Jack's Modern Family Doctor. London: T. C. and E. C. Jack, Ltd., 1923.

Joannitius (Hunayn ibn Ishaq al-Ibadi). Some writings included in the Latin Venetian edition of *The Canon*, 1608.

Jones, Eli M. *Medical Times*, 1918, March 9. Boston, MA: Therapeutic Publishing Co., Inc, 1911.

Khan, Inayat. *Diwan*. Gayan.

Khan, Inayat. *Hindustani Lyrics*. Inner Life, etc.

Khan, Inayat. *In an Eastern Rose-garden*.

Khan, Inayat. *The Mysticism of Sound*.

Khan, Inayat. *Various Writings and Sayings*. Southampton: Sufi Publishing Society, 1915-1929.

Kuhne, Louis. *The New Science of Healing*. (From a German book). New

Jersey: Benedict Lust, 1917.

Kuhne. Louis. *The Science of Facial Expression*. New Jersey: Benedict Lust, 1917.

Laloy, Louis. *La musique chinoise*. Paris: H. Laurens. (no date).

Lane's translation of the *Arabian Nights*. New York: Aldus Edition de luxe. (no date).

Lasance, F. X. *Thoughts on the Religious Life*. New York: Benziger Brothers, 1907.

Lasance, F. X. *Blessed Sacrament Book*. New York: Benziger Brothers, 1907.

Lavater. Essays on Physiognomy, 1855.

Leclerc, L. *Histoire de la medicine arabe*. Quoted by Campbell in Arabian Medicine and Its Influence on the Middle Ages.p. 153, endnote.

Legge, James. *The Sacred Books of China*. Oxford: Clarendon Press, 1899.

Lepicier. *Tractatus de prima hominis formatione*. Rome: 1909.

Li Ki. Translated by S. Couvreur, S. J. Catholic Press: Ho Kien Fou, 1913.

Lindley and Moore. *Treasury of Botany*. London: Longmans, Green and Co., 1876.

Lindsay, W. Lauder. *Mind in the Lower Animals*. 2 vols. London: Kegan Paul and Co., 1879.

Macfie, Cmapbell. *The Romance of the Human Body*. London: Wells Gardner, Darton and Co., Ltd, 1917.

Maher, Michael, S. J. *Psychology*. Stonyhurst Philosophical Series. Longmans, Green and Co., 1925.

Markam, Sir Clements. *Colloquies on the Simples and Drugs of India, of Garcia da Orta*. London: Sotheran and Co., 1913.

Martin, Alfred. *Deutsches Badewesen in vergangenen Tagen*. Jena: Eugen Diederich, 1906.

Massignon, L. *La Passion d'al-Hallaj, Martyr Mystique de l'Islam*. 2 vols. Paris: Geuthner, 1922.

Maugham, W. Somerset. *On a Chinese Screen*. Traveller's Library, no. 31.

McGonagh, S. Dominicana, Dec. 1928, p. 299.

McNabb, Vincent, O. P. *The Catholic Church and Philosophy*. Calvert Series. Burns, Oates and Washbourne, Ltd., 1927.

Mehren, M. A. F. *Traites Mystiques d'Abon Ali al-Hosain b. Abdallah b. Sina ou d'Avicenna*. 4 fascicules. Leyden: E. J. Brill, 1889-1899.

Mercier, Cardinal. *Manual of Modern Scholastic Philosophy*. London: Kegan Paul, Trubner and Co., 1921.

Meyerhoff, Max, M. D. *The Book of the Ten Treatises on the Eye Ascribed to Hunain Ibn Ishaq* (809-877 AD). Cairo: Government Press, 1928.

Mih King. Ten volumes on the pulse by Wang Shuh-Ho. Montreal. McGill Library.

Miles, Eustace. *Self-health as a Habit*. London: J. M. Dent and Sons, Ltd., 1923.

Mo hsueh ch'i cheng. *The Science of the Pulse*. Printed during the Ming Dynasty.

Muther. *Practitioner*. June, 1916, 613.

Naegeli. *Allgemein Konstitutionslehre, in naturwissen-schaftlicher und medizinischer Betrachtung*. J. Springer, 1927.

Nash. J. T. *Evolution and Disease*. Bristol: J. Wright and Sons, 1915.
Nasr, Seyyed Hossein. *Islamic Science: An Illustrated Study*. World of Islam Festival, 1976. Distributed by KAZI Publications, Chicago. 1976.
Nasr, Seyyed Hossesin. *Science and Civilization in Islam*. NY: Barnes & Noble, 1992. Distributed by KAZI Publications, Chicago.
Nasr, Seyyed Hossein. *Three Muslim Sages*. Delmar, NY: Caravan Books, 1964. Distributed by KAZI Publications, Chicago.
Nicholson, R. A. *Selected Poems from the Divani Shamsi Tabriz*. Cambridge: Cambaridge University Press, 1898.
Nicholson, R. A. *The Idea of Personality in Sufism*. Cambridge: Cambridge University Press, 1923.
Nicholson, R. A. *The Literary History of the Arabs*. London: T. Fisher Unwin, 1907.
Nicholson, R. A. *The Mystics of Islam*. London: Bell and Sons, 1914.
Nicholson, R. A., translator. *Kitab al-luma fi'l tasawwuf*. Gibb Memorial Publications. London: Juzac and Co., 1914.
Nicholson, R. A. *Studies in Islamic Mysticism*. Cambridge: Cambridge University Press, 1921.
Nicholson, R. A. *Studies in Islamic Poetry*. Cambridge: Cambridge University Press, 1921.
O'Leary, De Lacy Evans. *Arabic Thought and Its Place in History*. London: Trubner's Oriental Series, 1922.
Paracelsus. *Hermetic and Alchemical Writings*. Translated by A. E. Waite. 2 vols. London, 1894.
Paracelsus: Summary of Teachings. See Hartmann, F.
Pareira. *Materia Medica*. London: Longmans, Green, 1850.
Pater, R. *Mystic Voices*. London: Burns, Oates and Washbourne, 1923.
Paulus Aegin. *Optimistic Medicine*. Philadelphia: F. A. Davis Co., 1924.
Pearson and Wyllie. *Recent Advances in Diseases of Children*. Churchill, 1928.
Pegues, R. P. T., O. P. *Catechism of the Summa Theologica of St. Thomas Aquinas*. London: Burns, Oates and Washbourne, 1922.
Plopper, C. H. *Chinese Religion Seen Through the Proverb*. Shanghai: China Press, 1926.
Poulain. *The Graces of Interior Prayer*. London: Kegan Paul, Trench, Trubner and Co., Ltd., 1921.
P'u Sung-Ling, *Seltsame Geschichten*. Berlin. Alf. Hager, Verlag, 1924.
Randall, A.G. *Optimistic Medicine*. Philadelphia: F. A. Davis Co., 1924.
Renaudot, Eusebius. *Ancient Account of India and China*. London, 1733.
Rickaby, Joseph, S. J. *Moral Philosophy*. Stonyhurst Philosophical Series. Longmans, Green and Co., 1912.
Rickaby, Joseph, S. J. *Of God and His Creatures*. London: Burns and Oates, 1905.
Roger, G. H. *Introduction a l'etude de la Medicine*, Collection de Precis Medicaux, Masson et Cie. Paris: 1922.
Rumi, Jalal al-Din. *Mathnawi*. Translated by E. H. Whinfield. London: Kegan Paul, Trench, Trubner and Co., Ltd., 1898.
Sajous, C. E. *The Internal Secretions and the Principles of Medicine*. Philadelphia: 1922.

Sandford, Alex. E. *Pastoral Medicine: A Handbook for C. Clergy*. New York: J. F. Wagner, 1904.
Sauter, C. Avicenna: *Bearbeitung der Aristotelischen Metaphysik*. Herder, Freiburg im Breisgau, 1912.
Schade. Munch. Med. Woch, 1909, 5, etc.
Schlimmer. *Terminologie Medico-pharmaceutique*. Francaise-Persane, Tihran, 1874.
Shabistari, Mahmud. *Gulshan-i raz: The Mystic Rose Garden*. Translated by E. H. Whinfield. London: Trubner and Co., 1880.
Singer, C. and D. *The Scientific Position of Girolano Fracastoro*. Annals of Med. History, 1918.
Stedman's Medical Dictionary. Illustrated. 22nd edition. Baltimore, MD: Williams and Wilkins Co., 1972. Completely revised by a staff of 33 editors covering 44 specialities and sub-specialities.
Sontheimer. *Zusammengesetzte Heilmittel der Araber*. Herder, Freiburg im Breisgau, 1845.
Stanton, M. O. *An Encyclopedia of Face and Form Reading*. Philadelphia: F. A. Davis and Co., 8th edition.
Stoddart. *The Mind and Its Disorders*. London: H. K. Lewis and Co., Ltd., 1926. 5th edition.
Susuki and Carus. *T'ai Shang Kan Yin P'ien*. Chicago: Open Court Publishing Co., 1906.
Susuki, D. T. *A Brief History of Early Chinese Philosophy*. London: Probsthain and Col, 1914.
Susuki, D. T. *Essays in Zen Buddhism*. London: Luzac and Co., 1927.
Swindells, B. J. *Life and Its Origins*. R 83, Cath. Truth Society Pamphlets.
Tagore, Sir Rabindranath. *Gitanjali and Other Works*. 1920, etc.
Tanquery, Ad. *Precis de Theologie Ascetique et Mystique*, 5th ed. Paris and Rome: Desclee et Cie, 1923.
Thomas a Kempis. *Imiitatio Christi*.
Vallery-Radot. *Precis de Pathologie Medicale*. Paris: Masson et Cie, 1922.
Vassal-Phillips, O. R., C.. SS. R. *The Supernatural Life*. Catholic Truth Society (Do. 85).
Vilarino, P. R. S. J. *Devocionario de religiosos*. Bilbao, 1924.
Vonier, Dom Anscar, O. S. B. *Life of the World to Come*. London: Burns, Oates and Washbourne, 1926.
Vonier, Dom Anscar. *The Human Soul*. London: B. Herder, 1920.
Wan K'an t'ang: 1056-1064 A.D. Complete guide to the human pulse. 80 volumes. Reprinted at Peking, 1923.
Watson, J. K. *A Handbook for Nurses*. London: Scientific Press, Ltd., 1921.
White, King, Sir Lucas. *Tayyibat: Odes of Sadi*. London: Luzac and Co., 1926.
Wieger, L., S. J. *History of Religious Beliefs*. Translated by E. C. Werner. Hsien-hsien Press, 1927.
Wilhelm, Richard. I Ging, *Das Buch der Wandlungen, aus dem chinesischen*. Jena: Eugen Diederich, 1924.
Wilson, G. *Religio Chemici*. Macmillian, 1862.
Withington, E. T. *Medical History from the Earliest Times*. London: 1894.

General Index